Dec 17/86

To Mary La Fore with best wishes
for a great year with us.

Bill Moss —

Radiation oncology

RATIONALE, TECHNIQUE, RESULTS

Radiation oncology

RATIONALE, TECHNIQUE, RESULTS

WILLIAM T. MOSS, M.D.

Chairman, Department of Radiation Therapy,
University of Oregon Health Sciences Center,
Portland, Oregon

WILLIAM N. BRAND, M.D.

Director, Radiation Therapy Center,
Northwestern Memorial Hospital;
McGaw Medical Center of Northwestern University,
Chicago, Illinois

HECTOR BATTIFORA, M.D.

Department of Pathology,
Northwestern Memorial Hospital;
McGaw Medical Center of Northwestern University,
Chicago, Illinois

FIFTH EDITION

with 338 illustrations

The C. V. Mosby Company

ST. LOUIS • TORONTO • LONDON   1979

FIFTH EDITION

Previous editions copyrighted 1959, 1965, 1969, 1973

Printed in the United States of America

The C. V. Mosby Company
11830 Westline Industrial Drive, St. Louis, Missouri 63141

Library of Congress Cataloging in Publication Data

Moss, William T
    Radiation oncology.

    Includes bibliographies and index.
    1. Cancer—Radiotherapy. 2. Oncology. I. Brand,
William N., 1934-   joint author. II. Battifora,
Hector, joint author. III. Title. [DNLM: 1. Neoplasms
—Radiotherapy. QZ269.M913t]
RC271.R3M68   1979   616.9′94′0642   79-14367
ISBN 0-8016-3556-X

GW/CB/B   9 8 7 6 5 4 3   01/B/070

To

our **wives** and **children**

Preface

Recent knowledge has had a major impact on the contribution of radiation therapy to the care of the cancer patient. This new knowledge has led to a better understanding of the dose-time-volume relationships to acute and late tissue changes, to a more accurate appreciation of patterns of spread and extent of specific cancers, more precise clinical dosimetry, better equipment for dose delivery, and the coordination of radiation therapy with surgery and chemotherapy. In this fifth edition of *Radiation Oncology* every attempt has been made to incorporate this new knowledge into the process of patient care.

Aims of the previous editions have otherwise remained unchanged—to serve as an introduction to selected clinical problems in the care of cancer patients and to express a philosophy involving the use of radiation therapy that will lead to improved patient care. Rationale, technique, and results are discussed as well as the value of competitive modalities.

Obviously, our reviews of the literature had to be selective, and they are to some degree shaped by our prejudices. However the principles of radiation therapy which we propose have been crystallized from a variety of perspectives and so far as we can evaluate are directed toward the best current radiation therapy.

For all of their gracious help and advice, we wish to thank our many associates and residents at Northwestern University Medical Center and the University of Oregon Health Sciences Center. We especially wish to thank Ms. Paula Jenkins for her endless patience and generous help in preparation of the manuscript.

William T. Moss
William N. Brand
Hector Battifora

Contents

Radiation oncology

RATIONALE, TECHNIQUE, RESULTS

1

Introduction to radiation oncology

The beginning of radiotherapy was no different from that of any other medical specialty. A dependable method of measuring tissue dose was not available; even if it had been, optimum dose-time relationships were not understood. The physical and biologic mistakes that were certain to follow were often fatal. Recurrences from underirradiation and necroses from overirradiation were the natural consequences of this ignorance. Cancers totally unsuited for radiotherapy were irradiated by physicians who had almost no understanding of the tool they were employing. Unlike many modalities used in medicine, an early evaluation of the results of irradiation is rarely possible. Mistakes in judgment often cannot be recognized for years. Once a decision is made to change a faulty technique, case material must be accumulated, the patients must be treated, and the results of treatment must be followed; this, too, takes many years. Because of this time-consuming process of evaluation, every patient treated should be considered a research prospect and all possible clinical and physical data recorded to make future evaluations more meaningful. It may take hundreds or even thousands of patients with a specific type and clinical stage of cancer to detect meaningful differences in morbidity or survival between two techniques. In a lifetime no single physician may see such a volume of patients. To detect such differences within a reasonable time and thereby speed technical improvement, joint collaborative efforts involving many institutions are essential. Cooperative groups (Radiation Therapy Oncology Group [RTOG], Gynecologic Oncology Group [GOG], Southwest Oncology Group [SWOG], and the like) have undertaken major randomized clinical trials to define optimum techniques. However, this must limit neither individual initiative nor clever innovations, which are the real sparks of progress. Most important is that we remember that the *protocol* cannot relieve us of the responsibility of caring for each patient as an individual each day.

DEFINITION OF RADIATION ONCOLOGY

The administration of ionizing radiations to patients is only a part of the specialty of radiation oncology. The pretreatment definition of extent of the cancer, evaluation of patients for irradiation, care during irradiation, and posttreatment care and follow-

1

up examinations are vital to good radiotherapy, which, of course, means good patient care. Such a specialty demands a thorough knowledge of the origin and clinical evolution of the disease and the efficiency of alternative methods of treatment, an appreciation of the clinical aspects of radiophysiology and radiobiology, and a knowledge of the pertinent physical characteristics of the radiations used. Once the clinical distribution (stage), clinical evolution, and growth characteristics of cancer are understood and the radiation tolerances of the associated normal tissues are appreciated, the techniques of irradiating the *volume of interest* (the volume to be considered for irradiation [pp. 21 and 28]) are problems of geometry, physics, and mechanics. However, the day-to-day care of the patient during this period requires that the radiation oncologist identify and care for radiation responses, previously unidentified manifestations of the disease, and complications of the disease and provide general supportive care.

GENERAL CONCEPTS IN RADIATION ONCOLOGY

There is nothing worse in cancer therapy than being only half certain of the anatomic extent of the cancer and of the histologic diagnosis and proceeding with treatment. This not only delays adequate treatment, but also prejudices future adequate irradiation. The histologic diagnosis must be established if at all possible, and the clinical extent of the cancer must be determined with as much precision as is practical. Full treatment is then undertaken with an acceptable risk. If after every reasonable effort the diagnosis cannot be verified, one must proceed with the most likely diagnosis. If after weighing the data it is decided that irradiation is indicated, the dosage should be as if the suspected diagnosis were proved. In the same vein, irradiation can rarely remedy all the harm resulting from ill-advised surgery. All too often patients are referred to the radiation oncologist after having been told by the surgeon, "We took out all we could, and we are going to add a little irradiation to finish the job." Irradiation given after such inadequate surgery is at times the best possible course, but combinations of treatment modalities are most effective after careful pretreatment consideration of all factors affecting prognosis and the application of both modalities in the most effective manner.

High-dose radiation therapy of large volumes is associated with rather well-defined risks of damage to normal tissue. Reduction of these risks by improving dose-time relationships, reducing irradiated volumes whenever possible, improving beam quality, and the use of precision techniques have been major steps leading to reduced damage of normal tissue. However, the fear of serious normal tissue damage is the most common cause of undertreatment. All oncologists become frustrated when they recognize that cancer is recurring because of their attempts to spare the patient morbidity.

In addition to its curative usefulness, radiotherapy is one of the most valuable palliative tools available. Many cancerous masses that are not curable by any means are made to regress or are held in check by irradiation. Irradiation can make infected, bleeding cutaneous or mucosal ulcers heal, obstructing pressure-producing masses shrink, and painful bone-destroying metastases regress. In fact the great palliative value of radiotherapy sometimes masks its curative usefulness. The large proportion of hopelessly ill patients whose suffering is relieved by radiotherapy must not lead the radiation oncologist to lose sight of the curative possibilities of this modality. However, the tremendous palliative value of radiotherapy has resulted in an association of radiotherapy with inoperability, or even incurability, that is difficult to overcome. The image of radiation therapy as a curative modality has greatly improved with its serious administration by dedicated radiation oncologists using excellent equipment.

Inoperability per se is never an indication for irradiation. For patients with inoperable cancer an assessment of tumor size and extent, cell type, and goal of treatment should be made carefully and deliberately. Furthermore, the pathologist's report alone cannot guide one to a decision about irradiation. Even the slowly growing, well-differentiated cell types may be helped by irradiation in certain circumstances, whereas the more undifferentiated cell types may not always benefit from irradiation. A referring physician may suggest the use of radiotherapy for the psychologic boost it gives terminally ill patients. Faking radiation therapy or giving radiation therapy for psychologic reasons alone is poor psychotherapy and even worse radiotherapy. Instead, the physician must accept his real responsibility in the care of these terminal patients. Neither cytotoxic agents nor radiations should be administered to render some vague psychotherapeutic effect.

To avoid the unnecessary association of our armamentarium with failure, the radiation oncologist should select patients for palliative treatment just as carefully as he selects those for curative treatment. To withhold treatment that will likely relieve suffering is inexcusable, but to administer irradiation with no hope of producing relief is likewise the practice of poor medicine. In the selection of patients for irradiation it is much more difficult to withhold than to administer radiotherapy. As in any other field, it often takes wide clinical experience coupled with courage to render the best care to the patient. It may sound paradoxic, but palliative irradiation usually requires more mature judgment and more personal involvement by the radiation oncologist than curative irradiation.

In the chapters that follow, recent published results as well as some classic studies are cited. The statistical validity of these results may be justifiably challenged. However, such data must serve as the radiation oncologist's guide until better figures become available.

Similarly, a statement of optimum dose can almost always be criticized because of obvious inaccuracies. Optimum doses, by necessity, are based on clinical experiences extending back as far as 25 years. In this period dosimetry was crude by contemporary standards. However, many of the dosage guides now used for cancer control and normal tissue response are based on these data. Radiation oncologists have nothing better from which to extrapolate for today's optimum techniques. Currently available computer-aided techniques show us the magnitude of heterogeneity of dose within the volume of interest. Precise treatment planning assists in delivering the desired dose distribution to the selected volume. The size and number of fractions, volume of the cancerous mass, volume encompassed, total number of days, and total dose are parameters that also influence the likelihood of local control and local complications. These are inseparable from consideration of the correct "total dose," which is too often used as the sole criterion for adequate irradiation.

Special attention should be given to obtaining the histologic diagnosis. Without expert guidance from a well-qualified surgical pathologist, all cancer therapy, whether radiotherapeutic, surgical, or chemotherapeutic, will be on uncertain ground. Without such guidance the radiation oncologist will be uncertain as to what he is treating and, if he cures the patient, he will not know what he has cured or why he has been successful. In addition, the microscopic cell type is frequently critical in determining whether the treatment will be surgical, radiotherapeutic, chemotherapeutic, or a combination. If the treatment is to be irradiation, the microscopic diagnosis will be one of the more important factors determining the time-dose-volume relationships. If the diagnosis were malignant lymphoma rather than well-differentiated squamous cell carcinoma, we would advocate more generous fields and lower total doses. A careful gross and microscopic examination of the surgical specimen is a good measure of the adequacy of excision. The diagnosis of "inadequate excision," or "narrow margins," may well justify vigorous irradiation with a curative aim before there are clinical signs of recurrence. If the pathologist thinks that the excision has been adequate, careful follow-up with no irradiation may be the best policy.

It is imperative that a close collaboration exist between the pathologist and the radiation oncologist. The pathologist should convey to the radiation oncologist his findings in more detail than simple pathologic coding. Not only must he describe cell type and degree of differentiation, but also the type of invasive growth and presence or absence of vascular permeation. The type of host response to the tumor is also an important contribution to treatment planning. Since standard nomenclature is not uniformly agreed on, even by pathologists themselves, the pathologist must make every effort to clarify his interpretation, especially in uncommon cases. A candid and open-minded approach is necessary when dealing with cases of doubtful or controversial nature. The need for further diagnostic measures and the means by which to obtain them can then be mutually agreed on.

Aside from these immediate contributions of the surgical pathologist to the conduct of clinical radiotherapy, it is through careful study of autopsy and operating room material that the radiation oncologist can learn the origin, routes of spread, and extent of infiltration and metastases. He learns the frequency with which certain lymph node groups will be involved and thus can justify treatment or no treatment of specific volumes on such data. He discovers the reasons for treatment failure and may change his technique to remedy the defects. The pathologist, better than anyone else, can assist the radiation oncologist in defining tolerances of deep tissues and high-dose sequelae.

If the radiation oncologist is fortunate enough to have a pathologist sympathetic to his problems, he must be aware of the pathologist's capabilities and understand what he means by his interpretations. Frequent discussions of problems with the pathologist will assist him in understanding them and will enable him to contribute greatly to patient care. This type of cooperative approach permits the pathologist to realize the satisfaction of playing a more direct role in patient care.

The other two major modes of treatment, that is, chemotherapy and surgery, may of course be used alone, in combination with each other, or with radiation therapy varying with anatomic site, clinical stage, and histologic type. However, with few exceptions local control is dependent on radiation therapy or surgery or a combination of the two, whereas chemotherapy is usually directed toward growth restraint or widespread metastases. The participation of the radiation oncologist, surgeon, and chemotherapist in the treatment decision process for each patient presupposes similar levels of oncologic background, clinical judgment, and dedication to good patient care. Such a balance in expertise is infrequent. Nevertheless, the concept of "multidiscipline" consultation is an essential of optimum treatment for a wide variety of cancers.

The cancer patient often seeks the advice of the primary care physician before the diagnosis is made. This cancer-conscious primary care physician often has the responsibility of making an early diagnosis, and it is to him that we must look for major progress in shortening the interval from onset to diagnosis. If these primary care clinicians are acquainted with the indications for irradiation and the characteristics differentiating good from poor radiotherapy, they can refer cancer patients in a direction that will assure their most effective care.

Patients in age periods in which cancer most commonly occurs also have a relatively high incidence of cardiovascular, pulmonary, and renal diseases. Not infrequently the successful administration of radiations will depend on simultaneous treatment for these degenerative diseases. The internist can provide vital help with his special knowledge of hematology, infectious diseases, and circulatory and renal diseases. During such collaborative efforts each physician must at all times appreciate the other's aims. It is for these reasons that the internist must appreciate good radiotherapy and work with the radiation oncologist. The reverse is equally true.

RADIOBIOLOGIC CONCEPTS IN CLINICAL RADIATION ONCOLOGY

The clinically important physiologic and morphologic changes produced by radiations are presented in the discussions of each anatomic site. No review of these changes need be presented here. However, certain radiation-induced changes common to all cells and tissues and certain concepts important in discussing clinical radiation responses are pertinent. The superficial abbreviated description that follows is intended to emphasize the *impact* of radiation biology on clinical radiation therapy technique. A huge number of studies with cell cultures and laboratory animals have been done to define modes of action, optimum fractionation patterns, various aspects of cellular kinetics, and the like. These exciting and highly valuable studies can be almost overwhelming to the beginning clinically oriented trainee.

For this reason we have provided selected references and limited discussions of areas that have direct impact on clinical practice. For radiobiology presented specifically for residents in clinical radiation oncology see Pizzarello and Witcofski, Duncan and Nias, Hall, and the provocative paper by Alper.

Cellular radiation responses

Radiation-induced changes in tissues and organs are the sum of changes in the constituent cells. The various types of mammalian cells, both normal and malignant, show similar patterns of response provided the cells are in comparable phases of their growth cycle and have comparable growth cycles. Many malignant and nonmalignant mammalian cells can be grown and studied in tissue culture with a technique similar to that used for bacteria (Puck and Marcus). In such studies the cell's reproductive capability is used as a measure of its viability and growth potential. Thus the number of colonies or clones that grow after irradiating a known number of viable cells is an index of the radiosensitivity of the reproductive mechanism. The typical dose-response curve plots the log of the percentage of cells surviving against various doses of radiations (Fig. 1-1). The slope of the curve varies with the radiosensitivity of the particular cell type, its environment during irradiation, the type and the method of administration of radiations, and the biologic state of the cells. This curve has a char-

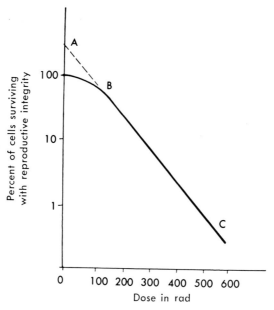

Fig. 1-1. Typical dose-response curve. Proportion of cells retaining reproductive integrity after a given dose of radiations is plotted. A curve is drawn through series of points obtained with various doses. Slope of *BC* varies with radiosensitivity of particular cell type and its environment during irradiation. Length of line from *A* to 100% survival point is apparently a measure of average number of targets in a cell that must be hit within a relatively short period of time to cause cessation of reproduction.

acteristic "shoulder" followed by a straight line. The more resistant the cell, the broader the shoulder and the less steep the slope. The shoulder represents the accumulation of damage and subsequent repair (Elkind recovery).

There is no totally satisfactory single interpretation of this recovery process, although there are two types of models that should be considered.

The *multiple-target single-hit model* is widely accepted and the most popular. Following is a summary of this model.

When considering the injurious effects of radiations, cells are pictured as containing certain critical structures that play essential roles in their reproductive capacity. These structures are called *targets* and are generally accepted as being DNA molecules in genes. Radiation-induced damage to a DNA molecule (target) may trigger a sequence of serious cellular changes. However, if this type of DNA damage occurs singularly, it is rapidly repaired. Mammalian cells are said to have several such targets, which must be hit within the same short period to end cellular reproduction. By contrast haploid cells, such as bacterial cells, may require only one hit. The shoulder of the cell survival curve (Fig. 1-1) is thought to be a graphic demonstration of this accumulation of sublethal, repairable damage to critical targets in mammalian cells. With a single low dose very few mammalian cells will have all targets hit. Therefore survival will be high. With a higher dose most cells will have some critical targets hit. Some will have all targets hit, and only they will fail to reproduce. Finally, with still higher doses, many cells will have accumulated sufficient hits in a short period of time so that only one additional hit will be necessary to destroy reproductive capacity. At this dose and above, the relationship between dose and reproductive capacity is exponential, that is, it is shown by a straight line on a semilog plot (Fig. 1-1).

The shape of the shoulder depends in part on the number of critical targets in the cell. This number of targets is determined by extrapolating up along the straight part of the curve to the point of intersection with the ordinate (Fig. 1-1). The length of the ordinate between this intersection and the 100% survival point is called the *extrapolation number (N)* and is a measure of the average number of critical targets in each cell. The number of critical targets varies with physiologic conditions, presence or absence of oxygen in the cell, phase of the cell in its life cycle, and unknown factors.

Repair models have been proposed as alternatives to the multiple-target single-hit model. An excellent discussion of the need for such alternatives has been published by Alper (1977). This concept may be summarized as follows: radiations produce potentially lethal lesions which are rapidly repaired by a process that is limited or by a material that is depleted in the process of repair. Sinclair called this the *Q-factor*. The presence of such a factor could satisfactorily explain some radiobiologic phenomena not explained by the multiple-target single-hit model. Thus the diffusion of such a factor from one cell to an adjacent cell might explain why cells in contact with other cells seem to have a larger N than the same cells irradiated singly. Other examples are mentioned by Alper.

The cell survival curve illustrates that the larger the volume, that is, number of cancer cells, the higher the dose of radiations necessary to eradicate it. This assumes either that every tumor cell must be killed by the radiations or that a certain minimum number of cells are essential for tumor viability. This curve also illustrates that most mammalian cells seem capable of recovering from a substantial part of the radiation-induced injury in a matter of a few hours.

Radiosensitivity and radioresponsiveness

The radiosensitivity of cells in a culture is expressed by the slope of the cell survival curve (Fig. 1-1). It is also expressed in terms of D_0, that is, the single dose of radiations necessary to kill 63% of the cells using the straight part of the curve. The magnitude of intracellular repair is measured by the broadness of the shoulder denoted by D_q (Fig. 1-5). However, these definitions are not readily applied to a clinical situation.

From a clinical standpoint the terms *radiosensitive* and *radioresponsive* have been used in such a variety of circumstances that confusion results from clinical application of the terms. The most unfortunate consequence of this confusion has been the delay in application of radiations to various malignant diseases. For instance, adenocarcinoma of the prostate and many of the soft tissue tumors until recently were only infrequently treated with radiations because of their slow response (shrinkage), thus falsely implying their insensitivity and resulting radioincurability (Gagnon).

Clinically these terms are of limited value, but it is nevertheless important to distinguish between them. Our oncologic colleagues base many of their treatment decisions on interpretations of the different characteristics of tumors as well as normal tissue. For this reason the terms *radiosensitivity* and *radioresponsiveness* should be understood.

As mentioned before, our radiobiology colleagues have attempted to define radiosensitivity on the basis of cell survival data. Cell death and loss of reproductive integrity are good endpoints to choose because these are the critical biologic changes related to the radiotherapeutic control of cancer. But it must be remembered that radiosensitivity is always a relative property. Tumor location, as well as its size, cell type, blood supply, general condition of the host, presence of infection, and the like influence radiosensitivity to some degree. The following restatement of definition was developed by Gagnon. *Radiosensitivity can be defined as the ability of radiations to biologically change* (biologic change may mean cell killing or a destruction of reproductive integrity) *cells comprising a tumor or other tissue.* These changes will ultimately manifest themselves clinically as an alteration in structure or function.

Radioresponsiveness refers to the time required for these changes to occur and *can be measured in terms of the rate at which clinical manifestations of radiation-induced biologic change take place.* A tumor that shrinks rapidly following administration of any amount of irradiation would be rapidly radioresponsive. One that shrinks less rapidly would be moderately or even slowly radioresponsive. Any or all of these tumors could be radiocurable and therefore would have to be radiosensitive,

Table 1-1. Examples of use of terms*

Tumor type	Radiosensitivity	Radioresponsiveness	Radiocurability
Acute leukemia	High	Rapid	Poor to none
Small cell undifferentiated carcinoma of lung	High	Rapid	Poor to none
Hodgkin's disease	High	Rapid	Excellent
Squamous cell carcinoma of tonsillar fossa	Moderate	Moderate	Good
Adenocarcinoma of prostate	Moderate	Slow	Fair to good
Glioblastoma multiforme	Low	Slow	Poor
Glomus jugulare	Low	Slow	Good

*From Gagnon, J.: Personal communication, Nov., 1978.

despite their differences in radioresponsiveness. The curability of a tumor is therefore related to its radiosensitivity regardless of its responsiveness. *Radiocurability is defined then as the ability of radiations to reduce the number of malignant cells below a critical level such that no further clinical manifestation of their presence will occur during the remaining lifetime of the host.*

Table 1-1 illustrates how these definitions allow for use of these terms. It can be seen that a high degree of radiosensitivity and rapid radioresponsiveness are not absolute requirements for the radiocurability of some tumors. Therapy then must not be based on any outmoded idea that a cancer is incurable by irradiation because it responds so slowly.

A cancerous mass or a normal organ shrinks when cell death, cell loss, and absorption exceed new cell production. At least three cellular changes are necessary. Mitosis must be slowed or arrested. At the same time the existing nonmitotic cells may or may not die at an increased rate, and they must be absorbed either by autolysis or phagocytosis. Shifts in any or all of these rates may modify the rate of tumor shrinkage. Cell turnover rates of the irradiated cells are important determinants. In some cancerous masses, such as large nodes in the neck, a high proportion of the cells are necrotic, nearly necrotic, or nonproliferating. In such a situation, in which circulation is poor, coagulative necrosis occurs, and the necrotic tissue may not be removed for months. If dead cells or coagulative necrosis occupies a large proportion of the tumor, the tumor may shrink very little, even if all of the remaining cells are killed. Other factors that modify shrinkage of a cancer are integrity of phagocytic processes and rate of proliferation of the cancer cells or normal cells between fractions. Thus the rate of shrinkage of a cancerous mass may be misleading if it is regarded as an index of response as is done in both radiation therapy and chemotherapy. The possibility of a poor correlation between rate of tumor shrinkage and ultimate control of a cancerous mass has been stressed by Suit and associates, and by Fazekas and associates. Yet it must be emphasized that large masses with extensive necrosis are the most likely to remain indurated at the completion of radiotherapy, and these same large masses are the most likely to have persistent viable cancer. It is not surprising, therefore, that clinical support exists relative to the prognostic significance of persistent induration at the completion of irradiation. Indeed, this constitutes one of the radiobiologic justifications for *boosting doses* that are delivered to residual masses after large-port irradiation.

In a normal organ with a recognized cell renewal system there is a spectrum of cellular radiosensitivities. These sensitivities are related to the proliferative activity of the cells in question, that is, whether they undergo mitosis frequently, occasionally, only after unusual stress, or never. The same spectrum of cells exists in cancers. The response of a given cancer to irradiation is related to the proportion of cells ordinarily destined to undergo early and frequent mitosis as well as the proportion that is destined to a long survival in a more mature nonmitotic state. Bergonie and Tribondeau described this in 1906 in their "law," which states that the effect of radiations on cells is proportional to the cells' functional and morphologic differentiations.

It is not likely that the current fractionation scheme of 150 to 200 rad per day, 5 days a week to a total dose of 6000 to 6500 rad is optimal for all types of squamous carcinoma. Preirradiation knowledge of cellular kinetics of each cancer might assist in tailoring a more efficient fractionation. However, even within a given patient, metastasis may show different doubling times, and the doubling time in a given metastasis may increase as it enlarges. Thus the practical use of cell kinetics in tailoring optimum fractionation patterns is not yet within reach.

The slope of the cell survival curve varies with the cellular oxygen tension (Fig. 1-2). Both in vitro and in vivo studies confirm that for a given lethality anoxic cells require two to three times the dose required for well-oxygenated cells (Fig. 1-3). The ratio of the former dose to the latter is called the oxygen enhancement ratio (OER); its importance is found in the fact that cell clusters of more than a few millimeters in diameter undoubtedly contain hypoxic cells. Because of their decreased radiosensitivity, hypoxic tumor cells could account for a proportion of local cancer persistences. To enhance the effect of radiations, dissolved oxygen must be in the cell near the site of the radiation-produced free radical. The enhancement is presumed to be a consequence of oxygen combining directly or indirectly with free radicals split from critical cell targets by radiations. In this way oxygen reduces the chances that recombination of free radicals with critical targets will occur and thus reduces the chances of restoring the integrity of the critical targets. From a practical standpoint the enhancement is effective over a limited range of oxygen partial pressures (Fig. 1-2).

The survival curve for irradiated oxygenated cells is steeper than for hypoxic cells. Furthermore, the curve will show a larger extrapolation number and a sharper shoulder (Fig. 1-3). When the extrapolation number as well as slope changes with oxygenation, the OER will vary. Thus OER will be one value when measured on the straight part of the two curves and another value when measured at the shoulders of the two curves. It is important to measure OER at the dose levels to be used and to presume that it is different at different dose levels in the shoulder regions. In Fig. 1-3 it can be seen that to reduce the surviving fraction of aerobic cells to 1% requires about half the dose required to reduce the surviving fraction of anoxic cells to 1%. If the oxygen tension within a cancerous mass remains constant during irradiation,

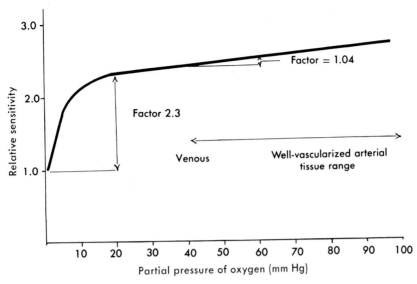

Fig. 1-2. Variation in relative radiosensitivity with variation in tension of dissolved oxygen. As oxygen tension increases, radiosensitivity increases but at a decreasing rate. It should be emphasized that this curve was constructed on data obtained at room temperature. (Modified from Gray, L. H.: Br. J. Radiol. **30:**403-423, 1957.)

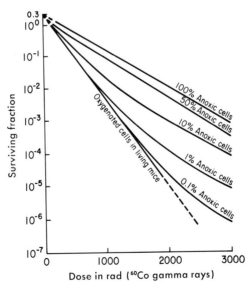

Fig. 1-3. Survival curves for mouse leukemia cells with various proportions of the cells anoxic at time of irradiation. (Modified from Hewitt, H. B., and Wilson, C. W.: Br. J. Cancer **13:**675-684, 1959.)

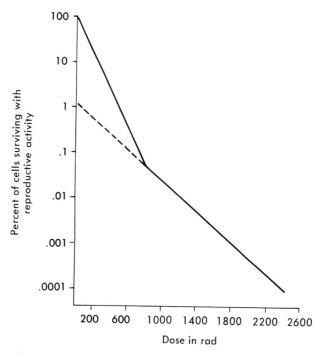

Fig. 1-4. Survival curve for lymphosarcoma cells of the mouse. Tumors 1 to 2 cm in diameter were irradiated with single doses in vivo while the animal was breathing air. After irradiation the tumors were minced, cells were diluted, and a known number were injected into similar living mice after the method of Hewitt. The dilution that gave tumor takes 50% of the time was proportioned to the fraction of cells surviving. Presumably the oxygenated cells were killed selectively. Anoxic cells with less radiosensitivity then predominated to form the lower part of the curve with less slope. It should be noted that single doses were used to obtain this curve. There is evidence that with fractionation of dose under favorable circumstances a significant proportion of anoxic cells become sufficiently well oxygenated to be destroyed. (Modified from Powers, W. E., and Tolmach, L. J.: Nature **197**:710-711, 1963.)

there is a relative sparing of the hypoxic fraction. Even though the hypoxic fraction may initially be small, it may eventually comprise a major fraction of the surviving cells (Figs. 1-4 and 1-5). Thus, with a single dose of radiations or with a few large, closely spaced fractions, the hypoxic cells of a cancer are selectively spared. When small fractions are given over a period of weeks, presumably not all the hypoxic cells remain hypoxic. As sensitive cells are killed, lysed, and absorbed or phagocytized with each small fraction, some hypoxic cells are shifted to the well-oxygenated group to become more radiosensitive. The relationship of the size of the hypoxic fraction to the size of the tumor mass is illustrated graphically in Fig. 1-5.

The concern that hypoxic cells might be a major source of postirradiation recurrences has stimulated extensive research aimed at reducing their potential impact. Such research has included varied patterns of fractionating dose; clinical trials irradiating patients under hyperbaric conditions; the use of beams of atomic particles including neutrons, protons, pi mesons, and stripped nuclei; chemical modifiers

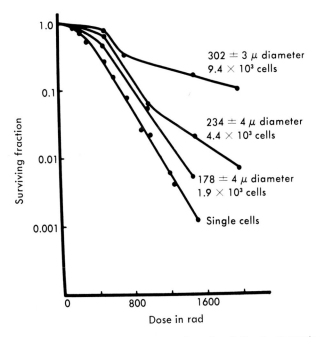

Fig. 1-5. Survival curves for cell masses of various sizes. Irradiation in atmospheric oxygen, ^{60}Co beam, 135 rad/min. Compare with Fig. 1-4. The proportion of hypoxic cells increases dramatically as this particular cell mass increases from 178 to 302 μ in diameter. Note that as size of mass increases, the shoulder quickly broadens. This experimental model suggests that clinically employed initial fractions are too small for efficient cell killing in large tumor masses. Although the D_0 for oxygenated cells does not shift significantly as a function of tumor mass, the D_q is markedly influenced by tumor size. (From Sutherland, R. M., Inch, W. R., and McCredie, J. A.: Int. J. Radiat. Biol. **18:** 491-495, 1970.)

such as electron affinic compounds; and combinations of hyperthermia with radiations. These will not be discussed here, since they are still largely experimental.

A greater clinical exploitation of the shift of hypoxic cells to the oxygenated compartment has been suggested by Elkind and may be summarized as follows:

1. In most cancers of palpable dimensions, a relatively large initial dose fraction will kill a large proportion of the well-oxygenated tumor cells but will spare a large proportion of the hypoxic cells.

2. These killed cells must be lysed and absorbed before the spared hypoxic cells can shift to become well oxygenated.

3. An estimate is that several days are required for this type of killing, lysis, and absorption. The optimum interval is likely to be longer than 24 hours, but it would vary, being shorter with rapidly shrinking tumors and longer with slowly shrinking tumors.

4. In this interval, additional dose fractions could conceivably do more harm than

good. The factors responsible for hypoxic tumor cells would persist. Little additional tumor would be killed, yet considerable normal tissue injury would be likely.

5. Resumption of proliferation of tumor cells is slight in the interval of several days required for lysis and absorption.

Elkind's proposal for a rather large initial fraction followed by an interval of several days of no irradiation is an interesting and rational recommendation. This proposal, along with variation of the initial dose and length of interval, probably justifies clinical trials. It must be remembered, however, that in certain cancerous masses such as large cervical lymph node metastasis only a very small proportion of the total cells present are eligible for killing with this initial dose. In such cases there is not likely to be early visible or palpable change. This concept is outlined not so much to recommend its immediate clinical application as to emphasize how basic radiobiologic concepts might be used to design clinical treatment patterns.

The feasibility of high-pressure oxygen in clinical radiotherapy was proved by Churchill-Davidson, Wildermuth, Atkins and associates, Van den Brenk, and Glassburn and associates. The contribution of this technique to the cure of cancer was at best marginal and for the most part has been abandoned.

Induced normal tissue hypoxia has also been considered potentially useful for therapy. When available oxygen is decreased, the normal tissues have a greater loss of dissolved oxygen than do the already hypoxic cancer cells; this reduces the radiosensitivity of normal cells more than that of the already hypoxic cancer cells. In this way therapeutic ratio can be improved (Comas; Suit and associates). However, these patients—many of whom have borderline adequate coronary and cerebral vessels—cannot tolerate significant systemic hypoxia. The experimental use of this method was therefore limited to the treatment of lesions of the extremities. This also has been abandoned after little, if any, benefit was observed.

Radiosensitivity varies during the different phases of the cell cycle. The apparently contradictory laboratory data on this subject are related in part to the parameter being measured, that is, chromosomal aberrations or cell survival (Fig. 1-6). However, in the absence of synchronized cell populations, no clinical use has been made of these variations in sensitivity other than the fact that rapidly cycling cells are in a sensitive phase more often.

In the comparison of cell culture studies with clinical findings, several factors should be considered. Cells growing in clumps are more resistant to radiation-induced killing than cells of the same variety growing singly in a culture media (Durand and Sutherland). In addition, cells studied in tissue culture are stimulated to reproduce. Their mitotic rate is frequently greater than exists in vivo. In vivo, those tissues normally showing sparse mitotic figures are pictured as being less easily destroyed by radiations than those tissues showing greater mitotic activity. Of course not all body cells require a reproductive capability to maintain their functions. In this category are neurons of the central nervous system and cardiac muscle fibers. The limitations of using reproductive capacity as a measure of viability of normal tissues are immediately obvious. However, one of the more serious injuries

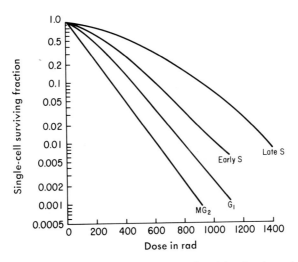

Fig. 1-6. Survival curves for Chinese hamster cells irradiated in vitro in various phases of cell cycle. At low dose levels difference in sensitivity between cells in the most sensitive phase (MG₂) and the most resistant phase (late S) is greater than difference between anoxic and well-oxygenated cells. (Modified from Sinclair, W. K.: Time dose relationships in radiation biology as applied to radiotherapy, Publication 50203 (C-57), p. 97, Brookhaven National Laboratory, New York.)

is to the cell's reproductive mechanism (and all cancer cells and many normal tissues must undergo mitosis or disappear). It is to be expected that tissues with high mitotic activity will be affected the most. When the integrity of a given normal tissue is dependent on a high mitotic rate of its cells, and when it is realized that the reproductive capability of a cell is suppressed by relatively low doses of radiations, early and dramatic radiation-induced effects in the tissue are expected. On the other hand, when integrity of a tissue is not highly dependent on frequent mitoses of its constituents, only minor early changes are expected. Thus the fact that a single dose of 500 rad destroys the reproductive capability of a high proportion of many different cell types in tissue culture is not incompatible with our conventional concept of the apparent different radiosensitivities between these very same cell types in vivo, where they exhibit widely differing reproductive cycles and are always clumped with other cells. Physiologic demands for cellular replacement vary. For example, a previously irradiated tissue may serve its function well until trauma or infection demands of it a response that, because of its radiation-induced injury, it cannot supply. Obviously, cellular replacement is such a response. When this is the case, late radionecrosis may be the result.

Clinically, we are confronted not only with the number of cells capable of reproduction but also with the number of cells actually present. Clones developing from previously irradiated populations are frequently smaller than those from unirradiated populations. If the clinical endpoint is the restoration of a tissue—that is, epithelial surface of the gut or skin—not only the number of clones but also their rate of growth are important. Within limits, the higher the dose, the more slowly the subsequent

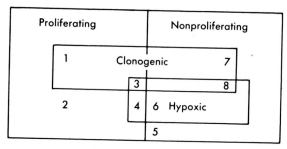

Fig. 1-7. Simplest current tenable model of a cancerous mass. Cancer cells are classified as proliferating or nonproliferating, clonogenic or nonclonogenic, oxygenated or hypoxic. Category 1 contains the most commonly pictured cancer cells that are proliferating, clonogenic, and oxygenated—that is, a very small squamous cell carcinoma of the tongue with metastasizing capabilities. Category 2 contains oxygenated, proliferating, but nonclonogenic cells. These cells contribute to tumor growth but cannot divide indefinitely. Categories 3 and 4—hypoxic proliferating cells with or without clonogenic capabilities—may not exist if conditions that render the cells hypoxic also prevent them from proliferating. Categories 5 and 6 contain nonproliferating, nonclonogenic, oxygenated, or hypoxic cells. In some types of tumors the largest fraction of cells may be in these categories, especially if necrotic areas are present. Electrode measurements of tissue oxygen tension and response to hyperbaric conditions would be misleading if taken from Category 6. Categories 7 and 8 contain nonproliferating clonogenic cells. These are cells that for some reason are not proliferating at time of radiotherapy and therefore will not be affected by cycle-related sensitivities of irradiation. The hypoxic nonproliferating cells are critical to question of hyperbaric oxygenation. (Modified from Mendelsohn, M. L.: Radiation effects in tumors. In Radiation research 1966, Amsterdam, 1967, North-Holland Publishing Co.)

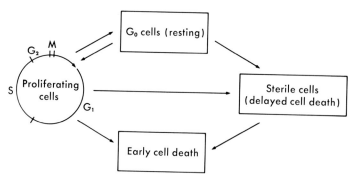

Fig. 1-8. Four functional compartments into which cells of a cancerous mass may be divided. (1) The growth fraction is represented by the cell cycle (proliferating cells). From here cells may pass into any of three states. (2) They may die. (3) They may become quiescent (G_0 cells resting). From here they may either lose reproductive capacity completely or be later recruited back into proliferating compartment by a homeostatic stimulus for increased proliferation. (4) Some proliferating cells may lose proliferating capacity permanently but otherwise remain alive for variable periods of weeks or months before dying. Proportion of cells in each of these four compartments may change as tumor mass enlarges and also during irradiation, thus making it difficult to predict tumor doubling times or precise patterns of radiation response. (Modified from Mendelsohn, M. L., and Dethlefsen, L. A.: Tumor growth and cellular kinetics in the proliferation and spread of neoplastic cells. Houston, 1967, M. D. Anderson Hospital.)

clone enlarges. Other factors affecting the time required for tissue restoration relate to the proportion of new cells proceeding to differentiation rather than continuing to proliferate, the duration of the various phases of the cell cycle, and the longevity of the newly formed differentiated cell. This fascinating study of rates of growth and rates of cell turnover or population kinetics is beyond the scope of this book, but the interested student can read Fowler (1966), Rubin and Casarett, and the many excellent papers included in the Carmel Conference of 1969.

The simplest current tenable model of a cancerous mass has been diagramed by Mendelsohn (Fig. 1-7). The problems rapidly become more complex in organs with multiple normal cell types and multiple functions. A useful growth fraction model is shown in Fig. 1-8.

Fractionation

When a given dose of radiations is divided into several increments and delivered over a period of several hours or days, the biologic effect is usually, though not always, less than if the radiations had been given in a single dose (Fig. 1-9). This decreased response with daily fractionation appears to be related to cell recovery occurring between increments and to the capability of surviving cells to adapt to radiation-

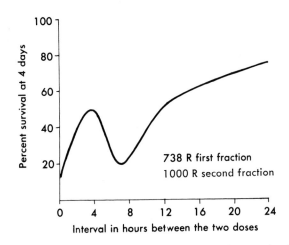

Fig. 1-9. Lethality of two fractions of radiations as their interval of separation is varied. Recovery from injury of crypt cells of the small bowel of the mouse was used as end point. At the 0 interval there is no separation between the two fractions. As the fractions are separated there is at first a sharp rise in percentage of survival. This is attributed to "prompt recovery" after the first fraction. Subsequent oscillations in survival are attributed to the changing sensitivity of cells as they pass into the various phases of the mitotic cycle. At an interval of about 24 hours the curve nearly flattens. The surviving cells reproduce between the two fractions. Presumably the split-dose curves for cancer cells and selected normal cells differ. Exploitation of such differences could define the optimum timing for fractions. (Modified from Hornsey, S., and Vatistas, S.: Br. J. Radiol. **36**:795-800, 1963.)

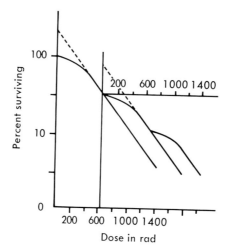

Fig. 1-10. Typical dose-response curve is reproduced with each fraction spaced 24 hours apart. Recovery leads to the reproduction of the shoulder with each daily fraction.

induced alterations of the surrounding tissues. The dependency of biologic effectiveness on degree of fractionation is classically referred to as the *dose-time relationship* in radiotherapy. Elkind found that cells which survived the acute effects of an irradiation repaired their damage in less than 24 hours. When such cells are subsequently reirradiated, clones grow in the same percentage as following the initial irradiation. However, as we shall see later, clones developing from irradiated cells grow more slowly. With conventionally fractionated irradiation given in daily increments, injuries are repaired daily, and the shoulder is therefore duplicated with each daily fraction (Fig. 1-10). The response is thus highly dependent on the number of shoulders or fractions and to a somewhat lesser degree on the interval between fractions as long as the interval is at least 24 hours. This type of recovery accounts for most of the increased dose necessary with the usual fractionation of about 4 weeks. The daily duplication of the shoulder is obviously not an efficient use of energy as far as suppression of reproduction of a single cell type is concerned. For a given total dose, a single massive dose with only one shoulder would be more efficient. Yet a part of the superiority of fractionated irradiation is thought to occur because of different rates of recovery between different cell types.

The type of rapid recovery just described is known as Elkind recovery and is to be distinguished from the classic concept of tissue repair occurring during and after a course of fractionated irradiation. The classic concept of tissue repair includes recovery from the immediate effects in addition to cellular proliferation. With short treatment periods (daily fractions for about 4 weeks), Elkind recovery seems to account for most of the decrease in biologic effect seen with fractionation of a given dose. With longer treatment periods, the classic concept of tissue repair seems significant (Fowler and Stern).

In addition to repairable sublethal cellular injury described above, nonrepairable cell injury occurs. This is caused by the densely ionizing "tail" of the electron tracks, which are in fact components of high linear energy transfer (LET) radiations. This component is present in small proportions in all beams of low LET photon radiations. Its relative importance depends in large part on the size and number of daily fractions and the capacity of the cells to repair sublethal injury. Thus, with daily fractions that do not "reach" the exponential part of the survival curve, most of the sublethal injuries will be repaired, and the small number of nonrepairable injuries are significant. On the other hand, if a few large fractions are given and the exponential portion of the curve is "reached" with each fraction, the high LET component is relatively insignificant.

Finally, as far as can be determined in vitro and in vivo, there is no systematic difference in the survival curves of cancer cells and normal cells. The differences observed in clinical radiation therapy are more likely related to normal tissue regeneration and differences in radiation-induced changes in the cell cycles.

The classic concept of tissue repair includes the resumption of mitotic activity in normal tissue. The "split" course of fractionated irradiation exploits this type of repair. Radiation-induced cell death initiates a feedback mechanism that activates a reparative process. This has been called the homeostatic stimulus to normal tissue repair. Malignant cells are as a rule less affected by the stimulus. Presumably an interruption in a course of fractionated irradiation permits this reparative process in noncancerous tissue to proceed unhampered. The cancer cells also recover and multiply, but at a much slower rate. (Some tumors have been observed to enlarge after cessation of irradiation, but after a delay of 2 to 3 weeks [Withers].) Fibroblastic proliferation and reepithelization can be seen in the interval. Reseeding of the irradiated zone with normal cells occurs with some cell types. Improvement in the patient's general condition usually parallels this healing process. Furthermore, in the interval of a split course the cancerous mass continues to shrink as the dead cells are cleared from the area. As described previously, this leads to improvement in oxygen tension in the remaining cells. Thus there are several reasons to justify the concept of a split course radiotherapy. However, the optimum factors of dose-interval-dose and total dose are not known. Sambrook, Holsti, and Scanlon and associates have all reported on the clinical aspects of this technique, but meaningful clinical trials have not been reported. A nationwide randomized clinical study is underway to test the value of this technique.

Since fractionation of dose was first introduced, radiation oncologists have needed a means of comparing and summating tissue effects produced by different patterns of fractionation. The very nature of fractionation with its associated normal tissue recovery, the dynamic changes within the tumor, and modification of the patient's general status limit the validity of most methods of comparison. A nominal standard dose has been used as a guide in the absence of a more meaningful concept. The nominal standard dose (NSD) is that single dose producing a clinical reaction somewhat similar to that produced by a given fractionated dose. Ellis proposed that the

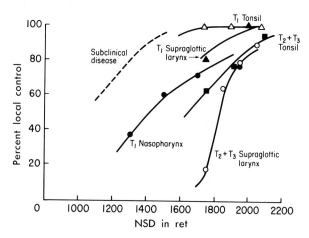

Fig. 1-12. Graph of dose (NSD)-related control rates illustrating effects of anatomic site and tumor volume. Curve for control of subclinical disease is primarily taken from experience with lymph nodes in neck. (Modified from Shukovsky, L.: Clinical applications of time-dose data to tumor on the time-dose relationships. In Caldwell, W. L., and Tolbert, D. D., editors: Clinical radiotherapy, Madison, Wis., 1975, Radiotherapy Center of Wisconsin Clinical Center. Data for nasopharyngeal lesions from Moench, H. C., and Phillips, T. L.: Am. J. Surg. **124:**515-518, 1972. Data for other curves includes data from Fletcher, G. H.: Br. J. Radiol. **46:**1-12, 1973.)

intercellular contact and growth fraction alterations, also contribute to the increased resistance of larger cell masses. The reason cells in contact with other cells have enhanced capacity to repair is unknown (Durand and Sutherland, 1972).

Clinically, this decreased radiocurability with increased volume is widely recognized. However, for clinical situations there are far too many unknowns to specify on mathematical grounds alone the increase in dose necessary for a measured increase in volume. Nevertheless, clinical experience has provided us with useful guidelines (Figs. 1-11 to 1-13). For example, clinically occult metastases to lymph nodes in the neck from squamous cell carcinoma of the oral cavity are destroyed readily with total doses of 4500 to 5000 rad in 4 to 5 weeks. When the metastases are palpable (1 to 2 cm), total doses of 6000 to 6500 rad in 6 weeks are necessary. When the metastases are 4 to 6 cm, total doses in excess of 6500 (boosting doses to the node) are considered. Metastases 6 cm or larger are difficult to control with the usual tolerated doses. Cancers of different cell types may show different time-dose relationships (Figs. 1-12 and 1-13). This relationship between dose and volume of cancer has been reviewed by Fletcher (1978).

It is a uniform observation that tolerance decreases as the irradiated volume of normal tissue increases. The most obvious example of this is seen with skin reactions. The skin dose necessary to produce a given reaction of the skin is inversely proportional to the cube root of the diameter of the irradiated field (Cohen). We recognize similar though less easily measured relationships in all tissue. This increased severity of reaction with the increased irradiated volume is not explained entirely by the in-

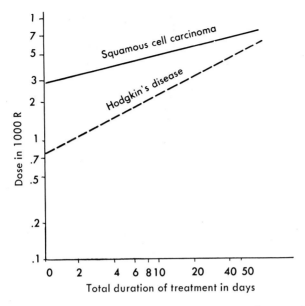

Fig. 1-13. Comparison of time-dose relationships for different types of cancer. Data for Hodgkin's disease were taken from Scott and Brizel and that for squamous cell carcinoma from Andrews and Moody. The difference in their radiosensitivity becomes relatively less with greater fractionation.

creased recovery time described previously. Cohen points out that the surface area per unit volume decreases as the volume increases. Small volumes have comparatively greater surface areas than large volumes. With a given dose the surface area of an irradiated volume would have an effect on the severity of the injury under several circumstances. Whether there is a diffusable injurious substance produced in the tumor bed by radiations or an ameliorative healing substance or migrating normal cells available from surrounding tissues has not been proved. However, the area-volume relationship discussed by Cohen helps to explain an otherwise apparent radiobiologic inconsistency.

Since normal connective tissue tolerance to radiations decreases as the irradiated volume increases, the NSD must be lower for large volumes than for small volumes. However, fractionation patterns from which the NSD concept was developed did, by necessity, bear a relationship to volume. In these data, small volumes were generally treated in fewer days than large volumes, and doses were adjusted accordingly. In this sense the NSD concept does take volume into account when the usual fractionation patterns are followed.

Summary

The differences between the cellular responses to a single dose and those to a fractionated dose involve four factors that Withers has termed "the 4 R's" (Withers, 1975).

1. *Repair (intracellular).* This is the Elkind recovery from sublethal injuries men-

tioned earlier. It takes place within the first 24 hours. The capacity for this type of recovery is measured by the split-dose technique illustrated in Fig. 1-8. So far as we can determine there is no systematic difference in the survival curves of cancer cells and normal cells.

2. *Repopulation through regeneration of the stem cells.* Mitotic activity is resumed after a dose-dependent interval between fractions. The restoration of the pre-irradiation pattern of cellular differentiation and rate of mitosis is complex and may require several days. It has been commonly accepted that there is little or no homeostatic stimulation of tumor regrowth following radiation-induced cell killing (as occurs in many normal tissues). However, some animal tumors have shown rapid spurts of regrowth after initial radiation-induced shrinkage. This rapid regrowth may be delayed more than that seen in many stem cell populations of normal tissues. In any case, it is still accepted that the differences in regenerative capability account, in part, for the selective destruction of malignant tumors.

3. *Reoxygenation.* This is discussed later.

4. *Radiation-induced synchrony.* The response of cells to a dose of radiations depends on their stage in the cell cycle (Fig. 1-6). Cells in the most sensitive stage are killed in large numbers, leaving a viable population that resumes its modified progress through the cycle from a more nearly common starting point—thus the concept of radiation-induced synchrony. One of the more dramatic demonstrations of this radiation-induced synchronization is seen in the type of "2-fraction" survival graphs shown in Fig. 1-9. The extent to which synchrony is established and is maintained is uncertain, and the impact it has on response to more than a fraction or so is debated (Fowler). Attempts to exploit these fluctuations in cell sensitivity as might be suggested by Fig. 1-9 have not met with any clinical success. Yet it is likely that radiation-induced redistribution of cancer cells in the cell cycle is a major factor in the selective destruction of malignant tumors.

The more obvious advantages of fractionation of dose can be summarized as follows:

1. There is a significant component of hypoxic cells in any palpable cancerous mass. The initial fractions of a course of fractionated irradiation reduce the number of hypoxic cells. Cater and Silver used the polarographic technique to measure tumor oxygen tensions before and after fractionated irradiation. Tumor oxygen tensions invariably increase after irradiation. Changes in normal tissue oxygen are slight or absent. This reduction in hypoxic cancer cells is a result of three changes.

    a. The absolute number of cancer cells is reduced by the initial fractions with the initial killing of well-oxygenated cells. If the available oxygen remains constant and there are fewer cancer cells, then the oxygen per remaining cell increases.

    b. Blood vessels compressed by a growing cancer are decompressed as the cancer shrinks. This permits better oxygenation of both the cancer and vasculoconnective tissues. The blood vessels themselves are injured by the radiations (Chapter 9). Thus there are changes in capillary permeability, blood flow, local thrombosis, hemorrhage, and, eventually, vascular occlusion. The timing of these changes is, of course, critical to radiation response. The dominant change might well depend on the factors of fractionation.

   c. The distance oxygen must diffuse through tissue is reduced with each fraction. Capillaries are actually measured to be closer together after the initial fractions of a series of treatments.

   2. Fractionation of dose increases the relative significance of the densely ionizing (high LET) electron "tails" during *photon* beam absorption and the significance of nonrepairable cellular injury. Although this is a minor contribution, it is of importance in the killing of hypoxic cells when each fractionated dose is small.

   3. Fractionation exploits the differential recovery rates between normal tissues and neoplastic tissues. This is thought to be largely caused by the selective response of normal tissue to homeostatic influences and not differences in Elkind recovery. Thus the epidermis of the skin recovers much more rapidly than the cells of the squamous cell carcinoma of the skin. Bowel mucosa recovers much more rapidly than adenocarcinoma of the bowel. Malignant cells are not under the influence of all the usual growth regulatory mechanisms, but normal cells are. Radiation-induced death of normal cells activates homeostatic factors and a reparative process. Fibroblastic proliferation and reepithelization of a denuded area are actually seen during a long fractionated irradiation. Furthermore, it is entirely possible that the irradiated zone is reseeded by normal cells migrating from outside the treated zone.

Radiation-induced redistribution of cells within the cell cycle tends to sensitize proliferating tissues. Obviously this can be exploited only by fractionation of dose.

   4. The initial increments of a course of fractionated irradiation will often produce enough benefits—that is, cessation of hemorrhage, reduced infection, and improved nutrition—so that the remaining fractions are better tolerated.

   5. Very high single doses produce local edema that in some sites can threaten life, increase the incidence of late sequelae, or produce major discomfort. These sequelae can be reduced or eliminated by a technique of fractionation.

   6. The discomfort and malnourishment of radiation sickness may demand a more fractionated technique.

   7. Fractionation permits greater flexibility in that higher doses can be given to volumes requiring and tolerating more, whereas lower doses can be given to volumes needing or tolerating less. For example, after a dose judged adequate for occult foci of cancer in a large volume, boosting doses can be given to a more limited volume of known disease. This sound radiobiologic principle should be practiced whenever feasible.

In an effort to improve the therapeutic ratio, many clinical studies have been made of various fractionation patterns, that is, massive single doses, prolonged fractionation patterns of Baclesse, 2 fractionations daily, 1, 2, 3, and 5 daily fractions per week (Caldwell and Tolbert, 1975; Wiernik and associates, 1978). There is no clear-cut evidence that a given fractionation pattern is optimum for all sites nor is one likely to emerge. We can anticipate that the optimum fractionation of pelvic irradiation (in which large and small bowel are in the high-dose volume) will be different from that of neck nodes or carcinoma of the breast. Also, it may vary with clinical stage and histologic type. Some of the problems are discussed by Fowler (1971), Ellis (1967, 1971), and Withers (1975). The generally accepted fractionation patterns will be given for the various clinical situations as they are presented. However, these patterns are almost certain to change as knowledge is accumulated.

Reirradiation

Previous irradiation, if it has been intense, will seriously alter radiation response to reirradiation. In fact, inadequate dosage can so alter radiation response that a cancer which was initially radiocurable can be rendered radioincurable. Several important changes occur after partial irradiation. If there are cells of different radiosensitivities in a given tumor, a greater proportion of the more sensitive ones will be destroyed. It has been postulated that the surviving cells grow to produce a more resistant tumor. It has also been suggested that a part of this decreased radiosensitivity might be a result of radiation-induced mutations with the production of a more resistant cell type. Probably the most important changes leading to decreased tumor response and curability are changes in the tumor bed. After irradiation, subendothelial connective tissues proliferate in blood vessels. Vessels are narrowed, the blood supply to the surrounding tissue decreases, and fibrosis develops throughout the soft tissues. These changes contribute to the decreased available oxygen and nutrition for the malignant cells. Even though the malignant cells have already received some radiations, they respond poorly to further irradiation in their new bed. It is for this reason that, in any curative attempt, full cancerocidal doses should be delivered with the first irradiation. It also emphasizes why, in many radiation failures, radical surgery is more likely to be successful than reirradiation.

CLINICAL GUIDES TO DOSAGE AND TREATMENT PLANNING
General condition of the patient

It is not without good reason that the general physical condition of the patient as denoted on the Karnofsky performance scale (Table 1-2) has become an integral part of the patient's pretreatment evaluation (American Joint Committee). In fact, survival rates of patients with cancer of certain anatomic sites seem more closely correlated with the patients' Karnofsky performance rating than any other pretreatment finding.

The patient's general physical condition also plays a major role in his tolerance to irradiation. A declining nutritional status with anemia is a common early finding in cancer patients. The causes for this are many and varied and need not be reviewed here. Under such circumstances normal tissue tolerance is decreased, and wound healing is slowed. The larger the treated volume, the more important the restoration of tolerances and healing to normal. An example of this has been reported by Evans and Bergsjo for carcinoma of the cervix. Patients with low hemoglobin at the onset of treatment showed a lower survival rate than those with near normal hemoglobin. This was true even when allowances were made for possible differences in stage of advancement.

Table 1-2. "Performance status" (Karnofsky scale)*

Criteria of performance status (PS)

Able to carry on normal activity; no special care is needed	100	Normal; no complaints; no evidence of disease
	90	Able to carry on normal activity; minor signs or symptoms of disease
	80	Normal activity with effort; some signs or symptoms of disease
Unable to work; able to live at home and care for most personal needs; a varying amount of assistance is needed	70	Cares for self; unable to carry on normal activity or to do active work
	60	Requires occasional assistance but is able to care for most of his needs
	50	Requires considerable assistance and frequent medical care
Unable to care for self; requires equivalent of institutional or hospital care; disease may be progressing rapidly	40	Disabled; requires special care and assistance
	30	Severely disabled; hospitalization is indicated although death is not imminent
	20	Very sick; hospitalization necessary; active supportive treatment is necessary
	10	Moribund; fatal processes progressing rapidly
	0	Dead

*From Karnofsky, D. A., Abelmann, W. H., and Carver, L. F.: Cancer **1:**634-656, 1948.

Our studies indicate that an anemia or polycythemia that is corrected to normal immediately after a single high dose of radiations does not in itself modify therapeutic ratio (O'Brien and associates). By contrast, an uncorrected anemia and negative nitrogen balance impair healing of radiation-induced injuries, just as they impair healing of other types of tissue destruction.

A severe decline in general condition may precipitate late radiation necrosis. We have seen patients several years after high-dose curative irradiation subjected to sudden severe hemorrhage from an unrelated cause. Massive tissue necrosis of the irradiated zone appeared within 24 hours.

In animals, irradiated blood vessels respond to subsequently acquired hypertension by developing profound hypertensive vascular damage (Asscher and Anson). This damage is much more severe than in unirradiated tissue of the same organ. Asscher and Anson pointed out that hypertension from any cause developing in a patient who previously had vital tissues irradiated—that is, brain, spinal cord, bowel, or lung—can, because of the exaggerated vessel response to the hypertension, lead to the development of vascular necrosis in the patient, thus leading to heretofore unexplained sequelae.

When one recommends certain doses of radiations for a given disease, it must be realized that, just as with any other type of medication, individual needs and tolerances vary widely. Individualization of therapy should be routine. The principles involved in individualization of therapy are the same as those involved in any good medical care. This begins with a meticulously taken history and a thorough physical examination, a review of the radiographs, a review of the biopsy material and a discussion with the pathologist of its possible and probable implications, a review of pertinent laboratory data, and, when possible, inspection and palpation of the lesion. There will be enough uncertainties without increasing their number by incomplete pretreatment examinations and studies. Every patient must then be evaluated as an individual problem, using all available data to determine the volume likely to contain the cancer, or, as we call it, *the volume of interest.*

Within this volume of interest will lie normal organs. We must know their tolerance to doses that might be expected to produce the desired results. Finally, we must know the total body effects. If it is advisable to irradiate a relatively large volume with a curative aim, the patient's general condition must be good. This may require that it be improved just as for any major surgical procedure. If the patient is anemic, the sooner his hemoglobin is restored to its normal level the better. It is likely that with a slowly developing anemia the growth of the cancer will be modified in keeping with the limited oxygen. Transfusion with early irradiation could conceivably be critical in the cure of such a cancer. If there are nutritional deficiencies, appropriate diets supplemented with vitamins should be given. Tissue healing is delayed with a negative nitrogen balance. Necrosis and infection are decreased with adequate nutrition. The degenerative diseases that so frequently limit surgery in aged patients also limit vigorous irradiation. The general principle of vigorous supportive care cannot be emphasized too strongly. Specific preirradiation preparation for lesions of the oral cavity, antrum, bladder, and so forth are also important, and specific suggestions in this regard are made in the discussion of each disease. During the period of treatment, reevaluation of the patient's local and systemic tolerances occasionally justifies changes in daily doses and even field sizes. The development of symptoms referable to a previous undetected metastasis or other factors that modify anticipated longevity may result in a radical change of aim of treatment. Local swelling or edema may demand decreased daily dose. An increasing blood uric acid, an unpredicted drop in blood counts, nausea and vomiting, diarrhea, dysuria, and dysphagia may signal an unusual response in a sensitive individual. Many other reasons justifying daily attention by the radiation oncologist will be mentioned later. He will be looking for signals not familiar to the usual referring physician. This daily attention and the adjustment of technique in keeping with the observed response demand time and experience but are essential to good patient care.

Curative irradiation, like curative surgery, usually implies radical treatment. In radiotherapy radical treatment usually means vigorous irradiation of the volume suspected to contain all tumor. Early, intense cutaneous and mucosal reactions may be mandatory. Late cutaneous changes, bone damage, and fibrotic changes in deep organs may of necessity be the price of curative treatment. There are actually few instances in which the chief indication for curative irradiation is that it is a less demanding procedure.

If the treatment has been given rapidly, it is not unusual for maximum mucosal and skin reactions to appear after completion of treatment. Such fractionation obviously requires postirradiation care by the radiation oncologist. However, it is important that follow-up be continued for years postirradiation, not only to treat recurrences the moment they appear but also to evaluate tumor and normal tissue response and tolerance. It is from these follow-up data that rational changes in treatment are justified. Radiation therapy based on the principles discussed is not a treatment administered by a technician and supervised loosely by an already overworked radiologist. The ideal arrangement calls for a well-trained radiation oncologist to supervise the complete care of many of the patients during and immediately after the period of treatment. Other patients require collaborative efforts of the entire team.

In a way it is unfortunate that under a good teacher few complications of overtreatment will be seen by the trainee. Not infrequently, the newly certified resident, like his surgical counterpart, is convinced that better results will follow more radical treatment. With megavoltage beams it is easy and tempting for the new radiation oncologist to increase field sizes and doses and to extend the indications of and doses from interstitial implants. He launches his career by producing an increased number of radiation necroses without increasing control rates. Slowly and painfully he appreciates the skill and advice of his teacher.

Radiation oncology as presented in the preceding discussion is the clinical practice of medicine. It places the full responsibility of pretreatment evaluation on the radiation oncologist. It demands that he plan his treatment in keeping with the known routes of infiltration and metastases. It demands that he carry the dose to a level ensuring maximum cure rates or palliation but producing a minimum of serious sequelae. He must accept the full responsibility for his successes and his failures.

Selecting an optimum dose

The many factors that guide us in selecting an optimum dose, including the parameters of volume, fractionation, and total treatment time, have been mentioned throughout this chapter. When the term *optimum dose* is used, it includes the parameters previously mentioned. These factors have been analyzed in a variety of ways throughout the history of radiotherapy and are summarized briefly here. The aim of optimization of dose is to obtain maximum cure rates with minimum sequelae. There is no single optimum for all cancers of a given cell type, of a given anatomic site, or of a given volume. Optimum values must be determined by clinical trials, although recently our knowledge of cellular radiobiology has suggested the directions in which we should search.

Cancers of different anatomic sites respond differently even when they appear to be of similar histologic types and of similar sizes. Squamous cell carcinomas of the lip are much more easily controlled than similar-sized cancers of the piriform sinus. The reason for this difference is unknown, although we can speculate about the differences in proportion of hypoxic cells and in cellular kinetics.

The gross morphology of cancers, that is, whether they are exophytic, necrotic, deeply infiltrating, or superficial, are clinical manifestations of differences in cellular nutrition, oxygenation, cellular kinetics, host reaction, and undoubtedly other factors modifying response to radiations. Clinical staging systems such as the TNM system cannot remain practical and still take into account all these variations in morphology. Yet we recognize a spectrum of response associated with gross morphology. The necrotic lesions respond least because they contain the greatest proportion of hypoxic cells, whereas the exophytic lesions respond most quickly.

The reasons why the size of the cancerous mass affects optimum dose have already been discussed. A large mass of cancer cells respond less well to a given dose than does a small mass of cells. This difference in response applies equally well to primary cancers of different sizes and to metastases of different sizes. Certain general principles and observations should be noted.

1. For a large cancerous mass, initiate treatment with large ports, and then after a dose judged adequate for well-oxygenated occult peripheral cancer cells, deliver a boosting dose to the residual mass through a reduced portal.

2. Small cancerous masses require less dose for control and can be controlled with fewer sequelae than large cancerous masses.

3. Clinically occult disease, whether it be metastases in lymph nodes or after inadequate surgery, requires less dose for control and can be controlled with fewer radiation-induced sequelae than clinically obvious cancerous masses.

Optimum dose varies with cell type. There is a spectrum of responses ranging from the lymphomas to the epithelial carcinomas to the soft tissue sarcomas and osteosarcomas. It is not known why this type of variation exists, although we relate it to the response of the tissue of origin and the cellular kinetics of those tissues. These differences and similarities are discussed in the chapters to follow.

Paramount in determining optimum doses are the tolerances of normal tissues and organs encompassed in the volume of interest. Examples of this are seen for many cancers in many areas of the body. The tolerance of the larynx is very near the dose required for maximum control of carcinoma of the glottis. Similarly, the tolerance of the rectum is a major factor in determining the dose and technique used for treating carcinoma of the cervix. For almost every anatomic site there are limiting normal organs that prompt a specific technique and dose. This is more noticeable for those cancers that require high doses in anatomic sites easily damaged.

Thus the definition of optimum dose is sometimes a highly complex determination, balancing the fear of persistence of cancer with the hazards of radiation-induced sequelae. Dose alone is only a part of this complex determination.

General aspects of treatment planning and dose selection

As mentioned previously, in evaluating a given patient for irradiation, one either consciously or intuitively considers three factors.

1. The site of origin and routes of spread (This defines the location and size of the volume to be considered for irradiation—the volume of interest.)

2. The dose necessary to produce the hoped-for result (This would be the dose necessary to achieve either palliation or control depending on the clinical circumstances. The dose necessary to accomplish a given change will vary with anatomic site, histologic type, volume of tumor masses, dose rate, and type of fractionation.)

3. Radiation tolerance of the neighboring organs to the contemplated dose and of the patient as a whole to the procedure (Once the location and size of the volume are determined and the required dose is defined, the advisability of the entire procedure can be assessed from the standpoint of both local and systemic reactions.)

Although in subsequent discussions we have tried to define each of these three factors for each tumor type, clinical experience alone can equip the physician with the skill required to assess these three factors. The steps involved in treatment planning are not presented as a recipe to be followed but rather as an outline to assist the trainee in organizing the procedure into a rational routine.

Treatment planning is ordinarily pictured as the construction of a patient's contour, the selection and direction of beams, the summation of isodose curves, and the mechanics of "setting up" and reproducing the treatment each day. We object to this concept of treatment planning because it implies a simplicity that does not exist. As previously indicated, to create a treatment plan, the volume requiring irradiation must be defined, the radiosensitivity and radiocurability of the cancer must be considered, and the tolerance of adjacent normal tissues must be respected.

1. Definition of the volume of interest. Tumor localization is the weakest point in treatment planning. It is the end product of a good history and physical examination, pertinent films, and a host of specifically indicated specialized studies varying from isotope scans to lymphangiograms, computed tomography, and surgical exploration. The extent of the cancer thus visualized and palpated establishes the basis for clinical staging. However, this alone does not define the volume to be irradiated. Once the distribution of the detectable cancer is defined, the natural history of that particular cancer must be considered. The usual behavior of that cell type of that anatomic origin and clinical stage constitutes the basis on which we predict occult extension. If the statistics suggest that there is sufficiently frequent occult extension, then clinically uninvolved volumes must be encompassed in the high-dose distribution. This extension of the volume of interest is a recognition of the limitations in tumor localization techniques. The size, shape, and location of the volume to be considered for irradiation are thus defined. Tumor localization is not a one-time job. The radiation oncologist is concerned here with biologic material. The flat contour of yesterday's abdomen may be rounded by today's gas. Patients may lose from 15 to 20 pounds during irradiation. Skin fields sag, and a viscus may change in size and shape. Repeated verification films are a great teacher.

The definition of the precise volume to be irradiated also depends on the sensitivity and importance of neighboring structures. By necessity, a volume may be restricted to exclude a sensitive critical organ such as the kidney but not restricted over a more resistant or expendable organ.

Thus the definition of the volume of interest is a judgment based in part on objective evidence and in part on experience and statistics. The judgment must balance precautions for encompassing likely cancer with the fear of injuring normal organs.

2. Radiosensitivity of the primary cancer and its extensions. This defines the minimum dose necessary to accomplish either cancer eradication for cure or growth restraint for palliation. The complexities of radiosensitivity and radioresponsiveness have already been presented on p. 8. The minimum dose necessary to accomplish one's aim is less well defined than the maximum dose tolerated. Therefore, at least for the more radiosensitive cancers, overdosage occurs often. Clinical experience has established certain guidelines, but numerous uncertainties exist as to the minimum necessary dose in all of the many clinical situations.

3. Radiation tolerance of neighboring organs. In terms of tissue damage what price is the patient to pay for the radiation oncologist's curative or palliative efforts? What price is justified? For known palliative aims few if any injuries are justified. On the other hand, major injuries may be justified if such injuries are also necessary to obtain a maximum cure rate. For example, a young girl's ovaries may be sacrificed if irradiation of nearby lymph nodes will increase the cure rate 5%. Jaw necrosis in 20% of the cured patients may be acceptable if it is an unavoidable part of a technique that cures 10% more patients than any other technique. This balancing of radiation-induced sequelae against increased benefits can be one of our most difficult judgments.

4. The specification of dose. The intention of some treatment plans is to enclose the cancer in a uniformly dosed volume. When any of the numerous exceptions to this are encountered (cancer of the cervix, the need for boosting doses, separate treatment of primary site and nodes), the variation in doses should be clearly defined and in keeping with the radiobiologic justifications discussed earlier. In either case the treatment plan should reduce the dose to the nontumor-containing volume to a minimum. What degree of precision is necessary and what degree of precision is clinically practical? Even a moderate degree of precision by the physicist's standards demands good equipment and time-consuming calibration, to say nothing of the clinical requirements. If a homogeneous distribution of dose is desired, is a ±10% variation of dose in the volume of interest acceptable? Is a ± 5% variation in does necessary? What is the best we can expect in day-to-day clinical practice?

The interrelationships between dose, time, and volume have been mentioned several times and will be stressed repeatedly throughout subsequent chapters. It can be misleading to discuss one of these factors without recognizing its relationships with the other two. An examination of the *ret* doses required to control various sizes of cancerous masses attempts to incorporate all three factors and has been used by Shukovsky, Fletcher, Moench and Phillips, and others. Fig. 1-12 illustrates the relationships of local control to ret dose for some common anatomic sites. Several important conclusions are possible from such graphs.

1. Local control rates are dependent on the ret dose.

2. For a given rate of local control a large cancerous mass, that is, a nodal metas-

tasis 5 cm in diameter, requires higher ret doses than a small cancerous mass, that is, a mass 1.5 cm in diameter.

3. Small changes in ret doses produce large changes in local control rates for T2 and T3 supraglottic cancers, but much less changes in local control rates for T1 lesions of the nasopharynx.

Thus one must add the variable of anatomic site to the complex relationship of time, dose, and volume.

Fig. 1-12 may also give us a measure of the relative importance of precision in selecting and delivering a given dose to a given volume of cancer in a specific anatomic site. Small errors in dose selection or dose delivery could be critical in the irradiation of T2 and T3 lesions of the supraglottic larynx (Herring and Compton, 1970). The same degree of error seems to be relatively less critical in the irradiation of limited cancers of the tonsil or nasopharynx.

Similar variations in optimum dose-time-volume relationships undoubtedly exist for other anatomic sites but are generally less precisely defined.

Herring and Compton assembled similar data in an effort to define the increment of dose necessary to trigger necrosis of normal tissues. Here, too, more than a simple statement of total dose is involved, but dose is the one yardstick that has been analyzed. Stewart showed that the probability of laryngeal necrosis increased from near zero after 5500 rad to 6% after 5750 rad (Fig. 1-14). Thus 250 rad, or about one treatment, triggered a significant incidence of laryngeal necrosis. Finally, Fletcher and associates pointed out that with their adoption of the rad as the clinical unit of dose they proceeded to administer the same number of rads as they had been giving

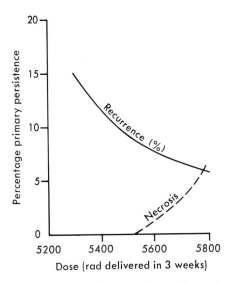

Fig. 1-14. Plot showing decreasing local persistence rate with increasing dose. With doses above 5500 rad incidence of necrosis rose sharply. (Modification of Herring's plot of Stewart's data; from Herring, D. F., and Compton, D. M.: Report No. EMI-216 [Enviro-Med] pp. 10-11, 1970.)

of roentgens when that was their unit of dose. Since 1 roentgen of ^{60}Co radiations equals 0.93 rad, they actually gave a 7% higher dose. This apparently small increase in dose increased the incidence of massive laryngeal edema from near zero to 10%. A similar increase in rectal reactions was produced by the same change in treating cancer of the cervix.

It is now obvious that when high-dose irradiation is necessary for cure as for carcinoma of the larynx and cervix, the dose producing maximum cures is very near the dose producing prohibitive sequelae. As little as 500 rad above or below the optimum is significant. In our opinion a variation of dose 10% above or 10% below the optimum dose is excessive, whereas a variation of dose no more than 5% above or 5% below the optimum may be difficult to achieve in many clinical situations. This level of precision is not so critical when low-dose palliative techniques are required or when high doses are not necessary for cure.

Most correlations of doses with responses have been made by the summation of central axis depth doses. There are obvious limitations to using this single number to define dose in a large heterogeneously irradiated volume. Computer-aided dosimetry can provide a practical, almost instantaneous summation of isodose curves with correction for oblique incidence and can provide, in certain circumstances, corrections for nonhomogeneity of tissues. Dose can be readily expressed in a number of ways, but great care must be taken when such changes are made. It seems reasonable to use the modal dose, that is, that dose which is most widespread in the treated volume provided the minimum and maximum doses to the volume of interest are also given. However, it must be remembered that in most instances the modal dose will be lower than the summation of the central axis doses. Substituting the modal dose for the dose that had heretofore been accepted as optimal would result in giving an 8% to 10% higher dose. From previous discussions in this chapter, the sequelae of such an oversight are predictable.

REFERENCES

Alper, T.: Elkind recovery and "sub-lethal damage": a misleading association? Br. J. Radiol. **50**:459-467, 1977.

Asscher, A. W., and Anson, S. C.: Arterial hypertension and irradiation damage to the nervous system, Lancet **2**:1343-1346, 1962.

Atkins, H. L., Seaman, W. B., Jacox, H. W., and Matteo, R. S.: Experience with hyperbaric oxygenation in clinical radiotherapy, Am. J. Roentgenol. **93**:651-663, 1965.

Caldwell, W. L., and Tolbert, D. D.: Proceedings of Conference on the Time-Dose Relationships in Clinical Radiotherapy, Madison, Wisconsin, Oct. 4 and 5, 1974, Middleton, Wis., 1975, Madison Printing & Publishing Co.

Cater, D. B., and Silver, I. A.: Quantitative measurements of oxygen tension in normal tissues and in the tumours of patients before and after radiotherapy, Acta Radiol. **53**:233-256, 1960.

Churchill-Davidson, I.: Oxygen effect on radiosensitivity, Proceedings of the Conference on Research of the Radiotherapy of Cancer, New York, 1961, American Cancer Society, Inc.

Cohen, L.: Radiation response and recovery: radiobiological principles and their relation to clinical practice. In Schwartz, E. E., editor: The biological basis of radiation therapy, Philadelphia, 1966, J. B. Lippincott Co.

Comas, F. V.: Comparative changes in radiosensitivity between bone marrow and a rat tumor irradiated under anoxia, Radiology **83**:528-534, 1964.

Duncan, W., and Nias, A. H.: Clinical radiobiology, Edinburgh, 1977, Churchill Livingstone.

Durand, R. E., and Sutherland, R. M.: Effects of intercellular contact on repair of radiation damage, Exp. Cell Res. **71:**75-80, 1972.

DuSault, L. A.: The time-dose relationship in radiotherapy. In Buschke, F., editor: Progress in radiation therapy, New York, 1958, Grune & Stratton, Inc.

Elkind, M. M.: Cellular aspects of tumor therapy, Radiology **74:**529-542, 1960.

Elkind, M. M., and Sutton, H.: Radiation response of mammalian cells grown in culture, Radiat. Res. **13:**556-593, 1960.

Elkind, M. M.: Reoxygenation and its potential role in radiotherapy. In Brookhaven National Laboratory: Proceedings of Conference on Time and Dose Relationships in Radiation Biology as Applied to Radiotherapy, Carmel, Calif., 1969, BNL50203 (C-57).

Ellis, F.: Fractionation in radiotherapy. In Deeley, T. J., and Wood, C. A., editors: Modern trends in radiotherapy, vol. 1, New York, 1967, Appleton-Century-Crofts.

Ellis, F.: The relationship of biological effect to dose-time-fractionation factors in radiotherapy. In Ebert, M., and Howard, A., editors: Current topics in radiation research, ed. 4, New York, 1968, John Wiley & Sons, Inc.

Ellis, F.: Nominal standard dose and the ret, Br. J. Radiol. **44:**101-108, 1971.

Evans, J. C., and Bergsjo, P.: The influence of anemia on results of radiotherapy in carcinoma of the cervix, Radiology **84:**709-717, 1965.

Fazekas, J. T., Green, J. P., Vaeth, J. M., and Schroeder, A. F.: Postirradiation induration as a prognosticator, Radiology **102:**409-412, 1972.

Fletcher, G. H.: The evolution of the basic concepts underlying the practice of radiotherapy from 1949 to 1977. Radiology **127:**3-19, 1978.

Fletcher, G. H., Tongpoon, W., and Rutledge, F. N.: Whole pelvis irradiation with 4,000 rads in Stage I and II cancers of the uterine cervix, Radiology **86:**436-443, 1966.

Fowler, J. F.: Radiation biology and radiotherapy. In Howard, A., and Ebert, M., editors: Current topics in radiation research, vol. 2, Amsterdam, 1966, North-Holland Publishing Co.

Fowler, J. F.: Fast neutron therapy—physical and biological considerations. In Deeley, T. J., and Wood, C. A., editors: Modern trends in radiotherapy, vol 1, New York, 1967, Appleton-Century-Crofts.

Fowler, J. F.: Experimental animal results relating to time-dose relationships in radiotherapy and the "ret" concept, Br. J. Radiol. **44:**81-90, 1971.

Fowler, J. F., and Stern, B. E.: Dose-time relationships in radiotherapy and the validity of cell survival curve models, Br. J. Radiol. **36:**163-173, 1963.

Gagnon, J.: Personal communication, Nov., 1978.

Glassburn, J. R., Brady, L. W., and Plenk, H. P.: Hyperbaric oxygen in radiation therapy, Cancer **39:**751-765, 1977.

Hall, E. J.: Radiobiology for the radiologist, New York, 1973, Harper & Row Publishers, Inc.

Herring, D. F., and Compton, D. M.: The degree of precision required in the radiation dose delivered in cancer radiotherapy, Enviro-Med. Report No. EMI-216, pp. 10-11, 1970.

Holsti, L. R.: Split-course megavoltage radiotherapy: one year follow-up, Br. J. Radiol. **39:**332-337, 1966.

Los Alamos Scientific Laboratory of the University of California: Proceedings of Conference on Particle Accelerators in Radiation Therapy, LA-5180-C, Los Alamos, N. M., 1972.

Mendelsohn, M. L.: Radiation effects in tumors. In Radiation research, 1966, Amsterdam, 1967, North-Holland Publishing Co.

Mendelsohn, M. L., and Dethlefsen, L. A.: Tumor growth and cellular kinetics in the proliferation and spread of neoplastic cells, Houston, 1967, M. D. Anderson, Hosp., p 200.

Moench, H. C., and Phillips, T. L.: Carcinoma of the nasopharynx, Am. J. Surg. **124:**515-518, 1972.

O'Brien, P. H., Moss, W. T., Louwenaar, K., May, J., and Peterson, L.: The effect of acute anemia on the radiosensitivity of V_2 rabbit sarcoma, Radiology **91:**1159-1162, 1968.

Orton, C. G., and Ellis, F.: A simplification of the use of the NSD concept in practical radiotherapy, Br. J. Radiol. **46:**529-537, 1973.

Pizzarello, D. J., and Witcofski, R. L.: Medical radiation biology, Philadelphia, 1972, Lea & Febiger.

Puck, T. T., and Marcus, P. I.: Actions of x-rays on mammalian cells, J. Exp. Med. **103:**653-666, 1956.

Puck, T. T., Morkovin, D., Marcus, P. I., and Cieciura, S. J.: Action of x-rays on mammalian cells. II. Survival curves of cells from normal tissues, J. Exp. Med. **106:**485-500, 1957.

Rubin, P., and Casarett, G. W.: Clinical radiation pathology, Philadelphia, 1968, W. B. Saunders Co.

Sambrook, D. K.: Theoretical aspects of dose-time factors in radiotherapy technique, Clin. Radiol. **14:**290-297, 1963.

Scanlon, P. W., Devine, K. D., Woolner, L. B., and McBean, J. B.: Cancer of the tonsil: 131 patients treated in the 11-year period 1950 through 1960, Am. J. Roentgenol. **100:**894-903, 1967.

Scott, R. M., and Brizel, H. E.: Time-dose relationships in Hodgkin's disease, Radiology **82:** 1043-1048, 1964.

Shukovsky, L. J.: Dose, time, volume relationships in squamous cell carcinoma of the supraglottic larynx, Am. J. Roentgenol. **108:**27-29, 1970.

Sinclair, W. K.: Cell cycle dependence of the lethal radiation response in mammalian cells. Curr. Top. Radiat. Res. **7:**264-285, 1972.

Sinclair, W. K.: N-Ethylmaleimide and the cyclic response to x-rays of synchronous Chinese hamster cells. Radiat. Res. **55:**41-57, 1973.

Stewart, J. G.: Late effects of radiation—the radiotherapists' problem, Br. J. Radiol. **42:**797-798, 1969.

Suit, H. D., and Shalek, R. J.: Response of anoxic C3H mouse mammary carcinoma isotransplants (1-25 mm. 3) to x-irradiation, J. Natl. Cancer Inst. **31:**479-495, 1963.

Suit, H. D., and Shalek, R. J.: Response of spontaneous mammary carcinoma of the C3H mouse to x-irradiation given under conditions of local tissue anoxia, J. Natl. Cancer Inst. **31:**497-509, 1963.

Suit, H., Lindberg, R., and Fletcher, G. H.: Prognostic significance of extent of tumor regression at completion of radiation therapy, Radiology **84:**1100-1107, 1965.

Sutherland, R. M., Inch, W. R., McCredie, J. A., and Kruuv, J.: A multicomponent radiation curve using an in vitro tumour model, Int. J. Radiat. Biol. **18:**491-495, 1970.

Van den Brenk, H. A. S.: Hyperbaric oxygen in radiation therapy: an investigation of dose-effect relationships in tumor response and tissue damage, Am. J. Roentgenol. **102:**8-26, 1968.

Whitmore, G. F.: Some radiation effects on mammalian cells in tissue culture. In Kallman, R. F., editor: Research in radiotherapy, Washington, D. C., 1961, National Academy of Sciences—National Research Council, Publication 888.

Wiernik, G., Bleehan, N. M., Brindle, J., Bullimore, J., Churchill-Davidson, I. F. J., Davidson, J., Fowler, J. F., Francis, P., Hadden, R. C. M., Haybittle, J. L., Howard, N., Lansley, I. F., Lindup, R., Phillips, D. L., and Skeggs, D.: Sixth interim progress report of the British Institute of Radiology fractionation study of 3F/week versus 5F/week in radiotherapy of the laryngo-pharynx, Br. J. Radiol. **51:**241-250, 1978.

Wildermuth, O.: Hybaroxic radiation therapy in cancer management, Radiology **82:**767-776, 1964.

Wildermuth, O.: Clinical hybaroxic radiotherapy after five years, Radiology **93:**1149-1154, 1969.

Withers, H. R.: Capacity for repair of normal and malignant tissue. In Brookhaven National Laboratory: Proceedings of Conference on Time and Dose Relationships in Radiation Biology as Applied to Radiotherapy, Carmel, Calif., 1969, BNL50203 (C-57).

Withers, H. R.: The four "R's" of radiotherapy. In Lett, J. T., and Adler, H., editors: Advances in radiation biology, vol. 5, New York, 1975, Academic Press.

2
Combinations of radiotherapy and surgery

The rationale for combining irradiation and surgery to achieve maximum loco-regional control rates is presented below. The specific clinical problems of combining these two modalities are presented in subsequent chapters.

Radiotherapy and surgery may be combined in a variety of ways in the management of malignant neoplasms. The importance of each modality varies from disease to disease and indeed from patient to patient. The sequence and the aim of each modality is also highly dependent on the patient in question. The primary lesions of some malignant neoplasms are best treated by one modality, whereas their lymph node metastases are best treated by the other modality. For example, in the treatment of seminoma of the testicle, the primary lesion is removed and the iliac and para-aortic lymph node metastases are irradiated. In the management of carcinoma of the tongue, this sequence is often reversed; the primary lesion is irradiated and the cervical lymph node metastases, especially if large, are excised by a radical neck dissection. In both instances the planned combined therapy has a curative aim. The area treated by one modality may not be retreated by the other modality. The second portion of the treatment is given with the conviction that the first portion of treatment has succeeded in its aim. The literature provides us with ample data to confirm the value of this type of combined therapy in selected cancers. This is not considered preoperative or postoperative irradiation. The terms *preoperative* and *postoperative irradiation* are applicable when both irradiation and resection are used in the same anatomic site.

Fundamental in the rationale of combining the two modalities is the recognition that some aspects of loco-regional control are best accomplished with irradiation and some are best accomplished with excision. The need for the combination is seen in the technical limitations of surgery and the radiobiologic limitations of radiation therapy. Thus radiocurability of a given cancerous mass is, in part, dependent on the volume of the mass. Small or subclinical foci of cancer may be readily eradicated by irradiation, whereas large masses of the same cell type in the same anatomic site may not be controlled by acceptable doses. Coupled with this is the common observation that surgical excision of a large cancerous mass may fail because of residual subclinical foci of cancer at the operative site. For these reasons combinations of irradiation and surgery may achieve loco-regional control rates that neither modality alone can achieve.

Two other observations have encouraged the combination of these modalities. Histologic types heretofore often considered "radioresistant" may in fact be eradicated by irradiation when the tumor volume is small. This is especially true for soft tissue sarcomas. The use of postoperative irradiation is now almost "routine" in such patients. Also concern for surgical disruption of the "tumor bed" has been a long-standing argument for preferring preoperative irradiation over postoperative irradiation. We now recognize that in many instances there are little or no clinically discernable surgically induced effects detrimental to the response of the tumor bed to irradiation. This depends on early wound healing, little or no postoperative infection or edema, and in the case of the pelvis, an acceptable risk of bowel damage. In such patients the surgeon finds postoperative irradiation a useful complement with an acceptable risk.

PREOPERATIVE IRRADIATION

In selected sites the high incidence of local persistence after irradiation alone or after surgery alone has naturally led to the trial of a great variety of combinations of the two modalities. Locally advanced cancers in all sites are likely to persist regardless of their initial method of treatment. Especially frustrating in this regard have been advanced cancers of the oral cavity, upper air passages, breast, bladder, lung, and rectum. By their location, postsurgical local persistences have more or less been accepted as a consequence of cancer transection. The possibility that cells migrate to the suture line from beyond the line of excision cannot be excluded (Gricouroff). Irradiation, whether preoperative or postoperative, has been given primarily to decrease the incidence of persistence.

Combinations of irradiation and surgery are necessary and effective only in selected circumstances. Thus, if the entire cancer is resectable by the anticipated surgery, preoperative irradiation is unnecessary. If the cancer has already metastasized distantly or invaded beyond the irradiated volume, preoperative irradiation will not contribute to cure. To increase the cure rate, preoperative irradiation must either prevent critical iatrogenic metastases produced at the time of surgery or destroy cancer limited to the region adjacent to the anticipated surgical wound. The cancer adjacent to the anticipated surgical wound may be clinically obvious or occult, but the principles of preoperative irradiation will be the same.

Aims of preoperative irradiation

In addition to rendering a locally nonresectable cancer resectable, preoperative irradiation has been given with three other aims—the aims of rendering nonviable any malignant cells that happen to be implanted in the wound or circulatory system during surgery, the aim of increasing the resistance of normal tissues to tumor cell implants and further tumor invasion, and, finally, in certain anatomic sites one

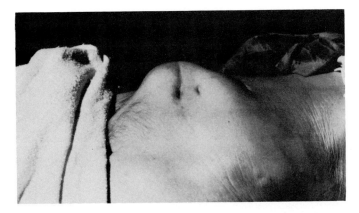

Fig. 2-1. Wound implantation of a transitional cell carcinoma of the bladder into suprapubic area.

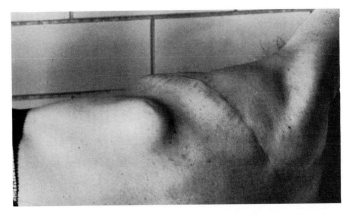

Fig. 2-2. Bronchogenic carcinoma implanted in stab wound in which a drain was placed post-operatively.

method of therapy may be recognized as more effective against limited cancer whereas another method would be preferred if the lesion were known to be advanced. If it is impossible or impractical to determine the extent of spread before treatment, and if the application of both modalities of treatment is not associated with a major increase in morbidity or mortality, it may be advisable to apply both modalities to most patients.

Once viable cancer has been transected and gross recurrence has developed, the task for irradiation becomes more difficult (Figs. 2-1 and 2-2). It was formerly thought that when both irradiation and surgery were to be used, irradiation should be used preoperatively rather than postoperatively. The validity of this concept is supported by the study of Perez and Olson. They found that for a lymphosarcoma in mice, preoperative irradiation given in single doses up to 3000 rad produced a higher control rate than similar doses given postoperatively. However, the sequence of the two modalities varies according to tumor and anatomic site. These will be discussed later.

CONVERSION OF A NONRESECTABLE CANCER TO A RESECTABLE ONE. One of the most frequently given justifications for preoperative irradiation has been the conversion of a locally nonresectable lesion into a resectable one. This justification demands that the portion of the tumor producing nonresectability must be eradicated by irradiation, and it implies that a second part of the same tumor, incurable by irradiation, must be removed.

As a cancerous mass enlarges, its supporting connective tissue and blood vessels are incapable of maintaining the usual oxygen and nutritional requirements. Centrally located cells develop hypoxia, and they even necrose. Similar but less severe changes develop within cellular columns throughout the mass. By contrast, the less crowded peripheral cells are well oxygenated, well nourished, and mitotically active. These peripheral cells push along lines of least resistance to points beyond the palpable tumor borders. Since such peripheral fingers of cancer cannot usually be clinically detected, the unsuspecting surgeon transects them. Microscopically these peripheral fingers are recognized as perineural sheath permeation, extension along muscle planes, or between fat lobules. They are presumed to be the most common source of postoperative local persistence.

It is now generally accepted that the better oxygenation of the peripheral fingers makes them more radiosensitive than the central mass of cells. On this assumption alone rests the most common rationale of using modest doses preoperatively. The fingers, with their greater sensitivity, may thus be sterilized in a significant proportion even though the hypoxic central mass is not. This concept, then, assumes that a double standard of radiosensitivity exists in the nonresectable primary cancer. It implies that a cancer, nonresectable because of a well-oxygenated but nonresectable periphery, may indeed be rendered resectable by preoperative irradiation. It implies that large-field, modest-dose preoperative irradiation might destroy the occult peripheral fingers of a cancer and thus prevent their accidental transection. A spectrum of animal studies support this concept, that is, studies on malignant lymphoma (Powers and Tohmach), mammary carcinoma and carcinosarcoma (Inch and McCredie), melanoma (Powers), and hepatoma (Nakayama and associates). Generally, with these animal tumors, 500 to 2000 rad given in single doses 1 to 6 days before surgery decreases the incidence of local persistence. Similarly convincing studies with low doses have not been done in man.

The idea that peripheral fingers of a cancer are more susceptible to radiation death than the central mass is widely accepted. However, Goldman and Friedman suggest this may not always be true. After tissue doses of 5500 rad in 6 weeks they found tiny, apparently viable foci of cancer cells scattered well beyond the main mass of the primary. They challenged the classic concept that radiation-induced cancer shrinkage is from the periphery to the point of origin. The persistence of scattered foci emphasizes the need for surgery in these cancers even when there is no palpable or visible residual tumor. The distribution of the foci emphasizes the hazard of doing a limited resection for what was initially an advanced cancer (Goldman and Friedman; Galante and associates).

The rationale of irradiating subclinical regional metastases is quite similar to that of irradiating subclinical peripheral extensions from the primary lesion. However, systematic or "prophylactic" irradiation of regional nodes is not in the true sense preoperative or postoperative irradiation. The rationale for it is presented in the discussion of each anatomic site.

The correlation of dose of radiation required to dependably eradicate cancerous masses of various volumes has been reviewed by Fletcher. In addition, specific dose requirements are presented in the discussion of each anatomic site.

PREVENTION OF IATROGENIC METASTASES. The finding of cancer cells in washings from the surgical incision and the development of cancer regrowth in wound edges implicate the surgeon in the act of cancer dissemination (Figs. 2-1 and 2-2). Whether dissemination in the wound is a result of transecting cancer or the emptying of vessels is not clear (Gricouroff). Preoperative irradiation, even in low doses, produces changes both in the cancer cells and in the wound edges, which could be beneficial to the patient.

Effect on wound edges. Doses of 500 to 3000 rad delivered to normal tissues comprising the wound edges will decrease the incidence of take of subsequently implanted nonirradiated cancer cells (Vermund and associates; Summers and associates; Hewitt and Blake). Whether this effect is secondary to blood vessel or lymph vessel damage or related to cell death in connective tissues is not known. The effect of higher doses may last for months. If viable cancer is transected, however, the remaining cancer will grow into the irradiated zone after the period of "diminished cancer viability."

Although irradiation of some normal tissues as described will decrease the incidence of take of subsequently implanted cancer cells, other normal tissues do not respond in this fashion. Preinjection irradiation of the lung does not decrease the incidence of hematogenous pulmonary metastases from cancer cells injected intravenously after irradiation of the lung (Dao and Yogo). The route of administration of cancer cells is thus important.

Effect on cancer cells. Preimplantation irradiation of tumor cells decreases the incidence of take. Hoye and Smith irradiated mouse tumors in vivo with low doses of x rays (170 to 2000 R single dose). These doses did not in themselves stop the growth of the primary tumor. The researchers found that the growth of such an irradiated tumor subsequently injected into nonirradiated tissue (intravascularly, intramuscularly, and into an axillary wound) was decreased by more than 90%. Similar studies by Smith and Godbee show that preimplantation in vivo irradiation of cancer cells can reduce the number of lung metastases resulting from subsequent intravenous injection of these cells. The most obvious explanation of the decrease in incidence of take is found in the fact that a critical number of viable tumor cells must be implanted to produce a tumor take. This minimum number of required cells varies from tumor to tumor and from host resistance to host resistance. There is no reason to believe that in this regard man differs from the laboratory animal. Preimplantation irradiation reduces the number of cells capable of subsequent continued mitotic activity; it does this without immediately removing such cells from the population counted for implantation. It is likely that many sublethal radiation injuries—combined with the trauma of implantation in an environment that may not be ideal—culminate in a cytolethal effect. Thus cell death and a loss of reproductive integrity of many transplanted cancer cells reduce the incidence of local persistence.

The number of cancer cells in a tumor (usually measured by the tumor volume) affects its radiocurability (Chapter 1). Since radiation-induced cell death is exponentially related to dose, the greater the number of cancer cells, the greater the dose required to cure (Figs. 1-5 and 3-14). It is at least theoretically true, then, that a reduction in tumor volume, however slight and however accomplished, would indeed reduce the statistical chance of persistence. From a clinical viewpoint one must apply this fact with caution. This line of reasoning has led to the misconception that a significantly smaller dose of radiations is adequate even if gross tumor is transected, that is, "debulking" the tumor with gross tumor left behind. There are sometimes other reasons for debulking such a cancerous mass, but as long as gross cancer has been left behind, the dose of radiations required will have been reduced very little if at all. In addition, the hazards of an inadequate resection will have been inflicted on the patient.

PRIMARY CANCERS OF UNCERTAIN EXTENT. The application of both modalities to the same primary lesion with the hope that one treatment will cure more patients with limited cancer and the other will cure more patients with advanced cancer smacks of shotgun therapy and has not been frequently analyzed or practiced. The potential merits of this type of combined therapy are more obvious in the treatment of carcinoma of the endometrium than in most other sites. Thus surgery can easily control all lesions truly limited to the corpus, provided, of course, that the patient is a good operative risk. There is no question but that a few of these small lesions that are easily cured by surgery are resistant to radiations. On the other hand, the more invasive lesions that remain confined to the pelvis may be controlled by radiations even if their lateral infiltrations or vaginal spread should place them beyond the scope of the usual surgical approach. This was well demonstrated by Lampe, Kottmeier, and Landgren and associates when they reported cure rates of 20% to 27% by using radiotherapy alone on the inoperable patients.

Thus there are some lesions curable by irradiation that would not be controlled by the usual surgery, and there are lesions curable by surgery that would not be controlled by the usual irradiation. When this is true, and when the extent of disease is uncertain, both methods can and should be applied, provided, of course, that mortality and morbidity rates are acceptable. We can confidently predict an improved cure rate by administering vigorous preoperative irradiation to the apparently resectable cancer that has undetected or occult local extension beyond the limits of the proposed operation. Unfortunately, the only means by which such occult, local extension can be treated before transection and dissemination is to treat all such patients at reasonable risk preoperatively. The same reasoning can be applied equally well to other sites and has been tried for carcinomas of the lung (Collaborative National Study; Paulson; Shields and associates), bladder (Whitmore), oral cavity (Buschke and Galante; Galante and associates), breast (Montague), pharynx and larynx (Goldman and Friedman; Silverstone and associates), cervical lymph nodes (Henschke and associates; Milburn and Hendrickson), and esophagus (Nakayama and associates; Doggett and associates).

Finally, one of the more obvious dangers of preoperative irradiation is found in the delusion that low or modest doses of radiations may actually justify a less radical operation. Occasionally this may be true; indeed, the value of preoperative irradiation depends on its ability to increase the effectiveness of a given operative procedure, that is, conservative hysterectomy following whole pelvic irradiation for a barrel-shaped cancer of the cervix or the excision of a residual jugular node after irradiation of the neck. At this stage of our knowledge, however, preoperative irradiation does not ordinarily justify a less radical operative procedure. This is particularly important if the dose of preoperative radiations has been low.

OPTIMUM PREOPERATIVE DOSE OF RADIATIONS. The optimum preoperative dose of radiations has been difficult to define. Optimum preoperative irradiation should yield the maximum cure rate compatible with an acceptable postoperative morbidity. Clinical trials have not established the value of preoperative irradiation in most anatomic sites, much less established optimum doses. Animal studies have shown that, within limits, the higher the preoperative dose of radiations, the lower the incidence of postoperative residual cancer (Perez and Powers). Few satisfactory randomized clinical trials have been completed that compare the relative value of low-dose with high-dose preoperative irradiation. Hendrickson and Liebner reported finding no difference between 2000 rad in eight treatments and 5000 rad in twenty treatments, but their series was too small and showed a definite clumping of advanced cases in the latter option.

It seems likely that the optimum dose will vary with anatomic site and cell type. It also seems likely that, when the dose is sufficiently high to kill all cancer cells at or beyond the margins of excision, a still higher dose can produce no further improvement in local control. Subclinical foci of cancer cells, whether squamous cell carcinoma or adenocarcinoma, seem to require doses of about 5000 rad in 5 weeks for their eradication. We therefore recommend doses of this level when preoperative irradiation is to be given for these cancers. Although this dose undoubtedly slows wound healing, it has not produced a serious increase in the incidence of complications in most anatomic sites.

OPTIMUM INTERVAL BETWEEN PREOPERATIVE IRRADIATION AND SURGERY. There are competing factors in the selection of an optimum interval between preoperative irradiation and surgery. Obviously the radiation oncologist wants the normal tissues to recover sufficiently from radiation damage in order that wound healing will proceed uneventfully. Yet he does not want the cancer cells to recover and to proliferate to the point that any benefit from tumor shrinkage is lost. Differences in cellular kinetics of normal tissues and cancer cells are such that a single optimum interval for all anatomic sites and all cell types is highly unlikely. For example, the optimum interval between irradiation and resection may be different for large bowel, breast, hypopharyngeal, and endometrial cancers. The consequences of poor healing of an irradiated bowel that is to be anastomosed are entirely different from those related to slow healing of the chest wall or head and neck tissues. In addition, the magnitude of the preoperative dose is a vital factor in defining the optimum interval. By necessity, higher doses demand longer intervals.

Animal studies have done little except to confirm the complex nature of this problem. A preoperative dose of 1000 rad to a lymphosarcoma in mice was most effective in reducing regrowths if surgery was done immediately rather than 1, 3, or 7 days postirradiation (Perez and Powers). This finding is supported by the work of Belli and associates. Yet Inch and associates (1970) found that a preoperative dose of 2000 rad to an adenocarcinoma in mice was most effective in reducing tumor persistence if surgery was done on the sixth postirradiation day rather than on the first or twelfth day. Thus the optimum interval between irradiation and surgery likely varies according to cell type. Data relative to the optimum interval for wound healing are lacking, although for head and neck tumors a 15-day interval seemed appropriate (Powers and associates). Silverstone and associates used higher total doses and recommend an interval of 21 to 42 days. For most tissues a 3-week interval after cancerocidal doses is minimal and 6 weeks is probably optimum. Shorter intervals can be used after smaller fractionated doses. Single doses of more than 1000 rad followed in 24 hours by resection are particularly damaging to wound healing (Ketcham and associates).

Summary of arguments for preoperative irradiation

Peripheral extensions of a cancerous mass are more radiosensitive than the more central cells. If these peripheral extensions account for nonresectability and are indeed more sensitive, preoperative irradiation may convert a nonresectable cancer to a resectable one.

Certain animal studies support the clinical use of preoperative irradiation. Preexcision irradiation of selected animal cancers decreases the incidences of take of its subsequently implanted cells. Also, irradiation of many normal tissues decreases the incidence of take of subsequently implanted cancer cells. Finally, radiations can probably reduce the number of viable cancer cells to below the critical number required for take.

Summary of arguments against preoperative irradiation

Radiations impair wound healing. The higher the dose the greater the impairment. Preoperative irradiation implies a delay in curative surgery. Whether this delay provides an additional opportunity for metastasizing is speculative, but the fear that the delay of definitive surgery is detrimental cannot be ignored. Locally advanced cancers have frequently already developed occult distant metastases. Preoperative irradiation cannot modify cure rates in the large segment of patients in which this has occurred. Also, gross shrinkage of the cancerous mass may tempt the surgeon to perform a less radical resection or radiation-induced shrinkage of the cancer may provoke the patient to delay or even to refuse attempts at curative resection. Finally, preoperative irradiation increases costs to the patient, interrupts the usual sequence of care, and requires more detailed scheduling.

Thus we have a variety of arguments from clinical experience and from animal and cell culture studies that justify clinical trials combining irradiation and surgery. However, despite numerous studies of a variety of anatomic sites, there is still no convincing clinical evidence that preoperative irradiation often contributes to cure. The benefits, if any, should be most obvious in those cancers that show frequent postoperative local persistence.

Principles of preoperative irradiation

Preoperative irradiation is that irradiation given prior to an anticipated surgical excision within the irradiated zone. The principles usually followed in giving preoperative irradiation are summarized:

1. For the time being at least, preoperative irradiation as a planned procedure should be applied chiefly to the apparently resectable cancers. (Exceptions to this are obvious for carcinomas of the ovary.)

2. The zone of irradiation should be larger than the anticipated surgical excision. This places the surgical incision through irradiated tissue. If the cancer has not shrunk to within the limits of the excision, there is still the advantage that the incision is through damaged cancer that has its viability greatly decreased. The advantages of this were presented previously.

3. The dose is rarely of a curative level, and there is rarely an intent to cure the patient by preoperative irradiation alone, even though residual cancer may not be found in the operative specimen.

4. Multiportal megavoltage or ^{60}Co beams should be used when the location of the irradiated volume permits. In this way superficial tissue will be spared and postoperative complications will be reduced.

5. An interval of 3 to 6 weeks is usually allowed between the two procedures.

6. Preoperative irradiation delays definitive surgery. The delay is not detrimental. On the contrary, the interval is necessary for proper administration of radiations and for optimum benefit from their use.

On examining the operative specimen after preoperative irradiation, the pathologist may or may not return a report of "persistent viable cancer." It is difficult if not impossible for the pathologist to correctly predict whether or not an injured cell will continue to reproduce indefinitely (Suit). Soon after the completion of irradiation, cells that appear surprisingly normal may reproduce once or twice and then die. It should also be understood that the absence of tumor cells in the operative specimen does not assure complete sterilization of the tumor. Careful clinical follow-up alone can measure the value of these combined procedures.

The use of preoperative irradiation is discussed with each anatomic site in the chapters to follow.

With preoperative irradiation we have a method of destroying the more sensitive peripheral cancer cells of a mass. The method is locally applicable. With radiations we have the unique capability of regulating dose in a given volume, in a given time, and in a given amount. It does not seriously affect the morbidity rate if appropriate precautions are taken. It has promise in reducing the incidence of local recurrence and decreasing morbidity in selected patients with locally advanced cancers.

POSTOPERATIVE IRRADIATION

Transection of viable cancer is rarely an intended procedure, and the hazards of "debulking" a tumor mass were mentioned before. Therefore, if the extent of a cancer were precisely definable prior to operation, postoperative irradiation would be only occasionally necessary. The optimist might anticipate a progressive decrease in the need for postoperative irradiation as our knowledge and surgical skill advance. There are no immediate prospects for improvements in this regard, but a review of cancers frequently requiring local postoperative irradiation does define those situations most likely to benefit from preoperative irradiation. The inaccuracies of assessing tumor extent preoperatively and of determining resectability in certain relatively inaccessible cancers assure a continuing need for more effective postoperative irradiation.

Postoperative irradiation has its chief indication when local residual cancer is suspected or known to be present. Under such circumstances, once the surgical wound is healed, the sooner the irradiation is administered, the more effective it is likely to be. Furthermore, with a knowledge that cancer is present, full cancerocidal doses can be justified and the risks associated with such doses can be accepted. Finally, a study of the surgically removed specimen sometimes assists the radiation oncologist in selecting the size, shape, and position of the volume requiring irradiation. This enables the administration of postoperative irradiation with a more detailed knowledge than is available for preoperative irradiation.

A program of planned preoperative irradiation does not necessarily prohibit the use of supplemental postoperative irradiation. In fact there are definite theoretical advantages to the so-called "sandwich" technique when large-port, preoperative irradiation is supplemented by additional small-port postoperative boosting dose of radiations directed to a specific persistence.

Factors influencing the conduct of postoperative irradiation

1. Surgically treated cancers are not usually particularly radiosensitive cancers. This means that high doses of radiations are generally necessary postoperatively if cure is the aim.

2. As a group, patients referred for postoperative irradiation have advanced

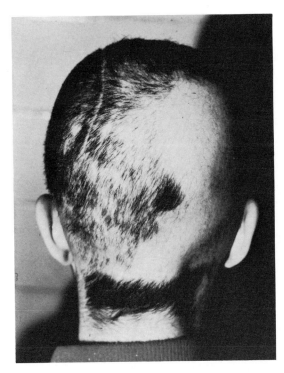

Fig. 2-3. Patient was given identical doses through right and left lateral occipital portals. Note decreased epilation in vicinity of operative site. Presumably this is a result of scalp hypoxia produced by the surgery.

cancers that for one reason or another extend beyond the anticipated limits. Thus the extensions are usually vague, and the act of transection may have disseminated cancer cells throughout the operative sites. The need for generous portals is obvious, but because of these large portals, limitation on high dose is equally obvious.

3. Resection reduces the number of cancer cells requiring irradiation. This rather small improvement in statistics is masked by disturbances of the tumor bed (Fig. 2-3). It seems likely that the normal healing process produces connective tissues with limited ability to recover from the insult of vigorous irradiation. The transected cancer encased in the connective tissue scar may be somewhat protected by hypoxia. Thus a less favorable therapeutic ratio may be created by the surgery. This problem can be partially overcome by starting postoperative irradiation as soon as wound healing permits.

4. In view of the points mentioned in paragraph 3, it is accepted that irradiation within a week or two of surgery is more likely to succeed than that given when regrowth is clinically obvious. However, so-called "prophylactic postoperative" irradiation must be given just as if cancer were known to have been left behind. Doses should be tailored to the volume of the suspected residual disease as well as the anatomic site, cell type, etc. (See Chapters 1 and 4.)

The charge for curative postoperative irradiation is a difficult one—that is, the eradication of one of the less sensitive cancers that has been transected and has been spread throughout the operative site. Large-port, high-dose techniques are called for often in a volume with known decreased tolerance of normal tissue.

These factors weigh heavily against postoperative irradiation contributing greatly to cure rates. This should not deter curative efforts under selected circumstances. We have all seen postoperative persistent cancers of the skin, head and neck, breast, pelvic organs, and testicle, and Wilms' tumors, gastric lymphomas, and the like cured by postoperative irradiation.

Techniques are the same as those used for primary irradiation. With the larger volume and decreased tolerance, greater fractionation is usually necessary. The details of postoperative irradiation in each anatomic area are covered in the chapters to follow.

COMPLICATIONS OF COMBINATIONS OF IRRADIATION AND SURGERY

There is uniform agreement that anything more than minor combinations of irradiation and surgery, regardless of the sequence, increases problems related to healing. Previous radical surgery increases the incidence of postirradiation sequelae, just as previous high-dose irradiation increases the incidence of postoperative complications. The nature of these complications varies with site, type of procedure, and age and general condition of the patient. These additional risks are generally accepted by both the patient and the physician if there is a reasonable increase in the probability of cure.

Radiations suppress cellular proliferation. Obviously this affects wound healing. Wound tensile strength is delayed in reaching its maximum, especially if the dose of radiations has been high and the interval short (Nickson and associates; Powers and associates; Ketcham and associates). Lower fractionated doses have not been found to decrease tensile strength of the bowel anastomoses seriously (Heupel and associates; Crowley and associates) and have been accepted in most clinical situations. Tildon and Hughes reported damage of normal lung by preoperative irradiation, but this has not been confirmed by others. The point is clear that preoperative irradiation does carry some risk of morbidity that varies with anatomic site and is greater the higher the dose and the larger the volume.

Intervals of many months between curative doses of radiations and surgery are associated with much more frequent complications. A previously irradiated tissue may serve its function well until trauma such as surgery demands a response such as an increased rate of cellular replacement. When the irradiated tissues cannot meet this demand, necrosis follows.

Multiportal megavoltage and ^{60}Co techniques permit subcutaneous vasculoconnective tissues to retain much of their healing ability. These factors have accounted for a notable decrease in radiation-induced wound complications and are largely responsible for our ability to give significant doses yet expect good wound healing.

Table 2-1. Incidence of postoperative complications with and without previous high dose ^{60}Co irradiation*

	After ^{60}Co irradiation	No ^{60}Co irradiation
Neck dissection	7/36	0/40
Buccal mucosa	5/8	1/25
Oropharynx	4/12	1
Larynx	6/12	2/14

*Modified from Rodier, D., and Herdly, J.: Bulletin du Cancer **52**:63-68, 1965.
Tissue doses of 4200 to 7000 rad at about 1000 rad/week. Surgery was done at varying intervals after irradiation when recurrence became obvious.

In our own experience and in that of Ditchek and Lampe, of MacComb and Fletcher, of Buschke and Galante, of Mill, and of Silverstone and associates, radical surgery after curative doses of radiations is possible with an acceptable although increased incidence of wound complications. One institution's experience is shown in Table 2-1.

SUMMARY

In radiations we find an agent that is uniquely localizable, one that is always under complete control as to dose and duration of therapy, and one with the means of adjusting treated volume to any desired size or shape. For certain cancers the dissatisfaction with the results of surgery alone, the results of combinations of radiations with excision in laboratory animals, and the availability of skin-sparing radiation beams have justified reevaluation of clinical combinations of radiations and surgery. The rationale of these combinations has been presented. Their contribution in specific sites has been mentioned and will be discussed in the following chapters.

REFERENCES

Belli, J. A., Dicus, G. J., and Nagle, W.: Repair of radiation damage as a factor in preoperative radiation therapy. In Vaeth, J. M.: The interrelationship of surgery and radiation therapy in the treatment of cancer, Baltimore, 1970, University Park Press.

Buschke, F., and Galante, M.: Radical preoperative roentgen therapy in primarily inoperable advanced cancers of the head and neck, Radiology **73**:845-848, 1959.

Collaborative National Study: Preoperative irradiation of cancer of the lung, Cancer **23**:419-429, 1969.

Crowley, L. G., Anders, C. J., Nelsen, T., and Bagshaw, M.: Effect of radiation on canine intestinal anastomoses, Arch. Surg. **97**:423-428, 1968.

Dao, T. L., and Yogo, H.: Enhancement of pulmonary metastases by x-irradiation in rats bearing mammary cancer, Cancer **20**:2020-2025, 1967.

Ditchek, T., and Lampe, I.: Radical surgery after intensive high-energy irradiation, Arch. Surg. **86**:534-539, 1963.

Doggett, R. L. S., III, Guernsey, J. M., and Bagshaw, M. A.: Combined radiation and surgical treatment of carcinoma of the thoracic esophagus. In Vaeth, J. M.: The interrelationship of surgery and radiation therapy in the treatment of cancer, Baltimore, 1970, University Park Press.

Fletcher, G. H.: The evolution of the basic concepts underlying the practice of radiotherapy from 1949 to 1977, Radiology **127**:3-19, 1978.

Galante, M., Benak, S., Jr., and Buschke, F.: Radical preoperative radiation therapy in primarily inoperable advanced cancers of the oral cavity. In Vaeth, J. M.: The interrelationship of surgery and radiation therapy in the treatment of cancer, Baltimore, 1970, University Park Press.

Goldman, J. L., and Friedman, W. H.: Investigative aspects of preoperative irradiation for advanced carcinoma of the larynx and laryngopharynx. In Vaeth, J. M.: The interrelationship of surgery and radiation therapy in the treatment of cancer, Baltimore, 1970, University Park Press.

Gricouroff, G.: Pathogenesis of recurrences on the suture line following resection for carcinoma of the colon, Cancer 20:673-676, 1967.

Hendrickson, F. R., and Liebner, E.: Results of pre-operative radiotherapy for supraglottic larynx cancer, Ann. Otol. 77:222-229, 1968.

Henschke, U. K., Frazell, E. L., Hilaris, B. S., Nickson, J. J., Tollefsen, H. R., and Strong, E. W.: Value of preoperative x-ray therapy as an adjunct to radical neck dissection, Radiology 86:450-453, 1966.

Heupel, H. W., Veinbergs, A., and Humphrey, E. W.: The effect of preoperative roentgen therapy upon the tensile strength of rectosigmoid anastomoses in dogs, Radiol. Clin. 35:129-140, 1966.

Hewitt, H. B., and Blake, E. R.: The growth of transplanted murine tumors in preirradiated sites, Br. J. Cancer 22:808-824, 1968.

Hoye, R. C., and Smith, P. R.: Effectiveness of small amounts of preoperative irradiation in preventing the growth of tumor cells disseminated at surgery, Cancer 14:284-295, 1961.

Inch, W. R., and McCredie, J. A.: Effect of a small dose of x-radiation on local recurrence of tumors in rats and mice, Cancer 16:595-598, 1963.

Inch, W. R., and McCredie, J. A.: Concentrated preoperative irradiation. In Rush, B. F., and Greenlaw, R. H.: Cancer therapy by integrated radiation and operation, Springfield, Ill., 1968, Charles C Thomas, Publisher.

Inch, W. R., McCredie, J. A., and Sutherland, R. M.: Effect of x-radiation to tumor bed on local recurrence. In Vaeth, J. M.: The interrelationship of surgery and radiation therapy in the treatment of cancer, Baltimore, 1970, University Park Press.

Ketcham, A. S., Hoye, R. C., Chretien, P. B., and Brace, K. C.: Irradiation 24 hours preoperatively, Am. J. Surg. 118:691-697, 1969.

Kottmeier, H. L.: Carcinoma of the corpus uteri: diagnosis and therapy, Am. J. Obstet. Gynecol. 78:1127-1140, 1959.

Lampe, I.: Combined surgical and radiological treatment for carcinoma, Proceedings of the

Second National Cancer Conference, New York, 1954, American Cancer Society, Inc.

Landgren, R. C., Fletcher, G. H., Delclos, L., and Wharton, J. T.: Irradiation of endometrial cancer in patients with medical contraindications to surgery or with unresectable lesions, Am. J. Roentgenol. Radium Ther. Nucl. Med. 126:148-154, 1976.

MacComb, W. S., and Fletcher, G. H.: Planned combination of surgery and radiation in treatment of advanced primary head and neck cancers, Am. J. Roentgenol. 77:397-414, 1957.

Milburn, L. F., and Hendrickson, F. R.: Initial treatment of neck metastases from squamous-cell cancer, Radiology 89:123-126, 1967.

Mill, W. A.: Cancer of the larynx: laryngectomy after radiotherapy, Proc. R. Soc. Med. 49:73-84, 1956.

Montague, E. D.: High dose preoperative irradiation for breast cancer. In Rush, B. F., and Greenlaw, R. H.: Cancer therapy by integrated radiation and operation, Springfield, Ill., 1968, Charles C Thomas, Publisher.

Nakayama, K., Orihata, H., Yamaguchi, K.: Surgical treatment combined with preoperative concentrated irradiation for esophageal cancer, Cancer 20:778-788, 1967.

Nickson, J. J., Lawrence, W., Rachwalsky, I., and Tyree, E.: Roentgen rays and wound healing; fractionated irradiation; experimental study, Surgery 34:859-862, 1953.

Paulson, D. L.: The role of preoperative radiation therapy in the surgical management of carcinoma in the superior pulmonary sulcus. In Vaeth, J. M.: The interrelationship of surgery and radiation therapy in the treatment of cancer, Baltimore, 1970, University Park Press.

Perez, C. A., and Olson, J.: Preoperative irradiation and chemotherapy in the cure of a mouse lymphosarcoma, Radiology 92:136-142, 1969.

Perez, C. A., and Olson, J.: Preoperative versus postoperative irradiation: comparison in experimental animal tumor system, Am. J. Roentgenol. 108:396-404, 1970.

Perez, C. A., and Powers, W. E.: Studies on the optimal dose of preoperative irradiation and time for surgery in the cure of a mouse lymphosarcoma, Radiology 89:116-122, 1967.

Powers, W. E.: Preoperative and postoperative radiation therapy for cancer, Proceedings of the Sixth National Cancer Conference, New York, 1970, American Cancer Society, Inc., pp. 33-38.

Powers, W. E., Ogura, J. H., and Palmer, L. A.: Radiation therapy and wound healing delay: animal and man, Radiology 89:112-115, 1967.

Powers, W. E., and Palmer, L. A.: Biologic basis

of preoperative radiation treatment, Am. J. Roentgenol. **102:**176-192, 1968.

Powers, W. E., and Tohmach, L. J.: Preoperative radiation therapy: biological basis and experimental investigations, Nature (London) **201:** 272-273, 1964.

Prout, G. R., Jr., Slack, N. H., and Bross, I. D. J.: Preoperative irradiation as an adjuvant in the surgical management of invasive bladder carcinoma, J. Urol. **105:**223-231, 1971.

Shields, T. W., Higgins, G. A., Jr., Lawton, R., and others: Preoperative x-ray therapy as an adjuvant in the treatment of bronchogenic carcinoma, J. Thorac. Cardiovasc. Surg. **59:**49-61, 1970.

Silverstone, S. M., Goldman, J. L., and Ryan, J. R.: Combined high dose radiation therapy and surgery of advanced cancer of the laryngopharynx. In Vaeth, J. M.: The interrelationship of surgery and radiation therapy in the treatment of cancer, Baltimore, 1970, University Park Press.

Smith, R. R., and Godbee, G. A.: Alteration of tumor cell implantability by preoperative irradiation. In Rush, B. F., and Greenlaw, R. H.: Cancer therapy by integrated radiation and operation, Springfield, Ill., 1968, Charles C Thomas, Publisher.

Suit, H. D., and Gallager, H. S.: Intact tumor cells in irradiated tissue, Arch. Pathol. **78:**648-651, 1964.

Summers, W. C., Clifton, K. H., and Vermund, H.: X-irradiation of the tumor bed, Radiology **82:**691-703, 1964.

Tildon, T. T., and Hughes, R. K.: Complications from preoperative irradiation therapy for lung cancer, Ann. Thorac. Surg. **3:**307-326, 1967.

Vermund, H., Stenstrom, K. W., Mosser, D. G., and Johnson, E. A.: Effects of roentgen irradiation on the tumor bed. II. Inhibiting action of different dose levels of local pretransplantation roentgen irradiation on the growth of mouse mammary carcinoma, Radiat. Res. **5:**354-364, 1956.

Whitmore, W. F., Jr.: Preoperative irradiation with cystectomy in the management of bladder cancer. In Vaeth, J. M.: The interrelationship of surgery and radiation therapy in the treatment of cancer, Baltimore, 1970, University Park Press.

3

The skin

RESPONSE OF NORMAL SKIN TO IRRADIATION

With few exceptions, all radiation therapy techniques by necessity entail skin irradiation. For this reason, until the widespread use of megavoltage beams, skin reactions were the most common of all tissue reactions. This and the facts that skin reactions are easy to observe and that the skin does provide a spectrum of radiation-induced responses have made it a common subject for radiobiologic research. It is understandable that early workers used skin reaction as a unit for measuring dose, that is, the erythema dose. An understanding of the pathogenesis of these reactions and an appreciation of skin tolerance are paramount in radiation oncology. With megavoltage beams, an accurate statement of surface dose or dose at the germinal layer of the epidermis is usually difficult to establish. The depth and magnitude of the maximum dose is more significant. Megavoltage radiations diminish the limitations imposed by skin reactions and for most lesions decrease their importance. Paradoxically, irradiation of superficial lesions such as those of the skin, breast, and superficial lymph node regions entails more serious skin reactions than does irradiation of deeper tissues.

TYPES OF REACTIONS. Radiation reactions in the skin, as in other tissues, may be divided into early or acute changes and delayed or chronic changes. The severity of either phase depends on dose-time-volume factors—that is, the greater the skin dose the shorter the time, and the larger the surface area the more severe the reaction. Every acute reaction is followed by some degree of permanent or late change, although it may be slight and clinically insignificant. Some changes such as erythema, pigmentation, or even dry desquamation have been called "reversible." It must be realized that these transient signs of skin damage do not, on their disappearance, signify complete recovery of the skin, since the skin never completely recovers. By alteration of quality and fractionation, it is possible to minimize some features of skin reaction and to exaggerate others. Thus high total doses of poorly filtered, highly fractionated radiations may produce very few, if any recognizable signs of acute radiation reaction. Yet severe late changes, including ulceration and radiation-induced carcinoma, may develop (Figs. 3-9 and 3-10).

Early erythema is often unrecognized but may appear from 1 to 24 hours after a single dose of about 450 rad (200 kv, 1 mm Cu hvl). This erythema is short-lived (2 to 3 days) and is followed by little or no pigmentation. The more commonly observed erythema appears about 8 days after a single dose to the skin of 800 rad (factors same as above) and may require another 8 days to reach its peak. The time of onset, duration, and intensity are dose related. Pigmentation usually follows.

Fractionation of dose causes an overlapping of these various reactions. A skin dose of 3000 to 4000 rad in 3 weeks through a 10 × 10 cm field, using radiations with a half-value layer of 1 mm Cu delivered to the cervical skin, will usually produce a brisk acute reaction followed by moderate late changes. During the second week of administering a daily skin dose of 300 rad per day, 5 days a week, a second erythema appears and increases in intensity as the fractionated irradiation continues. If the irradiation is sufficiently intense, the erythema reaches its peak with the onset of the desquamation to be described. A capillary congestion develops and persists after complete desquamation, giving the denuded deep red area a purplish hue. With such doses the dermal circulation probably never returns to its normal state. The reparative process that follows is associated with progressive fibrosis and vascular subendothelial hyperplasia. Whether these two changes bear a cause-and-effect relationship is unknown, but telangiectasia, slow healing, and necrosis are the clinical manifestations of a permanent vascular insufficiency.

CHANGES WITHIN THE EPIDERMIS. The cells composing the epidermis consist of a rapidly multiplying germinal layer of columnar cells that serve as the source of supply for the overlying nondividing squamous cells. The squamous cells in turn become the elements that form the cornified layer. Since the cornified layer is brushed or washed off during the usual everyday activities, a normal epithelium is dependent on a mitotically active germinal layer to replace cells of the cornified layer at a rate in keeping with their loss. Like most rapidly dividing cells, the basal cells of the epidermis are quite sensitive to radiations. Their superficial position makes them susceptible to injury by very soft radiations, even of the ultraviolet range, as well as more penetrating beams. Low doses of 200 kv radiations (1000 rad or less in 10 days) decrease their rate of mitosis, which in turn produces a temporary thinning of the epithelium. Doses of an intermediate level will kill many, but not all, basal cells. If the surviving cells multiply to replace the dead cells before a 3- to 4-week period, a dry desquamation or "peeling" follows. The cells become quite dark and at times almost black before they flake off. This dark color is from melanin produced by a radiation-induced increase in a specific enzymatic activity in the melanocytes. From their location at the junction of the basal layer and the dermis, the melanocytes pass this increased pigment into the newly formed squamous cells. They in turn carry it until they are shed from the skin surface.

Doses of levels necessary to control skin cancers kill all cells of the basal layer. Within a 4-week period all the squamous cells existing at the initiation of irradiation have become cornified and in turn have been shed. In the absence of new cell formation, the dermis is then exposed and serum oozes from the surface. This is called a moist desquamation. Certain epithelial cells of the hair follicles are definitely more

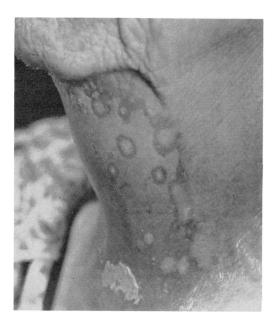

Fig. 3-1. Moderately severe, moist reaction produced by 5400 rad (skin) (280 kv; hvl, 2 mm Cu) in 22 days through a 9 × 12 cm field. Reepithelization is initiated at the periphery and from hair follicles. These islands of eipthelium enlarge and coalesce to cover area much faster than could be accomplished by healing from periphery alone.

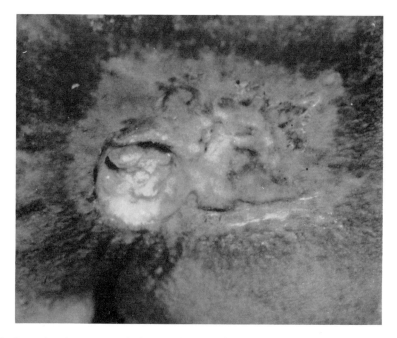

Fig. 3-2. Extensive tissue necrosis in sacral region from excessive irradiation. Dose unknown. Such areas may never heal if left alone. Surgical excision and repair are usually required.

resistant to radiations than are the basal cells described. If the dose has not been too high or has not been given too quickly, they proliferate to cover the denuded surface around the follicles (Fig. 3-1). These islands of epithelium coalesce to cover the dermis in a much shorter time than would be possible by healing from the periphery alone. At first the new epidermis is very thin and pink; although it thickens, it never attains the normal thickness. It appears atrophic, is smoother than normal, and is unable to form pigment if the dose has been sufficient to kill the melanocytes. The new skin has little or no hair and contains few or no sweat or sebaceous glands. This thinner epithelium is more easily broken, has less tolerance to further irradiation, and recovers poorly, if at all, from all types of injuries—infectious, chemical, or physical (Fig. 3-2).

The germinal cells of the epidermis can proliferate to cover unusual sites when the anatomy permits; for example, after vigorous irradiation of an ectropic eyelid the epidermis may extend over the free edge of the lid to cover the mucosal surface of the lid (Fig. 5-1).

The skin, like all other tissues, decreases in radiosensitivity during hypoxia (Suit). This is demonstrated clinically after surgery when blood supply to one skin flap has been impaired (Fig. 2-3). It is also demonstrated with skin grafts, which are discussed later in this chapter.

RADIATION-INDUCED PIGMENTATION OF SKIN. After ultraviolet or roentgen irradiation, an increased amount of melanin is found in the cells of the basal layer. As these cells "mature," they carry the melanin into the more superficial layers of the epidermis and give the skin a darker color. Ultraviolet and roentgen irradiation stimulate melanoblasts located at the junction of the epidermis and dermis to produce melanin pigment. This occurs when radiations activate tyrosinase to convert tyrosine to melanin. The melanocyte then passes the melanin to the basal cell. In the dermis, particularly in areas of normally greater pigmentation—that is, anus and areola—dermal chromatophores are found that contain large granules of pigment. The pigment content of the chromatophores also increases with x-irradiation. However, the distribution of these cells in the dermis is such that they could hardly contribute significantly to the pigmentation developing after ultraviolet or roentgen irradiation. Doses of radiations of a cancerocidal level frequently destroy the melanocytes so that a previously irradiated skin may be unable to form pigment. Thus the term *radiation-induced achromia* is applicable. Such an area will be easily sunburned and will be noticeable when the surrounding skin is tanned.

Often during a course of radiation therapy the zone immediately around each hair will be the first to show pigmentation, and the skin will present dozens of millimeter-sized brown specks. This is thought to be a result of the end-on view of the cylinder of pigmented epidermis as it invaginates to form the hair follicle (Fig. 3-3).

Although pigmentation from ultraviolet irradiation shields the basal layer from subsequent injury by ultraviolet radiations, it obviously can have no shielding effect against roentgen or gamma rays. In fact the presence of roentgen-induced pigmentation is a clinical sign that tolerance will be less.

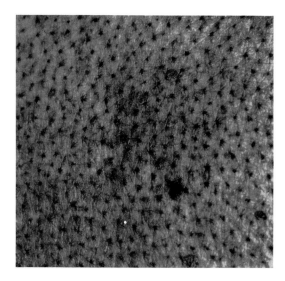

Fig. 3-3. Perifollicular pigmentation seen frequently near the middle of therapy—that is, after 2 to 3 weeks of irradiation. This is the end-on view of the epidermis as it invaginates to form the follicle.

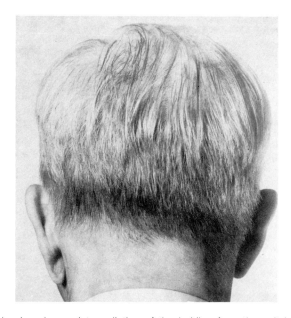

Fig. 3-4. Patient developed complete epilation of the hairline from the exit beam used to treat an advanced carcinoma of the antrum and ethmoids. Calculated exit dose was 2200 rad in 6 weeks with telecobalt. The new hair was black, in contrast to its previous gray color.

An erythema is not a prerequisite for pigmentation. Apparently the cellular damage responsible for pigment production and the vascular changes responsible for erythema are unrelated physiologic processes. Doses producing erythema will usually, but not always, produce pigment. On the other hand, multiple suberythema doses may produce pigment.

The skin changes described that are so characteristic of cancerocidal doses of 100 to 200 kv radiations are not usually seen after megavoltage or ^{60}Co therapy. Except for folds of skin or for tangential beams, the epidermis no longer receives a seriously high dose. Because the sites of more serious reactions are frequently hidden from view, skin changes are not reliable as guides in assessing tolerance for either initial treatment or retreatment.

EPILATION. For our purpose it should be recalled that the hair follicle represents a modification in the epidermis. The papilla at the root of the hair is similar to a dermal papilla. Over its surface are the rapidly dividing epithelial cells that produce the numerous layers around the developing hair. The shaft of the hair is formed by a process comparable to the formation of the cornified layer of the epidermis. Just as an appropriate dose of radiations may produce a dry or moist desquamation, so an appropriate dose can produce a shedding of hair. A low dose will produce a temporary decrease in growth rate in both diameter and length of the hair without causing epilation. A high dose may produce complete and permanent epilation. Within the first hour after a single dose of 500 rad to the hair follicle, mitotic activity of the germinal cells of the follicle is interrupted. Shortly thereafter the hair root separates from the papilla. About 3 weeks later the shaft of the hair separates from the neck of the follicle and the hair is shed. After this dose regrowth starts in 8 to 9 weeks.

Many factors have been shown to alter the ease of epilation. The more rapidly growing the hair, the more radiosensitive the hair follicle. In order of decreasing sensitivity, Lacassagne and Gricouroff placed the hair of the scalp, male beard, eyebrows, axilla, pubis, and, last, the fine hair of the body. They also pointed out that many fur-bearing animals that shed and grow their fur seasonally show seasonal variations in the radiosensitivity of their fur. Their fur is most sensitive when it is growing most rapidly.

After epilation hair may grow again but never with its former growth rate or density. Occasionally there is a radiation-induced defect in pigment development that results in a change in the color of the hair. In Fig. 3-4 is shown a change in hair color that occurred after radiation-induced epilation for treatment of carcinoma of the maxilla. A change in hair color is so constant in a certain strain of mice that the final hair shade is a biologic measure of dose. Hair that was originally straight may, after irradiation, grow curly. New hair is always finer than the previous hair (Fig. 3-5).

Epilation is usually an unavoidable sequela of irradiation for a malignant tumor. It rarely causes any concern except on the scalp, and in this age of inexpensive wigs even the loss of scalp hair is not regarded seriously. Depending on technical factors, regrowth of hair frequently completely covers the portals. Roentgen removal of

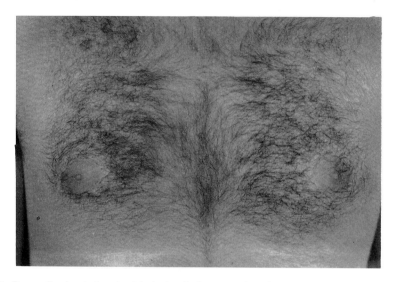

Fig. 3-5. Regrowth of anterior chest hair. Irradiation was given for Hodgkin's disease in the mediastinum. The skin dose was in excess of 3500 rad in 4 weeks through a field 11 × 16 cm using telecobalt. The new hair is sparse and fine.

hair on women's legs and upper lip was formerly practiced rather widely, but the caustic high dose required for complete permanent epilation and the frequent accidents associated with this practice led to many serious sequelae, including carcinoma of the skin. This procedure is mentioned only to condemn it.

SWEAT GLANDS. Clinically, we can best observe the radiosensitivity of sweat glands after irradiation of the axilla for Hodgkin's disease or metastatic carcinoma of the breast. Dryness is one of the characteristic features of irradiated skin. Heavily irradiated axillary skin (whether irradiated directly with a 200 kv beam or tangentially with a megavoltage beam) does not perspire. Such dryness is less noticeable but equally true of skin in other regions.

The sweat glands are in the dermis 2 to 3 mm below the skin surface. The cells lining the glands and ducts have relatively long lives and only occasionally undergo mitosis. These cells are not destroyed in the production of sweat (merocrine), and their turnover time is several weeks. Complete and permanent destruction of sweat gland function demands doses of near cancerocidal levels (greater than 3000 rad in 3 weeks). Microscopic examination of skin even after such doses may show the remnants of functionless sweat glands and their ducts. The ability of radiations to suppress formation of perspiration has no therapeutic indication.

SEBACEOUS GLANDS. Sebaceous glands are more radiosensitive than sweat glands. This is obvious when one examines irradiated skin microscopically. The sensitivity may be explained in part by the fact that the cells of the sebaceous gland are destroyed and used in the production of sebum (holocrine) and need continuous replacement through cellular proliferation. This proliferation occurs in the region of the duct, and with time the newly produced cells are moved into the depth of the gland.

The changed texture of irradiated skin is related in part to this absence of sebaceous glands. This is also true of the ceruminous glands. Although it has been suggested that it is this suppressing effect on sebaceous glands activity that makes radiations a useful tool in the treatment of acne vulgaris, it must be realized that many other types of infection are also beneficially affected by irradiation. Also, sebaceous cysts are not benefited by irradiation. In fact, when they happen to be in the irradiated field and are given high doses, they tend to become inflamed. The loss of oil from the skin leaves it dry and susceptible to fissuring. This contributes to the ease of infecting irradiated skin, which may lead to late necrosis. Regular application of a bland ointment such as petroleum jelly keeps the skin pliable and reduces fissuring.

DERMIS. The effect of radiations on the dermis is dependent on the quality and quantity of radiations considered and on the physical distribution of the ionization they produce. Ultraviolet radiations that have a caustic effect on the epidermis hardly affect the dermis. In contrast, megavoltage radiations of appropriate wavelengths may produce little epidermal damage but produce severe dermal changes. In addition to the effects of radiations on the glandular structures of the dermis already presented, there are both acute and late connective tissue and vascular changes. The erythema that was mentioned previously is a result of dermal capillary engorgement. Definite increase in blood flow through the dermis makes the irradiated field warmer. If the dose has been low, the capillaries apparently recover their normal tone. If the dose has been high (at least 1500 rad single-dose low-kilovoltage radiations or its biologic equivalent), the capillaries will lose some of their tone and will respond poorly to stimuli. It is debatable whether the capillary congestion is a result of direct capillary damage or is secondary to damage of the surrounding connective tissue. The erythema is cyclic, becomes intense and then fades, and recurs somewhat less intensely. This, too, remains unexplained. (See Chapter 9.)

Within the dermal connective tissues a dose of 1000 rad produces signs of acute inflammation—that is, edema and leukocytic infiltration. If the dose has been high, the permeability of the capillaries permits diapedesis of erythrocytes into the connective tissue. Fibroblasts show nuclear swelling and unequal nuclear divisions.

This acute reaction shades into a late dermal reaction, consisting of fibrosis that may give the skin a woody texture and the development of subendothelial fibrous hyperplasia in blood vessels. The latter is associated with the development of telangiectasia. Megavoltage radiations of the 2 to 6 mev range possess excellent epidermis-sparing characteristics. As mentioned previously, their maximum ionization occurs deep to the epidermis. At times the reaction of the subepidermal tissues to this high dose takes the form of a violent woody fibrosis underlying a nearly normal appearing epidermis. Certain areas show this type of reaction more often than others. The lower abdominal wall, the upper cervical and the paramandibular areas are particularly susceptible (Fig. 3-6). Obese patients seem to be especially prone to

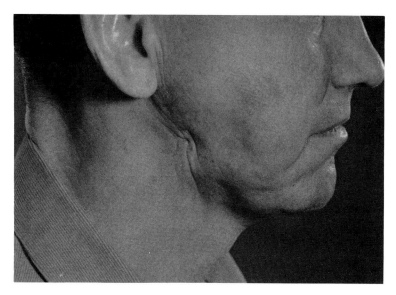

Fig. 3-6. Subcutaneous fibrosis sometimes seen after high-dose telecobalt therapy. The patient was treated with parallel opposing ports. Calculated skin dose was 5700 rad in 5 weeks.

develop this fibrosis. Clinically significant subcutaneous fibrosis occurs in 5% of all patients irradiated with ^{60}Co (Liegner and Michaud). The incidence of subcutaneous fibrosis can be reduced by several simple steps:

1. Use an adequate number of ports for the depth of lesion requiring radiation therapy.
2. Treat through each port each day, thus reducing the overall biologic effect on cutaneous and subcutaneous tissues in the beam.
3. Use beams of sufficient kv (adequate depth dose).
4. Do not exceed a maximum dose of 4000 rad in 4 weeks to the skin and subcutaneous tissues if alternate portals can be reasonably used.
5. Avoid overlapping portals on the skin and subcutaneous tissues. This includes the contribution of the exit dose of a contralateral beam.

The skin-sparing characteristics of megavoltage beams are decreased, of course, with tangential beams, beams directed through folds of skin, or treatment through bolus or dressings.

Although some dermal fibrosis is an expected late response to irradiation, the development of excessive amounts of scar (keloid) formation can be prevented by appropriately timed low-dose irradiation (Fig. 3-7). This fact has led to the frequent early prophylactic irradiation of wounds in a person in whom it is known that keloid forms. A dose of 1500 rad given as a single dose or preferably 500 rad every other day for three doses is advocated. (See Chapter 23.)

IRRADIATION OF SKIN GRAFTS. Skin grafting is a common necessity in cancer surgery. If cancer is known to have been left behind or if persistent cancer is mani-

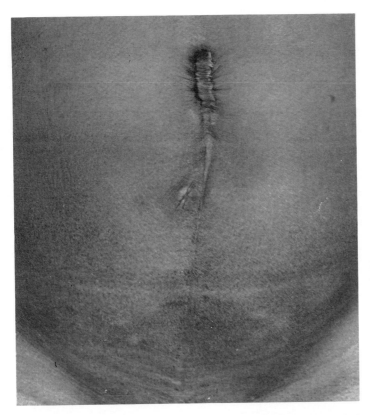

Fig. 3-7. Demonstration of effectiveness of irradiation in suppressing keloid formation. On laparotomy the patient proved to have an inoperable carcinoma of the endometrium. During subsequent lower abdominal irradiation only half of the recent incision was included in the field. Large keloid formed in the upper unirradiated portion. No keloid formed in the irradiated lower portion. Skin dose was 2500 rad in 5 weeks (much higher than is actually necessary for keloid prevention). (W. U. neg. 53-1993.)

fested deep under or adjacent to the graft, irradiation of the graft may be necessary. We are faced with this situation most often after radical mastectomy and after excision of cancers of the skin. The radiation response of grafted skin is not only dose-dependent but is also dependent on the stages in graft union to host tissues (Rubin and Grise). Irradiation of a new graft will suppress vessel and connective tissue proliferation vital in a successful take of the graft. The administration of high doses at this critical period is rarely essential. After several weeks, capillaries are formed and connective tissue proliferation has united the graft firmly to the recipient site. From this point on the graft tolerates radiations about as well as does the surrounding normal skin.

With the popularity of preoperative irradiation, the surgeon is occasionally confronted with the problem of skin grafting an area that has been recently irradiated. Doses up to 2000 rad in 10 fractions to the bed do not decrease the incidence of take.

Doses of 3000 rad produce a decreased incidence of take, but we believe grafting is still worth trying. With the facts given previously relative to the sensitivity of skin, the futility of grafting irradiated skin should be obvious. Single doses of 2000 rad to the donor skin prevent the skin from growing on either an irradiated or unirradiated bed (Elkin and associates).

USE OF RADIATIONS IN TREATMENT OF BENIGN DISEASES OF THE SKIN

In the evolution of our current practice radiations have been advocated for hundreds of benign diseases of the epidermis and dermis. Some of these diseases (keloids and hemangiomas) are discussed in Chapter 23. The mechanisms of the action of radiations in other skin diseases are pointed out elsewhere in this chapter. However, we must admit that the mechanisms of the action of radiations in most dermatologic diseases are unknown.

Certain skin diseases run a prolonged chronic course, and others tend to recur frequently over a long period. The use of radiations as a routine treatment is discouraged in patients with such chronic recurring benign diseases. Pioneer radiologists discovered early that such patients consulted one physician after another until they found someone who would treat them and make the condition temporarily better. They found that these patients soon accumulated dangerously high skin doses. Severe late skin damage and even skin cancer resulted.

One can never be certain just what part he is contributing to this cumulative damage. In this category of skin diseases are fungus infections of the feet and hands, psoriasis, acne, pruritus of the anus, and chronic dermatitis of a great variety of etiologies.

National attention has been focused on the use of radiations for *benign* diseases in "A Review of the Use of Ionizing Radiation for the Treatment of Benign Diseases," 1977. Certain guidelines have been developed regarding the use of radiations in treating *benign* lesions of the skin:

1. The potential risk must be recognized, and safer, acceptable methods should not be available.

2. The techniques of irradiation should be optimal relative to the prevention of late skin damage and injury to underlying organs.

3. Children should be irradiated for benign skin lesions very rarely.

In clinical practice the use of radiations for noncancerous diseases has greatly diminished, and the aforementioned guidelines are widely recognized.

CARCINOMA OF THE SKIN (SQUAMOUS CELL AND BASAL CELL CARCINOMA)

Carcinoma of the skin is, of course, the most accessible cancer. The diagnosis is readily made, and the limits of the lesion are usually easy to define. Basal cell carcinoma of the skin almost never metastasizes, and squamous cell carcinoma does so rarely. Although these facts make carcinoma of the skin the most curable cancer, the fact that it can kill and the fact that it occurs frequently make it important nonetheless. Ultraviolet radiations are the most important etiologic agents, but there are other physical as well as chemical agents that are occasionally responsible. Usually lesions arising in x-irradiated skin and in burn scars should be excised, but the etiology does not otherwise play a role in the determination of treatment (Figs. 3-8 and 3-9).

As mentioned previously, the accessibility and easily defined limits of carcinoma of the skin make it curable in a high proportion of patients. Whether squamous cell or basal cell in type, these carcinomas are sufficiently radioresponsive to be controlled in most instances by doses that are well tolerated. There are reports of success with roentgentherapy, radium therapy, scalpel excision, cautery excision, electrocoagulation, escharotics, as well as chemotherapeutic agents. Certainly no single method is best in all circumstances, and the careless application of any method can produce a poor cosmetic result or render a previously curable lesion incurable. We believe that all carcinomas of the skin can be handled very well either by roentgentherapy or by surgical excision. Actually, if the sole criterion of success is control

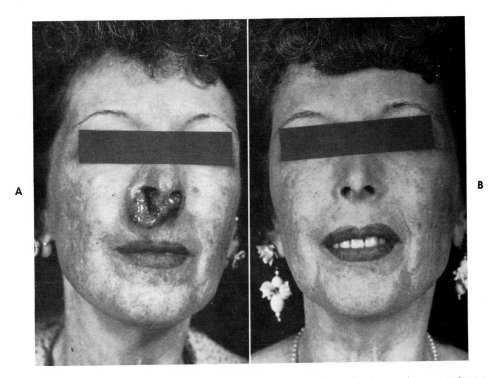

Fig. 3-8. A, Hazards of repeated local exposure to x rays. This patient was given an unknown number of x-ray treatments for severe acne 20 to 25 years previously. In addition to the carcinoma, the skin is leathery, dry, and without hair. The patient refused the recommended surgery. She was given 5000 rad (skin) in 5 weeks (220 kv; hvl, 2 mm Cu; TSD, 50). (W. U. neg. 53-1681.) **B,** Same patient 1 year later. She remains asymptomatic 5 years after treatment. (W. U. neg. 53-3719.)

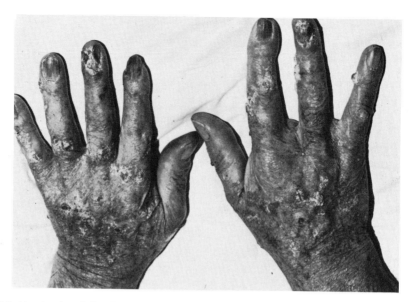

Fig. 3-9. Hands of a distinguished diagnostic radiologist. The total dose is unknown but changes are classic—a dry, easily fissured skin with many hyperkeratotic and precancerous lesions. Right middle finger was amputated for a squamous cell carcinoma of the skin.

of the lesion, either surgery or roentgentherapy adequately employed will yield similar results. But the use of either of these methods to the point of exclusion of the other is certain to yield less satisfying cosmetic and functional results than using each where it is best suited. If the possibility of control at a given site is equal by the two methods, the one yielding the best cosmetic or functional result should be selected. Should control be equal and cosmetic results similar by the two methods or should cosmetic results be relatively unimportant, the most expeditious treatment is preferred. Thus the choice between surgery and irradiation depends on tumor site, extension, previous treatment, and the significance of probable cosmetic and functional results (Fig. 3-10).

If a carcinoma of the skin is to be eradicated by irradiation, it has been found that a dose producing a moderate moist reaction is usually necessary and adequate. If properly fractionated, such a dose preserves the dermis and underlying structure. Postirradiation epithelization occurs quickly if the dose has not been too caustic. "Radiotherapy will be indicated because of its ability, when adequately applied, to destroy the carcinomatous tissue selectively without mutilation or dysfunction and with little or no visible sequelae; in other cases radiotherapy will be indicated because the extension of the lesion and its infiltration of deep structures make its treatment by any other method entirely impossible"* (Fig. 3-11). By reason of this selec-

---

*From del Regato, J. A., and Spjut, H. J.: Ackerman and del Regato's cancer: diagnosis, treatment, and prognosis, ed. 5, St. Louis, 1977, The C. V. Mosby Co.

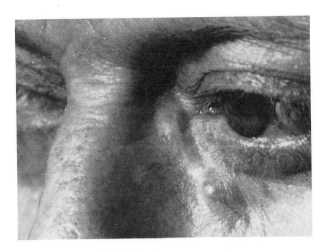

Fig. 3-10. Basal cell carcinoma, postoperative recurrence. An economical excision was attempted to avoid necessity of a skin graft. Six months later, recurrence appeared as a dumbbell-like induration at each end of incision. The justification for radiation therapy for lesions of this area is obvious.

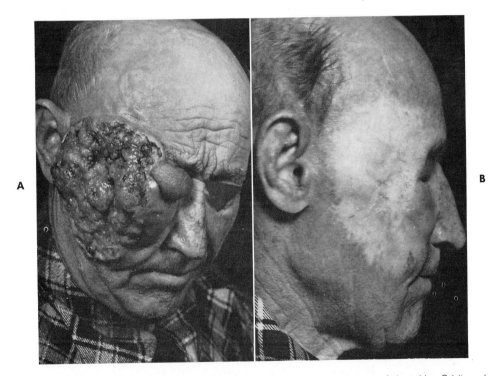

Fig. 3-11. **A,** Extensive infiltrating low-grade squamous cell carcinoma of the skin. Orbit and maxillary antrum were invaded. Patient was given 7200 rad (skin) in 64 days (220 kv; hvl, 2.5 mm Cu; TSD, 50). (W. U. neg. 52-2499). **B,** Same patient 1 year later. He died without recurrence 4½ years after irradiation. (W. U. neg. 53-2680.)

tivity, radiotherapy is usually indicated in the treatment of lesions of the eyelids, canthi, pinna, nose, and preauricular and postauricular regions and extensive or diffusely infiltrating lesions elsewhere. For certain large destructive lesions, it may be obvious from the onset that some type of posttreatment plastic repair will be necessary. It may then be better to treat such a patient with surgery from the beginning so that the plastic repair will not be performed in a heavily irradiated field.

TECHNIQUES. The only real superiority of irradiation over excision is its greater preservation of uninvolved tissues. When such tissue preservation is not important, surgery is usually more expeditious and is the treatment of choice. When preservation of normal tissue is important, the best available irradiation technique should be used. This means fractionation for any port over the eyelid or over cartilage and any port greater than 1 cm in diameter in other regions. We have used roentgentherapy and both radium and radon as molds and interstitially. As far as the irradiation of skin lesions is concerned, there can be no question but that roentgentherapy provides the greatest flexibility in adjusting quality, field size, and fractionation. In addition, roentgentherapy is the most convenient technique for most radiation oncologists and entails considerably less radiation hazard. Radium or radon used interstitially is contraindicated in the canthi, eyelids, and lesions over cartilage. In other sites the high dose immediately surrounding these sources falls off rapidly, resulting in a less homogeneous distribution of energy than can be obtained with roentgentherapy. Radium used in molds has no advantage over roentgentherapy, and the proper preparation of molds is much more time consuming. Although the radiation hazards are not serious with such molds, they do exist.

Carcinomas of the skin overlying the pinna and the nasal cartilages require special mention. Such cancers are seldom excised without a skin graft or removal of some cartilage. The administration of poorly fractionated, high-dose, contact therapy to the skin overlying these cartilages results in frequent painful chondritis that may require excision. However, carefully fractionated irradiation using a good quality of rays rarely results in chondritis and does not produce the deformity of an excision (Parker and Wildermuth; del Regato and Vuksanovic; Avila and associates). We enthusiastically recommend irradiation for such cancers if cartilage destruction has not been so great as to require plastic repair regardless of the method of therapy.

The radiation oncologist must estimate the extent of a given lesion of the skin by the same method that a surgeon uses to decide on the extent of excision. This is by inspection and palpation and must be a three-dimensional determination. Although most skin lesions are relatively superficial, it is generally unsafe to assume even with small lesions that penetration is less than 1 cm in depth. For this reason one usually must deliver a substantial dose to at least 1 cm depth. Since this is true, one rarely has occasion to use unfiltered low kilovoltage radiations (contact therapy). Such low kilovoltage radiations without a filter can undoubtedly control many lesions of the skin, but the high surface dose given in the process of delivering an adequate dose to 1 cm depth unnecessarily destroys much of the superficial tissue. The resulting deformity is greater from this rather striking nonhomogeneity. Most lesions require

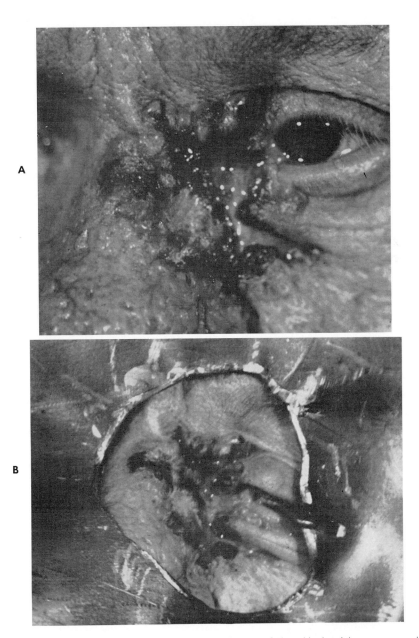

Fig. 3-12. A, Extensive superficial basal cell carcinoma of the skin involving upper and lower eyelids and bridge of nose. Treatment of this lesion entails irradiation of the nasolacrimal duct and generous portion of the eyelids. The patient was given 5200 rad (surface) in 32 days (220 kv; hvl, 1.25 mm Cu; TSD, 50). **B,** Same patient. Eye shield deep to eyelids and overlying lead shield in place. Eye shield protects lens and at the same time permits irradiation of entire thickness and width of lids. Overlying lead shield protects remainder of lower and upper lids and limits field to suspected area of involvement.

fields at least 2 cm in diameter and adequate doses to 1 cm in depth. For such lesions we have used radiations produced at 110 to 120 kv with a filter equivalent to about 0.25 mm Cu and 1 mm Al. For lesions requiring fields of 4 cm or larger with a corresponding infiltration, radiations produced at 200 kv and filtered with 0.5 mm Cu plus 1 mm Al are recommended. In the radiotherapy of advanced lesions that have infiltrated cartilage or bone, a still better quality of radiations is a necessity if frequent necroses are to be avoided.

The width of the border of apparently normal tissue to be included in the field will vary. For tiny lesions a 1 cm border will obviously be excessive, whereas for large infiltrative lesions 1 cm may appear inadequate. In the irradiation of lesions of the eyelids, special shielding is necessary to prevent damage to the lens and cornea (Figs. 3-12 and 3-13). This is easily accomplished with a local anesthetic and curved lead shields placed in the fornices. With large ports over the cheek, intraoral lead may be used to shield the tongue and gingiva.

DAILY DOSE. Much work has been done in an attempt to define optimum time-dose-volume relationships for carcinoma of the skin. For several reasons it is impossible to give rigid rules for these lesions. First, a small lesion of the cheek or neck can be treated quickly and in a more or less caustic fashion without significant risk of serious late sequelae. However, a similar small lesion on the tip of the nose or

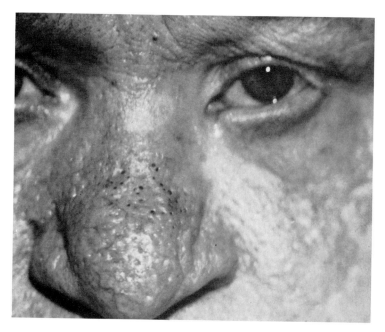

Fig. 3-13. Same patient as shown in Fig. 3-12. Appearance of treated area 6 months later. There is no disturbance in nasolacrimal function or in function of lower eyelid. The medial half of lower eyelash is lost. Cosmetic result is excellent.

lower eyelid will require an entirely different technique if serious cosmetic and functional sequelae are to be kept to a minimum.

The size of the lesion is a second important factor affecting technique. Large lesions definitely require higher doses than do small lesions (Fig. 1-10). However, the larger the irradiated area, the less the tolerated dose (Fig. 3-14). By more highly fractionating the irradiation, it is possible to deliver the required dose more frequently without exceeding tolerance.

The reports on dose-time relationships have rarely included an evaluation of the site and size of the lesion. The classic data published by Strandqvist are composite in that they include the average of skin lesions of many sites and sizes. As discussed in Chapter 1, small cancers respond to radiations as if they were more sensitive than large cancers. They are certainly more curable and, regardless of location, there is less risk of necrosis (Fig. 3-14). Strandqvist's data are of limited usefulness when a specific lesion in a specific site is being considered. It is difficult to define the average

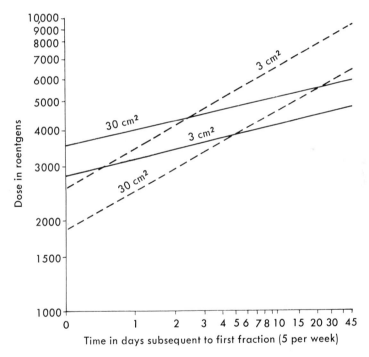

Fig. 3-14. Time-dose-volume relationships for fractionated irradiation of carcinoma of the skin. Solid lines are isoeffect curves for 99% tumor regression for cancers 3 cm² and 30 cm². Broken lines are isoeffect curves for 3% skin necrosis for skin areas of 3 cm² and 30 cm². Curves for tumor regression have less slope than those for skin tolerance. Unlike the classic Strandqvist curves, cancers of similar sizes are grouped together, emphasizing that larger cancers require a higher dose than small cancers. Curves also emphasize that for given fractionation large volumes tolerate less dose than small volumes. Moving along graph from left to right, with increased fractionation the curves for necrosis and tumor regression cross, then diverge, emphasizing the benefits of fractionation. (Modified from von Essen, C. F.: Radiology **81**:881-883, 1963.)

size and site of carcinoma of the skin. von Essen (1963) has reported the results of dose-time studies for ports less than and greater than 10 cm². The need for higher doses and greater fractionation for the larger cancers is beautifully confirmed by his study of necrosis, recurrences, and cures (Fig. 3-14). In speaking of fractionation, we imply daily treatment five or six times each week. The importance of this practice was emphasized by Traenkle and Muloy. Single weekly doses of 1000 rad for a total dose of 4000 to 5000 rad produced four times as many necroses as 300 or 400 rad three times each week. We believe daily treatments decrease sequelae even further.

Because cancer of the skin is rarely life-endangering, it tends to be regarded lightly and treated hurriedly to minimize patient inconvenience. Large individual doses or the single massive-dose technique is popular. Such techniques are usually devised to fit the immediate needs of the patient and sacrifice the proved benefits of fractionation. The cosmetic result with the single dose technique approaches that obtained by cautery. It must be remembered that single doses are often given with poor-quality rays at short target-skin distances so that factors other than fractionation are to be considered. Results obtained by this method may be acceptable in a few sites, but for most lesions of the face, when the advantage of using radiotherapy is in preserving tissue, it seem ridiculous to use this more caustic single dose technique. For 2 cm ports not over cartilage and not on the eyelids, 4000 rad (skin) in 10 days is quite satisfactory, provided the factors mentioned previously are used and the lesion is not deeply infiltrating. In most of these cases a shorter treatment will result in a rounded, blanched area. We believe the linear scar of excision is preferable to such areas of achromia. For most lesions treated with 2 to 3 cm fields on the lids, on the canthi, and overlying cartilage, a dose of 4200 to 5000 rad (skin) in 3 to 4 weeks gives excellent control and excellent cosmetic results. Large lesions 8 to 12 cm in diameter that infiltrate underlying bone or cartilage are best treated with a good quality of radiations. An accumulated dose of 6500 to 7500 rad (skin) in approximately 8 weeks may be required. These doses are employed for both squamous cell and basal cell carcinomas.

Lesions of the unexposed parts of the body can be controlled by irradiation just as those of the face; but in areas where cosmetic results are of no great importance, surgery is more expeditious and is therefore the treatment of choice. Radiation-induced moist reactions on the back may be very slow to heal and often leave undesirable telangiectatic areas. Excision is preferred for such areas. Lesions on the dorsum of the hand can likewise be controlled by irradiation; however, when compared to a skin graft, the postirradiation thin skin withstands trauma poorly. Excision and skin graft are usually the treatments of choice in such cases. If the lesion has infiltrated deep between the tendons, we have used irradiation followed by early graft. As mentioned earlier, such a graft will take despite the previous irradiation, provided it is applied within 2 months of the treatment. In a few such cases the hand will be preserved. If the procedure fails, amputation is still possible.

Telecobalt beams can be used to irradiate selected cancers of the skin of the nose, pinna, and penis. Of course, a suitable bolus assuring electron buildup must be used, and there should be the indication for irradiating the entire tissue thickness. Such a technique has a cartilage-sparing characteristic that could be critical in large, deeply infiltrating skin cancers of the organs mentioned (Schroeder and associates).

Electron beams of appropriate low energy may be used in the same fashion as superficial x-ray beams for small cancers of the skin and yield similar results. However, the cost per treatment with electrons is several times that for superficial x-ray beam therapy, and therefore it is not usually justified. However, for larger cancers of the skin, the electron beam energy and size can be precisely tailored to the dose distribution requirements, and treatment with electrons is an excellent technique.

PROGNOSIS AND RESULTS. Control rates are but one measure of the efficacy of the treatment for carcinoma of the skin. Cosmetic and functional results are important and often sway one's decision as to the modality recommended. Lesions of the eyelids, nose, tragus, and cheek are shown in Figs. 3-15 to 3-22.

In collaboration with del Regato, we reviewed the results obtained by treating 1011 basal cell carcinomas and 613 squamous cell carcinomas of the skin at the Ellis Fischel State Cancer Hospital. Lesions of the nose, naso-orbital region, eyelids, retroauricular region, and chin were usually treated by irradiation. Lesions of the cheek, cervical region, dorsum of the hand, and scalp were generally excised. In other areas, surgery and radiotherapy were applied with nearly equal frequency, depending on the size of the lesion, relative importance of cosmetic result, and so forth. The type of selection carried out does not permit a comparison of radiotherapy and surgery in the treatment of cancer of the skin. Of the 1011 basal cell carcinomas, 821 were irradiated. Of this group, sixty of the patients had recurrences within 3 years, and in fifty-seven of these sixty, the recurrences were controlled by subsequent treatment, usually surgery. Twenty-two of the patients were lost to follow-up, and 145 died of intercurrent disease. Of the 190 basal cell carcinomas surgically excised, six of the patients had recurrences within 3 years, and in five of these six, the recurrences were controlled by subsequent treatment. None of the patients was lost to follow-up, and fifty died of intercurrent disease. As already mentioned, the cases selected for irradiation are not comparable to those selected for surgery. To illustrate the value of irradiation, data on some of the lesions in the more difficult sites are presented in Table 3-1. A special study made of the recurrent lesions shows that there is no tendency for any particular microscopic variant to be more prone to recur (Table 3-2).

Although the number and distribution of squamous cell carcinomas of the skin differ from the number and distribution of basal cell carcinomas, the control rate of the local lesion is almost exactly the same as that for basal cell carcinoma. Carcinoma of the skin overlying cartilage deserves special mention in view of the frequent misconceptions regarding the value of irradiation over cartilage. Maximum control with a minimum of sequelae will be obtained when a well-filtered beam from 100 to 140 kv equipment is given through the smallest practical port and is fractionated over 3 to 6 weeks. Optimum doses have just been outlined. Of fifty-six consecutive patients

Text continued on p. 80.

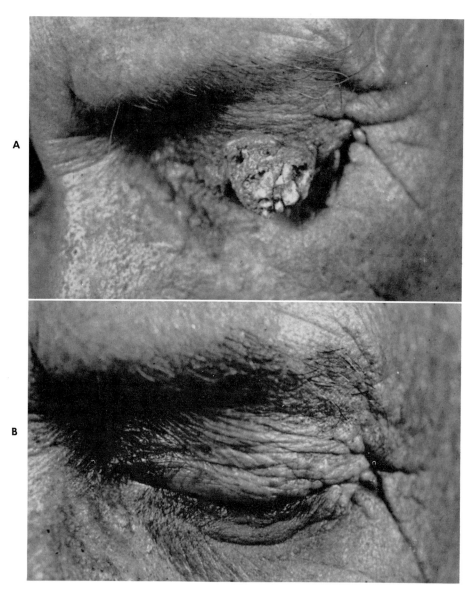

Fig. 3-15. A, Low-grade squamous cell carcinoma with large horn formation of upper eyelid. Patient was given 4800 rad (surface) in 3 weeks through a 2.5 cm port (110 kv filtered with 0.25 mm Cu and 1 mm Al). **B,** Same patient 1 year later. There is no trace of the previously treated lesion. Upper eyelash has been permanently epilated. Function is excellent.

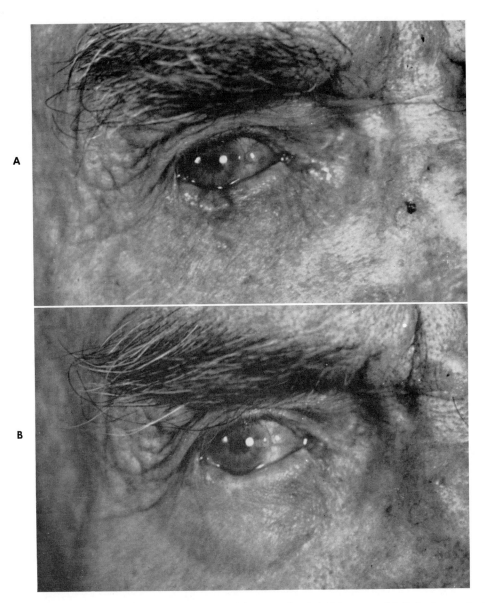

Fig. 3-16. A, Typical basal cell carcinoma of free margin of right lower eyelid. Patient was given 3700 rad (skin) in 12 days through a 1 cm port (110 kv filtered with 0.25 mm Cu and 1 mm Al). **B,** Same patient 3 years later, showing minimal depression of the free margin of lower lid with excellent function.

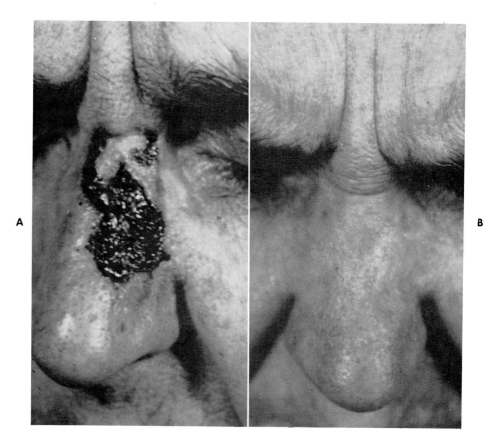

Fig. 3-17. A, Superficial basal cell carcinoma of bridge of the nose. Patient was given 4000 rad (skin) through a 4 × 2.5 cm port in 12 days (110 kv filtered with 0.25 mm Cu and 1 mm Al). **B,** Same patient 2 years later, with excellent cosmetic result.

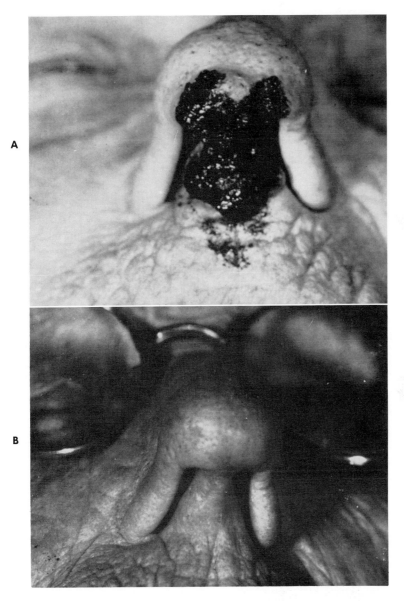

Fig. 3-18. A, Superficial basal cell carcinoma covering entire cutaneous surface of columella of nose. Patient was given 4400 rad (skin) in 3 weeks (110 kv filtered with 0.25 mm Cu and 1 mm Al). **B,** Same patient. Appearance of columella 2 years later.

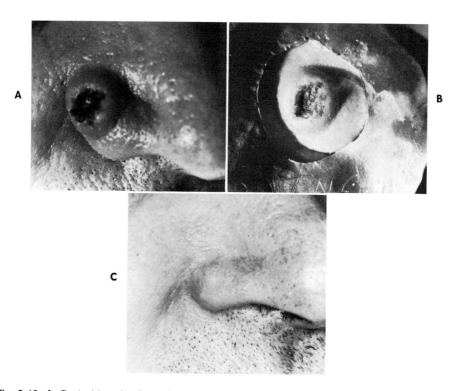

Fig. 3-19. A, Typical basal cell carcinoma of ala nasi. **B,** Lead cutout provides adequate margin. Lead strip is placed in nostril to shield septum. **C,** One year after administration of 4500 rad in 4 weeks (120 kv, hvl 4 Al, TSD 15 cm).

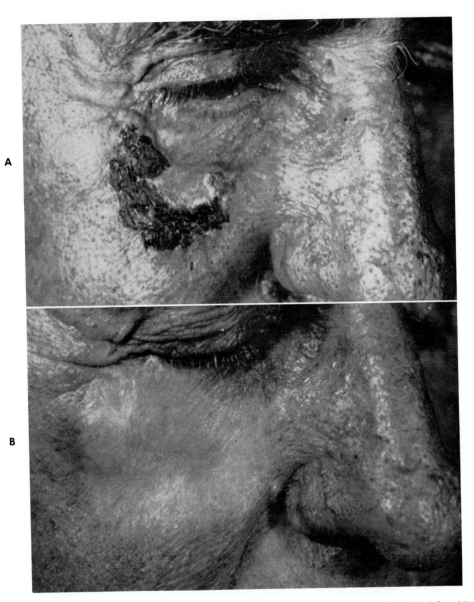

Fig. 3-20. A, Extensive superficial basal cell carcinoma of skin involving entire right infraorbital region. Induration extended into right lower lid. Patient was given 4700 rad (skin) in 3½ weeks through a 5 × 5 cm port, including outer half of lower eyelid (110 kv filtered with 0.25 mm Cu and 1 mm Al). **B,** Same patient 2 years later. Slight achromia and slight ectropion of right lower lid are evident. Cosmetic and functional results are acceptable.

Fig. 3-21. A, Squamous cell carcinoma of skin of the tragus and preauricular region. This lesion extended about 1 cm into external auditory canal. Patient was given 4700 rad (skin) in 4 weeks through a 4 × 4 cm port (110 kv filtered with 0.25 mm Cu and 1 mm Al). **B,** Same patient 3 years later, with some atrophy of irradiated skin and achromia. Results are satisfactory.

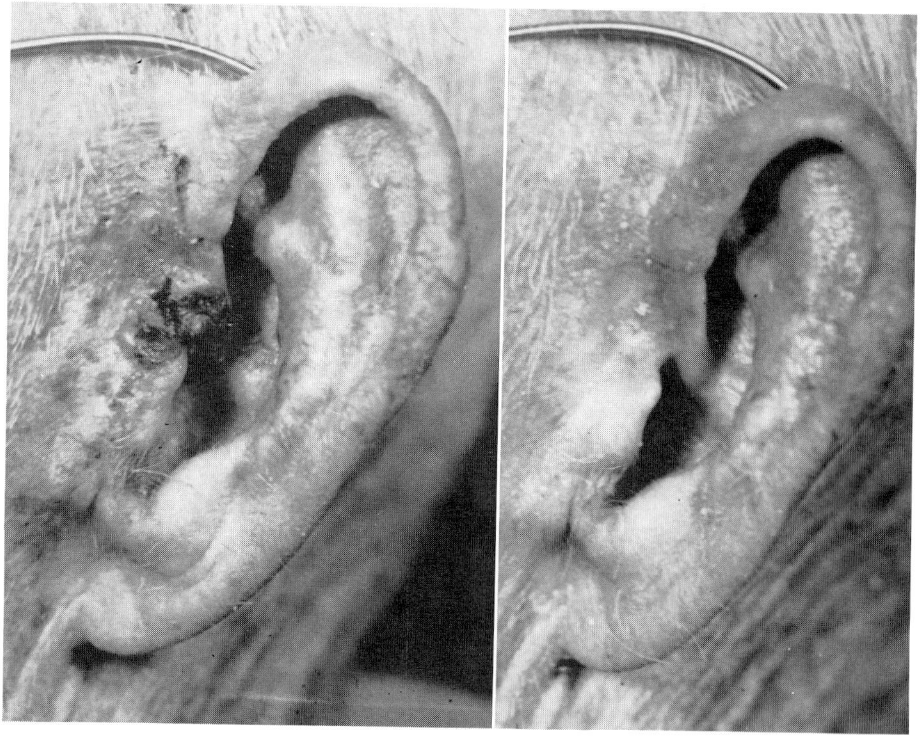

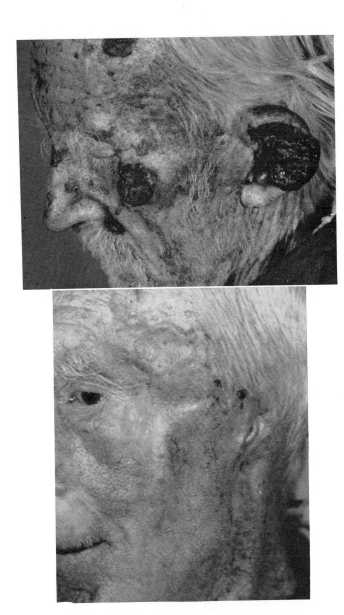

Fig. 3-22. Numerous carcinomas of skin in elderly farmer. Treatment of squamous cell carcinoma of the pinna, because of its very large size, consisted of surgical removal of ear. Other areas (forehead and malar and nasolabial regions) were treated with irradiation. Treatment of some lesions by irradiation and some by excision seemed to be the best treatment for this particular patient.

Table 3-1. Control of basal cell carcinoma of the skin

Site	Number irradiated	Number of recurrences	Number of recurrences controlled	Dead intercurrent disease	Lost	Well 3 years
Ear	32	2	2	10	1	21
Preauricular	36	1	1	7	3	26
Retroauricular	32	2	2	6	0	26
Nose	224	11	10	33	4	186
Eyelids and canthi (del Regato)	117	9	9	15	1	101

Only sites of special interest have been selected. Technique used was that outlined in text.

Table 3-2. Radiocurability of microscopic variants of basal cell carcinoma (The group studied was *devised* to contain equal numbers of recurrent and nonrecurrent lesions.)*

Growth pattern	Structure	Total recurrences
Infiltrating	Solid	25/12
	Degenerative cysts	8/2
	Adenoid	4/2
Circumscribed	Solid	19/11
	Degenerative cysts	8/4
	Adenoid	26/13
Special	Superficial spreading	3/1
	Diffuse infiltrating	6/2

*From Moss, W. T., and Johnson, R.: Unpublished data.
The microscopic slides of tissue from fifty-seven patients who later showed local recurrence of carcinoma were mixed with those of fifty-seven patients who showed no recurrence. The ratio of the total number of slides falling into each category over the number of slides from patients developing recurrence is shown. If a variant has no particular propensity for recurrence, the ratio should be 2:1.

with skin cancers overlying cartilages of the nose or ear, only three recurred, and all were subsequently controlled (del Regato and Vuksanovic). No cases of chondronecrosis developed. Cosmetic results were good. Parker and Wildermuth and Avila and associates have reported similar results.

Carcinoma of the eyelid is another site where roentgentherapy is of particular value and therefore justifies special mention. With carefully fractionated irradiation similar to that described previously for lesions overlying cartilage, the substance of the lid is preserved, and function is near normal. With the usual lead shield, the cornea and lens are not given a significant dose. Control rates are excellent (Table 3-1). Of ninety patients irradiated for such lesions, eighty-three were well at 3 years. Three of the seven recurrences were subsequently controlled (Fayos and Wildermuth). Similar results have been reported by McKenna and MacDonald.

Fitzpatrick and associates analyzed their results obtained by irradiating 477 can-

Table 3-3. Cosmetic and functional results of radiotherapy for cancer of the eyelid 1 year after treatment*

	Basal cell carcinoma	Squamous cell carcinoma
Excellent	294	19
Good	20	3
Fair	18	2
Poor	22	0
TOTAL	354	24

*From Fitzpatrick, P. J., Jamieson, D. M., Thompson, G. A., and Allt, W. E.: Radiology **104:**661-665, 1972.

Table 3-4. Metastasis of squamous cell carcinoma of the skin by region and the frequency of surgical control of metastasis

Site	Total number of patients	Number of patients developing metastasis	Controlled 3 years or more
Ear	94	14	3
Neck	57	2	1
Cheek	107	4	1
Nose	34	1	1
Hand	73	8	4

Average incidence of metastasis, 6.6%

cers of the eyelids. The doses and field sizes were the same for basal cell and squamous cell carcinomas. They used a spectrum of techniques from a single-dose technique (2000 rad single dose using 100 kv radiations) for the smaller, more superficial cancers to a more fractionated technique (4000 to 6000 rad in 3 weeks or more using medium-voltage beams) for the larger, more infiltrating cancers. Only 4.8% showed postirradiation persistence. The thirty squamous cell carcinomas were controlled as often as the 447 basal cell carcinomas. Cosmetic and functional results of their patients available for follow-up after 1 year are shown in Table 3-3.

Metastases of the squamous cell lesions do make the prognosis slightly worse, however. The incidence by site and the surgical curability of metastases by region are shown in Table 3-4. Pathologic grading was shown to be of little value in predicting the control of the primary lesion or the probability of development of subsequent metastases. Although we have seen several patients in whom biopsy-proved metastases in lymph nodes were permanently controlled by external irradiation, most of these metastases will be treated by surgery. Radiation therapy should be given special consideration in the treatment of metastases to preauricular nodes when adequate excision entails a risk of facial paralysis.

SUMMARY. Carcinoma of the skin is highly curable by a variety of means. Irradiation is indicated in those sites and situations in which preservation of normal tissues either for cosmetic or functional reasons is important. Roentgentherapy, because of its great flexibility, can be adapted to skin lesions of all sites and sizes. No single technique is best. The quality and quantity of radiations used and shielding precautions must be individualized. Control rates are good and cosmetic and functional results are excellent if this policy is followed.

REFERENCES

Avila, J., Bosch, A., Aristizabal, S., Frias, Z., and Marcial, V.: Carcinoma of the pinna, Cancer **40:**2891-2895, 1977.

del Regato, J. A., and Vuksanovic, M.: Radiotherapy of carcinomas of the skin overlying the cartilages of the nose and ear, Radiology **79:**203-208, 1962.

del Regato, J. A., and Spjut, H. J.: Ackerman and del Regato's cancer: diagnosis, treatment, and prognosis, ed. 5, St. Louis, 1977, The C. V. Mosby Co.

Dewing, S. B.: Radiotherapy of benign diseases, Springfield, Ill., 1965, Charles C Thomas, Publisher.

Elkin, M., Salvioni, D., and Binstock, M.: The effect of localised radiation on autologous skin transplants, Br. J. Radiol. **35:**235-240, 1962.

Fayos, J. V., and Wildermuth, O.: Roentgen therapy for eyelid carcinoma, Arch. Ophthalmol. **67:**298-302, 1962.

Fitzpatrick, P. J., Jamieson, D. M., Thompson, G. A., and Allt, W. E.: Tumors of the eyelids and their treatment by radiotherapy, Radiology **104:**661-665, 1972.

Lacassagne, A., and Gricouroff, G.: Action des radiations ionisantes sur l'organisme, Paris, 1956, Masson et Cie.

Liegner, L. M., and Michaud, N. J.: Skin and subcutaneous reactions induced by super-voltage irradiation, Am. J. Roentgenol. **85:**533-549, 1961.

McKenna, R. J., and MacDonald, I.: Irradiation for cancer of the eyelid, Calif. Med. **96:**184-189, 1962.

Parker, R. G., and Wildermuth, O.: Radiation therapy of lesions overlying cartilage, Cancer **15:**57-65, 1962.

Rubin, P., and Grise, J. W.: The difference in response of grafted and normal skin to ionizing irradiation clinical observations, Am. J. Roentgenol. **84:**645-655, 1960.

Schroeder, A. F., Scher, A. J., Brothers, W., and George, F. W.: Surface moulage treatment techniques utilizing cobalt[60] teletherapy: a follow-up study, Cancer **22:**968-972, 1968.

Strandqvist, M.: Time-dose relationship, Acta Radiol., supp. 55, p. 1, 1944.

Suit, H. D.: "Oxygen effect factor" of human skin, Radiology **79:**118-119, 1962.

Traenkle, H. L., and Muloy, D.: Further observations on late radiation necrosis following therapy of skin cancer. The results of fractionation of the total dose, Arch. Dermatol. **81:**908-913, 1960.

United States Department of Health, Education, and Welfare: A review of the use of ionizing radiation for the treatment of benign diseases, HEW Publication (FDA) 78-8043, Sept., 1977.

von Essen, C. F.: Roentgen therapy of skin and lip carcinoma: factors influencing success and failure, Am. J. Roentgen **83:**556-570, 1960.

von Essen, C. F.: A spatial model of time-dose-volume relationships in radiation therapy, Radiology **81:**881-883, 1963.

4

The oral cavity, oropharynx, and salivary and mucous glands

RESPONSE OF NORMAL WALLS OF THE ORAL CAVITY
AND OROPHARYNX TO IRRADIATION

BUCCAL MUCOSA. The stratified squamous epithelium lining the oral cavity is moderately radiosensitive. Coutard gave the first detailed description of the desquamation of such an epithelium, and he published data regarding the series of changes with respect to time and dose. He applied the term *radioepithelitis* to the reaction. The life span of the cells forming the mucosal epithelium is considerably shorter than that of cells forming the epidermis. It is to be expected that the epidermis would be slower in desquamating. Coutard found that after a given dose of radiations, mucosal epithelium is lost by the twelfth day. The same dose will produce a loss of the epidermis in 2 to 3 weeks. The mucosa will heal in 2 to 3 weeks, whereas the skin requires 5 to 6 weeks. However, the epithelium of the oral cavity does not respond in the same way in all locations. Coutard observed that desquamation of the soft palate usually occurs first, followed in order by desquamation of the mucosal covering of the hypopharynx, vallecula, floor of the mouth, cheeks, medial aspect of the mandible, laryngeal surface of the epiglottis, interarytenoid area, base of the tongue, vocal cords, and, last, the dorsum of the tongue. It will be seen later that the radioresponsiveness of cancers arising from these areas does not follow the order just listed. The cell of origin is but one of the important factors determining response. The bed in which the tumor cells grow is also important. Coutard believed originally that a dose of radiations sufficient to desquamate the mucosal epithelium was essential if the cancer was to be eradicated. He taught that the desquamation could be used as a valuable guide not only to the dose given but also to the adequacy of the port. If a false membrane completely encircled the tumor, both the dose and the port size were thought to be sufficient. These clinical guides are still valuable. However, Baclesse, and Buschke and Vaeth have shown that, with meticulous and prolonged fractionation, desquamation of the normal mucosal epithelium need not occur even with doses that will eradicate very small cancers. We have not utilized such a technique for cancer of the oral cavity, and indeed the application of this technique to any other than the laryngeal area is seriously ques-

83

tioned. The clinical guides to dosage as mentioned in Chapter 1 do not make direct use of mucosal reaction in judging adequacy of dose. After doses of radiations used to control cancer that are given with conventional techniques, the mucosa usually heals promptly. An exception to this may be seen after the irradiation of large tongue lesions, when a month or more may be required for healing. The newly formed epithelium is thin and fragile and may eventually appear pale and telangiectatic.

Postirradiation changes in the submucosa are inflammatory in appearance and are identical with those described for the dermis. In early stages there are capillary engorgement, edema, and leukocytic infiltration. Large multinucleated fibroblasts may appear, but this acute phase subsides after several weeks. Several months later a progressive fibrosis is apparent. Depending on the dose and the method of administration, this may vary from a barely noticeable induration to a stony hard fibrosis. Although the epithelium is thinner and more fragile, the subepithelial changes account for its pale appearance. All subepithelial tissues show the progressive fibrosis. Thus there is perivascular fibrosis and periglandular fibrosis. With time these fibrotic tissues contract to produce a shrinkage of the irradiated volume. (See Chapter 3.)

Symptoms produced by the immediate and late tissue responses will obviously vary with dose, anatomic site, and volume, to say nothing of the variation between patients. Acute reactions in the anterior portion of the oral cavity seem better tolerated than those in the oropharynx. On the other hand, late necroses develop in the floor of the mouth more often than in the buccal mucosa or the tongue.

SALIVARY GLANDS. The major salivary glands, as well as the small mucous glands of the mucosa, are frequently damaged in the process of irradiating lesions of the oral cavity. Although an early transient radiation-induced swelling of the salivary glands has been described (Bergonié and Speder), clinically it is seldom noticed.

The patient may complain that the evening after the first fraction a painful swelling developed. By the time the patient returns for his next treatment the swelling will have subsided. It may occur again after the second fraction, but rarely after the third or subsequent fractions. Whether this acute swelling is caused principally by interstitial edema or by duct obstruction is unknown; both are known causes. A few days later there is a marked reduction in parenchyma and a noticeable decrease in gland size (English and associates). Usually within the first week of treatment, and often within 2 to 6 hours, the patient will notice that saliva is scanty and thick (Kashima and associates). Others found that the secretions of the parotid gland are practically eliminated by two or three treatments of 200 to 225 rad each. The other salivary glands seem less responsive, but 5 daily fractions of 200 rad reduce *total* saliva by 40% and by the end of irradiation to 5% (Shannon and associates). By the end of treatment, the thick sticky saliva may be very bothersome. Saliva and solid food will be difficult to swallow, and the patient frequently will use liquid to wash down his food. If treatment has included all glands and has been vigorous, this difficulty will last for months. After therapy, secretions rarely return to a completely normal level. Lacassagne and Gricouroff explained the qualitative changes in saliva by the microscopic finding that serous acini appeared more seriously damaged than mucous acini. Several months after irradiation, however, more serous than mucous acini remain (Evans and Ackerman). Serum and urinary amylase are elevated by direct irradiation of the salivary glands. The magnitude of the response is related to the dose (Kashima and associates). Initially, serum amylase may be very high, but as radiotherapy progresses and most of the amylase-producing tissue is destroyed, serum levels may return to normal even with further irradiation (van den Brenk and associates). The administration of steroids before and after irradiation does not modify the magnitude of this reaction.

Microscopic changes are spotty and vary somewhat from gland to gland. Acinar cells of the sublingual and submaxillary glands are normally renewed every 60 to 65 days. Those of the parotid gland are renewed every 40 days. The cells lining the secretory tubules of the submandibular gland are renewed after 95 days (Glucksmann and Cherry). Thus variation in radiation response should be expected. A dose of 2000 rad given in 10 daily fractions destroys acinar cells but permits acinar repopulation and resumption of function in 7 months. Higher doses given with similar fractionation produce more severe and permanent injury. Regardless of the location of the gland, radiation-induced damage is greatest in the acini and least in the excretory ducts. With time the ducts enlarge, even while periductal fibrosis and vascular narrowing are progressing.

Four months or more after commonly given "curative" doses of radiations, the late changes described by Evans and Ackerman appear. There is patchy destruction of nearly all acini with a few serous acini remaining. The onset of these changes is seen within a few weeks. Thus by 6 weeks ducts are dilated and surrounded by inflammatory changes (Fig. 4-1). Fibrosis surrounds the ducts, lobules, and acini. When such changes take place in the submaxillary salivary glands, the glands feel hard, are enlarged, and may be confused with cervical lymph node metastases (Evans and Ackerman).

In contrast to direct radiation-induced damage of the gland, disturbance in function has been reported secondary to moderate doses of total body radiations. A single dose of 350 rad total body irradiation to the dog produces mild transient hypersecretion of several months' duration. A higher dose of 500 rad single dose produces a decrease in gland secretion. This type of dysfunction is thought to be due to a disturbance of the reflex regulatory mechanism but is otherwise not defined (Kurtisin).

Saliva performs several functions that assist in preventing dental caries. It dilutes foods, lubricates the oral cavity, buffers and dilutes acids produced by fermentation, and continuously washes food particles and organisms from the oral cavity. Irradiation of the salivary glands alters saliva both quantitatively and qualitatively. The thick, sticky saliva is less effective in each of these functions. If precautions are not taken, it is not surprising that caries appear soon after irradiation and destroy the crowns of many remaining teeth, making extractions necessary. Del Regato described

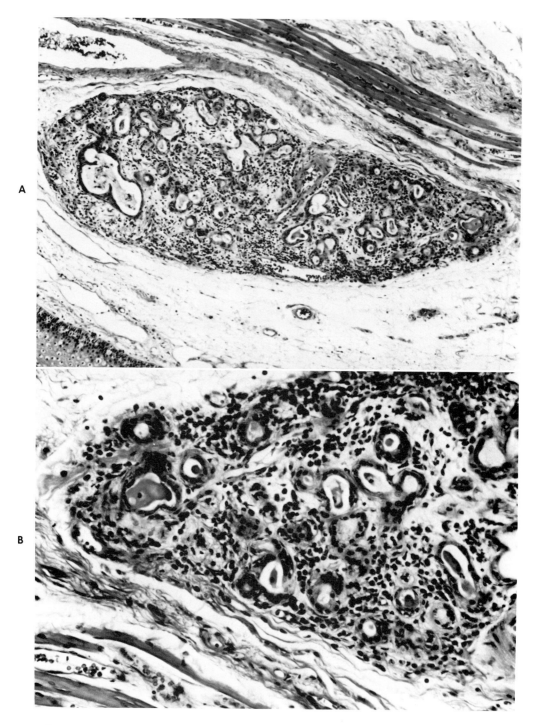

Fig. 4-1. A, Photomicrograph of minor salivary gland given 7000 rad in 7 weeks, 6 weeks prior to excision (magnification ×100). There is considerable atrophy of the acinar epithelium. Ducts appear dilated, contain inspissated secretions, and some display squamous metaplasia. A round cell stromal infiltrate is inconspicuous. **B,** Detail photomicrograph taken from same gland. Plasmocytic infiltrate of stroma and epithelial atrophy are clearly shown (magnification ×250). Fibrosis surrounds ducts, lobules, and acini.

these rather characteristic changes and pointed out that they appear even though the tooth or adjacent mandible has not been irradiated (Fig. 4-2). The point has been reemphasized by Frank and associates. As will be seen later, the incidence and severity of these caries can be greatly reduced by appropriate dental care. Extraction of such teeth in the presence of an irradiated mandible and gingival mucosa may trigger an osteonecrosis. Ng and associates confirmed this by experiments on dogs.

A saliva substitute has been developed and tested by Shannon and associates. The liquid mixture not only lubricates but also restores minerals and promotes remineralization of enamel. We now recommend this saliva substitute during and after irradiation in addition to the measures outlined on p. 90.

Taste. Irradiation of the oral cavity invariably modifies the patient's sense of taste. Indeed, this is often one of his most vigorous complaints. Radiations affect taste by damaging the taste buds and by modifying saliva. The perception of sour and bitter are suppressed more than that of sweet and salty (Bonanni and Perazzi). However, during the severe portion of an acute mucosal reaction many patients will complain that all foods have lost their flavor. Although much of this loss is

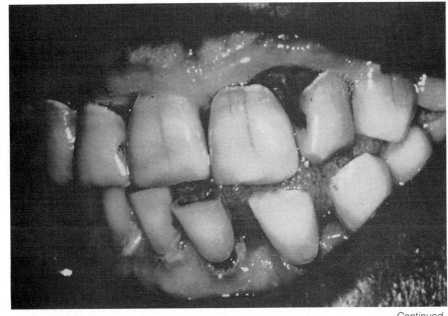

A

Continued.

Fig. 4-2. A, Patient received irradiation through parallel opposing ports for treatment of carcinoma of posterior half of lateral border of tongue. Both parotid glands were irradiated vigorously in the process of treatment. Teeth were in good condition at the time treatment was initiated. A tissue dose of 5300 rad in 6 weeks was delivered to middle of the tongue (1000 kv; hvl, 3 mm Pb). Three years later teeth show caries at gum level as described by del Regato. **B,** Same patient 8 years later. All teeth have extensive caries. Most have broken off at gumline. Roots remain in the mandible. **C,** Radiograph of teeth shown in **A** and **B** illustrating the characteristic location of the caries.

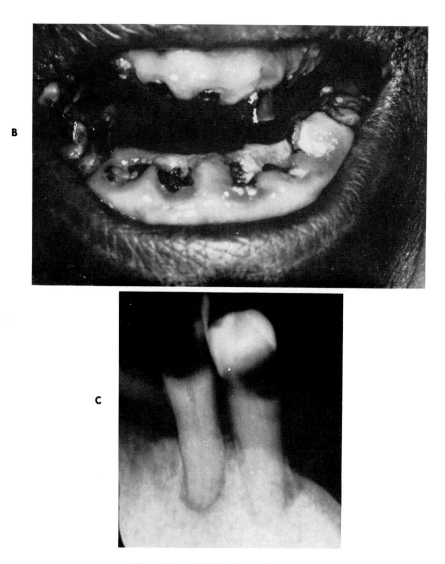

Fig. 4-2, cont'd. For legend see p. 87.

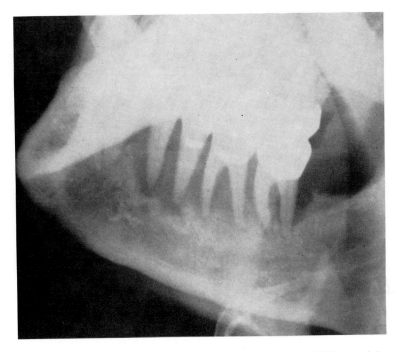

Fig. 4-3. Lower jaw was given calculated 6000 rad bone dose in 7 weeks (1000 kv; hvl, 3 mm Pb) for an adenocarcinoma of minor salivary gland in floor of mouth. Teeth were left in because they appeared to be in excellent condition. At time of this roentgenograph, 3 years later, the jaw showed extensive radiation changes. Teeth had to be removed at this time.

eventually recovered, some patients believe it is the worst sequela. The taste buds alone are relatively resistant to radiation damage. However, the changes in saliva and oral mucosa seriously modify the patient's ability to taste even though taste buds are nearly normal.

MANDIBLE. Regardless of the preirradiation precautions, a significant proportion of patients irradiated with a curative aim will sooner or later develop osteonecrosis (Fig. 4-1). The series of cellular changes within the bone leading up to osteonecrosis and sequestration is given in Chapter 21. Summarized briefly, these changes consist of damage to the haversian canal system of small blood vessels, killing of a large number of osteocytes, and serious injury to the periosteum. In addition, the connective tissues and mucosa covering the mandible will also have been irradiated and rendered less able to tolerate any type of insult. There is no single sequence of events leading up to necrosis, but infection or trauma often precede onset.

Wholesale dental extractions immediately prior to irradiation in a misguided effort to forestall future mandibular trauma does in fact increase the incidence of later mandibular necrosis. Some teeth may be spared and necrosis can be reduced by systematic preirradiation and postirradiation dental evaluation and care (Keys and McCasland; Shannon and associates), which includes the following:

1. Assessment of the patient's needs and prospects as related to disease and anticipated radiation therapy
2. Restoration of all salvageable teeth and initiation of a program for plaque control
3. Removal of only the nonsalvageable teeth using minimal trauma, smoothing the mandible, and closing the mucosa to assure optimum early healing
4. Training the patient in daily care of the teeth, including application of stannous fluoride and use of a saliva substitute (Shannon and associates)
5. Counseling the patient regarding diet and dental follow-up care

The incidence of mandibular necrosis is dose related. With the dental regimen mentioned before, mandibular necrosis rarely develops with doses less than 6000 rad in 6 weeks (Bedwinek and associates). It is uncommon (1.8%) with doses under 7000 rad in 7 weeks and reaches 9% with doses over 7000 rad. The overall incidence of mandibular necrosis will obviously depend on the location and size of the primary lesion. The incidence may be as high as 25% for patients irradiated for large cancers of the floor of the mouth.

Patients at high risk for necrosis include alcoholics, heavy smokers, and patients with chronically poor nutrition or poor oral hygiene. In these patients the irradiated fragile mucosa covering the mandible sloughs more often, and mandibular necrosis

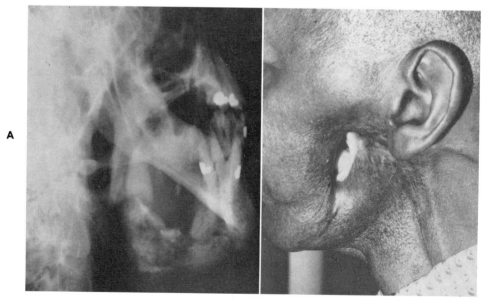

A

B

Fig. 4-4. A, Massive mandibular necrosis of an edentulous mandible 2 years after a calculated 6000 rad in 6 weeks given with telecobalt therapy. Entire angle of jaw has separated. **B,** Soft tissue and mandibular necroses have healed. Function is good. Patient refused any attempt at closure of fistula.

follows (Fig. 4-4). The first symptoms may be pain and tenderness of the gum or even of the entire mandible. The teeth may be suspected as the cause of the pain, and extraction may therefore be performed. There is no question that necrosis may be initiated occasionally by extractions (Ng and associates).

The process of sequestration usually requires months or years. The associated severe pain, malnutrition, and foul breath make the care of these patients one of the most difficult problems in radiotherapy. Instruction in oral hygiene, advice and encouragement as to nutrition, and medication for pain form the basis for their care. Surgical removal of the damaged bone usually results in large soft tissue losses. For this reason conservative management should be followed if at all possible.

The maxilla is not only much less frequently irradiated than the mandible, but it is also less dense than the mandible and it has a better blood supply (Hinds). Necrosis of the maxilla is unusual even when it is involved by cancer.

TEETH. The developing tooth, and to a less extent the adult tooth, both present constituent cells that exhibit proliferation, maturation, and secretion. These cell series are similar to those described for the epidermis. Both the developing tooth and the mature tooth have a complex interrelationship with the supporting mandible. After irradiation of the lower jaw, it is difficult to sort out the contribution of the several components to the specific changes under consideration. See Kimeldorf for a good summary of these changes.

Low doses of radiations (less than 1000 rad) arrest growth of the tooth bud. If the dose is much higher than 1000 rad, the bud will be completely destroyed. Depending on the stage of development when radiations are given, the tooth may remain abnormally small, may erupt rootless, or may show gross defects in dentin and enamel deposition.

The mature tooth is relatively resistant to direct radiation damage. Cancerocidal doses produce minimal damage to mature odontoblasts. It seems likely that most of the dental changes caused by direct irradiation of the adult tooth are due to radiation-induced obliteration of pulp vasculature. The periodontal membrane exhibits sensitivity similar to that of periosteum. Radiation damage of the periodontal membrane results in absorption of alveolar bone and a loosening and eventual loss of the tooth.

SUMMARY. In the process of irradiating cancers of the oral cavity and oropharynx, changes are produced in many tissues, including the salivary glands, mandible, teeth, and neighboring soft tissues. The interrelationship of these tissues in the maintenance of their integrity is complex. After radiation injury of a proportion of these tissues by "cancerocidal" doses, the changes may be compounded to produce major sequelae.

The incidence of mandibular necrosis can be greatly reduced by implementing a program of dental care, respecting the recognized dose limitations, shrinking the treatment portal or using interstitial sources whenever possible, and using modest daily doses.

CARCINOMA OF THE ORAL CAVITY

In this category of malignant tumors are a variety of gross and microscopic types. Only those types sufficiently radiosensitive to be thought of as radiocurable will be considered from a radiotherapeutic viewpoint. Over 80% of such a group will be keratinizing squamous cell carcinomas. Transitional cell carcinomas and lympho-epitheliomas, also referred to as nonkeratinizing squamous cell carcinomas, will make up a smaller variable proportion, depending on the site under consideration. The malignant tumors arising from the minor salivary glands or from glands within the mucosa will also form a small but important group. Although it may be of prognostic value to differentiate lymphoepithelioma and transitional cell carcinoma from squamous cell carcinoma, the treatment plan for the primary lesion will not vary significantly from that outlined for squamous cell carcinoma. However, the regional metastases of the former two are generally regarded as being more frequently radiocurable and are irradiated by preference. Other differences will be indicated in the appropriate sections.

A variety of clinical stage classifications has been proposed for carcinoma of the oral cavity. Therefore care must be taken in comparing so-called similar clinical stages. With the hope of achieving uniformity, we recommend use of the stage classification of the American Joint Committee (1978).

TNM CLASSIFICATION (Each anatomic site is considered separately.)*

T— Primary tumor

TX	Tumor that cannot be assessed by rules
T0	No evidence of primary tumor
TIS	Carcinoma in situ
T1	Tumor 2 cm or less in greatest diameter
T2	Tumor more than 2 cm but not more than 4 cm in greatest diameter
T3	Tumor more than 4 cm in greatest diameter
T4	Massive tumor more than 4 cm in diameter with deep invasion to involve antrum, pterygoid muscles, base of tongue, or skin of neck

N—Nodal involvement

NX	Nodes cannot be assessed
N0	No clinically positive node
N1	Single clinically positive homolateral node 3 cm or less in diameter
N2	Single clinically positive homolateral node more than 3 cm but not more than 6 cm in diameter or multiple clinically positive homolateral nodes, none over 6 cm in diameter
N2a	Single clinically positive homolateral node, more than 3 cm but not more than 6 cm in diameter
N2b	Multiple clinically positive homolateral nodes, none more than 6 cm in diameter
N3	Massive homolateral node(s), bilateral nodes, or contralateral node(s)
N3a	Clinically positive homolateral node(s) one more than 6 cm in diameter
N3b	Bilateral clinically positive nodes (in this situation, each side of the neck should be staged separately; that is, N3b: right, N2a; left, N1)
N3c	Contralateral clinically positive node(s) only

---

*From the American Joint Committee for Cancer Staging and End Results Reporting: Manual for staging of cancer, Chicago, 1978, Whiting Press.

M—Distant metastasis
> **MX**   Not assessed
> **M0**   No (known) distant metastasis
> **M1**   Distant metastasis present

HISTOPATHOLOGY

Predominant cancer is squamous cell carcinoma

GRADE

Well-differentiated, moderately well-differentiated, poorly to very poorly differentiated, or numbers 1, 2, 3-4

STAGE GROUPING

Stage I	T1 N0 M0
Stage II	T2 N0 M0
Stage III	T3 N0 M0
	T1 or T2 or T3, N1, M0
Stage IV	T4, N0 or N1, M0
	Any T, N2 or N3, M0
	Any T, any N, M1

Carcinoma of the lower lip

Carcinoma of the vermilion border of the lower lip constitutes about a fourth of all malignant lesions of the oral cavity. They are almost invariably squamous cell in type, are well differentiated, are diagnosed relatively early, metastasize in about 13% of all cases, and are highly curable by either irradiation or excision. When metastases occur, they are usually direct to the submaxillary or submental nodes. These nodes are rarely skipped. Of 519 patients, only one developed distant metastases (Gladstone and Kerr). Control of the primary malignant tumor is rarely a serious problem. However, ill-advised attempts at plastic repair will often leave much to be desired from the viewpoints of function and appearance. Similarly, irradiation using a poorly filtered beam or inadequate fractionation may leave an unsightly, malfunctioning lip.

To clarify the indications for irradiation and surgery for various lip lesions, the lesions have been divided into three categories. Control of the carcinoma is the primary consideration. If control is equal by two methods, the one yielding the better cosmetic and functional results should be selected. These factors being equal, the most convenient method is preferred.

1. For the small, well-defined lesions that would require irradiation or excision of less than a third of the lip (usually 1 cm or less), cosmetic and functional results are acceptable by either method. Irradiation, although slightly more time-consuming, gives equal results, however.

2. For the somewhat larger lesions in which destruction of the lip is relatively small but in which excision would necessitate a more complicated plastic repair, radiotherapy is definitely preferred. Both functional and cosmetic results are more satisfactory if such a practice is followed. Most carcinomas of the lip will fall in this category.

3. For certain large, highly destructive lesions, control may be equally good by excision or by radiotherapy. Regardless of which treatment is used, if plastic repair will be required, excision may be preferable. Then the plastic repair need not be carried out in a heavily irradiated field. It should be emphasized that it is a rare lip cancer that falls into this category. Indeed it is surprising how well the healing process apparently restores the substance of the lip. Lampe (1959) illustrated this beautifully in his series of sixty-seven patients irradiated for cancers 3.5 cm or greater in one diameter or another. Residual defects in the lip were relatively small despite considerable pretreatment tissue destruction.

There will be exceptions to indications for treatment as just outlined. Well-planned irradiation will almost always produce better results than poorly planned surgery. On a given patient, if either modality has been tried and has failed, the other method is usually tried. Areas already irradiated to cancerocidal levels cannot generally tolerate vigorous reirradiation, whereas lips that have had an unsuccessful excision will almost always require plastic repair after a second excision. For this reason irradiation of gross or occult postsurgical persistence is recommended.

TECHNIQUE. The teeth and mandible immediately posterior to the lip lesion should be evaluated routinely. Bad teeth that might serve as a source of irritation should be repaired or extracted. Since it is usually possible to protect the teeth and gums and only rarely necessary to irradiate a significant portion of the mandible or salivary glands, the teeth and mandible are not in danger of being damaged. In addition to the malignant lesion of the lip, if there are atypical keratoses, these, too, should be included in the field of irradiation. We frequently include the entire vermilion border of the lower lip when degenerative changes are seen on both sides of the carcinoma. Lesions involving the oral commissure should be evaluated with particular care, for their extensions along the buccal mucosa are easy to miss.

Many techniques have been used for treating cancers of the lip. "Roentgentherapy has the greatest adaptability to the peculiarities of the given case."* With x-ray therapy, the size of the field, the degree of protraction and fractionation, and the quality of the beam can be easily tailored to fit the problem at hand. A 1 cm width of apparently normal margin should be included in the field if the palpable borders of the lesion are sharp. A wider margin should be allowed if the lesion is infiltrative with vague borders (Fig. 4-5). Associated degenerative epithelial changes should be included in the irradiated volume.

When the volume to be treated has been determined, a simple lead cutout will not only define the margins of the beam but will also shield the teeth and gums from the exit radiations (Fig. 4-6). Radiations generated at 100 to 150 kv filtered with 0.25 mm Cu plus 1 mm Al will be sufficient for irradiated ports 3 cm or less in length and 2 cm in breadth. With this energy lesions up to 1 cm thick are irradiated adequately. Larger lesions require 200 kv radiations. The optimum time-dose ·factors vary with the dimensions of the irradiated field. Areas of the order of 1.5 cm in diameter

---

*From del Regato, J. A.: Roentgen therapy of carcinoma of the lower lip, Radiology **51**:499-508, 1948.

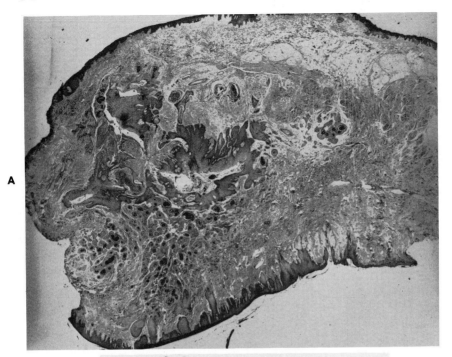

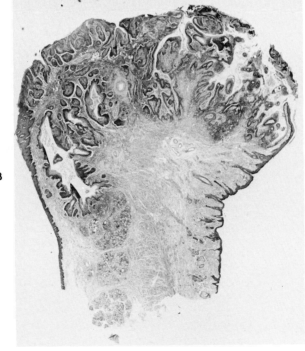

Fig. 4-5. A, Low-power photomicrograph revealing extensive infiltration in substance of the lip deep to a relatively small ulceration on the mucosa. Compare with **B,** well-differentiated squamous cell carcinoma of lower lip. Cancer involves the ducts of minor salivary glands with the formation of irregular cystic spaces. It remains well localized without extensive infiltration. (**A,** W. U. neg. 47-4764; courtesy Dr. L. V. Ackerman.)

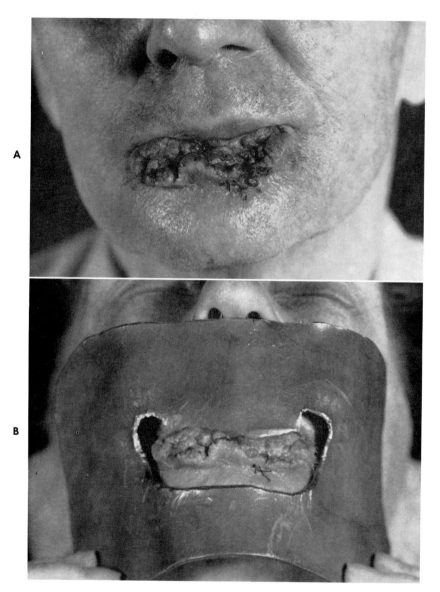

Fig. 4-6. A, Extensive deeply infiltrating carcinoma of lower lip extending from commissure to commissure and inferiorly to lower gingiva. **B,** Same patient with lead shield in place for irradiation. Note that central part of the lead is inserted between lip and lower gum to prevent unnecessary irradiation of intraoral structures. Special attention has been given to provide adequate margins in regions of the commissures. **C,** Same patient 8 months after treatment. He remained well over 5 years.

can be satisfactorily treated with 4000 rad (skin) in 10 days, although large lesions infiltrating the entire lower lip in thickness and breadth should be fractionated with doses of 5000 to 6000 rad (skin) in 4 to 6 weeks or more. Frequent cleansing and continuous petroleum jelly dressings assure prompt healing with a minimum of telangiectasia and fibrosis. The healed lip should be shielded from subsequent sunburn and tobacco irritation.

When possible, cervical lymph node metastases from carcinoma of the lip should be treated by radical neck dissection. The so-called prophylactic neck dissection performed in the absence of clinically suspicious nodes is not indicated in carcinoma of the lower lip (Lyall and Grier). Similarly, radiation therapy for occult metastases is not indicated. About 6% of the patients will have palpable nodes when first seen, and an equal number will develop metastases to the nodes subsequently. In either instance, radical neck dissection will control the metastatic disease in about 50% of the patients. When neck dissection is not advisable, or when it is refused, the patient should be evaluated for irradiation of the metastases. Such nodes can be controlled by irradiation. Irradiation in the treatment of squamous cell carcinoma metastatic to cervical lymph nodes is discussed later in this chapter.

RESULTS. As indicated previously, carcinoma of the lower lip is highly curable by both surgical and radiotherapeutic techniques. At least 80% can be controlled by either. Photographs of the before and after variety are often presented to illustrate the superiority of one or the other form of treatment. These selected results are naturally the better ones; the poor results are not likely to be publicized. Yet good aesthetic results can hardly be recorded by methods other than photography. Figs. 4-6 to 4-8 illustrate the before and after views of advanced lip lesions treated by roentgentherapy. The appearance is good and function is normal. In our experience,

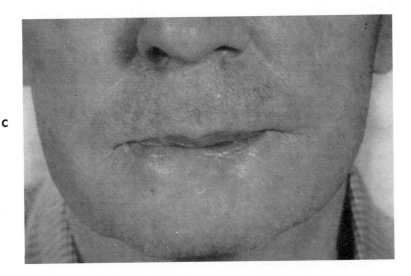

C

Fig. 4-6, cont'd. For legend see opposite page.

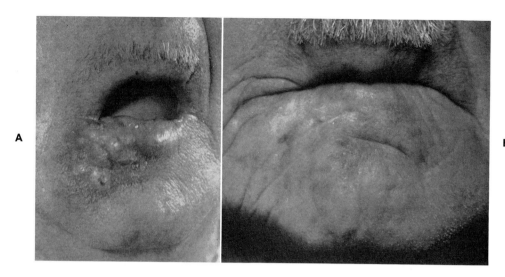

Fig. 4-7. A, Deeply infiltrating squamous cell carcinoma extending into substance of lip and chin. Patient was given 4800 rad through an 8 × 6 cm port over 24 days (280 kv; hvl, 2 mm Cu). **B,** Same patient 5 years later.

such results are the rule. Few lesions will recur after 3 years (Gladstone and Kerr; del Regato and Sala).

Lampe's results were cited previously. Hornback and Shidnia have also illustrated the excellent tissue-sparing potential of roentgentherapy in treating very advanced carcinomas of the lower lip. del Regato and Sala reported that of sixty-two cancers less than 2 cm in diameter and selected for roentgentherapy, there were no persistences with a minimum follow-up of 3 years. Of 129 cancers 2 to 12 cm in diameter and selected for roentgentherapy, twelve recurred. All persistent disease was subsequently controlled. Dick reported that of 287 patients selected for radiotherapy only five showed persistent cancer within 3 years. Good or very good cosmetic results were observed in 80%, fair results in 15%, and poor cosmetic results in only 5%. A comparison of these figures with surgical results obtained at the same institutions is not warranted because of the selection of cases for particular forms of treatment as outlined previously. However, of 1643 cases collected from the literature in which various means of treatment were used, the absolute 3-year control rate was 75% and the control rate in the determinate group was 83%. From life insurance tables, the expected 3-year survival in noncancerous patients of the same age group is 86% (Gladstone and Kerr). Thus it may be expected that less than 10% of these patients will actually die with their carcinoma uncontrolled (Krantz and associates).

SUMMARY. Carcinoma of the mucous membrane of the lower lip is highly curable by either irradiation or surgery. For limited lesions, surgery is as effective as irradiation, and cosmetic results obtained by surgery are acceptable. For moderately advanced cases, irradiation yields better cosmetic and functional results. For far-advanced cases in which bone is covered with cancer, or if massive postirradia-

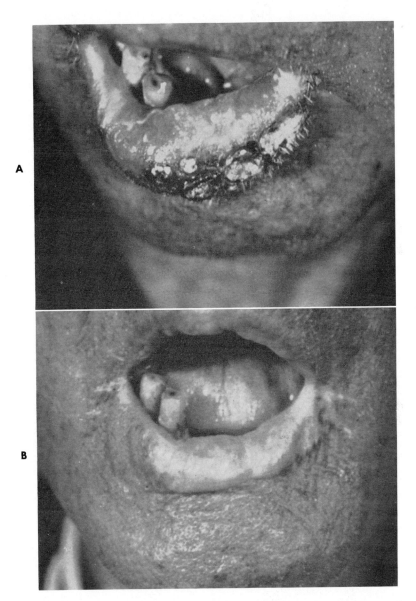

Fig. 4-8. A, Extensive squamous cell carcinoma of lower lip involving left commissure and extending inferiorly to gingiva. Patient was given 4700 rad in 30 days through a 6 × 2 cm port (100 kv filtered with 0.25 mm Cu and 1 mm Al). **B,** Same patient 3 years later, with satisfactory cosmetic and functional results.

tion plastic repair is anticipated, primary excision will not require the procedure to be carried out in heavily irradiated soft tissue. However, after irradiation, even very large cancers of the lower lip will usually heal and lead to good restoration of normal function with quite acceptable appearance. The optimum dose-time relationship for a given lesion will depend on its dimensions. Lymph node metastases should be treated by radical surgery when possible. If neck dissection is not possible and vigorous irradiation is warranted, some of these metastases can be controlled.

Carcinoma of the anterior two thirds of the tongue and the floor of the mouth

Carcinomas of the anterior two thirds of the tongue and the floor of the mouth have much in common. Their clinical courses and their treatments are similar, and very often both of these anatomic sites are involved even though the cancer may originate in only one site. Generally, the primary lesion is confined within the arch formed by the horizontal rami of the mandible. Infiltration of the musculature of the tongue and floor of the mouth occurs early (Fig. 4-9). However, swallowing and speaking are rarely affected until late in the course of the disease. Metastases to ipsilateral upper cervical nodes near the angle of the jaw and in the submaxillary region are common. Submental, posterior cervical, and lower cervical nodes are

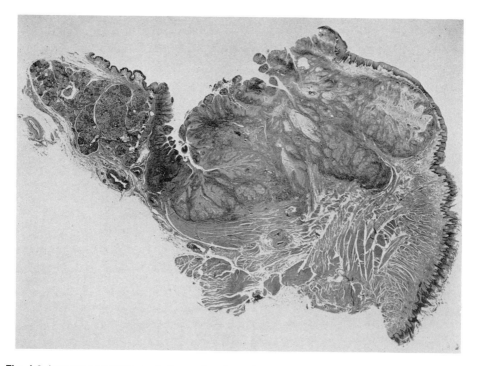

Fig. 4-9. Low-power enlargement of a section through a squamous cell carcinoma of lateral border of tongue showing deep infiltration between muscle bundles.

uncommon. Contralateral nodal involvement occurs about one tenth as often as ipsilateral nodal involvement. Palpable cervical metastases will be present in 35% to 40% of all patients when first seen, and an equal proportion will develop metastases subsequently.

Squamous cell carcinomas of the tongue and the floor of the mouth are not highly radioresponsive. However, the proliferative or exophytic lesions are usually more responsive than the infiltrative type. Histologic grading is of little value in helping one to decide the treatment of choice or, if irradiation is to be given, the technique. In any case, high doses of radiations are required for control of these lesions.

Verrucous carcinoma is a distinctive variant of epidermoid carcinoma predilecting the buccal mucosa, but also seen occasionally in the larynx and male and female external genitalia. A few cases have also been described in the uterine cervix. In a high percentage of cases the oral lesions are associated with tobacco chewing and poor oral hygiene. They invariably present as warty fungated masses of rather large size (2 to 10 cm) (Fig. 4-10). On section they are made up of bulbous papillary masses projecting from the surface epithelium with no great tendency to infiltrate the subjacent tissues (Fig. 4-11). Because of the lack of anaplasia and the orderly maturation of the epithelial cells of the tumor, the diagnosis is frequently missed until after several biopsies and the pathologist is made aware of the gross appearance of the lesion. The need for adequate, deep biopsies should be emphasized, for it is only at the base of the tumor that some degree of pleomorphism and, at times, tissue infiltration can be detected. Although the tumor seldom metastasizes, there have been several reports of anaplastic change and metastasis after radiotherapy for ver-

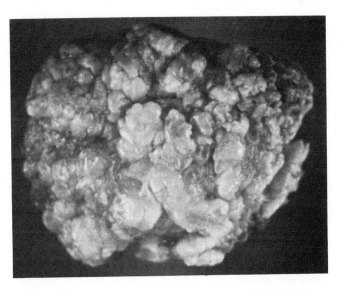

Fig. 4-10. Verrucous carcinoma excised from floor of mouth. Note bulbous papillary exophytic character of the growth.

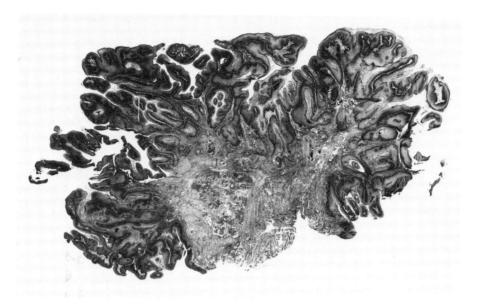

Fig. 4-11. Cross section through a verrucous carcinoma illustrating extreme exophytic nature of the papillary growths.

rucous carcinomas (Kraus and Perez-Mesa). The clinical staging is the same as given on p. 92.

TECHNIQUE. The treatment plan for cancers of the tongue and floor of the mouth depends on the following:

1. Microscopic diagnosis. Verrucous cancers respond poorly to radiotherapy and probably should be considered surgical problems from the beginning (Kraus and Perez-Mesa). Poorly differentiated cancers of the tongue and floor of the mouth will generally respond more dramatically to radiotherapy than will differentiated cancers.

2. Gross morphology. Exophytic lesions with well-delineated borders exhibit limited infiltration and usually require narrower borders than infiltrating lesions with vague borders.

3. Size of cancer and tissues invaded. Small lesions in selected patients are easily and successfully treated with peroral irradiation or interstitial techniques. Large cancers require external irradiation, either alone or in combination with interstitial irradiation (Fu and associates). When the gingiva is involved, the risk of jaw necrosis increases and cure rate decreases (Porter). These risks must be accepted or surgery must be considered.

4. Presence or absence of metastases to cervical lymph nodes. If adenopathy is present, neck dissection is usually recommended. However, there is good evidence that if the nodes are no larger than 2 cm, radiotherapy is equal to surgery in ability to control the metastases and it is much less demanding on the patient (Hanks and associates; Wizenberg and associates; Votava and associates). The irradiation of

neck nodes is discussed in detail at the end of this chapter. For patients with carcinoma of the tongue we recommend that neck dissection be performed when the adenopathy is greater than 2 cm maximum diameter but less than 6 cm and not fixed.

The problem in treating the primary cancer is one of homogeneously irradiating a volume of tissue between the horizontal rami of the mandible without irradiating the mandible excessively. The hazards of mandibular irradiation have been discussed previously. The necessary preirradiation precautions have also been discussed, and it is particularly important that those recommendations receive attention, since they apply to carcinoma of the tongue and floor of the mouth. Certain types of carcinomas of the tongue have been shown to respond poorly to irradiation. In this category are those rare carcinomas arising in syphilitic glossitis, lesions associated with more than minimal edema, lesions fixing the tongue to the mandible, and verrucous carcinomas. Since the advanced cancers of the tongue are also infrequently controlled by surgery, radiation therapy may render the best palliation. However, such patients should also be evaluated for resection.

A major prerequisite to proper planning of irradiation is a clear definition of tumor size and its relations to important neighboring structures. Often an ulcer that appears limited will be associated with an extensive infiltrating lesion. Not only the anteroposterior and lateral dimensions must be defined, but also proximity and fixation to the mandible. Bimanual palpation may reveal surprising inferior infiltration into submental tissues. There is no significant anatomic barrier to perineural extension or extension between the muscle planes.

The breadth of apparent normal tissue to be included in the adequately irradiated volume deserves special mention. If the irradiated margin is consistently excessive, the incidence of necrosis will be higher than necessary. Planned underdosage to reduce the incidence of necrosis leads to an increased persistence rate. An inadequate margin leads to marginal persistence. The fine line between these extremes is not easy to define. The guides to adequate margins vary with technique and characteristics of the cancer, and will be given in the following discussion.

PERORAL IRRADIATION. Peroral irradiation is highly useful for selected cancers. For small anterior lesions of the tongue, floor of the mouth, or gingiva, peroral roentgentherapy is as effective as any other method and far less traumatic than either interstitial sources or external irradiation (Fig. 4-17). High mandibular doses may be avoided, as are the pain and discomfort of an interstitial implant. Salivary glands are spared, and damage to remaining teeth is slight. Unfortunately, only a minority of lesions is sufficiently small for this excellent technique. An apparent margin of 1 cm around the lesion is essential. The patient must be sufficiently cooperative to remain in position. Malleable lead cones are much superior to the more common rigid cones. Such lead cones can be pressed into optimum shape and cut with shears for individualized positioning. A periscopic attachment assures accurate positioning and gives confidence with each setup. Tissue doses of 5500 to 6000 rad (200 kv radiations at short target-mucosa distance) in 4 weeks are well tolerated and are highly successful for these selected lesions. Lampe, a leading proponent of this technique, has recommended doses of 7000 to 7500 rad in 4 to 5 weeks (Fayos and Lampe, 1967). We believe this dose is high, however, and agree with Phillips that the lower dose decreases the rate of necrosis without seriously modifying the cure rate. Cancers selected for this technique will obviously be the smaller, favorably situated lesions. Doses somewhat higher than usual would therefore be tolerated, and high cure rates should be obtained. Griffin and associates selected eighteen patients with small superficially invasive cancers of the oral cavity for irradiation by this technique. Local control was obtained in 100% of the patients, and only one patient developed an easily excised necrosis.

Most carcinomas of the tongue and floor of the mouth will not fall into the category just described. The more advanced lesions that remain within the horizontal rami may be considered for either an interstitial implant alone or a combination of external irradiation plus an implant.

INTERSTITIAL SOURCES. Techniques making use of interstitial radium, radium substitute, or afterloading sources, evolved in three steps. Initially it seemed logical to space sources evenly throughout the volume of interest. Then, in a set of rules based on sound physical principles, Paterson and Parker defined patterns of insertion necessary to achieve the maximum practical homogeneity of dose. The original Paterson and Parker rules are published in Meredith's work on radium dosage. Cesium or afterloading of iridium 192 in amounts equivalent in intensity to the standard radium needles are now common. Finally, by computer-aided techniques the inhomogeneities of a given pattern can be defined. With this information, modifications of the Paterson and Parker rules have been recommended. The immediate postimplant dose distribution for every implant is now available as a guide to dosage (Fu and associates; Fletcher and Stovall).

A good implant starts with a meticulous evaluation of tumor size and position, together with specific plans for radioactive source size, number and arrangement. This must take place well before the patient has gone to the operating room. It will assure that proper sources are available. When radium is used, low-intensity needles (0.33 and 0.66 mg/cm length radium or its equivalent) should be arranged in the patterns recommended by Paterson and Parker. For special situations such as the sharply concaved planar implant and the very thin two-plane implant, modifications to improve dose distribution are advisable. The technical refinements of interstitial implants in the various sites within the oral cavity can be taught only through clinical contact and the analysis of individual computer printouts. Provisions should be made for uncrossed ends, optimum source length, and linear intensity for the volume in question. Facilities should be available for radiographs to be taken before the patient is moved from the operating table. Computer-aided dosimetry carried out before insertion of afterloading sources or while the sources are still in place defines hot and cold spots and assists in the decision relative to source removal (Fu and associates).

It is important to keep the volume of the implant as small as possible. Placement of sources 0.5 cm beyond the edge is a permissible extension of the volume if the lesion has sharp, easily palpated edges. However, 1 cm is permissible if the edges are vague and the lesion is deeply infiltrative. Sources should never be separated from each other by more than 1.5 cm. Since glossal edema may separate the sources, it is wise to insert sources at intervals of less than 1 cm. Once films taken in the operating room confirm a satisfactory implant, each radium source must be fixed in place. For afterloading sources this is simple. For needles, multicolor sutures are a help. A single-plane implant will suffice for superficial lesions of the borders of the tongue. A two-plane implant will be sufficient in 50% of the cases. For the remainder a volume implant will be necessary. Cobalt or cesium needles or iridium, yielding dose rates similar to low-intensity radium needles, produce identical results.

Most lesions of the floor of the mouth extend posteriorly to the junction of the tongue with the floor of the mouth. When this has occurred, an adequate posterior margin can be obtained only by inserting the sources through the dorsum of the tongue. Under these circumstances the entire implant should probably be made through the dorsum of the tongue. The tongue should be immobilized by suturing its tip to the gingiva.

The dose rate using low-intensity sources is such that a dose of 4500 to 7000 rad is delivered in 6 to 8 days. For small volumes (T1 lesions) a dose of 6000 rad in a week is usually satisfactory. For T2 lesions 6500 rad in a week seems adequate. Thus the larger lesions require higher doses; however, the larger volumes, especially if they include the floor of the mouth, do not tolerate the dose well. We seldom give doses greater than this with interstitial irradiation alone. Most T3 lesions will be irradiated initially with external irradiation. If this is to be supplemented with interstitial irradiation, the combined rad dose will be greater than 7000 rad.

Guides to time-dose-volume factors for interstitial therapy for cancer of the tongue have been critically reviewed by Fu and associates. All of their seven patients with T1 lesions had local control with implants that delivered at least 6000 rad. Only

Table 4-1. Relationship of incidence of necrosis to dose and volume for patients with carcinoma of the anterior two thirds of the tongue treated with interstitial radium implants alone or in combination with external irradiation*

Dose† (rad)	Incidence of necrosis (%) for various tumor volumes			
	V > 500 mm³	V > 750 mm³	V > 1000 mm³	V > 1500 mm³
>9000	11/55 (20.0%)	11/43 (25.6%)	11/43 (25.6%)	7/30 (23.3%)
>10,000	9/35 (25.7%)	7/23 (30.4%)	7/21 (33.3%)	4/10 (40.0%)
>11,000	8/24 (33.3%)	5/17 (29.4%)	4/13 (30.8%)	3/5 (60.0%)
>12,000	6/16 (37.5%)	4/12 (33.3%)	4/9 (44.4%)	2/3 (66.0%)
>13,000	4/10 (40.0%)	3/7 (42.9%)	3/4 (75.0%)	2/3 (66.0%)
>14,000	3/7 (42.9%)	3/4 (75.9%)	2/2 (100.0%)	
>15,000	3/4 (75.0%)	2/3 (66.7%)		

* Modified from Fu, K. K., Chan, E. K., Phillips, T. L., and Ray, J. W.: Radiology **119**:209-213, 1976.
† Dose = total dose from implant and external irradiation.

two of four were controlled if the dose was less than 6000 rad. Of eleven patients with T2 lesions, ten were controlled with implants that delivered at least 6000 rad. Only five of eleven were controlled if the dose was less than 6000 rad. It is clear from these data that selected small primary lesions (T1 and T2) can be controlled in a high proportion by interstitial implants. Dose levels must be modified in keeping with the volume of the tumor. There is no widespread agreement as to specific points or levels used to express dose. This problem has been emphasized by Fu and associates. We agree with them that for purposes of assessing cancer control one should select the *minimum* dose within the tumor volume by reviewing isodose curves through several levels of the implanted volume. One should be aware of this in the systematic application of their recommendations.

The incidence of necrosis of the tongue increases with dose (most likely it correlates closely with maximum dose rather than minimum dose in volume) and with the irradiated volume. This is demonstrated by Table 4-1.

Lesions of the floor of the mouth present many of the same problems as lesions of the mobile tongue. Because of their proximity to the mandible there is greater risk of bone necrosis than for lesions of the tongue. For T1 lesions radiation therapy usually consists of interstitial sources with doses of the same level as for the tongue. T2 lesions are usually given combined external irradiation and interstitial sources. Control of T3 lesions is poor with irradiation alone but good with preoperative irradiation and resection (Table 4-2). Insufficient dose is the most common cause of failure. Just as for lesions of the tongue, dose must be increased in keeping with the volume of the cancerous mass.

The patient can be administered a broad-spectrum antibiotic during the time of the implant, although we have not done this routinely. Liquid diet is usually well tolerated. Frequent mouthwash with half-strength hydrogen peroxide and cleansing with cotton applicators are important. Codeine is generally sufficient to control pain.

EXTERNAL IRRADIATION. When external irradiation is used in a curative effort, it is generally supplemented with interstitial or peroral irradiation or a boosting dose through reduced ports. External irradiation is used alone for the more extensive cancers of the tongue (T3) and floor of the mouth (T3). The technique must be tailored to reduce the normal tissue damage to a minimum. Parallel opposing ports with 30° wedges are satisfactory for extensive lesions of the floor of the mouth and mobile tongue. Lateral and anterior beams with 45° wedge filters are suitable for unilateral cancers in the oral cavity. This technique spares the contralateral mandible and salivary glands. When, for the more extensive cancers, external irradiation is the sole treatment method, 6500 rad in 6 weeks or its equivalent is the minimum dose. Split-dose techniques are valuable in decreasing the severity of the acute reaction in many of these aged debilitated patients with extensive cancers. The radiobiologic justification for the split-dose technique was discussed in Chapter 1. An initial dose of 4000 to 4500 rad in 4 weeks is used. Then after a 2-week interval of no irradiation an additional dose of 3000 to 3500 rad in 2 weeks through reduced ports is given. This technique or modifications of it has been widely used (Montana

Table 4-2. Control of cancer of the floor of mouth 2 years after various treatment modalities*

	Treatment modality						Salvage by		Ultimate control rate	
Stage	External radiotherapy	External radiotherapy + surgery	External radiotherapy + implant	External radiotherapy + cone	Cone	Surgery	Surgery	External radiotherapy	Number	Percent
T1 N0	19/23	1/1	0/1	3/4	7/9	11/13	4	1	46/51	90
T2 N0	18/28	2/2	2/3	0	0	8/9	4	0	34/42	81
T3 N0	2/7	4/4	0	1/1	0	0	1	0	8/12	67
T1 N1-3	0/2	0/1	0	0	0	1/2	1	0	2/5	40
T2 N1-3	3/11	3/3	1/1	0	0	2/2	2	0	11/17	65
T3 N1-3	4/21	2/2†	0/2	1/1	0	0	2	0	9/26	35
TOTAL	46/92	12/13	3/7	5/6	7/9	22/26	14	1	110/153	72

*Modified from Fu, K. K., Lichter, A., and Galante, M.: Int. J. Radiat. Oncol. Biol. Phys. **1**:829-837, 1976.

†One patient received methotrexate concurrently with external radiotherapy.

and associates) and in our opinion is the radiation technique of choice for extensive yet potentially curable carcinomas of the mobile tongue and floor of the mouth when an implant is inadvisable.

COMBINED EXTERNAL IRRADIATION AND INTERSTITIAL IRRADIATION. Although external irradiation permits a more homogeneous distribution of dose than does interstitial therapy, the mandible is invariably irradiated by the external irradiation. The dose to a segment of the mandible is about the same as that delivered to the cancer, and mandibular necrosis is feared when high doses are necessary. Interstitial irradiation produces a dose distribution that is highly variable. Indeed, the variation of dose within an ideal implant is much greater than would be accepted in external beam techniques. However, the very physical characteristics of an implant, which account for its nonhomogeneous distribution of dose, enable one to irradiate these carcinomas without delivering high doses to the mandible. The combined technique provides the maximum homogeneity permitted by the limitations of the mandible. Although the final distribution of dose is not as homogeneous as would be delivered by external irradiation alone, it does not vary to the extent of an inter-

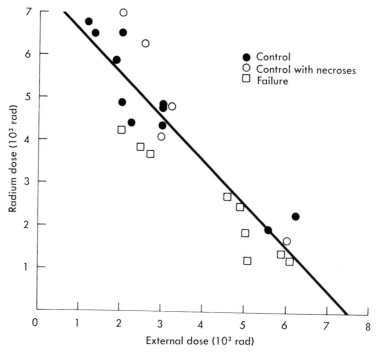

Fig. 4-12. Scattergram of local control and failures of T1, T2, and T3 lesions of the anterior two thirds of the tongue treated by combined external irradiation and interstitial implants. The larger tumor masses were generally given higher doses with external beams and less with interstitial sources. The smaller masses were given a large proportion of their dose with interstitial sources. The diminished control rate at right end of curve is expected in view of the high proportion of advanced lesions. (From Fu, K. K., Chan, E. K., Phillips, T. L., and Ray, W.: Radiology **119**:209-213, 1976.)

stitial implant alone. The different distributions of doses in these two techniques justify their use in combinations varying with the size of the primary cancer, that is, an occasional T1 lesion, about one third of the T2 lesions, and most T3 lesions. External irradiation is usually given first. For limited lesions, as little as 2000 to 2500 rad given by external irradiation is followed by giving 5000 to 7000 rad with an implant. For more extensive cancers 5000 rad given by external irradiation is followed by giving about 3000 to 3500 rad with an implant. An effort to balance the combination of these two modalities is illustrated in Fig. 4-12. Gross changes produced are shown in Fig. 4-13.

We have favored a combination of the two techniques if there is any uncertainty regarding the interstitial implant and for most larger lesions still confined within the mandibular arch (Fig. 4-14). Chu and Fletcher have emphasized the importance of such combinations in controlling primary cancers of the anterior part of the oral cavity.

It is to be expected that a higher incidence of necrosis and failure will be associated with external irradiation whether used alone or combined with interstitial sources. The reason for this is that *small* lesions are best irradiated with interstitial sources alone. Not only is the volume small, but the dose need not be high. Large lesions require external irradiation either alone or combined with interstitial sources.

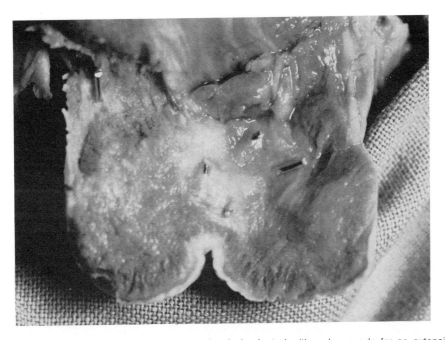

Fig. 4-13. Gross specimen of a tongue previously implanted with radon seeds for an extensive squamous cell carcinoma; 1 mc seeds were placed an estimated 1 cm apart in the involved volume. Note that the seeds are surrounded by areas of extensive fibrosis. (W. U. neg. 51-4253; courtesy Dr. L. V. Ackerman.)

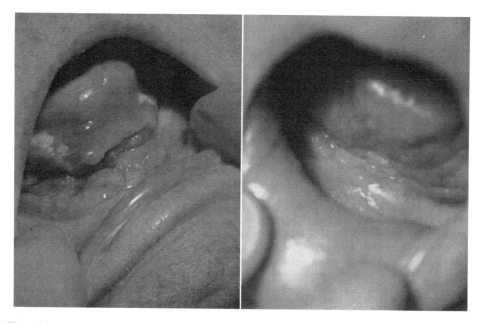

Fig. 4-14. Advanced squamous cell carcinoma of floor of mouth irradiated by a combination of external telecobalt (4000 rad in 4 weeks) followed by an interstitial volume implant through the tongue (3500 rad). Patient remained free of disease over 5 years.

The volume is large and the dose is justifiably high. A higher proportion of complications cannot be avoided (Table 4-1).

INDICATIONS FOR SURGERY AND IRRADIATION. The frequently encountered decision to resect large volumes in this area with no serious consideration for the contribution of modern radiotherapy may end with defects that might have been avoided. Radiotherapy, when successful, does spare soft tissues and bone at this important site. Function and appearance remain nearly normal. The risk of post-irradiation bone and soft tissue necrosis exists, but megavoltage techniques, together with wider use of wedged beams and controlled dosimetry in the use of interstitial sources, have reduced the risks of sequelae. We know which patients are most likely to develop postirradiation sequelae and which patients are less likely to be cured by irradiation. Unfortunately, these are generally patients with advanced cancer in whom resection is also less successful. Certainly for the lesions not involving the gingiva or mandible, when the tongue is not particularly edematous and syphilitic glossitis is not present, irradiation should be considered first.

Surgery is considered the treatment of choice in cancer of the tongue in patients with syphilitic glossitis. Such lesions respond poorly to radiotherapy. Surgery is also the treatment of choice in patients in whom the cancer is attached to the mandible or has extended into the gingival mucosa, since adequate irradiation will deliver a high dose to the mandible, and we believe such patients will likely develop mandibular necrosis. The third group of patients, those with even moderate edema of the tongue, will probably do equally poorly by either irradiation or surgery. When one accepts only advanced inoperable cancers of the tongue and floor of the mouth for high-dose irradiation, necrosis will be the rule and cure will be infrequent. Guides for treating the more limited lesions must not be based on such a disappointing experience.

Planned preoperative irradiation of cancers of the tongue and floor of the mouth has been reserved for the more advanced stages. No one has yet reported the results of its systematic use. However, Buschke and Galante as well as Benak and associates have shown that vigorous preoperative irradiation is feasible. They have given doses of 5000 to 6500 rad in 5 to 6 weeks and then surgery in 1 to 5 months, which has been well tolerated. This technique has recently been recommended by Fu and associates for T3 lesions. The rationale for this combination was presented in Chapter 2. When radical surgery has been the primary treatment for an advanced lesion and cancer has been left behind, postoperative irradiation of the primary site is often poorly tolerated, but is occasionally curative.

An occasional patient will have an "excision biopsy" of a carcinoma of the tongue or floor of the mouth. The margins of excision may be questionably adequate or obviously inadequate. In these circumstances treatment should not be delayed until there is clinical recurrence. Irradiation given soon after such an excision is almost uniformly successful in preventing recurrence. Of twenty-three such patients treated with interstitial radium (5500 to 6000 rad), all had local control and the incidence of complication was small (Ange and associates). For such patients elective irradiation of the clinically negative cervical lymph nodes is not usually indicated unless prior to surgery the original primary lesion was particularly infiltrative or measured 2 cm or more.

Metastases to cervical lymph nodes from lesions of the tongue or floor of the mouth should generally be treated by radical neck dissection. There is no longer any question about the ability of external irradiation to control metastases to cervical lymph nodes. Indeed there is some evidence that when the primary site is irradiated, simultaneous irradiation of the cervical nodes is as effective as surgery (Hanks and associates; Wizenberg and associates). There is also evidence that, at least for some sites, cure rates are doubled if vigorous postoperative cervical irradiation is given to those patients who, on radical neck dissection, are found to have several nodes involved (Lindberg and Jesse).

In our institution radical neck dissection is done only if nodes are clinically involved. For this reason radical neck dissection is frequently followed by postoperative irradiation of that side and elective irradiation of the contralateral side. If there are no clinically involved nodes when the patient is first seen, systemic elective irradiation is given to both lateral cervical lymph node chains. Details of this technique are discussed later in the chapter.

REACTIONS AFTER IRRADIATION OF THE TONGUE AND FLOOR OF THE MOUTH. Early reactions are similar to acute mucosal reactions seen in other sites. If the dose is given rapidly, a false membrane will be seen within the first week of treatment. The sequence of false membrane development in various anatomic sites has been given previously in this chapter. Although it has been possible to complete curative irradiation of cancer of the larynx without producing a false membrane (Baclesse; Buschke and associates), such has not been the case with cancer of the oral cavity. An intense false membrane near the end of irradiation is unavoidable. The saliva becomes thick and sticky soon after therapy starts. Swallowing is then painful and mechanically difficult. Special efforts to maintain nutrition are important during this period. Occasionally during treatment a patient will develop a mycotic infection of the mucosa. If not treated promptly with appropriate antibiotics, the combined trauma of irradiation and infection results in extreme mucosal reactions at a much lower dose than would have followed irradiation alone.

Late sequelae are less frequent than acute reactions but more serious. The major late complications of irradiation of the oral cavity are primarily related to the limited radiation tolerance of the mandible and soft tissues of the floor of the mouth. The tolerance of the mandible varies rather widely and, with certain exceptions, it is difficult to predict. If the cancer is extensive and adjacent to or invading the mandible, chances of necrosis after curative irradiation are high (about 70%). If the cancer is small and separated from the mandible by 0.5 cm or more, the chances of necrosis are greatly reduced. At first glance, modality of irradiation also appears related to the incidence of necrosis. We have never seen mandibular necrosis in a patient treated by peroral roentgentherapy alone. Interstitial irradiation alone is followed by fewer sequelae than the combination of interstitial irradiation and external irradiation. It should be emphasized that these various techniques actually reflect the stage of advancement. The more limited lesions are irradiated by peroral techniques, and the more advanced lesions are irradiated by a combination of techniques. The first does not require mandibular irradiation, whereas in the latter it cannot be avoided. One cannot therefore incriminate any specific technique without further qualification. It is rather the magnitude of the volume combined with the high dose.

As in other anatomic sites, the incidence of mucosal and soft tissue necrosis is greater the larger the treated volume and the higher the dose. The interval between irradiation and necrosis varies from a few months to several years. It is definitely more common in alcoholics and heavy smokers and after continued irritation from poorly fitting dentures. Such necrosis develops primarily as a result of the radiation-induced injury of the epithelium and underlying blood vessels. There is reduced ability of the thinned epithelium to recover from postirradiation injury. It lacks the normal response of cellular repair and replacement. In the submucosal tissue reparative fibrosis and restriction of the vascular bed compound the defect. Time of recovery from soft tissue necrosis varies from months to years. Energetic support of nutrition, strict avoidance of all irritants, and meticulous oral hygiene promote recovery. Of course, persistence of cancer must be decided by biopsy. Measures that will reduce the incidence of mandibular necrosis were discussed on p. 90. They are particularly applicable for the irradiation of cancers of the tongue and floor of the mouth.

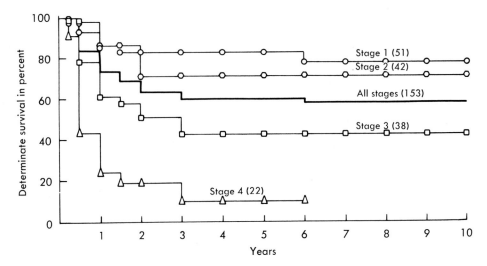

Fig. 4-15. Determinate survival rate by clinical stage of patients treated for cancer of floor of mouth. Initial treatment was irradiation alone in 114, surgery alone in twenty-six, and a combination in thirteen. Irradiation techniques included external beam alone in ninety-six, external beam combined with interstitial sources in seven, peroral cone alone in nine, and peroral cone combined with external beam in six. (From Fu, K. K., Lichter, A., and Galante, M.: Int. J. Radiat. Oncol. Biol. Phys. **1**:829-837, 1976.)

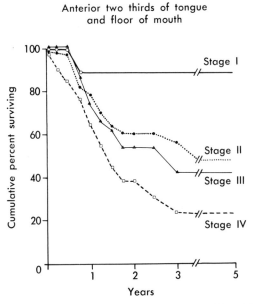

Fig. 4-16. Curves of survival rates for carcinoma of mobile tongue and floor of mouth at intervals after radiotherapy. Staging used is similar to that of the M. D. Anderson Hospital. Treatment methods employed were similar to those previously described. (Modified from Montana, G. S., Hellman, S., von Essen, C. F., and Kligerman, M. M.: Cancer **23**:1284-1289, 1969.)

Bothersome but less serious sequelae include dryness due to ablation of the salivary glands, edema, fibrosis similar to that following high-dose irradiation of any tissue, and finally atrophy and telangiectasia of mucosa. As mentioned on p. 87, artificial saliva is of great benefit in alleviating the symptoms related to a dry mouth.

PROGNOSIS AND RESULTS. The results of several recently reported series have been given in Tables 4-1 and 4-2. With the more precise definition of dose required for the various tumor sizes and the more precise delineation of the limitation of radiation therapy alone for these lesions, control rates have improved and will continue to improve. The currently available survival rates for cancer of the tongue and for the floor of the mouth are shown in Figs. 4-15 and 4-16.

Carcinoma of the base of the tongue

The base of the tongue is defined as that portion posterior to the circumvallate papillae. It forms the anterior wall of the vallecula and, in contrast to the anterior two thirds of the tongue, has limited mobility. Its lymph drainage goes almost directly lateral to upper cervical nodes (subdigastric). Bilateral metastases to lymph nodes are common.

Along with carcinomas of the nasopharynx and piriform sinus, carcinoma of the base of the tongue is frequently asymptomatic and is diagnosed after the metastases have made their appearance. Treatment is therefore usually given late in the course of the disease. Carcinoma of the base of the tongue infiltrates deeply into the substance of the tongue and may invade the glossopharyngeal sulcus and the lateral wall of the pharynx. Extension over the medial surface of the mandible is associated with a worse prognosis and increased incidence of postirradiation mandibular necrosis (Spanos and associates). Also the extension may progress anteriorly into the deep muscles of the anterior two thirds of the tongue (Fig. 4-17). However, it is to be differentiated from lesions arising in these sites. The lesion may be exophytic and readily visible or barely visible and detected only by palpation. Assessment of size and extent is accomplished by visualization and palpation. However, depth of infiltration into the tongue is difficult to assess accurately.

Cervical lymphadenopathy will be present in about 90% of all patients and will be bilateral in about 50% (Marcial). Despite the fact that this lesion often seems limited to the base of the tongue and upper cervical nodes, control by irradiation requires a high dose. Surgical excision of the base of the tongue is always associated with serious difficulties in swallowing and speech. Therefore, control by radiation therapy is of great practical importance.

TECHNIQUE. The volume to be irradiated is best determined by palpation of the base of the tongue and the cervical adenopathy. The primary lesion and the usual metastases can be included in parallel opposing lateral ports. A boosting dose with a 20 mev electron beam anteriorly may be useful (Spanos and associates). We have usually treated the cervical nodes with additional radiations through anterior and posterior tangential ports as described later in this chapter in the discussion of irradiation in the treatment of squamous cell carcinoma metastatic to cervical lymph

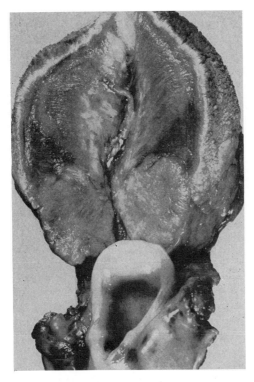

Fig. 4-17. Gross photograph of undifferentiated squamous cell carcinoma of base of tongue. (W. U. neg. 50-371; from Ackerman, L. V., and Rosai, J.: Surgical pathology, ed. 5, St. Louis, 1974, The C. V. Mosby Co.)

nodes. The time-dose-volume relationships related to the local control of these lesions have been analyzed by Spanos and associates. Their conclusions may be summarized as follows. Primary lesions 2 cm or less in diameter (T1) are controlled in more than 90% of patients given doses of 6000 rad in 6 weeks to 6500 rad in 6½ weeks. Lesions over 2 cm in diameter but not massive (T2 and T3) are controlled more than 80% of the time by a dose of 7500 rad in 7½ weeks. As expected, the incidence of complications (mandibular necrosis) increases the higher the dose and the larger the cancerous mass. The doses required to control lesions of the base of the tongue are somewhat higher than the dose required to control lesions of similar size in the glossopalatine sulcus. Our experience, like that of Dalley, has been that a good implant in most of the lesions of the base of the tongue is next to impossible. The sources that irradiate the posteroinferior margin of the tumor must be placed and sutured in the vallecula. The correct placement and crossing of such sources are usually unsatisfactory. Excision of persistent cancer is at times worthwhile (Ballantyne and Fletcher), but routine postirradiation excision of either the primary lesion or the nodes has not seemed necessary otherwise (Hanks and associates). Million and associates have emphasized the importance of irradiating the lower cervical

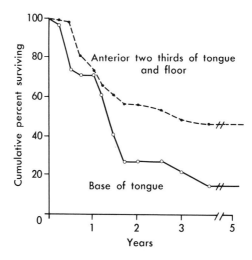

Fig. 4-18. Comparison of prognosis for carcinoma of anterior two thirds of tongue and floor of mouth with carcinoma of base of tongue. Techniques for therapy were similar to those previously described. (Modified from Montana, G. S., Hellman, S., von Essen, C. F., and Kligerman, M. M.: Cancer **23:**1284-1289, 1969.)

Table 4-3. Control of primary carcinoma of the base of the tongue according to "T" category*

"T" category	Number of patients	Primary controlled 2 years		Failure at primary	Died of other causes
		Number	Percent		
T1	32	23	71	3 (9%)	6
T2	49	23	47	14 (29%)	12
T3	64	33	51	14 (22%)	17
T4	29	6	21	14 (48%)	9

*Modified from Spanos, W. T., Shukovsky, L. J., and Fletcher, G. H.: Cancer **37:**2591-2599, 1976.

region, even in the absence of clinically positive lymph node metastases. This is now standard procedure for all patients with carcinoma of the base of the tongue.

PROGNOSIS AND RESULTS. It is often difficult to ascertain the site of lesions grouped under the heading of cancers of the base of the tongue. There are few recent series of patients treated by irradiation alone. Spanos and associates' results are shown in Table 4-3.

Fig. 4-18 compares the survival of patients with carcinoma of the anterior two thirds of the tongue with the survival of those with carcinoma of the base of the tongue. Table 4-3 gives the rate of controlling the primary lesions of various sizes.

Cure rates are good for limited lesions, but most lesions of this site are advanced when diagnosed.

Carcinoma of the lower gingiva

Patients with carcinoma of the lower gingiva will usually seek the advice of a dentist first. Patients may conclude that the ulcerated lesion is due to a defect in dentures, whereas other patients may suspect an infection of the gingiva. Thus the dentist plays a vital role in the early diagnosis of these lesions. Like lesions of other sites in the oral cavity, carcinoma of the lower gingiva may or may not arise in an area of leukoplakia. Although leukoplakia seems to be associated with multiple primary lesions, it is of no prognostic value otherwise and probably plays only an infrequent role in determining the type of treatment. We recognize two major clinical types of carcinoma of the lower gingiva. The verrucous type is strikingly exophytic, invades late, and metastasizes rarely (Kraus and Perez-Mesa). Much more commonly seen in the type that infiltrates and metastasizes frequently and that clinically may appear either exophytic and ulcerated or flat and infiltrating. The proximity of bone assures frequent osseous attachment, although invasion does not occur as often as one might expect. Even in those patients in whom bone invasion is not suspected clinically or is not demonstrable radiographically, the underlying bone must be treated as if it were involved. Of thirty-six surgically treated patients with carcinoma of the lower gingiva or buccal mucosa, 50% showed mandibular invasion (Modlin and Johnson; Swearingen and associates). Cervical lymph node metastases also appear frequently. Of 275 patients, 65% developed metastases. Most of these metastases will be to the submaxillary nodes or the upper cervical nodes near the angle of the jaw.

From the summary just given, it is obvious that a successful plan of treatment must include treatment of the underlying mandible and usually cervical lymph node metastases. A surgical approach means the loss of a segment of mandible plus an in continuity neck dissection. With a radiotherapeutic approach one must accept the relatively high risk of osteonecrosis with its associated pain and bone loss, plus a separately performed neck dissection if node metastases are suspected.

The factors related to mandibular necrosis have been discussed previously and should be reviewed in considering the treatment of these lesions. The infiltration and destruction of alveolar mucosa by tumor increase the risk of postirradiation mandible exposure. In our experience, if the lesion is deeply ulcerating and is more than 3 cm in palpable length, postirradiation mandibular exposure is almost a certainty. By contrast, papillary-like growths may be irradiated with much less risk of bone exposure and bone necrosis (Fig. 4-19). The mandibular complications may vary from an intermittent tenderness over the bone to an extensive osteonecrosis, depending on the irradiated volume and the technique and factors employed. We believe it is here that fractionation of a good quality of radiations is of particular importance in reducing the incidence and severity of this complication. It is this complication coupled with the frequent necessity of a neck dissection that accounts for the general acceptance of surgery for lesions of the lower gingiva. Because of the frequent complications that follow cancerocidal doses of radiations to large volumes in this region, we believe large lesions of the lower gingiva are best handled by

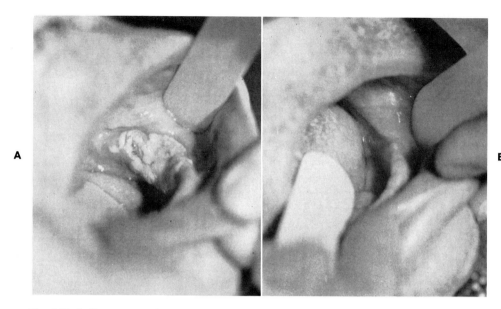

Fig. 4-19. A, Squamous cell carcinoma of lower gingiva. There was attachment to mandible but no evidence of bone invasion on radiograph. **B,** Same patient 4 years after peroral irradiation. Patient was given 6000 rad in 30 days through a 4 cm peroral cone (280 kv; hvl, 1 mm Cu).

surgery. This is not meant to imply that they cannot be controlled by irradiation but rather that surgery is probably less demanding on the patient. For lesions smaller than 3 cm and when no neck dissection is contemplated, we have preferred irradiation. Lampe has shown what can be accomplished by irradiating both limited and advanced lesions.

TECHNIQUE. When irradiation has been selected as the treatment of choice, pretreatment dental evaluation is essential, as mentioned before. The ideal technique would deliver a homogeneous dose to the diseased gingiva and that portion of the mandible suspected of being involved while sparing uninvolved tissues. An adequate interstitial implant is usually impossible because of the bone. The choice then lies between an external irradiation procedure, peroral roentgentherapy, or a mold technique. For larger infiltrating lesions, either of the latter two procedures is completely inadequate, and if radiotherapy is to be used, the only hope lies in external megavoltage irradiation, using wedge filters when possible.

Either peroral roentgentherapy or a radium mold can be used for small lesions of the anterior two thirds of the gingiva. For these we have preferred peroral roentgentherapy using radiations produced at 220 kv filtered with 0.5 mm Cu and 1 mm Al and a target–end of cone distance of 45 cm. A periscopic viewing mechanism is essential for proper placement of malleable lead cones. We have preferred an average surface dose of 5000 rad in 21 days when the cone tip was no greater than 4 cm in diameter (Fig. 4-19). Griffin and associates have also found this technique highly effective for selected small lesions.

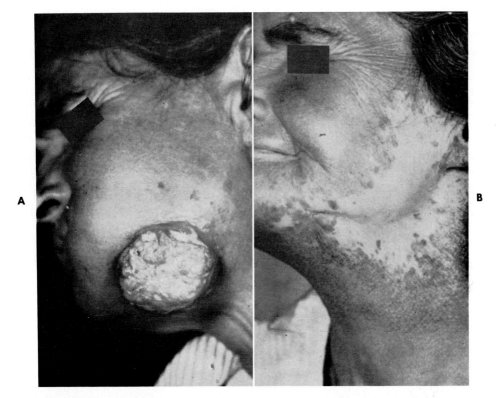

Fig. 4-20. A, Extensive low-grade squamous cell carcinoma of lower gingiva and buccal mucosa in patient who had used snuff for nearly 40 years. Lesion had destroyed almost entire width of lower jaw and had ulcerated by direct extension as shown. Irradiation was given through a direct lateral port measuring 12 × 10 cm with a skin dose of 6200 rad in 57 days. Supplementary irradiation was given during same period through an anterior port measuring 7 × 8 cm, with a skin dose of 4200 rad. Calculated minimum tissue dose was 5700 rad in 57 days (220 kv; hvl, 2 mm Cu; TSD, 50). **B,** Same patient 1 year later. The patient remained well for at least 2 years, during which time her lower jaw fractured spontaneously. This was asymptomatic.

As indicated previously, external irradiation is essential for the more advanced lesions. It has the undesirable feature of damaging a rather large segment of normal tissues both superficial and deep to the lesion. Also, a large portion of the mandible is unavoidably included. However, when large volumes are involved by more extensive lesions, adequate irradiation is not possible by any other technique. The rationale of following external irradiation with peroral irradiation to the center of the mass presumes that the center is less sensitive than the periphery and therefore requires a higher dose. Lampe's good figures would seem to support the use of such a combination. When the residual cancer cannot be encompassed with a peroral cone (as is usually the case), boosting doses through reduced external ports should be given.

For most larger cancers ^{60}Co or megavoltage radiations giving a tissue dose of 6500 rad in 6 to 7 weeks has been the maximum. Wedge filters should be used when the lesion involves less than half the floor of the mouth or the tongue. After this dose, control will be obtained in some patients, and high-dose sequelae will appear in some.

PROGNOSIS AND RESULTS. The method of selection practiced in the past makes it impossible to compare irradiation and surgery in the treatment of carcinoma of the lower gingiva. As stated previously, we believe surgery is probably the treatment of choice in most patients, but irradiation appears equally effective in patients with less advanced lesions. Some patients with advanced inoperable lesions have shown remarkable regression and even control (Fig. 4-20). Lampe reported that eleven of thirty-three patients irradiated were living 3 years or longer. Of these eleven, five showed radiographic evidence of bone invasion. Survival figures on patients who were free of cancer 5 years after treatment are shown in Table 4-4 and Fig. 4-21. Most recent reports have grouped surgically treated patients with irradiated patients, making an evaluation of irradiation alone impossible.

Table 4-4. Results obtained by irradiating carcinoma of the lower gingiva*

Author	Years included	Number of patients treated	Dead intercurrent disease	Lost	5-year control
Lampe	1940-1951	27	3	0	Corrected 8 (33.4%)
Fletcher†	1948-1962	120			Living 5 years (47%)

*Modified from Lampe, I.: Am. J. Roentgenol. **73:**628, 1955.
†Surgery performed in some patients.

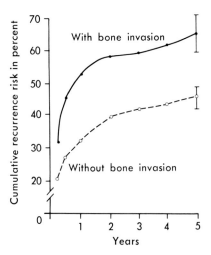

Fig. 4-21. Cumulative recurrence risks for patients irradiated for carcinoma of the gingiva (180 patients without bone invasion compared with seventy-one patients with bone invasion). Most patients were treated with megavoltage techniques. (Modified from Porter, E. H.: Clin. Radiol. **22:**139-143, 1971.)

Carcinoma of the hard palate and upper gingiva

From several aspects it is important to consider carcinoma of the upper gingiva and hard palate separately from carcinoma of the buccal mucosa and maxillary antrum.

1. Carcinomas of the hard palate and gingiva are generally better differentiated and spread more slowly than carcinoma of the antrum. The usual case of carcinoma of the upper gingiva or hard palate is diagnosed earlier, and the prognosis is better than for antral malignancy. Lesions of the upper gingiva and hard palate are preferably treated with surgery, whereas control of some antral lesions is accomplished with irradiation.

2. Although carcinomas of the upper gingiva and hard palate behave clinically like carcinomas of the buccal mucosa, they are closely related to bone. This alters the part irradiation plays in their treatment.

Surgical removal of a portion of the upper jaw is less deforming than surgery of the opposing segment of the lower jaw. A carefully fitted upper plate with an appropriate obturator is usually well tolerated and functions well. Irradiation of the upper gingiva or hard palate is followed by the same sequelae as irradiation of the lower gingiva. For these reasons surgery is usually given preference as the primary treatment. When for one reason or another a lesion is to be irradiated, we have used the same techniques and doses as described for carcinoma of the lower gingiva.

Any attempt to quote survival rates obtained by radiotherapy is meaningless in view of the scarcity of these cases.

LYMPHOMAS OF THE ORAL CAVITY

Lymphomas may arise in apparent extranodal lymphoid tissue in the buccogingival sulcus, gingiva, cheek, or similar tissues. These tumors are frequently large, but infrequently metastasize to cervical lymph nodes (Wang). If cervical lymphadenopathy is present, work-up is that of the usual non-Hodgkins lymphoma. If no cervical adenopathy is present, treatment should be given through large portals, and the total dose should reach 5000 rad in 5 weeks or its equivalent. We have favored irradiation of both cervical node chains even in the absence of lymphadenopathy. If no cervical nodes are present, the long-term disease-free survival rate will be about 70%. If cervical adenopathy is present the rate will be about 30% (Wang).

CARCINOMA OF THE TONSIL, PALATE, PALATINE ARCH, AND RETROMOLAR AREA

For this anatomic area the definition of site of origin is straightforward for limited cancers. However, the more advanced cancers often involve several sites, and it may be impossible to specify site of origin of the primary cancer. For this reason cancers of the faucial arch, retromolar trigone, and tonsillar fossa are frequently grouped together. Fletcher has analyzed the behavior and radiation response of cancers of these various anatomic sites. The radiotherapeutic management should be tailored to the clinical behavior if maximum control rates and minimum sequelae are to be obtained. In the discussion to follow we have used the irradiation of carcinoma of the tonsil as a model. Differences between carcinoma of the tonsil and carcinomas of the anterior pillar, retromolar trigone, and faucial arch are summarized at the end of this section.

Response of the normal tonsil to irradiation

The tonsils consist of bilateral, oval clumps of lymphoid tissue encased between the anterior and posterior pillars of the soft palate. They are covered by stratified squamous epithelium that invaginates into the fifteen or twenty crypts over the medial surface of the lymphoid tissue. In their superficial position the tonsils are subjected to frequent infections, some of which are secondary to inspissated debris in the crypts. The tonsils are normally large in children and begin their involution about puberty. Similar tissue is found at the base of the tongue and at the roof and lateral walls of the nasopharynx.

The lymphoid tissue at these sites responds to radiations as does similar tissue elsewhere. Doses as low as 200 to 300 rad produce massive death of the proliferating lymphocytes, and the organ shrinks. Use has been made of this fact in the treatment of chronically hypertrophied lymphoid tissue, particularly that near the eustachian tube orifices. The early abuse of this technique for hypertrophied lymphoid tissue in children contributed to the incidence of cancer of the thyroid. This fact plus the effectiveness of antibiotics has almost eliminated this need for radiations.

Carcinoma of the tonsil

Carcinoma of the tonsil comprises about two thirds of all malignant tumors of the tonsil. This lesion arises from the squamous epithelium, not the lymphoid tissue. Most of the carcinomas are undifferentiated and are usually exophytic and ulcerated. The lesion is only rarely confined to the tonsillar fossa; it will usually involve the anterior and posterior pillars. The anterior pillar extends anteroinferiorly to attach to the lateral border of the tongue and thus provides a pathway for infiltration of the cancer into the tongue. The posterior pillar extends inferiorly to the lateral wall of the oropharynx. The soft palate and the tongue will be involved in about half the patients. Between 70% and 80% of the patients will have developed cervical lymph node metastases on admission. In the advanced stages lower cervical nodes and nodes beyond the neck will become involved. By far the most commonly involved lymph nodes are the subdigastric nodes just posterior to the angle of the jaw. Submaxillary and mid and upper jugular chains are occasionally involved as is the upper posterior cervical chain. This latter group is not ordinarily encompassed in the ports used to irradiate the lateral cervical chains and may be overlooked in ports used for the primary lesion.

A primary lesion that is still confined to the tonsillar fossa is readily controlled by irradiation. Extension into the base of the tongue or laterally into the muscles of the jaw greatly diminishes the probability of local control. The American Joint Committee stages for cancer of the tonsil are like those of the oral cavity—"T" category is determined purely by dimension. The significance of invasion into tissues mentioned before should be considered in any clinical evaluation.

Analysis of results with special attention to factors affecting prognosis have shown that the clinical extent of the primary lesion and the presence or absence of cervical metastases are most important (Perez and associates, 1972; Fayos and Lampe, 1971). The histologic classification of the carcinoma and the age and sex of the patient modify prognosis very little. This emphasizes the importance of defining extent of the primary tumor.

TECHNIQUE. The total volume involved by the primary tonsillar lesion is usually small, and it alone will rarely require a field larger than 8×8 cm. Inspection and palpation are required to define the volume involved. Extension into the pillars, palate, or base of the tongue should be searched for specifically, since this warrants a poorer prognosis. The tendency of these carcinomas to recur in the base of the tongue calls for higher total doses or boosting doses. Ipsilateral lymphadenopathy is the rule. Treatment will therefore usually entail simultaneous irradiation of the primary lesion and the cervical lymph node chains. External irradiation is by far the best approach to the irradiation of this volume. An occasional small lesion in a cooperative edentulous patient may be treated by peroral roentgentherapy. For these small lesions a peroral tissue dose of 5000 to 5500 rad delivered at the rate of 300 rad per day, 5 days a week, will generally be sufficient.

For supplementing the external irradiation with interstitial sources, removable ^{192}Ir, permanent ^{125}I, or radon seeds have been tried sporadically for selected patients (Goffinet and associates; Perez and associates, 1970). The aims of such combinations are to spare salivary glands and diminish risks of jaw necrosis. One need only examine the depth and breadth of infiltration as demonstrated on the operative specimen to appreciate the type of implant required to encompass advanced T2 and T3 lesions of the tonsil. The ultimate advantage of and indications for interstitial tonsillar implants are yet to be demonstrated. In addition, the superb control rates obtained by both Shukovsky and Fletcher and by Perez and associates using external beam techniques (Table 4-5) demand that for the primary lesion competing techniques yield very high control rates.

Before starting external irradiation, one should recognize the fact that a segment of the parotid gland and a portion of the mandible will be included in the volume of treatment. Therefore the teeth should be evaluated for the reasons mentioned

Table 4-5. Control of cancer of the tonsillar fossa obtained according to T category and dose*

T category	Perez		Shukovsky		
	Dose	Control		Dose	Control
T1	5500	11/12		6500	8/8
T2	6000	20/28		7000	8/10
T3	7000	20/35	T3 and T4 {	7000	8/13
T4	7000	9/30		7500	12/13

*Dose usually given at a rate of 5 fractions per week, 200 rad per fraction.

earlier in this chapter. However, when the curative dose levels that are described in the following paragraphs are given, a few patients (less than 10%) will have major soft tissue and bone necrosis.

If the tonsillar lesion is small, ipsilateral wedged beams can be used with the aim of sparing the contralateral parotid gland. However, since most of these cancers will have extended well beyond the tonsillar fossa, parallel opposing beams will be used most often. As a group, carcinomas of the tonsil are considered the most radiore-sponsive squamous cell carcinomas of the entire head and neck region. Small lesions (T1) are highly curable with the doses tolerated by small volumes. Larger cancers requiring treatment of large volumes of the oral and pharyngeal mucosa tolerate less total dose and usually require longer overall treatment time using less daily dose or split-dose techniques.

Two excellent analyses of dose-time data are available to guide us in irradiating carcinoma of the tonsil (Shukovsky and Fletcher; Perez and associates). The critical clinical material of these two studies is summarized in Table 4-5. These data indicate that primary cancers of the tonsil, 2 cm or less in maximum diameter, are almost uniformly controlled by doses of 6000 to 6500 rad given in 6½ weeks. Primary lesions, 2 to 4 cm in diameter, will almost always be controlled by doses of 7000 rad in 7 weeks. Finally, lesions greater than 4 cm in diameter will require doses of 7500 rad in 8 weeks. Table 4-5 suggests that if the above doses are used, all T1,

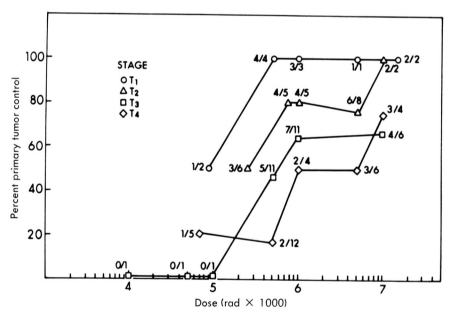

Fig. 4-22. Dose-response (control) curves for various "T" categories of cancer of the tonsil. (From Perez, C. A., Lee, F. A., Ackerman, L. V., Korba, A., Purdy, J., and Powers, W. E.: Int. J. Radiat. Oncol. Biol. Phys. **1:**817-827, 1976.)

almost all T2, and over three fourths of T3 lesions will be controlled. Fig. 4-22 emphasizes the dose-related aspect of local control.

Over 70% of these patients will have developed metastases to cervical lymph nodes by the time of diagnosis. The commonly involved nodes are those near the angle of the mandible. Nodes in this area are easily and effectively encompassed by the primary beam. Just as the size of the primary lesion has an important bearing on the required dose-time factors, so also does the size of a cervical lymph node metastasis bear on the dose required for its eradication (Schneider and associates; Perez and associates). Occult nodal metastases are uniformly controlled by 5000 rad in 5 weeks. Nodes up to 3 cm in diameter are controlled 95% of the time with doses of 6000 rad or greater in 6 weeks. Nodes larger than 2.5 to 3 cm may require very high doses, that is, 7500 rad or more in 8 or more weeks.

Clinical experience has shown us that the primary lesion and the lymphadenopathy are seldom the same size and often require quite different doses. A 1.5 cm primary lesion may be associated with lymphadenopathy at the angle of the jaw measuring 3 cm. The fact that this node is encompassed by the primary beam must not lead to an undertreatment of the node. Such an oversight no doubt accounts in part for the former misconception that metastases to cervical nodes are more "resistant" than the primary lesion.

A second word of caution appropriate in planning the treatment is in regard to encompassing the upper posterior cervical chain of nodes. A rather small square or rectangular parallel opposed pair of lateral beams can quite adequately encompass the primary lesion and any nodes near the angle of the jaw. An anterior beam is often matched to the inferior border of this beam to irradiate the cervical chain down to the sternoclavicular joint. This common combination often fails to encompass the ipsilateral upper posterior cervical chain of nodes. We have repeatedly seen the development of metastases in these nodes when this area has not been encompassed. This area justifies the same systematic elective irradiation as does the lower cervical chain. The technique of irradiation must respect the limited tolerance of the spinal cord. A single ipsilateral photon beam or preferably an electron beam of appropriate energy is satisfactory.

PROGNOSIS AND RESULTS. The 5-year control rate varies with the presence or absence of cervical metastases on admission and the degree of extension of the primary lesion. In addition, there can be no question but that cure rates for carcinoma of the tonsil have improved in recent years. Most of this improvement is a consequence of improved dosage because of the availability of megavoltage and ^{60}Co beams and because of our recognition that dose requirements vary with "T" and "N" categories, that is, the volume of the cancerous mass. The overall results of several series are shown in Tables 4-5 and 4-6 and in Figs. 4-22 and 4-23.

These types of control rates have more meaning if we are able to examine the relative proportion of limited and advanced lesions as shown in Fig. 4-22. Factors that affect prognosis were discussed earlier. Direct extension beyond the tonsillar fossa decreases cure rate in proportion to the magnitude of that extension. This is

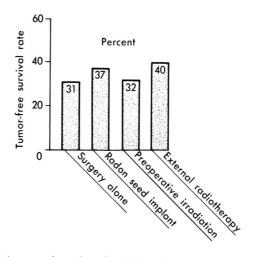

Fig. 4-23. Relative effectiveness of a variety of techniques for control of carcinoma of tonsil. As a rule, somewhat more limited cancers are more likely to be selected for surgery and radon seed implant. Yet external irradiation was superior. (Modified from Perez, C. A., Mill, W. B., Ogura, J. H., and Powers, W. E.: Radiology **94:**649-659, 1970.)

Table 4-6. Overall results of treatment of carcinoma of the tonsil*

Author	Years included	Number of patients	5-year control
Fletcher	1948-1962	96	35%
Fayos and Lampe (1971)	1955-1963	102	39.8% determinate
Perez and associates (1972)	1950-1967	57	40% absolute

*Lymphomas were excluded. Lymphoepitheliomas were generally included. Females showed a much better survival rate than males.

true if one specifies size of primary lesion in centimeters or in terms of involvement of neighboring structures.

Similarly, the presence of cervical adenopathy greatly reduces survival rate. When no cervical metastases are present, the cure rate is between 70% and 80%. When metastases are present, the cure rate is 40% or less (Perez and associates, 1972). When more than two or three enlarged nodes are present, the outlook is very poor. Perez and associates (1972) compared the various techniques of treatment and concluded external irradiation gave the best overall results (Fig. 4-23). Distant metastases develop in about 6% of all patients. The lungs and liver are most frequently involved. Of those patients dying before 5 years, local recurrence alone will develop in nearly a fourth. The patient should be evaluated for a radical resection of the recurrence, since a substantial proportion can be salvaged by surgery.

Lymphoepitheliomas of the tonsil are rare. We believe they should be treated as if they were squamous cell carcinomas despite their tendency to metastasize to lung, liver, and bone.

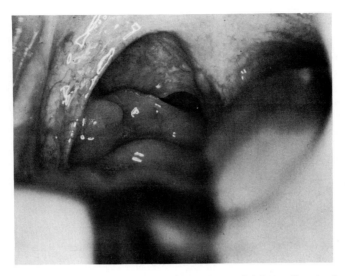

Fig. 4-24. Classic appearance of malignant lymphoma of right tonsil and vallecula.

Malignant lymphoma of the tonsil

Malignant lymphoma of the tonsil is about one sixth as common as carcinoma. Clinically it may appear markedly exophytic, nonulcerated, and even bilateral (Fig. 4-24). As in carcinoma, cervical metastases are the rule. The pretreatment evaluation should include a thorough search for nodal and extranodal extension beyond the neck. This includes the usual radiograms in addition to lymphangiograms, gallium scan, and marrow biopsy.

External irradiation with ^{60}Co or megavoltage beams is the treatment of choice for both the primary lesion and any regional metastases. Port arrangement can be the same as for carcinoma. However, generous margins of apparently normal tissue around the palpable tumor should be irradiated. The whole of Waldeyer's ring should be routinely encompassed (Wang, 1969). Although initial regression will be striking, one should not be deceived into giving a low tissue dose. The minimum dose to the volume of interest should be 4500 to 5000 rad with megavoltage beams in 4 to 5 weeks.

The question of irradiating ipsilateral or bilateral cervical areas in the absence of palpable adenopathy is answered in the same way as for other apparent localized lymphomas. We believe the next apparent uninvolved drainage area should be included in the treated volume. This usually implies irradiation of at least both cervical chains.

Patients free of disease for 5 years or longer will average between 30% and 64% (Berven; del Regato; Wang, 1969). Ennuyer and Bataini reported that of 150 patients treated, fifty-two were living and well after 5 years. In a survey of the literature reported by these authors, 147 of 531 patients were living after 5 years. Most of the patients who die will have developed generalized lymphoma without local recurrence, and about 60% of the total group will develop generalized lymphoma during or after treatment. Local recurrence alone is not infrequent (eleven of ninety-eight failures reported by Ennuyer and Bataini), but such failures are now recognized as a consequence of defective techniques (Wang, 1969). If the disease is apparently confined to the tonsil and upper cervical nodes, no systemic therapy is given. If lower cervical nodes or nodes beyond the neck are involved, the patient is evaluated for systemic treatment just as for any other non-Hodgkin's lymphoma of similar histologic type and stage.

Carcinoma of the soft palate and uvula

Carcinoma of the soft palate should be separated from that of the tonsil proper. Lesions of the palate are reported to be more resistant to radiations than those of the tonsil, but clear comparison is difficult. Lesions limited to the pillars are rare (twelve of 534 patients reported by Ennuyer and Bataini). The tonsil, walls of the nasopharynx, the tongue, or even the buccal mucosa may be involved. Lymph node metastases will be present in about 50% of these patients on admission. The lymph drainage and distribution of metastases resemble those from cancer of the tonsil except that spread to the upper posterior cervical nodes is much less common. The clinical staging used is the same as that given for carcinoma of the oral cavity.

TECHNIQUE. Lesions of the soft palate are treated similarly to lesions of the tonsil. Peroral roentgentherapy can be used for small, favorably placed lesions in cooperative patients, but extension into the tongue, onto the buccal mucosa, or onto the lateral or posterior pharyngeal wall requires external irradiation, preferably megavoltage or ^{60}Co beams. The dose probably should be somewhat higher than for primarily tonsillar carcinoma if the patient can tolerate it.

Metastases are usually palpable in upper cervical nodes near the angle of the jaw and should be treated just as described for metastases from carcinoma of the tonsil. Both sides of the neck will usually require irradiation (see p. 125).

PROGNOSIS AND RESULTS. The control rate will, of course, vary rather widely, depending on the degree of local advancement and the presence or absence of lymph node metastases. In 1956 Ennuyer and Bataini collected 325 cases reported in the world literature. Twenty-three percent of the patients were free of disease for 5 years or longer. In their own series of 121 patients, only nineteen were living and well after 5 years. Local recurrence was frequent in their patients, occurring alone in thirty instances and with cervical lymph node metastases in thirty-four. Failure to control cancer of the soft palate is more common than is supposed, but more recent experience shows a much improved rate of local control. Thus Gelinas and Fletcher (1973) were able to control all T1 lesions and all T2 lesions, that is, forty-eight patients in all. T3 lesions (greater than 4 cm in diameter) are more difficult to control (four of twenty-two recurred), and one half of all T4 lesions recurred. The overall 5-year disease-free survival rate of fifty-four patients was 49%. Multiple foci of origin are common. Superficial "inflammatory-like" extension of the cancer may extend well beyond the palpable limits. Many of the "marginal recurrences" are in fact manifestations of multiple foci of origin just at the edge of the treated volume.

Carcinomas of the anterior pillar and retromolar trigone

Carcinomas of the anterior pillar and retromolar trigone have many similarities to carcinomas of the tonsil, but differ as follows:

1. They are generally more differentiated and metastasize less frequently than cancers of the tonsillar fossa.

2. They rarely metastasize to contralateral cervical lymph nodes, submental lymph nodes, or the upper posterior cervical chain.

3. Their metastases have been found by some radiation oncologists to be less radioresponsive than those from carcinoma of the tonsil.

Other than omitting prophylactic radiotherapy of the contralateral cervical chain, we treat these cancers similarly to those of the tonsil. The upper posterior cervical chain need not be irradiated electively unless the digastric adenopathy is large or the primary lesion has infiltrated into the tonsillar fossa. Small metastases are radiocurable, but nodes larger than 2.5 cm should be removed with neck dissection.

IRRADIATION IN TREATMENT OF SQUAMOUS CELL CARCINOMA METASTATIC TO CERVICAL LYMPH NODES

For years radical neck dissection was the treatment of choice for metastases in cervical lymph nodes from primary cancers of the lip, tongue, floor of the mouth, gingiva, buccal mucosa, and palate. At the same time, radiotherapy has often been the recommended treatment for metastases to cervical lymph nodes from cancers of the nasopharynx and tonsillar region. The reason for this difference was based on reports and observations that some metastases seemed to respond incompletely, whereas others were radiocurable. With the development of skin-sparing beams and laryngeal and pharyngeal sparing techniques, substantial doses can be given to the entire right and left cervical lymph nodes chains with little patient discomfort and acceptable sequelae. The accumulation of clinical material necessary to evaluate this technique for all categories of metastases has been slow, but data from a variety of institutions are now available. Radiotherapy can control metastases in cervical lymph nodes in a proportion that challenges radical neck dissection in selected clinical circumstances (Hanks and associates; Wizenberg and associates; Northrop and associates; Votava and associates; Schneider and associates; Barkley and associates).

The most significant factor affecting radiocontrollability of cervical lymph node metastases is the size of the metastases. With acceptable doses nodes less than 2 cm in diameter are almost always controlled; nodes 2 to 3 cm in diameter are frequently controlled; nodes 4 to 6 cm in diameter are infrequently controlled. However, occasionally even large fixed or bilateral nodes may be controlled by radiotherapy (Votava and associates). In addition, it has been observed repeatedly that the primary lesion and the metastases of similar size respond similarly. With modern techniques it is unusual to control the primary lesion with radiotherapy and at the same time fail to control its metastases in cervical lymph nodes. The primary lesion and the regional metastases usually respond alike to radiotherapy except when the therapist fails to take their unequal size into account.

Much of what follows is summarized from the extensive analysis of patients treated at the M. D. Anderson Hospital by Fletcher and his associates. It makes use of sound radiobiologic principles in increasing the control rate and decreasing the deformity of radical neck dissection.

The management of cervical metastases should be tailored to the characteristics of spread peculiar to each primary site. In this regard we recognize four clinical situations.

1. *Treatment of occult metastases.* There are at least three arguments for treating metastases when they are in their earliest (occult) stage. First, the smaller the focus of cancer, the lower the dose required for its control. The reasons for this were given in Chapter 1. Occult metastases from squamous cell carcinoma or adenocarcinoma are almost always controlled by doses that are well tolerated, carry little risk, and leave few sequelae. Second, by controlling metastases early, one reduces the opportunity for more distant spread. Finally, control of occult metastases eliminates the risk of a subsequent deforming neck dissection should the nodes become larger than 2 cm, and such control eliminates the sequela of higher doses of radiations necessary to control large metastases in cervical lymph nodes.

After accepting the above, there are other data that must be examined before concluding that systematic prophylactic irradiation of cervical lymph nodes is justified.

    a. There should be a reasonable chance that the primary cancer has been or will be controlled. It is impractical to wait until we are assured of such control. It thus becomes a matter of judgment.

    b. There should be a reasonable chance that occult metastases are present. The question, "What is a reasonable chance?" cannot be answered with a simple percentage. The incidences of occult metastases for cancers of the oral cavity vary from 20% to 35% except for lesions of the buccal mucosa, for which it is about half of this figure. However, one must weigh demands and sequelae of the proposed treatment as well as compare results with competitive management before assessing these percentages as being reasonable.

    c. It should be proved that irradiation of occult metastases actually results in a higher cure rate than would have been obtained by treating only those patients who eventually develop clinically obvious metastases. Unavoidably related to the "wait and see" policy will be those patients who, because of the delay, develop large incurable cervical adenopathy or distant metastases.

    d. The morbidity of systematic prophylactic irradiation must be accepted for all patients, including those who did not have occult disease. Thus the treatment must be well tolerated, carry little risk, and leave few sequelae.

One might argue that where prophylactic radical neck dissection has previously been applied, prophylactic irradiation should now be substituted. In fact, irradiation, with its well-tolerated sequelae and the promise of avoiding the risk of a later deforming therapeutic neck dissection, should have somewhat broader indications than prophylactic radical neck dissection.

Systematic prophylactic irradiation of both lateral cervical chains is recommended for carcinomas of the nasopharynx, tonsillar region, anterior two thirds and base of tongue, and pharyngeal walls. Most cancers of the anterior two thirds of the tongue, floor of the mouth, and tonsillar pillars require ports that encompass a substantial porportion of the submaxillary and subdigastric tissues. This is especially true when parallel opposing lateral beams are required. Under such circumstances xerostomia is not significantly worsened by the addition of tangential beams to the cervical region. We have therefore used them freely with the full realization that their value is not statistically confirmed for all anatomic sites.

The technique is shown in Fig. 4-25. The dose delivered to the nodal chain is about 5000 rad in about 5 weeks.

2. *Treatment of small clinically suspicious nodes.* In this category are nodes that are 2 cm or less in diameter. Such metastases from primary cancers of the nasopharynx or tonsillar region have ordinarily been treated by irradiation, whereas those from the lips, tongue, floor of the mouth, gingiva, buccal mucosa, and palate have been treated by radical neck dissection. Our recent experience and the experience of others (Hanks and associates; Wizenberg and associates; Fletcher) proves

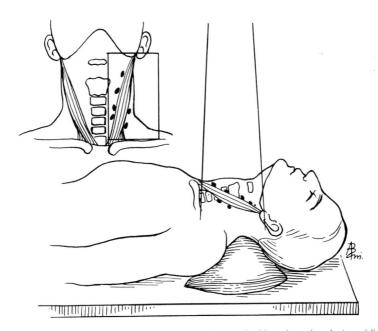

Fig. 4-25. Tangential telecobalt beam directed to include cervical lymph nodes, but avoiding midline structures. A parallel opposing posterior port can be added if nodes in the posterior cervical triangle are at risk.

that metastases of this size in cervical lymph nodes from squamous cell cancer of the head and neck can be controlled by radiotherapy in almost every instance in which the primary cancer is controlled. For this category, as for category 1, modern radiotherapy is the successor to radical neck dissection. If only ipsilateral adenopathy less than 2 cm in diameter is present, that entire cervical chain is irradiated with 6000 rad in 6 to 8 weeks; a preferable alternative is 5000 rad in 5 weeks to the entire chain with a boosting dose of 1500 rad through reduced ports to the region of the adenopathy. If, in the same patient, the contralateral chain is free of adenopathy, it should be given a dose suitable for occult metastases, that is, 5000 rad in 5 weeks.

3. *Treatment of movable (operable) adenopathy greater than 2 cm in diameter.* As metastases enlarge to a diameter greater than 2 cm, the total number of cells and the increasing hypoxia of tumor cells shift tumor response toward the borderline of radioincurability. Certainly some of these metastases can be controlled with radiotherapy alone. However, as the nodes enlarge the frequency of control by radiotherapy alone decreases. Postirradiation viable cancer frequently persists in nodes that were initially greater than 4 cm in diameter. There are three methods of managing this situation that deserve consideration.

    a. The classical method of management is radical neck dissection. It has been the unquestioned treatment of choice for 30 years.

    b. With the knowledge that radiotherapy can dependably control metastatic foci less than 2 cm in diameter, a sequence that was formerly considered heresy has been found effective and now justifies serious consideration. The entire cervical lymph node chain on the involved side is given 5000 to 6000 rad in 5 to 6 weeks. Six or 8 weeks later, limited surgery is performed for removal of residual masses. The rationale of this sequence is clear, and it has been used sufficiently to justify its cautious application. Diffuse infiltration by cancer should, when possible, be removed by radical neck dissection. The persistence of multiple large nodes after irradiation requires radical, not limited, surgery.

    c. When radical neck dissection is performed as the initial treatment and the operative specimen contains more than three or four positive nodes, the incidence of recurrent tumor growth in the neck is high (Table 4-7). Postoper-

Table 4-7. Comparison of posttreatment failure in neck surgery alone versus surgery plus postoperative irradiation (oral cavity, supraglottis, and hypopharynx)*

	Surgery alone	Surgery and postoperative irradiation
N1	13/94 (14%)	1/43 (2%)
N2 (a and b)	20/78 (26%)	4/43 (11%)
N3 (a and b)	10/29 (30%)	6/24 (25%)

*Modified from Jesse, R. H., and Fletcher, G. H.: Cancer **39:**868-872, 1977.

ative irradiation of the entire operative site is indicated. This reduces the incidence of recurrent growth in the neck in all categories but is relatively more effective in N1 and N2 categories. The contralateral neck should be treated for occult metastases as previously outlined.

4. *Treatment of fixed or large bilateral adenopathy.* Such metastases are generally accepted as inoperable. Yet, if the primary cancer can be controlled, a vigorous irradiation of the cervical metastasis is justified with a view of resecting residual masses with limited surgery not unlike 3a above (Votava and associates). A dose of 6000 rad in 6 weeks is used if limited surgery is to follow in 6 to 8 weeks. After this dose, if surgery is not advisable or the mass remains fixed, boosting doses through reduced ports are given. If the contralateral chain is clinically uninvolved, prophylactic irradiation is given to a dose of 5000 rad in 5 weeks.

At first glance these various recommendations seem complex. They are, in fact, the clinical application of current radiobiologic concepts, with a view toward increasing the control of metastases in the neck and of reducing the deformity of radical neck dissection. Just as for any other clinical recommendation, there will be exceptions and, with time, sharper definition of indications.

TECHNIQUE. The volume with which we are concerned is the same as that excised during a radical neck dissection. Cervical metastases do not usually occur as single nodes. For this reason we have advocated irradiation of the entire volume rather than a single palpable node. The volume usually extends laterally from the lateral edge of the trachea and from the clavicle to the mastoid. Depending on the

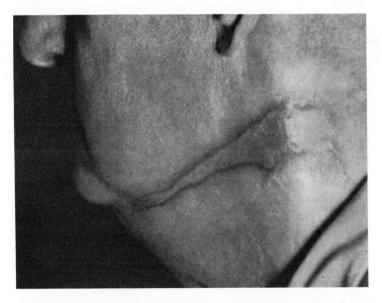

Fig. 4-26. Overlap occurred between upper lateral and lower anterior tangential beams because patient was treated in different positions for the two areas. This can be avoided by outlining the portals with skin ink and by carefully repositioning after each treatment.

anatomic site and size of the primary lesion, the risk of metastases to a specific nodal group varies considerably. Irradiation of this entire block of tissue to doses of 5000 rad or more at 1000 rad per week through a single lateral port carries the risk of chronic edema and irritation. Earlier, Baclesse used highly fractionated tangential medium-voltage x-ray beams with doses of 6200 rad in 70 to 80 days for undifferentiated lesions and up to 7200 rad in the same period for the more advanced differentiated metastases. He found that a dose of 5800 rad in this period to clinically palpable disease was usually followed by recurrence, and a dose of 4800 rad in this period was always followed by recurrence. With ^{60}Co or megavoltage beams, anterior tangential ports alone or a pair of parallel opposing anterior and posterior tangential ports are technically simple and well tolerated. All structures lateral to the trachea from the sternoclavicular joint to the mastoid bone are readily encompassed. The upper border of those beams must, of course, be adjusted to fit with the beams used to treat the primary cancer. Care must be taken to avoid overlap between the upper lateral and lower tangential beams (Fig. 4-26). Wedges can be used to improve dose distribution. The doses recommended for the various clinical situations were given previously. A daily dose of 180 to 200 rad five times each week to a total dose of 5000 rad has never, in our experience, produced a serious sequela. There are a significant number of patients who will develop bothersome fibrosis if the fractions are larger or if the total chain is carried to a dose considerably higher than 5000 rad. When higher doses are necessary, the risk of fibrosis must be accepted or reduced ports developed to increase the dose to the volumes justifying it.

SUMMARY. The treatment of metastases in cervical lymph nodes from cancer of the oral cavity and oropharynx cannot be considered separately from the treatment of the primary lesion. The management of the nodes is influenced in a major way by the treatment selected for the primary cancer.

Prophylactic irradiation of the cervical lymph node chains is the successor to prophylactic neck dissection. It is as effective as prophylactic neck dissection and carries less morbidity. Therefore it justifies somewhat broader indications. This is expecially obvious when considering the clinically negative contralateral lymph node chain when the ipsilateral chain is involved.

There is now clear cut evidence that radiotherapy of the clinically involved cervical lymph node chain in selected patients is an effective method of control. This is true not only for metastases from the nasopharynx, tonsil, base of the tongue, and supraglottic region, but also for other selected primaries. When the metastases are small, control of the metastases is usual. When the nodes are large, either radical neck dissection or limited surgery for postirradiation residual masses should be considered.

To diminish the chances of producing a serious "woody" neck after high doses and failures after inadequate doses, radiotherapy techniques must be adapted to the clinical findings both as to initial volume, reduced ports, and dose-time relationships.

POSTOPERATIVE IRRADIATION OF CERVICAL LYMPH NODE AREAS. When a surgeon realizes that he has left a portion of the disease behind, the only hope for cure remains with vigorous irradiation. Generally, this should be wide-port irradiation encompassing the entire operative field, that is, both the primary site and the area of the regional node dissection. Once cancer has been transected, the entire wounds may be seeded.

There are obvious radiobiologic arguments for proceeding with radiotherapy in the patient with known or suspected residual cancer rather than waiting for the disease to become clinically apparent. The smaller the foci of cancer cells, the greater the chances of radiotherapeutic control. Also, early irradiation lessens the opportunities for distant metastases. The superiority of early postoperative irradiation for high-risk patients has been shown for several anatomic sites, including head and neck cancers (Fletcher and Evers; Lindberg and Jesse). Thus when early or prophylactic irradiation was given to the patients with cancer transected at the margins of the specimen, 42% showed no evidence of disease subsequently. When irradiation was given for clinical recurrence, only 11% later showed no evidence of disease. Doses recommended depend on the clinical situation, but high doses are usually indicated for the primary site, that is, 5500 to 6500 rad in 6 to 7 weeks. Additional boosting doses through reduced ports are indicated when a bulky cancerous mass is known to have been left behind.

The contribution of postoperative irradiation of the cervical lymph node chains after radical neck dissection is dependent on the number and size of metastases the pathologist finds in the operative specimen (Table 4-7). There are many clinical situations in which information relative to the "adequacy of excision" is imprecise or unavailable. In such circumstances our decisions are based on very soft data, often impressions, or the wish of the surgeon to "play it safe." We must then select a dose-time schedule for this uncertain situation, that is, 5000 rad in 5 weeks for "occult foci," 6000 rad in 6 weeks because of the high risk of local recurrence of the primary lesion, 6500 rad in 6½ to 7 weeks because cancer was thought to have been transected, or 7000 rad in 8 weeks because we can define what we think is a focus of postoperative residual cancer. The titration of dose according to the volume of cancer being irradiated is a valid radiobiologic concept that demands more from us than we are always able to supply.

PREOPERATIVE IRRADIATION OF CERVICAL LYMPH NODE AREAS. A discussion of the various general aspects of preoperative irradiation has been presented in Chapter 2. In every respect that discussion is applicable to preoperative irradiation of cervical lymph node metastases and will not be repeated here. The aim of preoperative irradiation in this instance is to eliminate the more peripheral occult and therefore often transected extensions of tumor prior to surgery. The hope is that the more resistant residual is then excised by radical neck dissection with less risk of local recurrence.

The efficacy of preoperative irradiation for cervical lymph node metastases has not been settled. Henschke and associates attempted randomizing patients between preoperative and no preoperative cervical irradiation (2000 R air megavoltage beams in 5 days). Their two clinical groups were not equivalent (58.6% of the control group and 74.8% of the irradiated group had lymphadenopathy; also, fifty-eight patients fell into the group of those to be irradiated, but they were not irradiated). By 1 year, cervical recurrence developed in 33% of 146 control patients and in 23.1% of 111 patients given preoperative irradiation. Similarly, in a nonrandomized study Hendrickson reported that radical neck dissection alone controlled metastatic cancer in the neck for at least 2 years in 25% of 112 patients with proved metastases. Preoperative irradiation (2500 rad or more) followed by neck dissection controlled disease in the neck for at least 2 years in 90.2% of fifty-one patients.

Higher doses have also been tried. Jesse and Fletcher performed radical neck dissection 6 weeks after 4000 to 6000 rad to the neck nodes. Silverstone and Goldman performed radical surgery 3 to 6 weeks after 5500 rad in 5 weeks. The contribution of routine preradical neck irradiation remains to be defined. This must not be confused with the valuable contribution of irradiating the patient with multiple large or fixed nodes who, after irradiation, is benefited by limited resection of residual masses.

The concept of postirradiation limited surgery for residual masses was discussed earlier. It may provide a means for controlling advanced regional metastases without the deformity of a radical neck dissection.

METASTASES TO CERVICAL LYMPH NODES FROM AN OCCULT PRIMARY CANCER. Occasionally clinically imperceptible primary lesions of the head and neck will produce clinically obvious metastases in a cervical lymph node. The location of the adenopathy should be a clue to the site of the primary lesion, but there is sufficient inconsistency in this regard to create much uncertainty. The occult primary cancer will usually be in the base of the tongue, nasopharynx, tonsil, or piriform sinus. Repeated examinations and blind biopsies should be performed prior to considering treatment. In most cases the site of the primary lesion will eventually manifest itself.

However, if a vigorous search has failed to define a primary site of origin, we are faced with making decisions based on limited data. By necessity patients treated by radical neck dissection and a "wait-and-see" policy for the primary lesion are "selected." This selection determines the incidence and distribution of subsequently appearing primary sites. For this reason data acquired from this group are not strictly applicable to patients best suited for irradiation of the cervical lymph node chains or to the group as a whole. However, it is the most meaningful data available, and it illustrates important principles. Thus, of 104 patients treated with radical neck dissection and a "wait-and-see" policy for the primary site, twenty-one (20%) subsequently manifested a primary focus (Jesse and associates). Treatment at that point controlled the primary lesions in fourteen of the twenty-one. Thus seven patients died of uncontrolled primary lesions who might have benefited from earlier "prophylactic" irradiation of potential primary sites. However, only ten of the twenty-one primary lesions appeared in a site that would have been encompassed by the commonly irradiated volume, that is, nasopharynx, tonsil, and base of the tongue. These data are probably different from those which might be obtained from a group of patients referred for irradiation of the cervical nodes. Often patients with nodes anterior and lower are treated with a radical neck dissection; those with nodes higher and posterior are usually referred for irradiation.

If the nodes contain squamous cell cancer, are *anterior*, and do not exceed 4 cm in diameter, we have no hesitation in recommending radical irradiation to the entire ipsilateral chain from clavicle to mastoid and from the *midline* laterally. A dose of 6000 rad in 6 weeks is given using anterior and posterior tangential ^{60}Co beams. The ipsilateral piriform sinus, base of the tongue, and lower portion of the tonsillar fossa are encompassed by these beams. A primary lesion that cannot be detected is presumed to be very small and is controlled by a dose of 6000 rad in 6 weeks. If the node is more *posterior* and a primary cancer is suspected in the nasopharynx, parallel opposing lateral beams can be used to raise the nasopharynx to the dose of 6000 rad in 6 weeks. This technique will control occult disease in the cervical lymph nodes in almost every case. A boosting dose is given to palpable nodes in keeping with the discussion on pp. 131 to 135. If the node is large and persists after high-dose radiotherapy, it should be removed by limited surgery. The ultimate outcome is therefore dependent on whether there is cancer beyond the neck. A good proportion of these patients will be shown to have a primary cancer below the clavicle (Greenberg). When disease is not below the clavicle, the 3-year survival rate should be between 40% and 50% (McComb; Jesse and associates).

TUMORS OF SALIVARY AND MUCOUS GLANDS

Neoplasms of the salivary glands are uncommon, and for this reason some aspects of their management are uncertain. They may develop in the major salivary glands (parotid, submaxillary, and sublingual) or in any of the numerous small mucous glands of the mucosa of the oral cavity or upper air passages. A variety of cell types are recognized microscopically. The clinical behavior of these different cell types probably justifies considering each type separately, but the number of patients in each group is small so that differences are sometimes difficult to detect. As a general guide, adenoid cystic carcinoma, adenocarcinoma, and mucoepidermoid carcinoma respond with radiation-induced complete regression in about one half the patients (Rafla-Demetrious). Regression occurs slightly more often in ectopic sites or the small glands than in the major glands. Anaplastic cancers and the squamous cell cancers respond less well.

Benign mixed tumors

Mixed tumors of the parotid possess certain characteristics that are strongly tempting to the radiation oncologist. These tumors are relatively superficial in location and are not anatomically associated with radiosensitive vital structures. Excision of the area is limited because of the proximity of the facial nerve, the ear, and the mandible; postoperative recurrences have been frequently reported.

Despite these factors that appear to be favorable for irradiation of benign mixed tumors, vigorous irradiation as a *primary treatment* has been tried and found less effective than surgical excision. Doses producing serious changes in soft tissue frequently fail to eradicate the tumor. The reasons for this failure to respond are found in an examination of cell types and the large tumor mass often present. Benign mixed tumors of the salivary gland are derived from epithelial origin but contain elements that appear to be both epithelial and stromal. In such tumors well-developed glands, fibrous tissue, myxomatous stroma, cartilage, and rarely even bone are seen. None of these elements either alone or in mixture is particularly radiosensitive. Certainly some of these elements may be destroyed by vigorous irradiation. The growth rate of others can be decreased, and the disease can at times be permanently controlled. Two of thirty-three benign mixed tumors of the major salivary glands showed complete radiation-induced regression with high doses, whereas seven of eighteen benign tumors of the minor salivary glands showed complete regression (Rafla-Demetrious). These figures support the practice of using surgery as the treatment of choice in the benign mixed tumors. After high-dose radiotherapy, dense fibrous tissue and vascular changes may encase the tumor, and slow regrowth may result. However, if benign mixed tumors of the parotid were even moderately radiosensitive, surgery would not now play the major role in their management. For this reason even the most enthusiastic radiation oncologists agree that the primary treatment of these benign tumors should usually be surgery.

The question of postoperative irradiation invariably arises. Have we a right to expect any more of irradiation after surgery than of irradiation given without surgery? The radiobiologic fact that the fewer the cells present, the less the dose required for their destruction should strengthen the argument for postoperative irradiation for this benign tumor just as it does for many malignant tumors. However, this point is not easy to verify for benign mixed tumors of the salivary glands. Watson was able to show that doses of 5300 to 5700 rad in 5 weeks controlled *limited* postoperative residual benign mixed tumor in almost every instance. High doses are not justified routinely if the benign mixed tumor has been resected with a margin of apparently normal surrounding tissues. If, for one reason or another, complete excision is not done, radiotherapy should be considered. The overall results obtained by such management have been published by Watson and by Rafla-Demetrious, but the precise contribution of radiotherapy to longevity cannot be defined. Other interesting questions also remain unanswered. For example, can radiation-induced changes inhibit further neoplastic degeneration in the salivary glands? Can this decrease the incidence of apparent multiple foci of origin? Is the more actively growing tumor periphery more susceptible to radiation damage than the central bulk of a partially resected tumor?

Malignant tumors of salivary glands

Several histologic types of malignant tumors are sufficiently frequent to permit some conclusions regarding the role of radiotherapy in their management—malignant mixed tumors, cylindromas (adenoid cystic carcinomas), mucoepidermoid carcinomas, and undifferentiated cancers. The ease of local control and the incidence of distant metastases are very much dependent on the clinical stage of the disease. The American Joint Committee Stage Classification (1978) follows.

TNM CLASSIFICATION*

T —Primary tumor

TX	Tumor that cannot be assessed by rules
T0	No evidence of primary tumor
T1	Tumor 2 cm or less in diameter, solitary, freely mobile, facial nerve intact†
T2	Tumor more than 2 cm but not more than 4 cm in diameter, solitary, freely mobile or reduced mobility or skin fixation, and facial nerve intact†
T3	Tumor more than 4 cm but not more than 6 cm in diameter, or multiple nodes, skin ulceration, deep fixation, or facial nerve dysfunction†
T4	Tumor >6 cm in diameter and/or involving mandible and adjacent bones

N—Nodal involvement

NX	Nodes cannot be assessed
N0	No clinically positive node
N1	Single clinically positive homolateral node 3 cm or less in diameter
N2	Single clinically positive homolateral node more than 3 cm but not more than 6 cm in diameter or multiple clinically positive homolateral nodes, none over 6 cm in diameter
	N2a Single clinically positive homolateral node, more than 3 cm but not more than 6 cm in diameter
	N2b Multiple clinically positive homolateral nodes, none over 6 cm in diameter
N3	Massive homolateral node(s), bilateral nodes, or contralateral node(s)
	N3a Clinically positive homolateral node(s), one more than 6 cm in diameter
	N3b Bilateral clinically positive nodes (in this situation, each side of the neck should be staged separately; that is, N3b: right, N2a; left, N1)
	N3c Contralateral positive node(s) only

M—Distant metastasis

MX	Not assessed
M0	No (known) distant metastasis
M1	Distant metastasis present

HISTOPATHOLOGY

Mucoepidermoid, adenoidcystic, squamous cell, acinic cell, undifferentiated

GRADE

Well-differentiated, moderately well-differentiated, poorly to very poorly differentiated, or numbers 1, 2, 3-4

STAGE GROUPING

No stage grouping is recommended at present

This staging system has only recently been recognized, and results have not yet been reported using this classification.

The treatment of choice for resectable cancers has usually been radical surgery. If the cancer is apparently still localized but cannot be encompassed by excision, or if there is any question of adequate excision, vigorous postoperative irradiation

---

*From the American Joint Committee for Cancer Staging and End Results Reporting: Manual for staging of cancer, Chicago, 1978, Whiting Press.

†Applicable to parotid tumors only.

with a curative attempt should be considered. The anatomic restrictions to surgery in this area lead to frequent narrow or inadequate margins of cancer resection. The problem results from efforts to preserve the auditory canal, mandible, and facial nerve.

The value of postoperative irradiation for patients with questionably adequate or inadequate excision has been proven by several workers (Guillamondegui and associates; Fu and associates). Following are the indications for postoperative irradiation:

1. Obvious transection of cancer, questionably adequate or narrow margins of excision
2. High histologic grades
3. Cancer invasion of muscle, bone, nerves, or perineural lymphatics
4. Metastases in regional lymph nodes
5. Routinely following excision of recurrences
6. Primary lesion in or infiltration into deep portions of the gland
7. Decision made to spare facial nerve when the cancer is close to the nerve

Planned combinations of preoperative irradiation and surgery were discussed in Chapter 2. Carcinomas of salivary glands are often in critical sites and are notorious for direct extension beyond their palpable margins. These characteristics call for the advantages of combinations of preoperative irradiation and surgery, which has been recommended by Rafla-Demetrious. His arguments for preoperative irradiation are as follows:

1. Twenty-five of sixty-nine irradiated malignant tumors of the salivary glands regressed completely and did not require resection. Doses in some cases exceeded 6000 rad in 6 weeks.

2. Radiotherapy administered when the circulation is intact is more effective than after resection. This may be true, but there is now ample evidence of the effectiveness of radiotherapy given as soon as the operative wound has healed.

3. If radiotherapy is carefully fractionated, subsequent resection is not made more difficult. Deformity may be less than would have resulted from the use of surgery alone, since postirradiation resection will not always be necessary, and when it is necessary, a limited procedure may be adequate.

These promising concepts should be tested as they relate to carcinomas of the salivary glands. However, the scarcity of clinical material will make any such evaluation difficult. For the present, we accept the concepts in item 3 as a competitive alternative to primary radical resection when the cancer is marginally inoperable.

However, by far the most commonly used combination therapy consists of surgery *followed* in selected patients with postoperative irradiation as mentioned before. For known residual disease doses of 6500 to 7000 rad in 7 to 8 weeks are advocated. For so-called occult residual disease a midline dose of 5000 rad in 6 weeks is appropriate. We seldom recommend this low-dose technique for this anatomic site.

TECHNIQUE. Benign or malignant tumors of the parotid gland are usually near the skin; some of the malignant tumors will have invaded the skin. Depending on skin involvement, a single lateral megavoltage beam with or without thin bolus and a wobbled exit beam is the simplest adequate technique. An electron beam of appropriate penetration either alone or combined with a megavoltage beam permits partial sparing of the contralateral salivary gland. A wedged pair of beams can also be used to reduce irradiation of the contralateral parotid. However, care must be taken to avoid the contralateral eye and the brainstem. For an average port size of 8 × 10 cm, a dose of 5500 rad at 4 cm depth in 5 weeks seems well tolerated and is recommended for selected *benign* lesions which for one reason or another are not to be resected. Regrowth after lower doses is likely.

For malignant tumors ports will generally be wider and the total doses higher. There is no consensus as to the definition of adequate margins. Nerves may be invaded several centimeters beyond the obvious tumor margin. Deep infiltration cannot be accurately assessed by palpation. Thus *wide margins in all directions are important.* Unless there is good evidence that the tumor is confined to superficial tissues and all nerves are free of tumor, we systematically deliver at least 5000 rad to the midline through ipsilateral ports. Guillamondegui has emphasized that if the facial nerve is involved or if the patient has an adenoid cystic cancer, the mastoid bone must be irradiated. Also, if the auricolotemporal nerve is involved, the base of the skull must be included in the high dose volume.

The entire ipsilateral cervical node chain is irradiated even in the absence of adenopathy if the primary lesion is very large, recurrent, or of a high histologic grade. 5000 rad is given in 5 weeks to a depth of 3 cm through an anterior tangential cervical port. If a node dissection reveals metastases, a boosting dose of 1000 to 1500 rad is given to the areas of greatest concern. Both anterior and posterior tangential cervical ports may be necessary if the posterior chain of nodes is involved. Residual masses, whether at the site of the primary lesion or in the neck, are given doses similar to those described for masses of squamous cell carcinoma.

Irradiation of malignant salivary gland or mucous gland tumors at sites other than the parotid require but slight modification of techniques commonly used for squamous cell carcinoma of the same site. Here also wide margins of apparently normal tissue should be irradiated to compensate for the known tendency of these cancers to extend along fascial planes and nerves. Doses should be the maximum tolerated for the volume under consideration. Although cylindromas are said to be more radiosensitive than the other cell types, doses should not be decreased below those given for other histologic types.

RESULTS. When radiation therapy was used primarily and any residual cancer was excised, 43% of 104 cancers were controlled locally for 1 to 10 years (Rafla-Demetrious). Also of ninety-nine patients available for analysis after 5 years, he reported that 30% were living free of disease, whereas 19% were living with disease. King and Fletcher obtained local control above the clavicle in three fourths of seventy-one patients, and at 5 years there was no evidence of disease in 33.8%. Metastasis in cervical nodes developed in only two of forty-eight patients who had

Table 4-8. Effect of treatment modality on local control of cancer of the salivary glands*

| Histology | Treatment modality | | | |
	Surgery	Surgery + external radiotherapy	External radiotherapy only	Total
Adenocarcinoma	14/17	3/5	1/5	18/27 (67%)
Mucoepidermoid carcinoma	15/16	7/7	1/4	23/27 (85%)
Adenoid cystic carcinoma	3/10	9/10	1/2	13/22 (59%)
Undifferentiated carcinoma	3/5	2/2	2/5	7/12 (58%)
Squamous cell carcinoma	1/1	1/3	1/3	3/7 (43%)
Acinic cell carcinoma	3/3	2/2	0	5/5 (69%)
TOTAL	39/52 (75%)	24/29 (83%)	6/19 (32%)	69/100 (69%)

*Modified from Fu, K. K., Leibel, S. A., Levine, M. L., Friedlander, L. M., Boler, R., and Phillips, T. L.: Cancer **40:** 2882-2890, 1977.

Table 4-9. Effect of *postoperative* irradiation for cancer of the salivary glands on patients at high risk for local recurrence (4 years to unlimited follow-up)*

Histology	Number of patients	Number of recurrences
Malignant mixed carcinoma	3	2†
Mucoepidermoid (high grade) carcinoma	7	0
Adenoid cystic carcinoma	8	1†
Adenocarcinoma	4	0
Acinic cell carcinoma	1	0
Squamous cell carcinoma	4	1†
Undifferentiated carcinoma	1	0
Unclassified neoplasm	1	0
TOTAL	29	4 (14%)

*Modified from Guillamondegui, O. M., Byers, R. M., Luna, M. A., Chiminazzo, H., Jesse, R. H., and Fletcher, G. H.: Am. J. Roentgenol. Radium Ther. Nucl. Med. **123:**49-54, 1975.
†Recurrences at 21, 23, 44, and 64 months. All had definite postexcisional residual disease.

radiotherapy of an initially clinically normal neck. They could detect no difference in control rates of the various histologic types. More than 50% of those patients irradiated primarily or for known residual cancer died from distant metastases.

There will be a need for primary irradiation for a substantial proportion of patients with cancer of major and minor salivary glands. For such patients the results just quoted are the best that can be expected. However, the more common sequence of treatment for cancers of the salivary gland will be excision with postoperative radiation being considered for those patients with the indications listed on p. 140. The control rates for such patients obtained by Fu and associates are given in Table 4-8. The failure rates from irradiating these patients are given in Table 4-9. These data are meager, but they are the best we have, and they are adequate to support the argument for postoperative radiation in any patient with a recognized increased risk of local recurrence. We also recommend postoperative irradiation to the neck after radical neck dissection has been done for those patients who have clinical evidence of disease in the neck. There are no data to indicate the efficacy of this form of postoperative irradiation.

The principles of postoperative irradiation just described are also applied to cancers of the minor salivary glands, the oral cavity, paranasal sinuses, and the like. Some details of the management of these problems are discussed in those sections dealing with the particular anatomic sites.

Metastases from adenoid cystic carcinoma may occasionally grow very slowly and may produce few or no symptoms. At times they have shown surprising radiosensitivity. For this reason such metastases should be irradiated as they appear, with the appreciation that survival may extend for years (Lampe and Zatzkin). Doses of about 3500 to 4000 rad in 3 to 4 weeks have been sufficient.

REFERENCES

Ackerman, L. V.: Verrucous carcinoma of the oral cavity, Surgery 23:670-678, 1948.

American Joint Committee for Cancer Staging and End Results Reporting: Clinical staging system for carcinoma of the oral cavity, Chicago, 1977, The Committee.

Ange, D. W., Lindberg, R. D., and Guillamondegui, O. M.: Management of squamous cell carcinoma of the oral tongue and floor of mouth after excisional biopsy, Radiology 116:143-146, 1975.

Baclesse, F.: Carcinoma of the larynx, Br. J. Radiol., suppl. 3, 1949.

Ballantyne, A. J., and Fletcher, G. H.: Management of residual or recurrent cancer following radiation therapy for squamous cell carcinoma of the oropharynx, Am. J. Roentgenol. 93:29-35, 1965.

Barkley, H. T., and Fletcher, G. H.: The significance of residual disease after external irradiation of squamous-cell carcinoma of the oropharynx, Radiology 124:493-495, 1977.

Bedwinek, J. M., Shukovsky, L. J., Fletcher, G. H., and Daley, T. E.: Osteonecrosis in patients treated with definitive radiotherapy for squamous cell carcinomas of the oral cavity and naso- and oropharynx, Radiology 119:665-667, 1976.

Benak, S., Buschke, F., and Galante, M.: Treatment of carcinoma of the oral cavity, Radiology 96:137-143, 1970.

Bergonié, J., and Speder, E.: Sur quelques formes de reactions précoces âpres des irradiations rontgen, Arch. électr. Med. 19:241-245, 1911.

Bonanni, G., and Perazzi, F.: Variations of taste sensitivity in patients subjected to high energy irradiation for tumor of the oral cavity, Nunt. Radiol. 31:383-397, 1965.

Buschke, F., and Galante, M.: Radical preoperative roentgen therapy in primarily inoperable advanced cancers of the head and neck, Radiology 73:845-848, 1959.

Buschke, F., and Vaeth, J. M.: Radiation therapy of carcinoma of the vocal cord without mucosal reaction, Am. J. Roentgenol. 89:29-34, 1963.

Campos, J. L., Lampe, I., and Fayos, J. V.: Radiotherapy of carcinoma of the floor of the mouth, Radiology 99:677-682, 1971.

Cherry, C. P., and Glucksmann, A.: Injury and repair following irradiation of salivary glands in male rats, Br. J. Radiol. 32:596-608, 1959.

Coutard, H.: Sur les délais d'apparition et d'evolution des reactions de la peau, et des muqueuses de la boûche et du pharynx, provoquées par les rayons X, Compt. rend. Soc. de biol. 86:1140-1141, 1922.

Dalley, V. M.: The place of radiotherapy in the treatment of tumors of the base of the tongue, Am. J. Roentgenol. 93:20-28, 1965.

del Regato, J. A.: Dental lesions observed after roentgentherapy in cancer of the buccal cavity, pharynx, and larynx, Am. J. Roentgenol. 42:404-410, 1939.

del Regato, J. A.: Roentgen therapy of carcinoma of the lower lip, Radiology 51:499-508, 1948.

del Regato, J. A.: Cancer of the respiratory system and upper digestive tract. In del Regato, J. A., and Spjut, H. J.: Ackerman and del Regato's cancer: diagnosis, treatment, and prognosis, ed. 5, St. Louis, 1977, The C. V. Mosby Co.

del Regato, J. A., and Sala, J. M.: The treatment of carcinoma of the lower lip, Radiology 73:839-844, 1959.

English, J. A., Wheatcroft, M. C., Lyon, H. W., and Miller, C.: Long-term observations of radiation changes in salivary glands and the general effects of 1,000 R to 1,750 R of x-ray radiation locally administered to the heads of dogs, Oral Surg. 8:87-99, 1955.

Ennuyer, A., and Bataini, J. P.: Les tumeurs de l'amygdale et de la region vélopalatine, Paris, 1956, Masson et Cie.

Evans, J. C., and Ackerman, L. V.: Submaxillary irradiated and obstructed salivary glands simulating cervical lymph node metastasis, Radiology 62:550-555, 1954.

Fayos, J. V., and Lampe, I.: Radiotherapy of squamous cell carcinoma of the oral portion of the tongue, Arch. Surg. 94:316-321, 1967.

Fayos, J. V., and Lampe, I.: Radiation therapy of carcinoma of the tonsillar region, Am. J. Roentgenol. 111:85-94, 1971.

Fayos, J. V., and Lampe, I.: The therapeutic problems of metastatic neck adenopathy, Am. J. Roentgenol. 114:65-75, 1972.

Fletcher, G. H.: Textbook of radiotherapy, Philadelphia, 1973, Lea & Febiger.

Fletcher, G. H., and Evers, W. T.: Radiotherapeutic management of surgical recurrences and postoperative residuals in tumors of the head and neck, Radiology 95:185-188, 1970.

Fletcher, G. H., and Stovall, M.: A study of the explicit distribution of radiation in interstitial implantations, Radiology 78:766-782, 1962.

Frank, R. M., Herdley, J., and Phillippe, E.: Acquired dental defects and salivary gland lesions after irradiation for carcinoma, J. Am. Dent. Assoc. 70:868-883, 1965.

Fu, K. K., Chan, E. K., Phillips, T. L., and Ray, J. W.: Time, dose and volume factors in interstitial radium implants of carcinoma of the oral tongue, Radiology 119:209-213, 1976.

Fu, K. K., Leibel, S. A., Levine, M. L., Friedlander, L. M., Boler, R., and Phillips, T. L.: Carcinoma of the major and minor salivary glands, Cancer 40:2882-2890, 1977.

Fu, K. K., Lichter, A., and Galante, M.: Carcinoma of the floor of mouth: an analysis of treatment results and the sites and causes of failures, Int. J. Radiat. Oncol. Biol. Phys. 1:829-837, 1976.

Gelinas, M., and Fletcher, G. H.: Incidence and causes of local failure of irradiation in squamous cell carcinoma of the faucial arch, tonsillar fossa

and base of the tongue, Radiology 108:383-387, 1973.

Gilbert, E. H., Goffinet, D. R., and Bagshaw, M. A.: Carcinoma of the oral tongue and floor of mouth: fifteen years experience with linear accelerator therapy, Cancer 35:1517-1524, 1975.

Gladstone, W. S., and Kerr, H. D.: Epidermoid carcinoma of the lower lip: results of radiation therapy of the local lesion, Am. J. Roentgenol. 79:101-114, 1958.

Glucksmann, A., and Cherry, C. P.: Effects of irradiation on salivary glands in pathology of irradiation. In Berjis, C. C., editor: Pathology of irradiation, Baltimore, 1971, The Williams & Wilkins Co.

Goffinet, D. R., Martinez, A., Palos, B., Fee, W., and Bagshaw, M. A.: A method of interstitial tonsillo-palatine implants, Int. J. Radiat. Oncol. Biol. Phys. 2:155-162, 1977.

Greenberg, B. E.: Cervical lymph node metastasis from unknown primary sites: unresolved problem in management, Cancer 19:1091-1095, 1966.

Griffin, T. W., Gerdes, A. J., Simko, T. G., and Parker, R. G.: Peroral irradiation for limited carcinoma of the oral cavity, Int. J. Radiat. Oncol. Biol. Phys. 2:333-335, 1977.

Guillamondegui, O. M., Byers, R. M., Luna, M. A., Chiminzaao, H., Jesse, R. H., and Fletcher, G. H.: Aggressive surgery in treatment for parotid cancer: the role of adjunctive postoperative radiotherapy, Am. J. Roentgenol. Radium Ther. Nucl. Med. 123:49-54, 1975.

Hanks, G. E., Bagshaw, M. A., and Kaplan, H. S.: The management of cervical lymph node metastases by megavoltage radiotherapy, Am. J. Roentgenol. 105:74-82, 1969.

Hendrickson, F. R.: Radiation problems in integrated therapy of the orthopharynx and larynx. In Rush, B. F., and Greenlaw, R. H., editors, Cancer therapy by integrated radiation and operation, Springfield, Ill., 1968, Charles C Thomas, Publisher.

Henschke, U., Hilaris, B., Frazell, E., Tollefson, H., and Strong, E.: Preoperative radiation therapy and radical neck dissection. In Rush, B. F., and Greenlaw, R. H., editors: Cancer therapy by integrated radiation and operation, Springfield, Ill., 1968, Charles C Thomas, Publisher.

Hinds, E. C.: Dental care and oral hygiene before and after treatment, J.A.M.A. 215:964-966, 1971.

Hornback, N. B., and Shidnia, H.: Carcinoma of the lower lip, Cancer 41:352-357, 1978.

Jesse, R. H., and Fletcher, G. H.: Metastases in cervical lymph nodes from oropharyngeal carcinoma, Am. J. Roentgenol. 90:990-996, 1963.

Jesse, R. H., Perez, C. A., and Fletcher, G. H.: Cervical lymph node metastasis: unknown primary cancer, Cancer **31**:854-859, 1973.

Kashima, H. K., Kirkham, W. R., and Andrews, J. R.: Postirradiation sialadenitis; a study of the clinical features, histopathologic changes and serum enzyme variations following irradiation of human salivary glands, Am. J. Roentgenol. **94**:271-292, 1965.

Keys, H. M., and McCasland, J. P.: Techniques and results of a comprehensive dental care program in head and neck cancer patients, Int. J. Radiat. Oncol. Biol. Phys. **1**:859-865, 1976.

Kimeldorf, D. J.: Radiation-induced alterations in odontogenesis and formed teeth in pathology of irradiation. In Berjis, C. C., editor: Pathology of irradiation, Baltimore, 1971, The Williams & Wilkins Co.

King, J. J., and Fletcher, G. H.: Malignant tumors of the major salivary glands, Radiology **100**:381-384, 1971.

Krantz, S., Berger, I. R., and Brown, P. F.: Results of treatment of carcinoma of lower lip, Am. J. Roentgenol. **78**:780-789, 1957.

Kraus, F. T., and Perez-Mesa, C.: Verrucous carcinoma: clinical and pathologic study of 105 cases involving oral cavity, larynx, and genitalia, Cancer **19**:26-38, 1966.

Kurtisin, I. T.: Effects of ionizing radiation on the digestive system, New York, 1963, Elsevier Publishing Co.

Lacassagne, A., and Gricouroff, G.: Action des radiations ionisantes sur l'organisme, Paris, 1956, Masson et Cie.

Lampe, I.: Radiation therapy of cancer of the buccal mucosa and lower gingiva, Am. J. Roentgenol. **73**:628-635, 1955.

Lampe, I.: The place of radiation therapy in the treatment of carcinoma of the lower lip, Plast. Reconstr. Surg. **24**:34-44, 1959.

Lampe, I.: Radiotherapeutic experience with squamous cell carcinoma of the oral part of the tongue, Univ. Mich. Med. Center J. **33**:215-218, 1967.

Lampe, I., and Zatzkin, H.: Pulmonary metastases of pseudoadenomatous basal cell carcinoma (mucous and salivary gland tumor), Radiology **53**:379-385, 1949.

Lindberg, R., and Jesse, R. H.: Treatment of cervical lymph node metastasis from primary lesions of the oropharynx, supraglottic larynx and hypopharynx, Am. J. Roentgenol. **102**:132-137, 1968.

Lyall, D., and Grier, R. N.: Experiences with squamous carcinoma of the lip with special reference to the role of neck dissection, Ann. Surg. **152**:1067-1070, 1960.

Marcial, V., and Frias, Z.: Pilot study of dose fractionation in carcinoma of the base of the tongue: uninterrupted vs. split-course irradiation, Am. J. Roentgenol. **108**:30-36, 1970.

McComb, W. S.: Diagnosis and treatment of metastatic cervical cancerous nodes from an unknown primary site, Am. J. Surg. **124**:441-449, 1972.

Meredith, W. J., editor: Radium dosage, the Manchester system, ed. 2, Edinburgh, 1967, E. & S. Livingstone, Ltd.

Million, R. B., Fletcher, G. H., and Jesse, R. H.: Evaluation of elective irradiation of the neck for squamous cell carcinoma of the nasopharynx, tonsillar fossa, and base of tongue, Radiology **80**: 973-988, 1963.

Modlin, J., and Johnson, R. E.: The surgical treatment of cancer of the buccal mucosa and lower gingiva, Am. J. Roentgenol. **73**:620-627, 1955.

Montana, G. S., Hellman, S., von Essen, C. F., and Kligerman, M. M.: Carcinoma of the tongue and floor of the mouth, Cancer **23**:1284-1289, 1969.

Ng, E., Chambers, F. W., Ogden, H. S., Coggs, G. C., and Crane, J. T.: Osteomyelitis of the mandible following irradiation, Radiology **72**: 68-74, 1959.

Northrop, M., Fletcher, G. H., Jesse, R. H., and Lindberg, R. D.: Evolution of neck disease in patients with primary squamous cell carcinoma of the oral tongue, floor of the mouth, and palatine arch, and clinically positive nodes neither fixed nor bilateral, Cancer **29**:23-30, 1972.

Paterson, R.: Treatment of malignant disease by radiotherapy, ed. 2, Baltimore, 1963, The Williams & Wilkins Co.

Perez, C. A., Ackerman, L. V., Mill, W. B., Ogura, J. H., and Powers, W. E.: Malignant tumors of the tonsil, Am. J. Roentgenol. **114**: 43-58, 1972.

Perez, C. A., Lee, F. A., Ackerman, L. V., Korba, A., Purdy, J., and Powers, W. E.: Carcinoma of the tonsillar fossa. Significance of dose of irradiation and volume treated in the control of the primary tumor and metastatic neck nodes, Int. J. Radiat. Oncol. Biol. Phys. **1**:817-827, 1976.

Perez, C. A., Mill, W. B., Ogura, J. H., and Powers, W. E.: Carcinoma of the tonsil: sequential comparison of four treatment modalities, Radiology **94**:649-659, 1970.

Phillips, T. L.: Peroral roentgen therapy, Radiology **90**:525-531, 1968.

Pierquin, B., Chassagne, D., and Cox, J. D.: Toward consistent local control of certain malignant tumors, Radiology **99**:661-667, 1971.

Porter, E. H.: The local prognosis after radical

radiotherapy for squamous carcinoma of the alveolus and of the floor of the mouth, Clin. Radiol. **22:**139-143, 1971.

Rafla-Demetrious, S.: Mucous and salivary gland tumours, Springfield, Ill., 1970, Charles C Thomas, Publisher.

Scanlon, P. W., Devine, K. D., Woolner, L. B., and McBean, J. B.: Cancer of the tonsil: 131 patients treated in the 11 year period 1950 through 1960, Am. J. Roentgenol. **100:**894-903, 1967.

Scanlon, P. W., Soule, E. H., Devine, K. D., and McBean, J. B.: Cancer of the base of the tongue, Am. J. Roentgenol. **105:**26-36, 1969.

Schneider, J. J., Fletcher, G. H., and Barkley, H. T.: Control by irradiation alone of nonfixed clinically positive lymph nodes from squamous cell carcinoma of the oral cavity, oropharynx, supraglottic larynx, and hypopharynx, Am. J. Roentgenol. Radium Ther. Nucl. Med. **123:**42-48, 1975.

Shannon, I. R., Trodahl, J. N., and Starcke, E. N.: Remineralization of enamel by a saliva substitute designed for use by irradiated patients, Cancer **41:**1746-1750, 1978.

Shukovsky, L. J., and Fletcher, G. H.: Time-dose and tumor volume relationships in the irradiation of squamous cell carcinoma of the tonsillar fossa, Radiology **107:**621-626, 1973.

Silverstone, S. M., and Goldman, J. L.: Combined therapy, irradiation and surgery, for advanced cancer of the laryngopharynx, Am. J. Roentgenol. **90:**1023-1031, 1963.

Southwick, H. W.: Elective neck dissection for intraoral cancer, J.A.M.A. **217:**454-455, 1971.

Spanos, W. J., Shukovsky, L. J., and Fletcher, G. H.: Time, dose, and tumor volume relationships in irradiation of squamous cell carcinomas of the base of the tongue, Cancer **37:**2591-2599, 1976.

Swearingen, A. G., McGraw, J. P., and Palumbo, V. D.: Roentgenographic pathologic correlation of carcinoma of the gingiva involving the mandible, Radiology **96:**15-18, 1966.

van den Brenk, H. A. S., Hurley, R. A., Gomez, C., and Richter, W.: Serum amylase as a measure of salivary gland radiation damage, Br. J. Radiol. **42:**688-700, 1969.

Votava, C., Fletcher, G. H., Jesse, R. H., and Lindberg, R. D.: Management of cervical nodes, either fixed or bilateral, from squamous cell carcinoma of the oral cavity and faucial arch, Radiology **105:**417-420, 1972.

Wang, C. C.: Malignant lymphoma of the Waldeyer's ring, Radiology **92:**1335-1339, 1969.

Wang, C. C.: Primary malignant lymphoma of oral cavity and paranasal sinuses, Radiology **100:**151-153, 1971.

Watson, T. A.: Irradiation in the management of tumors of the head and neck, Am. J. Surg. **110:**542-548, 1965.

Wizenberg, M. J., Bloedorn, F. G., Weiner, S., and Gracia, J. R.: Treatment of lymph node metastases in head and neck cancer, Cancer **29:**1455-1462, 1972.

Wizenberg, M. J., Bloedorn, F. G., Weiner, S., and Gracia, J. R.: Radiation therapy in management of lymph node metastases from head and neck cancers, Am. J. Roentgenol. **114:**76-82, 1972.

5

The orbit

RESPONSE OF NORMAL ORBITAL STRUCTURES TO IRRADIATION

The composite character of the eye precludes a meaningful single statement about its radiosensitivity. The cornea, the ciliary apparatus, the lens, and the retina should be considered separately. In addition, radiation-induced changes in structures affecting vision indirectly, such as the eyelashes, eyelids, lacrimal glands, and the nasolacrimal apparatus, contribute significantly to the bulb changes. The cellular kinetics vary widely among these tissues, and the magnitude of damage is measured in terms of that tissue's usual function.

EYELASHES. The eyelashes serve as end organs of touch. Their contact with tiny particles initiates a blink that protects the eye. Irradiation epilates the lash and thus abolishes this protective reflex. The result is an increased irritation of the conjunctiva and corneal surfaces. Doses of the level of 2300 to 2800 rad in 2 weeks with 100 kv radiations will produce permanent epilation. The eyelash is spared by megavoltage beams so that it may remain at least partially intact even after maximum doses of 5000 to 6000 rad deep to the lid. Like hair elsewhere, an epilated lash may regrow a different color and in its new growth is frequently sparse and short. Although radiations could arrest the growth of troublesome hairs that turn inward to irritate the cornea, simpler and less risky means are available and should be used.

EYELID. The eyelid is covered by the thinnest skin in the body. The mucosa is similarly very delicate. This permits relatively effortless and rapid motion of the lid. Any inflammatory or fibrosing process will decrease the flexibility of the lid and thus decrease its effectiveness. Caustically applied high doses of radiations will produce contracture and deformity with all of their serious sequelae. In contrast, carefully applied fractionated irradiation can nearly always be carried to cancerocidal doses without serious permanent changes. Naturally, the frequency of serious permanent changes is decisive in selecting the treatment of choice. Irradiation of an ectropic lid produces the changes shown in Fig. 5-1. High doses given in the treatment of carcinoma of the lower lid produce acute changes similar to those seen in the mucosa of the oral cavity. An initial erythema is followed by false membrane formation well ahead of comparable skin changes. Healing of the mucosa occurs early, and usually there are no permanent gross changes marking the site of the treatment. Deformity

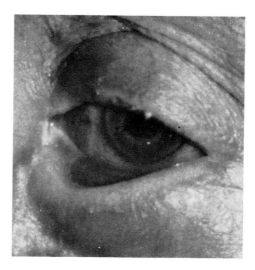

Fig. 5-1. Epidermatization of conjunctival surface of lower eyelid. The patient had a severe ectropion of the lower eyelid. Irradiation was given for an extensive basal cell carcinoma infiltrating the lid. In the process of healing, epidermis extended on to conjunctival surface. This is to be expected when an ectropion is present at time of treatment. It produces no additional symptoms.

of the lid margin may irritate the cornea and over a period of time produce serious damage. Changes in the upper lid are much more serious in this regard than changes in the lower lid. When the tarsus is included in the irradiated volume and given doses of 4000 to 5000 rad in 4 to 5 weeks, it gradually becomes thinner, but lid function is not significantly altered.

LACRIMAL GLAND. The lacrimal gland exhibits a radiosensitivity not unlike that of the salivary gland. In the rabbit, single doses of 3800 rad reduced the lacrimal gland to about half its original weight but produced no striking histologic changes (Cogan and associates). However, with whole orbital irradiation a cessation of or a decrease in lacrimal secretion does occur, and this is a much more serious sequela than alterations in saliva secretion (Hartmann and Fontaine). Tears not only lubricate the globe but also continuously wash its exposed surface. A dry eye deteriorates rapidly. Vision decreases within a short time, and pain may be so severe as to demand enucleation. In any case, corneal irritation that follows the loss of tears and loss of function of the numerous small lid glands leads to progressive corneal opacity. If the cornea is also in the treated volume, it may be difficult to define the relative contribution of direct corneal irradiation and lacrimal gland irradiation to the corneal changes. Loss of lacrimal gland function was formerly a major factor in the initiation of postirradiation corneal changes. Artificial tears greatly decrease the dangers and irritation resulting from a dry eye. In the earlier years of radiation therapy, the fact that irradiation could suppress tear formation was used clinically in the treatment of epiphora. Such a procedure is no longer indicated, and we have had no experience with it.

NASOLACRIMAL DUCT AND SAC. This drainage system for tears is lined with stratified squamous and pseudostratified columnar epithelium. After cancerocidal doses, desquamation of this epithelium and the associated inflammation may occasionally lead to duct obstruction. Such changes may occur subsequent to the irradiation of lesions of the medial canthus and the medial aspect of the lower lid or extensive lesions of the upper air passages. However, in our experience the production of this sequela by irradiation alone is infrequent. This has also been the experience of others (Renfer; Wildermuth and Evans). The ability to preserve duct function has been a rather strong argument in favor of the use of roentgentherapy in treating patients with malignant lesions near or involving the nasolacrimal duct and sac.

CORNEA. Blood vessels normally extend to the limbus but not into the cornea. The various layers of the cornea, including its outermost layer of stratified squamous epithelium and its thick connective tissue layer, are avascular. Therefore radiation-induced corneal changes do not depend on vascular injury but depend solely on disruption of mitotic activity in the epithelial and connective tissue layers. Clinical manifestations of injury are slow in appearing and require high doses. Severe radiation-induced corneal damage is characterized by inflammatory reaction of limbal vessels, punctate keratitis, corneal ulceration, and edema. Such damage is much more likely to occur if secondary infection is present, if there is simultaneous use of systemic 5-fluorouracil (Chan and Shukovsky), or if there is simultaneous damage to the lids or lacrimal glands. We have not seen such a reaction of the cornea in many years. There is no question but that the skin-sparing characteristics of ^{60}Co and megavoltage beams are corneal-sparing if in treating the orbit from the anterior aspect the patient keeps his eyes open. X rays produced by very low voltages (Grenz rays) and beta rays from ^{90}Sr confine almost all their effects to the cornea. With such beams damage to deeper structures is possible, of course, but only after corneal doses considerably beyond those usually recommended.

The epithelium covering the anterior surface of the cornea may develop tiny ulcers (punctate keratitis) after doses of 3000 to 5000 rad in 3 to 5 weeks. The keratitis may begin during or several weeks after irradiation. These areas can be seen when stained with fluorescein. The patient complains of irritation and lacrimation. The areas will usually heal in several weeks with appropriate ophthalmologic care. Rarely, these tiny areas coalesce to produce a corneal ulcer. Merriam and associates reported the development of three severe corneal ulcerations in twenty-five patients given 6000 rad to the orbital area in 5 to 6 weeks. These changes appeared 4 to 12 months postirradiation, and in two patients the cornea perforated.

Chan and Shukovsky reported that 6000 rad in 6 weeks (as given for cancer of the paranasal sinuses) produced corneal lesions in 15% of patients during a 2-year follow-up period. When systemic 5-fluorouracil was used in conjunction with the irradiation, all patients developed serious corneal ulceration.

Edema of the corneal stroma is highly variable and may appear after doses of 3000 to 5000 rad given in 3 to 5 weeks. With still higher doses (8000 rad in 8 weeks), the edema may be severe and prolonged. Usually, however, it is transient and subsides within a month.

Surface applicators and beta ray therapy. Doses from beta rays are naturally the surface doses and are also the maximum doses. Krohmer has made measurements on a variety of applicators and has emphasized the importance of calibrating each applicator in terms of rep at contact. This corrects for structural differences. The cornea is but 1 mm thick and is covered by an epithelium that is relatively radiosensitive. Mitotic activity of the corneal epithelium is interrupted with doses of 50 to 90 rad. Higher doses damage sensation of the corneal epithelium, and there is loss of sensitivity. A single dose of beta radiations of 1000 rad will produce superficial keratitis. This appears after a latent period of several weeks and will generally subside without being noticed clinically and without serious sequelae. Single doses up to 5000 rad produce punctate keratitis lasting 4 to 6 weeks (Merriam). Higher doses of 20,000 to 30,000 rad will produce the severe late changes of ulceration and still later keratinization and telangiectasis of the cornea. There will also be changes of the deeper structures, which are discussed later. The production of late corneal changes is never justified in the treatment of benign conditions. For this reason doses from beta plaques should remain below 5000 rad.

THE LENS. The lens is a highly transparent avascular, living organ. The fibers that compose its major portion, the lens cortex, are parts of living cells whose nuclei are near the lenticular equator and the anterior lens epithelium. Anteriorly, the fibers are covered by a single layer of cuboidal cells, and these are in turn covered by the capsule of the lens. The older, less viable cells near the periphery (equator) are shifted toward the center of the lens and there, after water loss and changes in chemical composition, form the more dense lens nucleus. The metabolism of the lens is unique, resulting from the fact that the lens is living tissue but does not actually perform work and is avascular.

The more centrally located cells of the anterior epithelial layer have the capacity to proliferate, but they normally seldom do so. By contrast, the more peripherally located cuboidal cells—those just anterior to the equator of the lens—show active proliferation that diminishes in rate from fetal life to old age. The newly produced daughter cells at this zone of proliferation migrate peripherally along the anterior surface of the lens toward the equator. After progressively elongating and turning so that their long axes are parallel to existing lens fibers, these cells are modified to become and function as fibers in the lens cortex (Fig. 5-2). As newer fibers are developed, the older fibers are pressed toward the center of the lens.

In most proliferating cell systems, dead or defective cells are removed either by shedding (epidermis) or by absorption (hemopoietic tissues). In the case of the lens, matured cells are retained within the lens capsule and form the important refractory elements of the lens. Defective fibers are not absorbed and have a low capacity for repair. Injuring them either by direct or indirect means may initiate cataracts.

Two mechanisms for radiation induction of cataracts have been considered. Irradiation of the proliferating cells near the equator almost certainly produces irreversible defects in those cells destined to become lens fibers. With low doses of radiations (less than 1000 rad single dose), the length of the latent period between irradiation

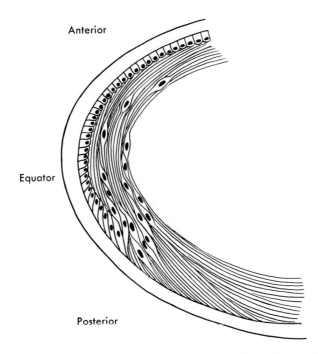

Anterior

Equator

Posterior

Fig. 5-2. Diagram illustrating cell pattern near equator of lens, which permits radiation-induced cell damage to be carried to interior of lens. See text.

and the appearance of defects suggests that injury to these cells is important in the sequence of cataract production. With higher doses, a "metabolic deficit" develops in the cortical fibers (Bateman). This is presumably secondary to injury of the anterior lens epithelium that normally serves as a portal of entry for the metabolic requirements of the lens fibers. Defects appear in such zones of metabolic deficit well before any damage to the germinal cell epithelium could account for them. With both of these mechanisms the defects mentioned are thought to be early steps in the development of cataracts.

Clinical observations. The observed clinical sequence of radiation-induced cataract formation has been supplemented and confirmed by animal studies. Much of the following is taken from the reports of Cogan and associates and Merriam and Focht. The first clinical sign of lens change is the appearance of many vesicles or discrete dots predominantly in the posterior cortex. These seem to be defects in the fibers and are dose related. Later on opacity appears near the posterior pole. It enlarges slowly as tiny vacuoles and granules appear in the surrounding fibers. The process may stop at this point or it may progress. In progressing, the opacity near the posterior pole enlarges to several millimeters in diameter, and additional vacuoles and granules appear in the anterior cortex. Later these defects seem to coalesce to form a single large opacity. The clinically recognized cataract is presumably composed of these various manifestations of injury.

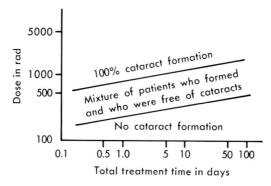

Fig. 5-3. Plot on log scale of the dose-time relationships for production of radiation-induced cataracts. (Modified from Merriam, G. R., Szechter, A., and Focht, E. F.: The effect of ionizing radiations on the eye. In Vaeth, J. M., editor: Radiation effects and tolerance, normal tissue, Baltimore, 1970, University Park Press.)

Table 5-1. Dose-time relationships for radiation-induced cataracts*

Overall time of treatment	Minimum cataractogenic dose	Maximum dose given without cataract formation
Single dose	200	175
3 weeks to 3 months	400	1000
Longer than 3 months	550	1100

*From Merriam, G. R., and Focht, E. F.: Am. J. Roentgenol. **77**:759, 1957.

In this same period the anterior lens epithelium near the anterior pole responds to radiation injury by localized cellular proliferation, thus producing a subcapsular haze.

Dose-time relationships for cataract formation. The higher the dose of radiations, the shorter the latent period between irradiation and the appearance of the cataract (Table 5-1 and Fig. 5-3). Merriam and Focht reviewed the literature and published their own material on this subject as related to man. Their data included all cataracts regardless of whether vision was impaired. The separation of their patients into many groups resulted in rather small samples. Even so, theirs are the best data available for man. They found the minimum cataractogenic dose of x rays in man to be 200 rad if given in a single irradiation, 400 rad if fractionated over 3 weeks to 3 months, and 550 rad if fractionated over 3 months. The latent period may be very long with these low doses.

We believe only a small proportion of all patients given doses of these levels will develop visual defects. About a third of all patients getting 750 to 950 rad to the lens fractionated over 3 weeks to 3 months will eventually develop visual defects due to cataracts. Many of these will be minor. A dose of 1150 rad after a sufficient latent period (sometimes many years) produces cataracts 100% of the time regardless of fractionation, but vision will not be totally lost.

The lens is definitely more sensitive in very young children than in adults. Thus for children the latent period is not only shorter for cataract development, but with a given dose the incidence of cataract development will be greater.

When comparing the cataractogenic properties of single-dose versus fractionated-dose irradiation, it is obvious that effects are diminished with fractionation (Fig. 5-3).

The study cited previously suggests that the lens is indeed highly sensitive to radiations, but to many persons this report has hardly seemed in keeping with our clinical impressions. Parker and associates could find but four radiation-induced cataracts in eighty-five lenses after doses of 2040 to 3900 rad given over 46 to 85 days. Only two of eighty-five eyes showed grossly diminished visual acuity. The doses of these two eyes were 3570 and 3900 rad. Doses of 6000 rad in 6 weeks produce serious vision-impairing cataracts in about 10% of the patients within 2 to 4 years. Of course, all such patients develop cataracts, but in the elderly, cataracts are slow to develop, and the latent period until vision loss is often several years. By contrast, within 2 years, over 50% of the patients who have 5-fluorouracil administered in conjunction with irradiation will have developed vision-impairing cataracts (Chan and Shukovsky). It is possible that total body irradiation may be sufficient to produce cataracts and yet permit survival. Thus among the survivors of the Japanese atomic bomb explosions, there were ninety-eight patients who developed cataracts. All but one patient had shown epilation, and most showed severe radiation reactions (Oughterson and Warren).

Beta rays from radioactive strontium are commonly used for selected benign corneal diseases. These electrons penetrate rather poorly, but at the periphery of the cornea about 10% of the surface dose reaches the lenticular equator. Surface doses of 5000 rad near the limbus may deliver a cataractogenic dose to the lens. Nearer the center of the cornea much less dose reaches the lenticular equator, and the risk of cataractogenesis is greatly decreased (Thomas and associates).

With these guides, lens changes can be predicted when eye irradiation is necessary and the requirements of lead shielding calculated when eye protection is possible. If it is necessary to irradiate the lens, cataract formation must be accepted as the price of the cure for cancer. If radiation-induced cataracts develop, they are amenable to the same type of surgery as other types of cataracts (Reese).

Neutrons are particularly cataractogenic (Evans), and as neutron therapy has become available, lens sensitivity has had to be reckoned with. The sensitivity is also of considerable importance to cyclotron workers and to workers in industry. Riley and associates and Upton and associates compared the relative effectiveness of neutrons and x rays in producing cataracts in mice. After establishing a standard degree of opacification, they found that a higher dose is required with x rays than with neutrons (Fig. 5-4). This ratio changes with the energy of the neutron and is variable among species. It is anticipated that use of neutron beams in radiotherapy will justify even more careful lens shielding than is now necessary with x rays or gamma rays.

RETINA. Although the retina is highly sensitive to electromagnetic radiations in

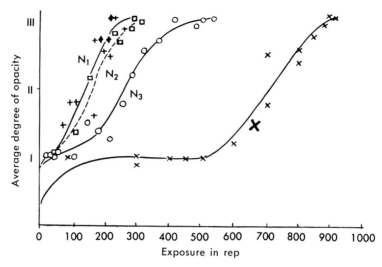

Fig. 5-4. Average degree of relative opacity observed 1 year after a single dose exposure to neutrons or x-radiations. N_1, "Low-energy" neutrons (diamonds = fission; plus signs = 37-inch cyclotron); N_2, "intermediate-energy" neutrons (squares = 60-inch cyclotron, 180 degrees); N_3, "high-energy" neutrons (circle = 60-inch cyclotron, beam center); X, 200 and 250 kvp x-radiations. (Redrawn from Riley, E. F., Evans, T. C., Rhody, R. B., Leinfelder, P. J., and Richards, R. D.: Radiology **67:**673-685, 1956.)

the visible light range, x rays and gamma rays are not perceived at the usual dose rates. Such radiations do, however, produce changes, first in the rods and later in the cones (Cibis and associates). A sensation of light does occur if the dose rate of radiations is sufficiently high. This sensation arises from the effect of x rays on the sensitive portion of the retina. Small changes may be produced in visual purple or in the neuron membranes. The electric response of the eye to illumination—the electroretinogram—is slowed by doses of x rays. Such changes are so small as to be unnoticed clinically. However, Gaffey was able to show that a single dose of 2000 rad promptly abolished the electroretinogram. Ophthalmoscopic examination revealed arteriolar constriction followed by a narrowing of retinal veins developing 6 to 8 hours after the electroretinographic changes.

In view of the greater sensitivity of rods in comparison to that of cones it might be expected that an appropriate dose of radiation would produce night blindness. This has not been described.

The optic tract requires about 100 times this dose to acutely block the response to a light stimulus. Late retinal changes have not been widely studied, primarily because the much more serious corneal and lenticular changes prevent adequate examination. With cancerocidal doses, narrowing of retinal vessels, together with chromatolysis of the ganglian cells, does occur (Cogan). The clinical importance of these changes is unknown. Late vascular changes in the retina are similar to those occurring in the skin and mucosa.

Retinal changes begin to appear with doses of 1000 to 3000 rad given in 1 week. Twenty percent of 119 patients given such retinal doses showed decreased visual acuity presumably secondary to blood vessel damage (Perrers-Taylor and associates). The injury is seen as vessel narrowing and with the dose levels mentioned above is usually of no clinical consequence. However, with higher doses the vessel narrowing may be protracted and may result in choroidal atrophy, modification of pigment distribution, and retinal degeneration; these are acceptable sequelae when retinal irradiation is unavoidable. The changes have not been a serious impediment to the use of the Stallard type of applicators, which deliver rather high doses to the retina in a few days. With doses of 5000 to 7000 rad, fragile telangiectatic vessels eventually form. Coughing or sneezing is frequently sufficient to rupture these vessels and to produce the retinal and vitreous hemorrhages often reported. These serious late sequelae with their resulting blindness were in part responsible for Reese's reduction of the dose recommended for retinoblastoma. At times it may be difficult to determine whether some of the changes such as retinal detachment are a result of the disease or of the irradiation.

The optic nerve and chiasma are encompassed in the high-dose volume used to irradiate cancers of the nasopharynx and nasal fossa. Radiation-induced changes in these critical structures are presented in Chapter 6.

UVEA. Irradiation to cancerocidal levels may produce an iridocyclitis resulting in an imbalance between aqueous production and absorption ending in glaucoma. Reese reported nine such instances. In selected patients, surgical procedures can relieve the tension and save the eye and vision. The severe pain may demand enucleation; if the eye is left in, spontaneous rupture of the globe with expulsion of the lens may occur. It should be remembered that an extensive tumor alone can produce glaucoma even if no irradiation is given. The pathogenesis of radiation-induced glaucoma has not been clarified, although it is thought to be related to changes in permeability of uveal vessels.

From the changes discussed previously, it is clear that when high doses to the orbit are necessary, radiation-induced damage to the eye and disturbance of vision are likely. However, even with doses of 5000 to 6000 rad in 5 to 6 weeks, years of useful vision may be retained if the dry eye and cataract can be cared for. Preirradiation enucleation is not justified purely on the basis of anticipated radiation damage. Tissues composing the eye do not seem to be prone to malignant change after irradiation. However, the same cannot be said for tissues forming the walls of the orbit. (See Chapter 21.)

DISEASES OF THE ORBITAL REGION TREATED BY IRRADIATION
Diseases of the eyelids

Diseases of the eyelids are discussed in Chapter 3.

Benign diseases of the cornea
CORNEAL VASCULARIZATION

The normal cornea contains no blood vessels or lymphatics. Its normal metabolic requirements are met chiefly by diffusion from the limbal capillaries and the aqueous humor. Most diseases of the cornea will result in some degree of its vascularization.

The new vessels begin as buds from the limbal loops and, depending on the etiologic factors, they may grow superficial or deep. The pattern of growth may likewise vary. Vessels may appear straight in interstitial keratitis or tortuous in keratoconjunctivitis. Once they have formed, they will always remain as evidence of the disease. Although there is considerable debate about their value as a healing aid, it is generally agreed that their presence decreases corneal transparency. Frequently the vessel ingrowth can be inhibited by appropriate irradiation. It is questionable, however, just how effective irradiation is in producing a regression of existing vessels (Michaelson and Schreiber). We believe that newly formed vessels may be quite sensitive and that vessels several weeks old are difficult to obliterate. If the corneal vascularization is just one manifestation of a generalized disease, irradiation is merely a part of the total patient care.

TECHNIQUE. Whether the newly formed vessels are superficial or deep in the cornea, the depths involved are minute compared to those usually encountered in therapeutic radiology. The cornea is but 0.95 mm thick in its center and 1.19 mm thick at its periphery. The anterior surface of the lens is slightly more than 2 mm from the posterior surface of the cornea. The lens usually measures 4 to 5 mm at its axis. These dimensions, with the relative penetration of various qualities of radiations, are shown in Fig. 5-5. In view of the proximity of the lens and the low dose required to produce a cataract, the need for special techniques is clear.

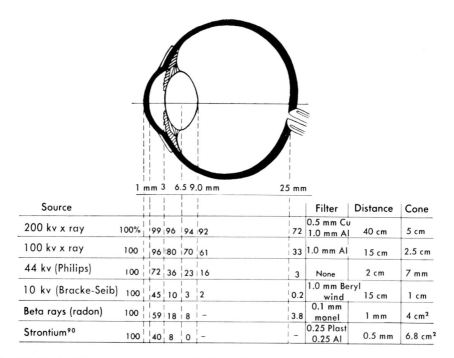

Source		1 mm	3	6.5	9.0 mm	25 mm		Filter	Distance	Cone
200 kv x ray	100%	99	96	94	92		72	0.5 mm Cu 1.0 mm Al	40 cm	5 cm
100 kv x ray	100	96	80	70	61		33	1.0 mm Al	15 cm	2.5 cm
44 kv (Philips)	100	72	36	23	16		3	None	2 cm	7 mm
10 kv (Bracke-Seib)	100	45	10	3	2		0.2	1.0 mm Beryl wind	15 cm	1 cm
Beta rays (radon)	100	59	18	8	–		3.8	0.1 mm monel	1 mm	4 cm²
Strontium⁹⁰	100	40	8	0	–		–	0.25 Plast 0.25 Al	0.5 mm	6.8 cm²

Fig. 5-5. Penetrability of various types of radiations with regard to the anatomic structures of the eye. (Modified from Sheie, H. G., et al.: Am. J. Ophthalmol. **33:**549-571, 1950.)

The distribution of dose essential for optimum corneal irradiation is almost ideally achieved with a beta ray plaque made of radioactive strontium. Its chief advantage is its lack of gamma radiations, making personnel protection simpler and lens dose less. The average energy of ^{90}Sr beta rays is 0.9 mev (including those of ^{90}Y). Their range in tissue is about 3.9 mm. With such plaques, surface doses up to 5000 rad have been recommended. We have used single doses of 500 rad weekly for 3 or 4 weeks.

Results are not uniformly good. Irradiation prevents or obliterates vessels after keratectomy and keratoplasty in about 40% of the cases. Ainslee and Snelling controlled corneal vascularization of corneal grafts in thirteen of sixteen patients by giving several doses of 400 to 500 rad 2 to 7 weeks postoperatively. Some radiations reach the lens, and if surface doses are above 5000 rad, the incidence of lens damage increases rapidly. From 3600 to 7200 rad, the incidence of lens changes is 20%; 7200 to 12,000 rad, 42.5%; and 12,000 rad or more, 73.3% (Thomas and associates). One must weigh these lens changes before administering doses above 5000 rad.

PTERYGIUM

An overall postsurgical recurrence rate of pterygium of 20% to 30% is common. Although routine postoperative irradiation is often mentioned (Van den Brenk), it is not commonly used in this country. Its major use is after the excision of a postoperative recurrence. Van den Brenk's experience indicates that 800 rad given at weekly intervals for 3 weeks is highly effective, that is, a recurrence rate of 1.4% in patients irradiated routinely after initial surgery and 6.1% recurrence in 115 patients irradiated after the excision of one or more postoperative recurrences. There seems to be rather wide flexibility in the radiation techniques. We have used 500 rad (surface dose with ^{90}Sr applicator) every other day for 3 days, but Van den Brenk's technique of 800 rad once a week for 3 weeks gives equally good results.

Exophthalmos of Graves' disease

Radiation therapy has been used to treat the exophthalmos of Graves' disease for 40 years. Such treatment is moderately effective in restoring vision and in diminishing the exophthalmos with little risk. There is general agreement that the exophthalmos is secondary to a massive collection of lymphocytes and fluid in the extraocular muscles. The etiology of this change is unclear, but it responds rapidly to irradiation. This supports the concept that it might be caused by an immune reaction to extraocular muscles with sensitized lymphocytes. Patients who develop exophthalmos acutely seem to respond more frequently to irradiation than those who develop it slowly (Donaldson and associates). Also a previous poor response to corticosteroid therapy is no indication that response to irradiation will be poor.

Radiation therapy of this disease consists of the administration of 2000 rad to the center of the orbits in 10 daily fractions. Small, individually shaped ports with secondary trimmers (ensuring minimal dose to both lenses) should be used. There may be a transient edema after the first few treatments, but symptomatic improvement occurs almost from the first treatment. Covington and associates reported improvement in five of seven patients, and Donaldson and associates reported excellent to good responses in fifteen of twenty-three patients (65%). Patients with long-standing exophthalmos and those with severe asymmetrical exophthalmos respond infrequently.

Malignant diseases of the orbital contents

With the exception of retinoblastoma, all primary intraocular malignant tumors are best treated surgically. The only possible excuse to irradiate eyes in patients with such lesions would be to preserve vision. This is not possible if the lesion is located in the anterior half of the bulb. Retinoblastoma is the only primary lesion of the posterior half of the bulb of sufficient radiosensitivity to permit eradication. Metastases of other cancers to the eye and orbit should be irradiated if their microscopic diagnosis suggests sufficient radiosensitivity. Extrabulbar orbital tumors are infrequent and invariably call for special techniques with individual tailoring for each patient.

CARCINOMA OF THE BULBAR CONJUNCTIVA

Carcinoma of the bulbar conjunctiva is a rather rare disease, but its treatment with irradiation is usually simple and effective. Nearly all lesions will be squamous cell in type, but an occasional basal cell carcinoma has been reported. Such lesions arise near or at the limbus and spread superficially to the sclera and less frequently to the cornea. Premalignant lesions may precede the development of cancer. The dense fibrous tissue that composes the sclera underlies these lesions. For this reason infiltration is regarded as a late manifestation. Usually the lesion will be superficial.

Either direct irradiation with 40 to 50 kv radiations or tangential irradiation with 100 kv radiations can control these lesions. By either technique, the entire thickness of the sclera can be irradiated to a cancerocidal dose without serious damage to the lens, lids, or lacrimal glands. Although a beta ray plaque has been advocated, it will obviously be inadequate if the lesion has any appreciable thickness. With low-voltage radiations, fractionated irradiation to doses of 5000 to 6000 rad in 3 weeks is usually sufficient. For thicker lesions, tangential beams using 100 to 120 kv radiations filtered with 0.25 mm Cu and 1 mm Al are preferable. Because of the greater homogeneity, somewhat lower surface doses are adequate. We have used 4500 to 5000 rad in 3 weeks, but Fayos and Wildermuth recommend doses of 3500 to 4000 rad in 4 to 5 days. Cure rates are good. By using tangential beams, Fayos and Wildermuth controlled six of seven small cancers for at least 5 years, and the seventh patient died without cancer. No cataracts developed. Less impressive control rates have been reported by simple excision; for example, Ash and Wilder controlled twenty-three of forty-eight cancers. Some of these cancers were more extensive, however. Surgery with enucleation is the only treatment for advanced lesions. Postoperative irradiation is indicated if the tumor has been transected.

TUMORS OF THE LACRIMAL GLAND

Histologically, tumors of the lacrimal gland are analogous to tumors occurring in the salivary glands. The method of treating tumors of the lacrimal gland is therefore usually surgical. The exceptions to this are lymphosarcomas, Hodgkin's disease, or transected carcinomas.

Although the surgical treatment of carcinomas of the lacrimal gland gives a disappointingly small proportion of cures, it is doubtful that radiotherapy could significantly improve the rate of control. However, there are no reliable data on this subject. We believe vigorous irradiation of the orbit is indicated in instances in which tumor is known to have been left behind. We have used the same dose as recommended for tumors of the salivary glands. Like carcinoma of the salivary glands, carcinoma of the lacrimal gland spreads along perineural spaces. Cancer may be well beyond the palpable margins of tumor. Ports with wide margins are therefore advisable. Irradiation of the clinically negative preauricular and cervical lymph nodes cannot be justified.

RHABDOMYOSARCOMA OF THE ORBIT

Rhabdomyosarcoma is the most common primary malignant tumor of the orbit during childhood. It is now recognized as being a radiosensitive and radiocurable tumor. The tumor tends to remain localized in the orbit more than rhabdomyosarcomas in other locations. Dose levels of 5000 rad in 5 weeks are adequate. The anterior and lateral ports are the most useful. Cassady and associates obtained a high incidence of local control, and a few patients were cured. (See Chapter 23.)

MALIGNANT LYMPHOMA OF THE ORBIT

Malignant lymphoma may involve the orbit primarily (Fig. 5-6), or it may involve the orbit as a part of generalized malignant lymphoma. It is bilateral in 15% to 30% of the patients (Kim and Fayos). When the disease is apparently confined to the orbits, the chances for long survival are good. About one half will have disseminated by the fifth year. Definition of tumor extent is usually impossible even after surgical exploration of the orbit. We have, therefore, used generous portals encompassing the entire orbit and a 2 cm margin. Anterior and lateral wedged beams are satisfactory. Every reasonable effort should be made to spare the vision. If possible, the lateral beam should be directed posteriorly to the lens, and a lens shield can be used with a wobbled anterior beam. A midorbital dose of 2500 rad in 2 to 3 weeks is adequate. The treatment of apparently uninvolved regional lymph node areas is not justified.

Survival in these patients has been good. Nine of ten patients lived at least 5 years in the series reported by Halman, and nine of nine patients lived at least 5 years in the series reported by Ahlstrom and associates. This long survival should be taken into consideration in planning treatment.

RETINOBLASTOMA

Retinoblastoma arises from the inner or the outer nuclear layer of the retina and expands into the vitreous or infiltrates into the retinal layers. Metastases to other structures within the bulb may occur through the vitreous. Spread beyond the bulb occurs chiefly by direct extension in the optic nerve through the lamina cribrosa (Fig. 5-7). This pathway permits extension to the subarachnoid space. Implants over

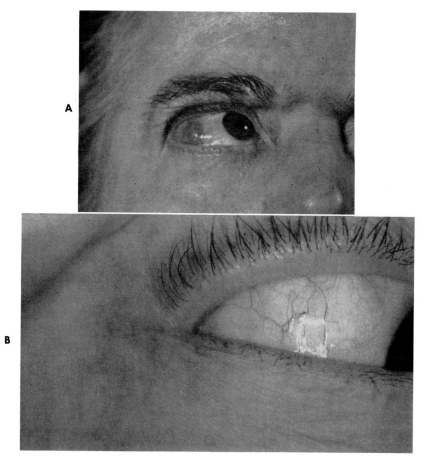

Fig. 5-6. A, Lymphosarcoma of the orbit also involving the sclera. This is highly radiosensitive. **B,** Four months after irradiation described in **A.** Vision was unimpaired at 6 months, although some future visual impairment is to be expected.

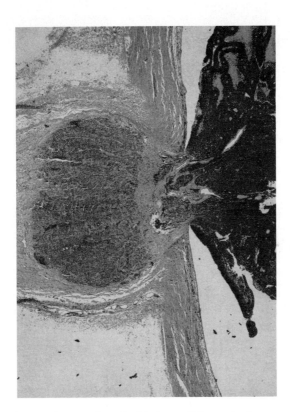

Fig. 5-7. Infiltration of the optic nerve by retinoblastoma. This emphasizes need for excision of as much of the nerve as is possible and importance of examining the cut end of the specimen. (From Smith, M. E.: The eyes and ocular adnexa. In Ackerman, L. V., and Rosai, J.: Surgical pathology, ed. 5, St. Louis, 1974, The C. V. Mosby Co.)

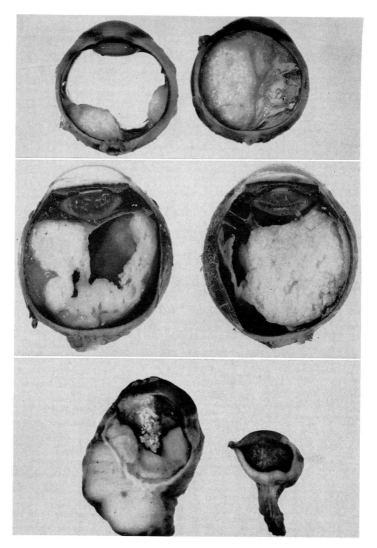

Fig. 5-8. Both eyes removed from three patients with bilateral retinoblastomas. Multiple foci of origin are present in the upper left section. The mass of tumor pushes the retina into the vitreous. Congenital defect of uninvolved eye is shown in the lower right. (From Hogen, M. J., and Zimmerman, L. E.: Ophthalmic pathology, Philadelphia, 1962, W. B. Saunders Co.)

the brain and spinal cord may follow. Spread may also occur through emissary veins to other orbital tissues. Multiple foci of origin are common (Fig. 5-8).

Generalized metastasis with or without extension to the brain is also common. Extracerebral metastases are most commonly seen in the subcutaneous tissues of the head and the preauricular lymph nodes (Gaitan-Yanguas). Reese found that of 116 eyes containing retinoblastoma, extension into the optic nerve occurred in thirty-two, or 27%. It was possible with surgery to encompass the optic nerve extension in

Table 5-2. Classification of retinoblastoma suggested by Reese* as related to survival from data as published by Tapley†

	Number of patients	Percent controlled
Group I: Very favorable	20	95
1. Solitary tumor, less than 4 disc diameter in size, at or behind equator		
2. Multiple tumors, none over 4 disc diameter in size, all at or behind equator		
Group II: Favorable	29	83
1. Solitary tumor, 4 to 10 disc diameter in size, at or behind equator		
2. Multiple tumors, 4 to 10 disc diameter in size, behind equator		
Group III: Doubtful	33	76
1. Any lesion anterior to equator		
2. Solitary tumors larger than 10 disc diameter behind equator		
Group IV: Unfavorable	17	71
1. Multiple tumors, some larger than 10 disc diameter		
2. Any lesion extending anteriorly to ora serrata		
Group V: Very unfavorable	59	32
1. Massive tumors involving over half of retina		
2. Vitreous seeding		

*Reese, A. B.: Tumors of the eye, New York, 1963, Harper & Row, Publishers, Inc.
†Tapley, N. duV.: Bilateral retinoblastoma combined treatment with irradiation and chemotherapy. In Vaeth, J. M., editor: Frontiers of radiation therapy and oncology, San Francisco, 1968, S. Karger A. G.

twenty-two of thirty-two. Autopsy on seventeen patients revealed the cause of death to be generalized metastases in seven, intracranial extension in nine, and extensive local infiltration in one (Merriam). Calcification within retinoblastoma is not uncommon. Most retinoblastomas will appear in children with no family history of retinoblastoma. However, parents who have been cured of retinoblastoma are very likely to find this disease in their children. Reese reported that eighteen survivors in his series had a total of thirty children, twenty-five of whom developed retinoblastomas. Manchester found that nineteen survivors had a total of thirty-six children, twelve of whom developed retinoblastomas. Proper examination of the offspring of these survivors should commence during infancy before symptoms appear. In the series of Bedford and associates the age at diagnosis was 8 months in those children with a positive family history compared to 17 months on the average for those with no family history. (For the hereditary aspects of this cancer see Knudson.)

If the disease is found in one eye, there is about a 20% chance that the other eye has or will develop a second retinoblastoma (Fig. 5-8). For the purpose of examination and follow-up, it is advisable to assume that the remaining eye is involved until proved otherwise. Since early treatment is of extreme importance, the children should be examined under general anesthesia with good pupil dilation. Size, number, and location of lesions all relate to prognosis (Table 5-2).

The usual lateral radiation beam is rarely carried anteriorly to the ora serrata unless there is obvious extension of retinoblastoma. Yet about one half of all postirradiation local recurrences are attributable to "occult" unirradiated tumor anterior to the ora serrata (Weiss and associates). This type of spread is very important in developing an optimum treatment plan.

TECHNIQUE, INDICATIONS, AND CONTRAINDICATIONS FOR IRRADIATION. The lesion is usually large when detected by the parent. The retina is more often than not rendered useless as far as future vision is concerned. At this stage radiotherapy would usually imply irradiation of the lens and uvea as well as the retina with little hope of useful vision. Under such circumstances surgery with excision of the longest possible section of optic nerve is indicated as the primary treatment of the extensive lesion. If the tumor is not cut through at the time of surgery, postoperative irradiation can hardly be justified. The chances are extremely remote that local tumor was unknowingly left behind (Reese).

If the tumor has been cut through, the orbit, the nerve stump, the region of the chiasma, and the whole brain should be irradiated (Fig. 5-9). The lateral and anterior beams with wedge filters will be most useful if the orbit only requires irradiation. A midorbital dose of 4500 rad in 4 weeks is adequate.

When a small retinoblastoma is found in the remaining eye or detected in the eye of a survivor's child, primary irradiation is indicated. Every technical effort should be made to spare the anterior third of the bulb in posterior lesions. With the single lateral port the lens can be shielded, the skin tumor distance is short, and the depth dose is high (Fig. 5-10). The dose to the most distant side of the eye is as previously mentioned. Meticulous beam definition, beam directioning, and patient immobilization are essential if the lens is to be spared while encompassing a maximum portion of the retina. An anterior beam as described by Weiss and associates should be used when the anterior one half of the retina requires irradiation. We have found ketamine a useful anesthetic for infants, but when used this requires a change from 5 to 3 fractions per week to avoid interference with nutrition. Bedford and associates, in a study of 139 cases of retinoblastoma, have emphasized the value of tailoring the treatment modalities to the degree of involvement of the retina, employing focal forms of therapy whether they be photocoagulation or ^{60}Co applicators for small lesions, ^{60}Co or megavoltage beams using a single anterior field for larger lesions or those showing multiple foci of origin or with vitreous seeding, and reserving enucleation only for those lesions with involvement of the optic nerve or failures of more conservative treatment. With external irradiation we employ a lateral beam only for those lesions with limited involvement of the posterior portion of the retina. It must be borne in mind that the effort to spare the lens, using a carefully positioned lateral beam, does indeed spare a portion of the retina and vitreous from irradiation. Concern for this unirradiated portion of the eye led Weiss and associates to develop a clever "central divergent lens block," which is positioned to cast a shadow over the lens during the use of an anterior beam. Combining such an anterior beam with the usual lateral beam eliminates the risk of having an unirradiated segment anteriorly. Fortunately, retinoblastoma is a relatively radiosensitive lesion. The effects of irradiation on the tumor are noticeable after 3 days of treatment, when the lesion

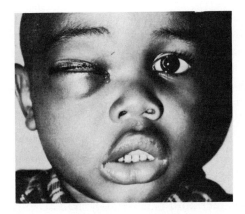

Fig. 5-9. Retinoblastoma recurrent in right orbit 3 months after enucleation.

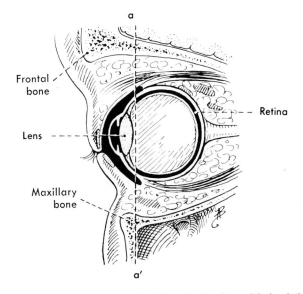

Fig. 5-10. Vertical section through the orbit showing bony landmarks and their relationship to lens and retina. Line **a--a'** marks anterior extent of retina. Note its proximity to posterior surface of lens.

becomes white. By 3 weeks, shrinkage is definitely noticeable. Regression continues slowly until only a flat white scar is left (Williams).

One might properly ask: "If irradiation with a view of sparing vision is optimum treatment for the patient who has already lost one eye, why is primary irradiation not optimum treatment for the initially involved eye?" As radiation oncologists have gained more confidence in the ability of radiations to locally eradicate this tumor, the indications for irradiating the initially involved eye have become stronger. Irradiation as the primary treatment of the initially involved, *potentially* useful eye is now indicated as the treatment of choice. The clinical picture is usually clear-cut, and no biopsy is necessary. We recommend radiotherapy primarily for either eye, provided there is a reasonable chance of useful vision. Bagshaw and Kaplan and Shidnia and associates have applied this concept with no increase of death rate and with definite increase in the proportion of useful eyes.

With a view of sparing normal tissues of the eye, surface applicators have been designed for placement on the sclera overlying the retinoblastoma (Rosengren and Tengroth; Stallard, 1966). Any possible superiority of such a surface applicator over external irradiation would depend on the following conditions.

1. The lesion must be unifocal.
2. No seeding must have occurred.
3. The maximum diameter of the lesion can be no greater than 10 mm.
4. The surface applicator must be accurately fixed over the lesion.
5. The dose to the anterior portion of the eye must be low.
6. If the lesion is near the optic disc, the ^{60}Co applicator cannot be used because of the risk of damaging the major retinal vessels.

Careful patient selection is essential. When irradiation was restricted to one lesion, multiple areas of involvement were seen in twenty-six of forty-three (60%) eyes (Stallard, 1966). Unfortunately, it is impossible to accurately compare the results obtained with the surface applicator with those obtained by modern external irradiation. Patients selected for treatment with the surface applicator have the more limited, favorable lesions, and they might be expected to do better than those treated by external techniques. Bedford and associates reported new tumors in twelve of sixty-three patients treated with surface applicators or photocoagulation and in five of the fifty-eight patients when the whole eye was irradiated. In view of the high incidence of multiple areas of involvement, we have favored external irradiation.

Technique for irradiating locally advanced retinoblastoma. Fear of the tragedy of total blindness has provoked an extension of the indications for radiotherapy. Involvement of the remaining eye has encouraged attempts at curative irradiation even though chances of residual vision seemed slim. At times shrinkage of the tumor will restore the retina to its previous position and expected vision will return. When the retinoblastoma involves the anterior half of the bulb, a straight anterior beam is used with the lens shield mentioned before. The lateral beam used with this is brought anteriorly as far as the lens will permit. The two fields are weighted 1:4.5 (anterior to lateral). The dose to the retina is usually 3500 rad in 3 weeks to 4500 rad in 4 weeks.

Of thirty patients in this advanced category, twenty-one (70%) were alive with some vision and were tumor-free at 18 months, two were dead from tumor, and three had their eyes removed because of recurrence (Skeggs and Williams).

The undesirable sequelae of vigorous irradiation might be deduced from the previous discussion of the effects of irradiation on the normal eye. The most common retinal changes are retinal exudates, retinal detachment, and retinal hemorrhage (Williams). In an attempt to decrease the undesirable sequelae of vigorous irradiation, combinations of systemic chemotherapy and irradiation were tried. None of these has any advantage over irradiation alone.

RESULTS AND PROGNOSIS. If all known local tumor is removed at the time of enucleation, the prognosis is good. Thompson and associates reported fifty of fifty-two patients surviving after enucleation, and thirty-seven of these patients were classed in Group V. It is thus obvious that the sole aim of nonsurgical therapy is the preservation of useful vision. Thompson and associates achieved this aim in twenty-four of thirty-four instances when irradiation was used. Only one patient in the group treated by irradiation died of metastases. (See Table 5-2.) In a national survey, Hansen and Miller concluded that 81% of children survive retinoblastoma. Bedford and associates reported success in all cases of Classes I and II, 86% of Class III, and 75% in Classes IV, V, and VI. (Their Class VI includes residual orbital disease or optic nerve involvement.) Shidnia and associates reported that of their thirty-two patients treated from 1967 to 1977 available for at least 2 years' follow-up, 100% were living, only one with disease.

If the tumor is cut through either in the optic nerve or in an emissary vein, the prognosis is much worse. Reese reported that where the tumor was thought to have been cut through, only five of twenty-one patients survived 14 months to 17 years after irradiation. However, of twenty-five patients developing palpable recurrence after surgery, none lived 5 years. Reese evaluated enucleation of the remaining eye in twelve patients who developed postirradiation recurrence. Five patients were free of disease subsequently.

As radiotherapy techniques have improved and as the diagnosis of involvement of the remaining eye is made earlier, the proportion of patients with useful vision increases. Reese reported useful vision in seventeen of nineteen treated patients. The effort to preserve vision has not led to an excessive mortality.

MALIGNANT MELANOMA

Malignant melanoma originating on the skin is classically regarded as relatively radioresistant, and surgery is accepted as the treatment of choice. However, when enucleation was refused for ocular melanomas and radiotherapy was accepted, some surprisingly good responses were observed. Frequent regression and control are obtained for melanomas of the conjunctiva and limbus. Similarly, it has been almost uniformly accepted that intraocular melanoma is sufficiently resistant to be radio-incurable. Yet of ninety-six patients treated with the Stallard surface applicator, sixty-one were controlled, twenty-three for over 5 years. This method is useful when, for any reason, surgery is inadvisable.

TECHNIQUE. Melanomas of the limbus or conjunctiva are usually early. At biopsy most of the bulk is generally removed. If the residual is flat and thin, beta ray therapy with a strontium applicator is desirable. A dose of 2500 rad weekly to 10,000 to 15,000 rad is recommended (Lederman, 1961). For infiltrating, thick, or widespread lesions, obviously the percentage depth dose will not be adequate. For such lesions of the medial or lateral conjunctiva, superficial x-ray therapy can be given with no direct irradiation of the cornea or lens. A lid retractor is used during each treatment. Surface doses of 6000 rad in 4 to 5 weeks to these small areas are tolerated.

When the Stallard surface applicator was used for the intraocular melanomas, the dose was 30,000 to 40,000 rad to the base of the lesion and 10,000 to 14,000 rad to the summit.

RESULTS. The control rate for radiotherapy of melanomas of the conjunctiva or limbus is excellent. Lederman reported control of disease in twenty-four of thirty-two patients. Smaller series report similar control. At the Christie Hospital, nine patients were irradiated for uveal tract melanomas limited to the orbit. Five of the nine were living at 5 years.

CHOROIDAL METASTASES

Cancers of any histologic type and any anatomic site of origin may metastasize to the choroid. However, by far the most common primary lesion is cancer of the breast (86%) with cancer of the lung being next most common. Occasionally the choroid will be the initial site of metastatic disease. Metastases will be in both eyes in about one third and unilateral in two thirds of the patients. In patients with the primary lesion in the breast the median survival is 10 months (Maor and associates), and concomitant brain metastases will be infrequent. Therefore simultaneous whole brain irradiation is indicated only if there is evidence of intracranial metastases.

Irradiation for choroidal metastases is accomplished with a simple lateral beam tilted slightly posteriorly to avoid the opposite eye. A choroidal dose of 3000 rad in 10 fractions is generally adequate. Chu and associates recommend the use of a 10 mev electron beam in order to avoid cross firing midline structures and the opposite eye. They use a dose of 4000 rad in 3 weeks. Improved vision follows irradiation in two thirds or more of the patients.

SUMMARY

The radiosensitivity of the eye is such that the dose of radiations reaching it must at all times be kept to a minimum. If the normal bulb must be included in the irradiated volume, specific changes can be predicted, most of which imply a decrease of visual acuity. The treatment of diseases of the cornea and sclera requires special techniques if the deeper structures of the eye are to be preserved. Retinoblastoma is sufficiently radiosensitive to be radiocurable. For this reason irradiation is indicated when surgery has not completely removed an advanced lesion or when a smaller lesion of the bulb can be vigorously irradiated without destroying vision. Selected melanomas have been cured by radiotherapy, permitting preservation of vision.

REFERENCES

Ahlstrom, S., Lindgren, M., and Olivecrona, H.: Radiologic treatment of orbital lymphoma, Acta Radiol. 3:441-448, 1965.

Ainslee, D., and Snelling, M. D.: Postoperative irradiation of corneal grafts, Lancet 2:954-956, 1961.

Ash, J. E., and Wilder, H. C.: Epithelial tumors of the limbus, Am. J. Ophthalmol. 25:926-932, 1942.

Bagshaw, M., and Kaplan, H. S.: Supervoltage linear accelerator radiation therapy. VIII. Retinoblastoma, Radiology 86:242-246, 1966.

Bateman, J. L.: Organs of special senses: eye and irradiation. In Berjis, C. C., editor: Pathology of irradiation, Baltimore, 1971, The Williams & Wilkins Co.

Bedford, M. A., Bedotto, C., and MacFaul, P. A.: Retinoblastoma, a study of 139 cases, Br. J. Ophthalmol. 55:19-27, 1971.

Cassady, J. R., Sagerman, R. H., Tretter, P., and

Ellsworth, R. M.: Radiation therapy for rhabdomyosarcoma, Radiology 91:116-120, 1968.

Chan, R. C., and Shukovsky, L. J.: Effects of irradiation on the eye, Radiology 120:673-675, 1976.

Chu, F. C. H., Huh, S. H., Nisce, L. Z., and Simpson, L. D.: Radiation therapy of choroid metastasis from breast cancer, Int. J. Radiat. Oncol. Biol. Phys. 2:273-279, 1977.

Cibis, P. A., Noell, W. K., and Eichel, B.: Ocular effects produced by high-intensity x-radiation, Arch. Ophthalmol. 53:651-663, 1955.

Cogan, D. G.: Lesions of the eye from radiant energy, J.A.M.A. 142:145-151, 1950.

Cogan, D. G., and Donaldson, D. D.: Experimental radiation cataracts. I. Cataracts in the rabbit following single x-ray exposure, Arch. Ophthalmol. 45:508-522, 1951.

Cogan, D. G., Fink, R., and Donaldson, D. D.: X-ray irradiation of orbital glands of the rabbit, Radiology 64:731-737, 1955.

Covington, E. E., Lobes, L., and Sudorsanam, A.: Radiation therapy for exophthalmos: report of seven cases, Radiology 122:797-799, 1977.

Donaldson, S. S., Bagshaw, M. A., and Kriss, J. D.: Supervoltage orbital radiotherapy for Graves' ophthalmopathy, J. Clin. Endocrinol. Metab. 37:276-285, 1973.

Evans, T. C.: Effects of small daily doses of fast neutrons on mice, Radiology 50:811-824, 1948.

Fayos, J. V., and Wildermuth, O.: Carcinoma of the ocular conjunctiva: its roentgen therapy, Radiology 79:582-587, 1962.

Friedell, H. I., Thomas, C. I., and Krohmer, J. S.: Description of an Sr^{90} beta-ray applicator and its use on the eye, Am. J. Roentgenol. 65:232-244, 1951.

Gaffey, C. T.: Biolectric sensitivity to irradiation of the retina and visual pathways. In Haley, T. J., and Snider, R. S., editors: Response of the nervous system to ionizing radiation, Boston, 1964, Little, Brown and Co.

Gaitan-Yanguas, M.: Retinoblastoma: analyses of 235 cases, Int. J. Radiat. Oncol. Biol. Phys. 4:359-365, 1978.

Halman, K. E.: Tumours of the eye treated by radiotherapy, Br. J. Radiol. 13:19-28, 1962.

Hartmann, E., and Fontaine, M.: Atrophie de la glande lacrymale avec irritation oculaire après radiothérapie de la face, Bull. Soc. d'opht. Paris, pp. 191-192, 1947.

Hyman, G. A., and Reese, A. B.: Combination therapy of retinoblastoma with triethylene melamine and radiotherapy, J.A.M.A. 162:1368-1373, 1956.

Jensen, R. D., and Miller, R. W.: Retinoblastoma: epidemiologic characteristics, J.A.M.A. 285:307-311, 1971.

Kim, Y., and Fayos, J.: Primary orbital lymphomas. A radiotherapeutic experience, Int. J. Radiat. Oncol. Biol. Phys. 1:1099-1105, 1976.

Knudson, A. G.: Retinoblastoma: a prototype hereditary neoplasm, Semin. Oncol. 5:57-61, 1978.

Krohmer, J. S.: Physical measurements on various beta-ray applicators, Am. J. Roentgenol. 66:791-796, 1951.

Lederman, M.: Some applications of radioactive isotopes in ophthalmology, Br. J. Radiol. 29:1-13, 1956.

Lederman, M.: Radiotherapy of malignant melanomata of the eye, Br. J. Radiol. 34:21-42, 1961.

Leinfelder, P. J., and Riley, E. F.: Further studies of effects of x-radiation on partially shielded lens of rabbits, Arch. Ophthalmol. 55:84-86, 1956.

Lenz, M.: International symposium on corneal surgery: radiotherapy for prevention and obliteration of corneal vascularization, Am. J. Ophthalmol. 33:46-52, 1950.

Manchester, P. T.: Retinoblastoma among offspring of adult survivors, Arch. Ophthalmol. 65:546-549, 1961.

Maor, M., Chan, R. C., and Young, S. E.: Radiotherapy of choroidal metastases, Cancer 40:2081-2086, 1977.

Merriam, G. R.: The effects of beta radiation on the eye, Radiology 66:240-245, 1956.

Merriam, G. R., and Focht, E. F.: A clinical study of radiation cataracts and the relationship to dose, Am. J. Roentgenol. 77:759-785, 1957.

Merriam, G. R., Szechter, A., and Focht, E. F.: The effects of ionizing radiations on the eye. In Vaeth, J. M., editor: Radiation effect and tolerance, normal tissue, Baltimore, 1972, University Park Press.

Michaelson, I. C., and Schreiber, H.: Influence of low-voltage x-radiation on regression of established corneal vessels, Arch. Ophthalmol. 55:48-51, 1956.

Oughterson, A. W., and Warren, S.: Medical effects of the atomic bomb in Japan, New York, 1956, McGraw-Hill Book Co.

Parker, R. G., Burnett, L. L., Woolton, P., and McIntyre, D. J.: Radiation cataract in clinical therapeutic radiology, Radiology 82:794-798, 1964.

Perrers-Taylor, M., Brinkley, D., and Reynolds, T.: Choriodoretinal damage as a complication of radiotherapy, Acta Radiol. 3:431-440, 1965.

Reese, A. B.: Tumors of the eye, New York, 1963, Harper & Row, Publishers, Inc.

Renfer, H.: The treatment of skin tumors of the inner canthus with regard to the function of the lacrimal ducts, Strahlentherapie 99:345-353, 1956.

Riley, E. F., Evans, T. C., Rhody, R. B., Leinfelder, P. J., and Richards, R. D.: The relative biological effectiveness of fast-neutrons and x-radiation, Radiology **67**:673-685, 1956.

Rosengren, B. O. H., and Tengroth, B.: A modified Cobalt 60 applicator for the treatment of retinoblastoma, Acta Radiol. **1**:305-313, 1963.

Shidnia, H., Hornback, N. B., Helveston, E. M., Gettlefinger, T., and Briglan, A. W.: Treatment results of retinoblastoma at Indiana University Hospitals, Cancer **40**:2917-2922, 1977.

Skeggs, D. B. L., and Williams, I. G.: The treatment of advanced retinoblastoma by means of external irradiation combined with chemotherapy, Clin. Radiol. **17**:169-172, 1966.

Stallard, H. B.: Multiple islands of retinoblastoma, Br. J. Ophthalmol. **39**:241-243, 1955.

Stallard, H. B.: Malignant melanoma of the choroid treated by radioactive applicators. In Fletcher, G. H.: Textbook of radiotherapy, Philadelphia, 1966, Lea & Febiger.

Tapley, N. duV.: Clinical results in the treatment of retinoblastoma with TEM and radiation. In Kallman, R. F., editor: Research in radiotherapy, Washington, 1961, National Academy of Science—National Research Council.

Tapley, N. duV.: Bilateral retinoblastoma combined treatment with irradiation and chemotherapy. In Vaeth, J. M., editor: Frontiers of radiation therapy and oncology, San Francisco, 1968, S. Karger A. G.

Tapley, N.: Retinoblastoma, Cancer in Childhood, Pediatr. Ann. **2**:35-38, 1974.

Thomas, C. I., Storaasli, J. P., and Friedell, H. L.: Lenticular changes associated with beta radiation of the eye and their significance, Radiology **79**:588-595, 1962.

Thompson, R. W., Small, R. C., and Stein, J. J.: Treatment of retinoblastoma, Am. J. Roentgenol. **114**:16-23, 1972.

Upton, A. C., Christenberry, K. W., Melville, G. S., Furth, J., and Hurst, G. S.: The relative biological effectiveness of neutrons, x-rays, and gamma rays for the production of lens opacities: observations on mice, rats, guinea-pigs, and rabbits, Radiology **67**:686-696, 1956.

Van den Brenk, H. A. S.: Results of prophylactic postoperative irradiation in 1300 cases of pterygium, Am. J. Roentgenol. **103**:723-733, 1968.

Weiss, D. R., Cassady, J. R., and Peterson, R.: Retinoblastoma: a modification in radiation therapy technique, Radiology **114**:705-708, 1975.

Wildermuth, O., and Evans, J. C.: The special problem of cancer of eyelid, Cancer **9**:837-841, 1956.

Wille, C.: Malign tumours in the nose and its accessory sinuses, Acta Otolaryngol., suppl. 65, pp. 44-54, 1947.

Williams, I. G.: Radiation therapy in the treatment of retinoblastoma, Am. J. Roentgenol. **77**:786-795, 1957.

6

The ear, nasopharynx, nasal fossa, and paranasal sinuses

Cancers of the nasopharynx, nasal fossa, and paranasal sinuses have a great deal in common. The carcinomas arise from respiratory epithelium, they are usually squamous cell in type, and they require rather high doses of radiations for eradication. Irradiation of the nasopharynx usually entails irradiation of the external and middle ear and the eustachian tube. Irradiation of the paranasal sinuses usually entails irradiation of the nasal fossa and frequently a part of the nasopharynx. The involvement of parts of the ear by these cancers and the irradiation of parts of the ear in the treatment of these cancers make it reasonable to consider them together.

THE EAR
Response of the normal middle ear and internal ear to irradiation

The columnar epithelium that lines the middle ear and covers the ossicles is actually desquamated by the doses used for control of cancers in this area. Edema of the mucosa and a collection of sterile fluid in the middle ear may appear after such irradiation. These changes are a result of direct damage to the mucosa and submucosal tissue of the middle ear as well as obstruction of the eustachian tube. We have termed this *radiation otitis media.* If severe reactions occur, the drum may rupture and hearing may be permanently impaired.

Shortly after doses of 4000 to 6000 rad to the ear in 4 to 6 weeks, about 50% of the patients note painless fullness in the ear. The mucosa of the middle ear shows edema with vascular and connective tissue changes described on pp. 83 and 190. Small submucosal hemorrhages may develop. The sensation of fullness signifies a loss of conduction. As the edema involves the eustachian tube and the mucosa covering all structures of the middle ear, fluid may collect in the middle ear. If the fluid becomes infected, serious damage to middle and internal ear functions may develop. Ordinarily the loss of hearing is mild, and some tinnitus may be present (Borsanyi). These symptoms usually clear spontaneously as the mucosa heals, but the patient may be more comfortable if he is given vasoconstricting agents and analgesics. If fever develops, suggesting secondary infection, the use of antibiotics is indicated.

Considerably lower doses of radiations have been reported to improve hearing

171

temporarily. Girden showed that this occurred in dogs but was unable to explain why. There are several changes that may contribute to this improvement in hearing, but the relative importance of each remains unknown. Lymphoid tissue, particularly that around the eustachian tube orifice, shrinks with such irradiation. The value of this response is widely appreciated and forms the basis for irradiating selected patients with hypertrophy of nasopharyngeal lymphoid tissue (Chapter 4). By such means tubal patency is reestablished, the middle ear becomes drier, air pressures equilibrate, and, as a result, hearing improves. Almost any of the chronic inflammatory processes will thus be helped both directly and indirectly by low-dosage irradiation. Whether changes occurring in the circulation, the tympanic membrane, or other structures contribute to increased auditory acuity in dogs is entirely speculative.

The magnitude of damage in patients and long-term effects of radiations on hearing in patients have been studied by Gamble and associates and by Dias. After the early reactions have subsided, most patients will show remarkably little hearing loss. Among those who show bothersome change, deafness is mixed in origin, some being related to tubal dysfunction, some to temporary vasculitis, some to the recruitment phenomenon, and some, rarely, to ossicle necrosis (Dias). In those instances in which permanent radiation-induced changes in hearing develop, tubal dysfunction is by far the most common cause. Most such defects will be in patients whose cancer modified tubal function prior to therapy.

As was implied in the previous discussion, the structures of the internal ear, the cochlea with the organ of Corti, and the semicircular ducts with their associated sensory hair cells are not clinically affected by the usual clinically employed doses of radiations (Table 6-1). Moskovskaya reported finding an increase in excitability of the labyrinth during radiation therapy, but this has not been confirmed. Gamble and associates reported that the endolymphatic spaces of the semicircular canals enlarge and become distended with single doses of 3000 rad. This was thought to be due to vascular changes but has not been reported with fractionated, clinically employed doses.

In the very young, hemorrhages and radiation-induced bone deformities may alter the development of the organ of Corti and the vestibular apparatus (Kelemen).

Table 6-1. Incidence of radiation-induced vestibulocerebellar lesions after various doses of radiations (200 kv, hvl 0.93 mm Cu) directed to one lateral half of the rabbit's skull (10 animals in each group)*

Labyrinthine dose	Vestibulo-cerebellar signs	Microscopic changes in cerebellum pons or nerves	Labyrinthine or auditory nerve damage
5400 R in 30 days	1	0	0
3000 R in 12 days	0	0	0
2000 R in one dose	9	9	5

*Modified from Berg, N. O., and Lindgren, M.: Acta Radiol. **56:**305-319, 1961.

Carcinoma of the ear

From the radiotherapeutic viewpoint, cancers of the ear are divided into the following three categories:

1. Lesions of the pinna, which are discussed in Chapter 2
2. Lesions of the outer two thirds of the external auditory canal
3. Lesions of the inner third of the external auditory canal, of the middle ear, and of the mastoid air cells.

CARCINOMA OF THE OUTER TWO THIRDS OF THE EXTERNAL AUDITORY CANAL

Carcinoma of the outer two thirds of the external auditory canal is rare. It is usually squamous cell in type, but adenocarcinoma of the ceruminous glands has been reported. In contrast to carcinoma of the middle ear, pain and suppuration are not prominent symptoms. Bleeding usually causes the patient to go to the physician. Extension may not occur until late, but it may then be superficial to the periauricular tissues or deep into the middle ear and its associated structures. Because of the difficulty in defining the limits of extension, it is advisable to treat a volume 1 to 3 cm in radius around the canal unless the lesion is obviously superficial. It is impossible to accomplish this with a central source of radium without necrosing the walls of the canal. If the cancer is confined to the concha and outer 0.5 cm of the canal, adequate irradiation can be accomplished without such necrosis by using fractionated irradiation with 200 kv radiations or an appropriate electron beam. If the cancer extends deeply into the canal, wedged megavoltage or ^{60}Co beams, beams with wobbled exits, or an electron beam are preferable.

No accurate time-dose data are available as guides in treating these lesions, but we believe that doses of the level of 5000 rad in 4 to 6 weeks will be well tolerated and effective in the more limited cases. For more infiltrative lesions 6500 rad in 7 to 8 weeks is necessary.

PROGNOSIS AND RESULTS. Unfortunately, most of these cases have been grouped either with those of the middle ear or with those of the concha. However, of twenty-six cases included in this group at the Christie Hospital, eleven of the patients were irradiated with a curative aim, and nine were living and well after 5 years (Boland and Paterson). Dalley reported six of eighteen patients were well at 5 years.

CARCINOMA OF THE INNER THIRD OF THE EXTERNAL AUDITORY CANAL, MIDDLE EAR, AND MASTOID AIR CELLS

Lesions of the inner third of the external auditory canal, middle ear, and mastoid air cells should be grouped together. They are usually advanced by the time biopsy is taken, and it is generally impossible to determine from which of these three sites the tumor originated. Although one may speculate that lesions of the mastoid air cells will extend early to deep osseous structures, and that lesions of the auditory canal will extend superficially, this has been of no practical value in managing these lesions. Most of the carcinomas will be squamous cell in type, arising by metaplasia from the columnar cells of the middle ear and air cells. Adenocarcinoma is rare.

The symptoms and signs of malignant lesions of this region differ from those of benign diseases only in degree (Lindahl). The most prominent symptoms are pain, which is frequently severe, bloody drainage from what appears to be granulation tissue, and, of course, suppuration. Depending on the type of extension, one may find deafness, signs of meningeal irritation, periauricular swelling, trismus, and paralysis of cranial nerves. Metastasis may occur by way of the peritubal lymphatics to pharyngeal nodes or to the periauricular or upper cervical nodes. Local node metastases are uncommon, and generalized metastases are rare but have been reported (Boland and Paterson). Regardless of the method of treatment, death is usually a result of extension through the petrous apex to involve the dura and then the brain. If extension is beyond the temporal bone, the prognosis is practically hopeless (Adams and Morrison).

TECHNIQUE. It has been impossible to prove the superiority of either surgery or irradiation or a combination of the two. The numbers of patients treated by the various modalities are too few. It is obvious, however, that radical surgery must be limited in depth because of vital structures. It is also obvious that once bone invasion has occurred the tumor is not particularly radiocurable. Preirradiation surgery does not significantly change the responsiveness to irradiation. From the limited data available, we have felt justified in advocating irradiation as an acceptable alternative, but a combination of surgery and irradiation is more commonly recommended.

It is often difficult to define the extent of these lesions and the volume to be irradiated. Palpation for induration is usually not helpful, and inspection into the canal reveals granulation-like tissue and edema. Neurologic examination may yield information relative to the route and degree of medial extension. Roentgenographic examinations (particularly in the submental vertex view), laminographic studies, and computed tomograms are helpful in defining bone destruction.

The volume to be irradiated is usually not large. It will be unilateral, and its medial margin will lie near the brain. External megavoltage and ^{60}Co beams are the only practical methods of delivering relatively homogeneous doses. The entire petrous portion of the temporal bone must be included, even in the apparently limited lesion. Sharply angled, wedged beams are excellent (Arthur and Wang). Special attention must be given to the medial margin of this heavily irradiated volume. Boland and Paterson reported at least one death from brain stem damage after the inclusion of the brain stem in the high-dose region (Chapter 22). Irradiation with a direct lateral portal was found to be associated with necrosis of the temporal bone if doses equivalent to an NSD of 2000 ret were given (Wang and Doppke).

We have advocated doses in the range of 6500 rad in 7 to 8 weeks if the brain can be excluded from the high-dose volume.

When radical surgery and irradiation have been combined, the sequence has usually been to use the irradiation postoperatively. Doses have been of the order of 6000 to 6500 rad in 8 or more weeks given through a pair of wedged beams.

PROGNOSIS AND RESULTS. The results of treatment are not good. This is attributed to the delay in diagnosis. The patients usually die as a result of cancer invading the brain.

Table 6-2. Summary of results in treatment of carcinoma of the middle ear*

Author	Number of patients	Survival
Surgery followed by radiotherapy		
Adams and Morrison (1955)	7	Mean survival, 3 years
		Range, 3-69 months
Frew and Finney (1963)		Not stated
Lederman (1965)	36	3-year survival, 39%
		5-year survival, 33%
		10-year survival, 15%
Tucker (1965)	57	3-year survival, 26%
Wang (1975)	20	5-year survival, 45%
Sinha and Aziz (1978)	15	5-year survival, 40% (6/15)
Radiotherapy alone		
Adams and Morrison (1955)	3	Average survival, 10 months
Holmes (1960)	22	2-year survival, 77%
Boland (1963)	18	5-year survival, 56% (10/18)
Frew and Finney (1963)	22	2-year survival, 33%
Lederman (1965)	29	3-year survival, 8%
		None survived 5 years
Sinha and Aziz (1978)	7	5-year survival, 14% (1/7)

*Modified from Sinha, P., and Aziz, H. I.: Radiology **126**:485-487, 1978.

Results collected from a variety of techniques are sumarized in Table 6-2. As can be seen, they vary widely and are not immediately suggestive of any preferable sequence.

Paraganglioma or chemodectoma

This category of tumors, also referred to as chemodectomas or glomus tumors, includes tumors arising from specialized neuroendocrine receptors generally referred to as paraganglia, which are associated with the carotid artery bifurcation (carotid body tumors), the tympanic nerve near the jugular bulb (glomus jugulare), and with the vagus nerve near the base of the skull (glomus intravagale) (Fig. 6-1). Microscopically these tumors present varying proportions of nerve epithelial and vascular elements in an organoid pattern. Some tumors present an epithelial or adenoma-like appearance, whereas in others the predominance of vascular endothelium may lead to confusion with vascular tumors. There are tortuous anastomoses between arteries and veins, and a bruit may be present.

Symptoms are dependent on the tissues compressed by the slowly expanding tumor. The growth may be very slow within a pretreatment history of 10 to 15 years. Lesions 0.5 cm in diameter may be symptom-producing at the jugular bulb, whereas a mass 10 cm in diameter may be almost asymptomatic at the carotid bulb. The tumor is usually encapsulated but may become bound to important adjacent structures (Palacios). Although rarely a paraganglioma of the head and neck may metastasize, these tumors are usually benign in the histologic sense. As they grow, they may erode bone by pressure and in some cases appear to actually invade bone.

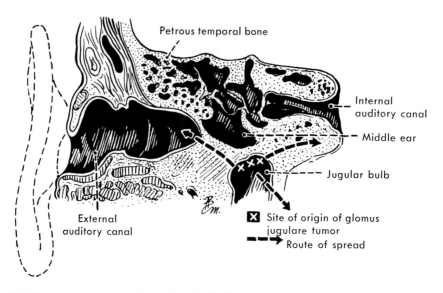

Fig. 6-1. Most common site of origin and route of infiltration of glomus jugulare tumor. The limitations of resecting this area are obvious. The danger of radiation damage to adjacent brain tissue is also obvious. (From Miller, J. R.: Radiology **79**:430-434, 1962.)

This tumor occurs more commonly in females than in males (3 to 1) and is usually unilateral but may be bilateral or, rarely, may develop in three or four sites. Occasionally there is a familial history. The many interesting clinical and diagnostic aspects of these tumors are reported by Palacios and by Rosenwasser. The value of angiograms, tomograms, and computerized tomograms in the diagnosis and definition of extent cannot be overemphasized.

In keeping with their recognized low growth rate, these tumors may shrink slowly following radiation therapy. Initially this slow rate of shrinkage led to the erroneous conclusion that these tumors were radioresistant. We now recognize that they respond well to doses of 4000 to 4500 rad in 4 to 5 weeks (Table 6-3). The deep location of these tumors, their firm attachment to important structures or proximity to non-resectable structures, and their frequent regrowth after attempted excision justify serious radiotherapeutic efforts. Thus Grubb and Lampe reported that 56% of the glomus jugulare tumors persisted after surgery alone. A similar figure was reported by Hatfield and associates and Newman and associates. There were few and sometimes no persistent growths if postoperative irradiation was used or with radiotherapy alone. Numerous other reports support these findings (Williams; Bradshaw; Maruyama and associates; Hudgins; Hatfield and associates; Tidwell and Montague; Simko and associates) (Table 6-4).

TECHNIQUE. Carotid body tumors are usually surgically removed and rarely require radiotherapy. By contrast, glomus jugulare and glomus intravagale tumors usually require irradiation. The technical problem is one of delivering a modest dose to the involved volume without producing brain, ear, or bone damage. Doses of 4000

Table 6-3. Definition of dose necessary to control chemodectomas (1000 rad in 5 fractions per week)*

Author	Total dose	Number of patients	Number recurrences
Hatfield and associates	Less than 4000 rad	5	4
	More than 4000 rad	16	0
Hudgins	4000-5000 rad	9	0
Tidwell and Montague	4200-5000 rad	17	1
Simko and associates	2800-6500 rad	14	2

*Modified from Tidwell, T. J., and Montague, E. D.: Radiology **116:**147-149, 1975.

Table 6-4. Frequency of response of chemodectoma to radiotherapy*

Author	Number of responders/total number	Percent
Williams (1957)	12/12	100
Hatfield and associates (1972)	16/16	100
Fuller and associates (1967)	43/43	100
Grubb and Lampe (1965)	14/14	100
Miller (1962)	13/14	93
Bradshaw (1963)	8/12	75
Tidwell and Montague (1973)	16/17	90

*Modified from Maruyama, Y., Gold, L. H., and Kieffer, S. A.: Acta Radiol. **10:**239-247, 1971.

to 5000 rad in 4 to 5 weeks are commonly used to control the disease (Table 6-3). The real risk of brain necrosis must be accepted if the dose is much higher than 5000 rad in 5 weeks and the volume of interest extends into the brain stem. Bradshaw reported a fatal brain necrosis after a dose of 5500 rad in 6 weeks, and Miller reported one after 5000 rad in 38 days. This dose is best delivered with converging wedged beams directed superoinferiorly or obliquely to avoid delivering a significant exit dose to the contralateral eye. The contralateral ear and salivary gland are likewise spared. Beams must be of such a size and angle as to avoid a high dose to the brainstem. This technique is illustrated by Tidwell and Montague. With such doses, tumor response is usual (Table 6-3).

RESULTS. The response to irradiation can be measured by the shrinkage of the visible mass and decrease or disappearance of pain (earache, headache, etc.), tinnitus, and rarely of the nerve paralysis. Appropriate 10-year follow-ups of patients irradiated by currently accepted techniques are few. Capps, Rosenwasser, and Fuller and associates indicated that well over half the patients will be living symptom-free at 5 years (Table 6-4). The natural course of the disease is long, and 10- to 15-year follow-up data are necessary to measure the ability of radiations to produce long-term control.

Serial angiography usually shows that in spite of almost uniformly good clinical responses, there are little, if any, radiation-induced changes in the appearance of angiograms (Maruyama and associates). It is presumed that at least part of the response depends on injury to small vessels below that of angiographic visibility. An occasional postirradiation microscopic examination confirms an increased fibrosis.

SUMMARY. Carcinomas of the middle ear and the external auditory canal are usually squamous cell in type. They are usually advanced when diagnosed and are neither easily excised nor particularly radiosensitive. We have felt justified in recommending vigorous irradiation as a primary treatment. By such means about half these tumors can be controlled.

Chemodectomas are not usually malignant in the histologic sense, although they may rarely metastasize or kill by severe hemorrhage or pressure on intracranial tissues. Prolonged beneficial growth restraint and control are produced by doses that carry an acceptable risk.

NASOPHARYNX
Malignant tumors of the nasopharynx

The nasopharynx is lined with ciliated columnar epithelium that, like respiratory epithelium elsewhere, contains numerous mucous and seromucous glands. The most frequent malignant tumor of the nasopharynx, squamous cell carcinoma, arises by metaplasia from this ciliated epithelium. Lymphoma, the second most common malignant tumor, arises from lymphoid tissue associated with the roof and, less frequently, with the lateral walls of the nasopharynx. Lymphoepitheliomas have a distribution similar to that of the lymphomas. Lymphoepithelioma is a poorly differentiated carcinoma diffusely infiltrated by lymphocytes. Ultrastructurally the tumor cells exhibit tonofibrils and desmosomes, both evidence of epithelial origin. In some of these cases electron microscopy is essential in distinguishing them from lymphoma. The rare adenocarcinoma of this region originates from mucous glands and presents types and characteristics common to carcinomas arising in minor salivary glands, as mentioned in Chapter 4.

Much of the difficulty in controlling lesions of the nasopharynx is a consequence of their relative inaccessibility and of their failure to produce early symptoms. The patient can neither see nor palpate the primary lesion. Unfortunately, the usual busy physician rarely suspects a malignant lesion of the nasopharynx until metastases to cervical lymph nodes are present or cranial nerve damage is obvious. Even then there may be a delay in establishing the proper diagnosis and initiating therapy.

A brief review of some of the anatomy of this region contributes greatly to an understanding of the routes of spread and of the signs and symptoms. This information is essential in defining the volume requiring treatment. The excellent description by del Regato and the detailed review by Lederman have been followed in the succeeding discussion.

The nasopharynx is bound by the first and second cervical vertebrae posteriorly, the declivity of the sphenoid posterosuperiorly, and the sphenoid sinus superiorly. A thin but rather tough layer of fascia shields these bones from early invasion by nasopharyngeal malignant tumors. Most of the lateral wall of the nasopharynx is composed of soft tissues into which tumor must infiltrate or through which it must

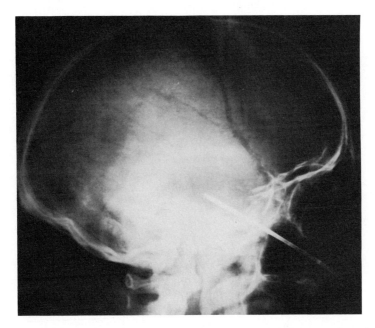

Fig. 6-2. This patient was being biopsied for a poorly differentiated squamous cell carcinoma of the nasopharynx when the suction tube passed without bony resistance into the cranial cavity. Destruction of the base of skull had been diagnosed earlier on the film of the base of skull. Patient was irradiated (5100 R in 33 days, 400 kv; hvl, 4 mm Cu) and was tumor-free at time of death from unrelated causes over 2 years later. (Courtesy Dr. G. Scott.)

metastasize to spread beyond the nasopharynx. A rather tough fascia extends from the foramen lacerum at the base of the skull inferiorly into the cervical region. This impediment to lateral infiltration and the similar barrier to posterosuperior infiltration leave the foramina in the base of the skull as the pathways of least resistance (Fig. 6-2). However, the fact that symptoms may not be produced by such extension usually demands that potential routes of infiltration and metastases be routinely treated, even in the absence of symptoms or signs. The relationship of the foramina to the nasopharynx is illustrated in Fig. 6-3. For a discussion of the anatomic relationships in the area see Lederman. Once extension through the foramina has occurred, adjacent important intracranial structures may be invaded. Extension may also progress anteriorly through the posterior nares, producing nasal obstruction.

More commonly, cervical adenopathy will cause the patient to go to the physician. The lymph drainage from the nasopharynx may be into the retropharyngeal nodes or more laterally into nodes of the upper posterior cervical region inferior to the lobe of the ear. The position of these metastases should suggest the nasopharynx as the primary site. Deeper metastases to nodes of the upper jugular chain may produce pressure paralysis of cranial nerves IX, X, XI, and XII. Cranial nerve paralysis may also be the sign causing the patient to go to the physician. A variety of cranial nerves may be involved in several different combinations, depending on the precise

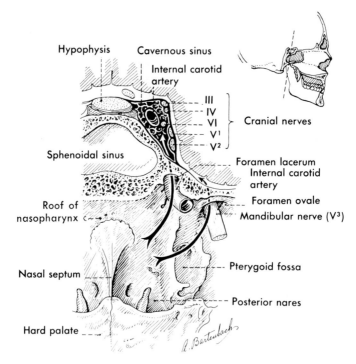

Fig. 6-3. Oblique view showing the base of skull and a cross section through sphenoidal sinus and hypophysis. For plane of section, see small figure in upper right. The arrows mark common routes of infiltration into cranial cavity and structures involved in such infiltration.

level of cancer extension. Godtfredsen lists ten such syndromes caused by various combinations of nerve paralyses.

From this discussion it is evident that nasopharyngeal cancers arise immediately inferior to the base of the skull and that with or without symptoms they may infiltrate into the nasal fossa or infiltrate laterally and superiorly into the cranial cavity by way of the basilar foramina. The cancer metastasizes posteroinferiorly to retropharyngeal nodes and laterally to the deep posterior cervical nodes near the base of the skull. The fact that any or all of this spread may occur without significant symptoms and with few positive signs demands that these areas of probable spread be routinely included in the irradiated volume.

CLINICAL STAGING. Although a variety of classifications for clinical staging of cancer of the nasopharynx have been proposed, none has been widely used. Therefore a comparison of end results has limited value. One must recognize the large categories such as the following:

1. The specific histologic type
2. The presence or absence of metastasis to cervical lymph nodes (unilateral or bilateral, movable or fixed)
3. The presence or absence of distant metastasis

4. The presence or absence of cranial nerve paralysis or the destruction of the base of the skull

Following are the definitions of TNM categories for cancer of the nasopharynx.

TNM CLASSIFICATION*

T—Primary tumor
TIS Carcinoma in situ
T1 Tumor confined to one site of nasopharynx or no tumor visible (positive biopsy only)
T2 Tumor involving two sites (both posterosuperior and lateral walls)
T3 Extension of tumor into nasal cavity or oropharynx
T4 Tumor invasion of skull or cranial nerve involvement, or both

N—Nodal involvement
NX Nodes cannot be assessed
N0 No clinically positive node
N1 Single clinically positive homolateral node 3 cm or less in diameter
N2 Single clinically positive homolateral node more than 3 but not more than 6 cm in diameter or multiple clinically positive homolateral nodes, none more than 6 cm in diameter
    N2a Single clinically positive homolateral node more than 3 but not more than 6 cm in diameter
    N2b Multiple clinically positive homolateral nodes, none over 6 cm in diameter
N3 Massive homolateral node(s), bilateral nodes, or contralateral node(s)
    N3a Clinically positive homolateral node(s), one more than 6 cm in diameter
    N3b Bilateral clinically positive nodes (in this situation, each side of the neck should be staged separately, that is, N3b: right, N2a; left, N1)
    N3c Contralateral clinically positive node(s) only

M—Distant metastasis
MX Not assessed
M0 No (known) distant metastasis
M1 Distant metastasis present

STAGE GROUPING
Stage I   T1   N0   N0
Stage II   T2   N0   M0
Stage III T3   N0   M0
Stage IV T1 or T2 or T3, N1, M0
            T4, N0 or N1, M0
            Any T, N2 or N3, M0
            Any T, any N, M1

TECHNIQUE. To define the volume to be irradiated, nothing helps more than adequate inspection of the nasopharynx, palpation of the neck, neurologic examination, and adequate radiographic examination. Inspection of the nasopharynx may be performed with a laryngeal mirror alone in a few patients. However, the majority of patients will require a good local anesthetic sprayed directly onto the soft palate and posterior pharyngeal wall and through each nostril onto the nasopharyngeal structures. A soft rubber catheter, No. 20 Fr. or smaller, passed through the nostril and brought out of the mouth pulls the soft palate forward effectively and permits

---

*From the American Joint Committee for Cancer Staging and End Results Reporting: Manual for staging of cancer, Chicago, 1978, Whiting Press.

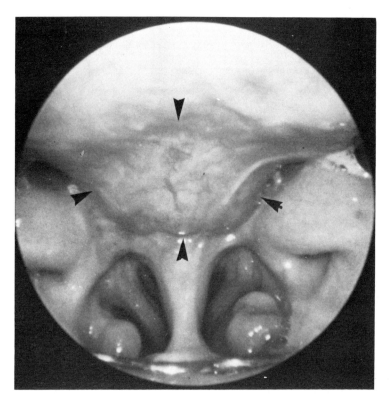

Fig. 6-4. Photograph of submucosal extension of a carcinoma of the roof of the nasopharynx. (From Chiang, T. C., and Jung, P. F.: Cancer **40:**2353-2364, 1977.)

thorough mirror examination of the nasopharynx (del Regato, 1970). Extension of the cancer into the nasal fossa anteriorly will require modification of lateral fields and more dose being given through an anterior field. For these reasons it is critical to clearly define the anterior margins of the cancer. Chiang and Jung have used a special photographing nasopharyngoscope to record the appearance of these lesions. Some of their illustrations are spectacular and are undoubtedly valuable in defining superficial extent (Figs. 6-4 and 6-5). In addition, the physical examination should include an evaluation of the status of all cranial nerves and the cervical sympathetic nerves. Special attention must be given to the cervical lymph node areas. A surprisingly large number of malignant tumors of the nasopharynx will metastasize beyond the cervical nodes. The general physical examination and roentgenographic studies should be done with this in mind.

Films of the base of the skull and neighboring sinuses should always be available to assist in determining whether bone destruction is present. The finding of bone destruction is of considerable prognostic value but is of little value in determining the volume to be irradiated. The base of the skull and adjacent brain are routinely included for reasons already given, although ports are larger for the more extensive

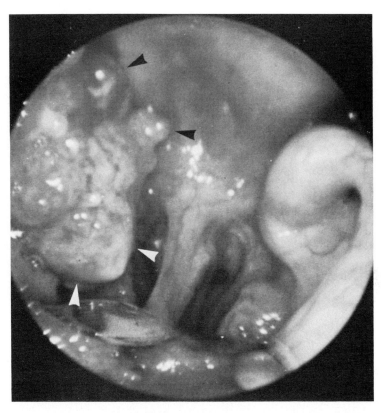

Fig. 6-5. Photograph of an ulcerated carcinoma of the patient's lateral nasopharyngeal wall. (From Chiang, T. C., and Jung, P. F.: Cancer **40:**2353-2364, 1977.)

lesions. A lateral roentgenogram using soft tissue technique is occasionally helpful in defining the pharyngeal extent of the tumor. The instillation of contrast media has been advocated, but we have not found that it contributes significantly to the diagnosis. Computed tomography (CT) scans are very useful in defining both lateral and superior infiltration, and we now obtain them as a routine part of the pretreatment evaluation.

We believe that bilateral parallel opposing beams combined with a single anterior beam are entirely adequate for the primary lesion. The single anterior beam is essential in those patients with cancer extending through the posterior nares into the nasal fossa, and it is highly desirable in most patients so that a lesser dose might be given through the lateral ports. This diminishes the risk of severe middle ear damage. With such a three-field arrangement, greater homogeneity can be obtained by using wedges for at least part of the dose given with lateral beams. We have found rotational techniques for this lesion neither necessary nor practical. It is often necessary to include at least a part of the middle ear and the eustachian tube and its medial orifice in the beam. If there is evidence of cranial nerve involvement or erosion of the base of the skull, the posterior margin of the lateral ports should

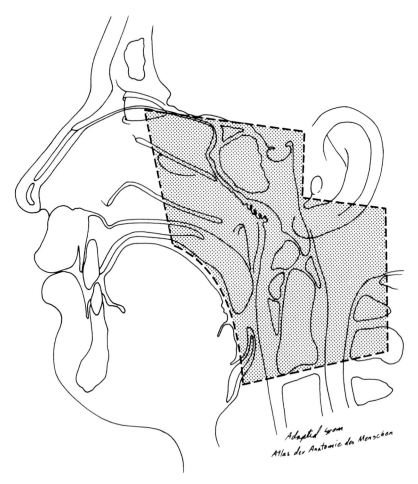

Fig. 6-6. Landmarks that serve as guides to beam placement. The base of skull should be included in irradiated volume. Beam size is not fixed for all patients but is tailored in keeping with clinical extent. Unnecessary corners of beams should be shielded.

encompass the entire foramen magnum (Fig. 6-6). Guides for port placement are shown in Fig. 6-6. Failure to use these guides is almost certain to be followed by recurrence (Fig. 6-7).

There are a variety of factors that support the inclusion of wide margins of normal tissue in the high-dose volume.

1. The majority of these tumors are either poorly differentiated, undifferentiated or lymphoepithelial.
2. Spread through the basilar foramina into the cranial cavity and to nodes at the base of the skull is not rare and may be asymptomatic.
3. Clinical experience has shown that small ports are associated with increased geographic misses and decreased local control rates (Hoppe and associates, 1976).

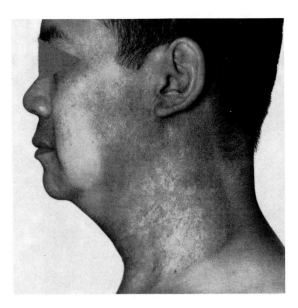

Fig. 6-7. Skin reaction marks size and position of previous irradiation and explains why there was persistence of cancer of the roof of the nasopharynx. Note that upper edge of the reaction is just below the tragus and therefore too low. Compare with outline shown in Fig. 6-6.

Techniques of irradiation and dose are not ordinarily varied with histologic types of carcinoma. This is related to the fact that most of the cancers are poorly differentiated and seem to require similar doses. The dose (NSD) to local control curve for all T1 carcinomas is shown in Fig. 6-8. From this analysis and other similar studies it is the consensus that primary carcinoma of the nasopharynx usually requires a minimum dose of 6500 to 7000 rad in 6½ to 8 weeks. Large primary lesions (T3 and T4) frequently recur, and a still higher dose to a large volume might seem indicated. However, the recognized tolerance of the brain stem and hypothalamus limits both dose and volume, thus making more aggressive irradiation inadvisable. For cervical lymph node metastases the dose should be tailored in keeping with the size of the mass as described in Chapter 4.

The dose to cervical lymph node metastases can never be safely raised to the required level by using *straight lateral* beams with the usual skin-source distances. The risk of damage to the larynx and spinal cord is too great. Anterior and posterior tangential beams or lateral electron beams are excellent for this purpose. The photon beams extend from the lower edge of the preauricular port to the sternoclavicular joint. Medially the beam should extend to the edge of the trachea, and the lateral limit is the skin. Since the frequently involved nodes are posterolateral, opposing posterior tangential beams are also recommended. The distribution of dose in tissue has been described by Million and associates, by Fletcher and Million, and by Hanks and associates (Chapter 4).

If an electron beam of appropriate energy is used to treat adenopathy in the

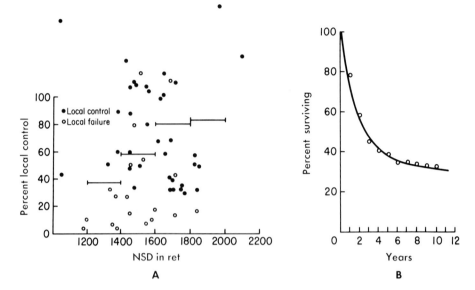

Fig. 6-8. A, Relationship of local control of T1 cancers of the nasopharynx to dose (NSD). **B,** Absolute survival rates for patients with carcinoma of the nasopharynx treated by radiation therapy. At 5 years the survival rate approaches 40%. (**A** From Moench, H. C., and Phillips, T. L.: Am. J. Surg. **124:**515-518, 1972; **B,** modified from Moench, H. C., and Phillips, T. L.: Am. J. Surg. **124:**515-518, 1972.)

posterior cervical triangle, spinal cord dose can be kept well below its "tolerance" levels.

The dose given for lymphadenopathy is tailored according to the size of the nodes (Fig. 6-9). (See Chapter 4.) There is perhaps no other group of patients so prone to severe fibrosis of the lateral cervical tissues. This is because of the rather wide distribution of the cervical adenopathy and the frequent need to deliver high doses through large tangential beams if the nodes are to be encompassed. A low daily dose of 180 rad diminishes the likelihood of severe fibrosis.

As mentioned previously, most of these patients will have cervical lymphadeno-pathy when first seen. For those not having lymphadenopathy, the radiation oncol-ogist is faced with the question of elective irradiation of the cervical areas. The results of Million and associates, of Fletcher and Million, and of Hanks and associates support its use. In a group of forty-two patients who had no clinically suspicious cervical nodes, twelve were not given "prophylactic" neck irradiation. Six of these twelve developed adenopathy on follow-up examinations. Of the thirty patients who were given "prophylactic" irradiation, none developed subsequent adenopathy (Moench and Phillips, 1972). We now advocate systematic elective irradiation of the cervical lymph node areas for squamous cell carcinoma, lymphoepithelioma, and lymphoma of the nasopharynx. The dose level is 5000 rad to a 3 cm depth in 5 weeks.

Because of their greater radiosensitivity, one might consider a lesser dose for the lymphoepitheliomas. However, the difference in required dose is small. We have generally given midline doses similar to those mentioned before.

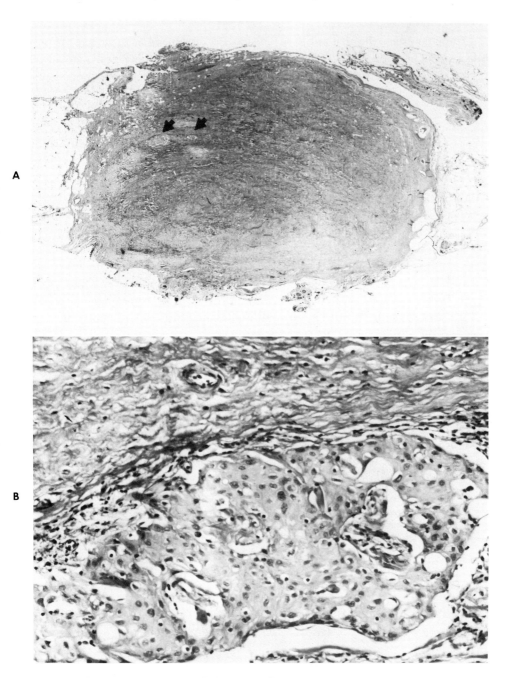

Fig. 6-9. A, Patient with squamous cell carcinoma of the nasopharynx had a metastasis to a cervical lymph node. Prior to irradiation the node measured 8 cm in diameter. Nodal dose of 7000 rad in 8 weeks reduced the mass to 1 cm in diameter. Excision of the 1 cm mass 6 weeks following irradiation revealed dense fibrous tissue and two small islands of tumor (arrows) trapped in the dense scar (magnification ×13). **B,** Detail from **A** of island of squamous cell carcinoma trapped in scar tissue (magnification ×475). The ultimate fate of such cancer cells is speculative.

LYMPHOMAS

Lymphomas may develop in the nasopharynx as a primary lesion and as the only site of involvement. The tumor may spread stepwise to upper and then lower cervical nodes before disseminating widely. The pretreatment examination should include a search for physical and radiographic evidence of spread beyond the neck. In addition to the obvious diagnostic procedures, a marrow biopsy, lymphangiogram, and spleen and liver scans should be performed. These will yield a certain proportion of abnormalities and in addition will provide a valuable "baseline" study to assist in follow-up evaluation.

When the disease has not spread beyond the neck, curative irradiation should be given, including generous parallel opposed lateral beams encompassing the nasopharyngeal primary site, along with the remainder of Waldeyer's ring, and anteroposterior cervical beams extending below the clavicles. If middle or low cervical nodes are enlarged, the mediastinum and probably the axillae should also be encompassed. A minimum dose of 4500 rad in 4 to 5 weeks should be delivered. If, on follow-up examination, widespread disease is found, the disease should be re-staged, then the patient treated as one with untreated widespread lymphoma.

PROGNOSIS AND RESULTS. Several studies have reviewed factors affecting prognosis (Table 6-5). Of the three major histologic types, squamous cell carcinoma carries the worst prognosis. The 5-year survival rate of patients with squamous cell carcinoma averages 30%, whereas the rate of those with lymphoepithelioma averages 43%, and the rate of those with lymphoma averages 57%. Younger patients have a relatively better prognosis than older patients. Patients over 70 have a very poor

Table 6-5. Factors influencing prognosis of cancers of nasopharynx (squamous cell, transitional cell, and undifferentiated cell cancers and lymphoepithelioma combined)

Factor	Author	Incidence of factor	Total	5-year survival (%)
No cervical lymphadenopathy	Chen Meyer Perez	7/18 31/47 11/23	49/88	55
Ipsilateral lymphadenopathy	Chen Meyer Perez	22/49 31/81 11/29	64/159	40
Bilateral or large fixed adenopathy	Chen Meyer Perez	21/76 4/26 1/12	26/114	23
Bone destruction or nerve paralysis or both	Chen Meyer Perez	8/39 12/46 7/27	27/112	24
Neither bone destruction nor nerve paralysis	Chen Meyer Perez	42/101 54/124 41/106	137/331	41

prognosis. Males have a worse prognosis than females, that is, 33/36.8 (Perez and associates) and 34/50 (Meyer and Wang). The effects of selected clinical findings on prognosis are summarized in Table 6-5. The failure to use a common clinical staging system makes a meaningful comparison of the various series difficult. When no cervical adenopathy is detected, 55% of the patients will be living at 5 years. If the primary lesion is small, it will be controlled 60% to 70% of the time. If there is no more than ipsilateral movable lymphadenopathy, the 5-year survival rate will be about 40%, whereas bilateral or fixed adenopathy decreases the survival to 23%. Roentgenographic evidence of bone destruction in the base of the skull or cranial nerve paralysis decreases the 5-year survival rate from 41% to 24%.

Cranial nerve involvement justifies a very poor prognosis. However, involvement of nerves I to VI signifying intracranial extension is worse than paralysis of nerves VII to XII, which usually occurs inferior to the skull (Scanlon and associates). The control rates obtained for squamous cell carcinoma are shown in Table 6-6.

Lymphoepithelioma may follow the same local routes of spread as squamous cell

Table 6-6. Results of radiotherapy in treatment of carcinoma of nasopharynx (squamous cell, transitional cell, and undifferentiated carcinoma)

Author	Number treated	5-year survival
Perez and associates (1969)	45	10
Meyer and Wang (1971)	131	49
Chen and Fletcher (1971)	83	23
Scanlon and associates (1967)	32	7
TOTAL	291	89 (30%)

Table 6-7. Overall results of radiotherapy in treatment of lymphoepithelioma of nasopharynx

Author	Number treated	5-year survival
Perez and associates (1969)	11	4
Meyer and Wang (1971)	39	17
Chen and Fletcher (1971)	60	27
TOTAL	110	48 (43%)

Table 6-8. Overall results of radiotherapy in treatment of malignant lymphoma (all histologic types)

Author	Number treated	5-year survival
Perez and associates (1969)	3	1
Chen and Fletcher (1971)	11	6
Wang and associates (1962)	8	5
Vaeth (1960)	4	3
TOTAL	26	15 (57%)

carcinoma, but it metastasizes hematogeneously more frequently. Most patients with such disease will die with metastases to the lungs, liver, and bones. Local control is perhaps easier, and prognosis is better (Table 6-7).

Malignant lymphoma of the nasopharynx is readily curable locally. The dose required to eradicate the primary lesion and cervical lymph node metastases is easy to give and is well tolerated. If the disease is confined to the head and neck, the chance of cure is good (Table 6-8).

The scarcity of cancer of the nasopharynx has made it difficult to collect data that reflect the differences in control as related to technical improvements. Wang and Meyer compared the survival rates of similar clinical stages treated before and after 1956. Their data indicate that aggressive high-dose irradiation controls a larger proportion of the advanced primary lesions, that is, 13% vs 22%, and systematic elective irradiation of the entire cervical nodal chains in patients with N1 disease increases disease-free survival rates from 20% to 40%. Finally, Moench and Phillips have shown that local control is dose related (Fig. 6-8, A), and the absolute 5-year survival may approach 40% (Fig. 6-8, B).

The major sequelae of radiotherapy of this region are those related to ablation of mucosal glands with the resulting dry mouth and those related to irradiation of the ears and eyes. Damage to the base of the brain, skull, cranial nerves, or spinal cord is rare. Radiation otitis media will probably develop near the end of therapy. The drum becomes reddened, and the external canal becomes edematous. Desquamation of the canal may follow. In spite of these changes, hearing improves if patency is restored to a previously obstructed eustachian tube. The long-term effects of this dose on hearing are usually acceptable, although an occasional serious late hearing loss may develop (Dias). Months after completing therapy the delicate epithelium of the external canal will be more readily infected and inflamed. Chronic external otitis is common. The eyes can usually be spared during the treatment of these cancers. However, one must be aware of the low dose necessary to produce cataracts and the fact that high doses damage retinal blood vessels and the optic nerve. In careful ophthalmologic examinations of thirty patients who had been irradiated 7 to 30 years previously for cancer of the nasopharynx and whose eyes had been shielded by the usual techniques, twenty-five developed lens opacities. Nineteen of these were similar to radiation-induced cataracts. Retinal changes were seen in eleven of fourteen patients whose retinas received over 2500 rad at a rate of 1000 rad per week (deSchryver and associates). This dose is well below that found by other workers.

These eye changes may be subdivided into three major categories (Shukovsky and Fletcher):

1. Macular and retinal degeneration described as multiple hemorrhages, neovascularization, exudates, and retinal atrophy with decreased vision from these occurring at 2 to 3½ years postirradiation and from doses exceeding 2000 rets

2. Optic nerve atrophy manifested by progressive loss of vision and a chalk-white nerve head (same doses as in 1)

3. Central retinal artery thrombosis manifested by sudden and complete loss of vision in the irradiated eye (doses about the same as in 1)

The macula seems to be the most sensitive part of the retina and the most commonly damaged by the aforementioned doses.

Finally, it must be remembered that the anatomic relationships are such that at times it is impossible to adequately irradiate advanced cancer of this area without encompassing the brain stem and the cervical part of the spinal cord. Serious cord damage may develop in such patients. Chen and Fletcher reported three such patients. A number of Boden's patients were treated for cancer of the nasopharynx. This complication has also been emphasized by Tan and Khor.

TREATMENT OF RECURRENT CANCER. Of 170 patients with cancer of the nasopharynx, fifty-three (31%) developed regrowth of the primary tumor (Meyer and Wang). These patients can usually be reirradiated to a high dose in spite of the initial curative effort. If the recurrence appeared 2 years or more after the initial irradiation, the average survival was 4.2 years after retreatment (Meyer and Wang), which is surprisingly good. Fu also noted that the prognosis with retreatment improved as the interval from first treatment to recurrence increased.

Similar salvage of patients with postirradiation recurrent cancer has been reported by Fu and associates. They used external irradiation and intracavitary radioactive sources, either alone or combined, to treat forty-two patients with recurrent nasopharyngeal cancer. Forty-one percent were alive at 5 years after their first recurrence. Doses were often high, and necrosis developed in nine. Such necroses seemed fairly well tolerated.

MAXILLARY ANTRUM
Carcinoma of the maxillary antrum

Of the carcinomas occurring in the maxillary antrum, more than 90% will be squamous cell in type and less than 10% will be adenocarcinomas. Lymphomas also occur in this region but are infrequent. The squamous cell carcinomas arise from the ciliated columnar cells. Since the lining mucosa is thin, malignant epithelial cells are but a millimeter or so from bone (Fig. 6-10).

For clinical staging purposes the maxillary antrum is divided into a suprastructure and an infrastructure. A theoretic plane joining the medial canthus with the angle of the jaw separates these two subdivisions. The American Joint Committee (1978) identifies the TNM categories as follows:

TNM CLASSIFICATION*

T— Primary tumor
- **TX** Tumor that cannot be assessed
- **T0** No evidence of primary tumor
- **T1** Tumor confined to the antral mucosa of the infrastructure with no bone erosion or destruction

---

*From the American Joint Committee for Cancer Staging and End Results Reporting: Manual for staging of cancer, Chicago, 1978, Whiting Press.

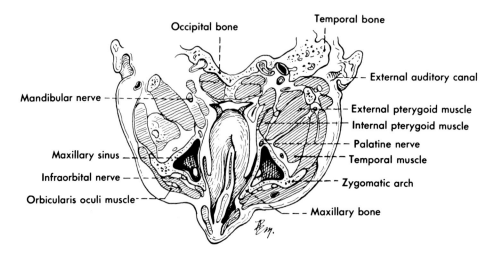

Fig. 6-10. Diagram of maxillary antrum illustrating reasons for early extra-antral spread. When this occurs posteriorly, superiorly, or superomedially, important tissues are involved yet extra-antral spread is not easily defined.

T2	Tumor confined to the suprastructure mucosa without bone destruction, or to the infrastructure with destruction of medial or inferior bony walls only
T3	More extensive tumor invading skin of cheek, orbit, anterior ethmoid sinuses, or pterygoid muscle
T4	Massive tumor with invasion of cribriform plate, posterior ethmoids, sphenoid, nasopharynx, pterygoid plates, or base of skull

N—Nodal involvement

NX	Nodes cannot be assessed
N0	No clinically positive node
N1	Single clinically positive homolateral node 3 cm or less in diameter
N2	Single clinically positive homolateral node more than 3 but not more than 6 cm in diameter or multiple clinically positive homolateral nodes, none over 6 cm in diameter
N2a	Single clinically positive homolateral node, more than 3 but not more than 6 cm in diameter
N2b	Multiple clinically positive homolateral nodes, none over 6 cm in diameter
N3	Massive homolateral node(s), bilateral nodes, or contralateral node(s)
N3a	Clinically positive homolateral node(s), over 6 cm in diameter
N3b	Bilateral clinically positive nodes (in this situation, each side of the neck should be staged separately; that is, N3b: right, N2a; left, N1)
N3c	Contralateral clinically positive node(s) only

M—Distant metastasis

MX	Not assessed
M0	No (known) distant metastasis
M1	Distant metastasis present

Early bone destruction is the rule. The diagnosis is not usually made until bone destruction is extensive. Wille found that on admission, 203 of 209 patients presented roentgenographic evidence of bone destruction. Although his series was weighted with some failures by previous treatment, it is obvious that bone destruction will be present in all but a few patients. In 197 of these patients more than two walls of the antrum showed bone destruction. About 40% of all patients will present a fistula from the antrum to the oral cavity, from the antrum through the cheek, or both. Invasion of the orbit with eye changes is present on admission in about 30% of all patients.

Regional lymph node metastases from carcinoma of the maxillary sinus have usually been described as infrequent and late. Yet Wille reported that 30% of the patients had lymph node metastases on admission and that an additional 5% developed them later. Pezner and associates found cervical adenopathy in thirteen of sixty-three patients (21%) on admission, whereas nine (18% of the remainder) had developed adenopathy by the time of the follow-up examination. It is thought that the retropharyngeal nodes are usually the first to be involved, but metastases to the upper cervical nodes may be the first to be detected clinically.

TECHNIQUE. Shocking signs of advanced cancer are unfortunately the rule. From these findings it is clear that, with the clinical material we now see, a successful result will usually depend on a mode of treatment adaptable to locally advanced cancer. The surgeon considers the hard palate, the orbital contents, and the lateral, anterior, and posterior walls with their associated soft tissues expendable structures, and the technique of radical resection is frequently discussed. However, the results of such procedures without associated irradiation are not good. Local recurrence is a common cause of failure.

The more commonly recognized clinical situations in which surgery is not recommended are extension into the frontal sinus, extension to the cribriform plate, extension into the walls of the nasopharynx or opposite antrum, bilateral or fixed nodes, distant metastases, and poor general condition (Beale and Molony, 1976).

In patients with limited lesions in which the anterior and superior walls are not involved, deformity after surgery need not be so severe, but we believe that in these selected patients similar cure rates are possible with irradiation, and the cosmetic and functional result will be better with irradiation. Neither in the more curable limited stages nor in the rarely controlled advanced stages has radical surgery *alone* been proved superior to carefully planned irradiation with resection of residual disease. It is probable that superior results are obtained by destruction of the peripheral part of this cancer by preoperative irradiation followed by excision of the centrally located more radioresistant nidus.

The relatively high incidence of postirradiation local recurrence is thought to be related to the fact that these primary lesions are often very advanced and of a large volume. Also the cancer is invariably in bone and muscle and often in perineural lymphatics. Of fifty patients with this cancer, forty-two or 84% were classified as T3 or T4 lesions (Cheng and Wang, 1977). It is not surprising that various combinations of radiation therapy, surgery, and chemotherapy are being tried with the hope of improving local control. Over the short-term interval we have been favorably impressed with local intra-arterial infusion of methotrexate and irradiation to a dose of 6000 rad or more in 6 to 7 weeks, followed by radical excision for patients with extensive primary lesions.

At the time of biopsy, an inspection of the antrum may assist in defining location

Table 6-9. Factors influencing prognosis in cancers of paranasal sinuses (treatment consisted of several techniques, some of which combined surgery and radiotherapy)*

Factors	Number of patients	5-year survival (%)
Localized to sinus (no bone destruction)	29	40.8
Bone destruction or ethmoids involved	63	28.9
Orbit involved	53	15.3
Regional metastases	43	8.8

*Modified from Holsti, L. R., and Rinne, R.: Acta Radiol. **6:**337-350, 1967.

Table 6-10. Causes of failure in patients irradiated and resected for cancer of paranasal sinuses (of 121 previously untreated patients, causes of failure in forty-four defined)*

Radiotherapy alone or combined with surgery	
1. Persistent cancer within irradiated volume	3
2. Persistent cancer at edge of irradiated volume	9
3. Persistent cancer in volume protected by eye shield	4
Surgery	
1. Persistent cancer at edge of resected volume	11
2. Cancer known to have been left behind	3
Planned palliation	14
TOTAL	44

*Modified from Boone, M. L., and associates: Am. J. Roentgenol. **102:**627-636, 1968.

and extent of the cancer. As much necrotic debris as is practical should be removed. If the patient is febrile, antibiotics should be used. This reduces the need for drainage.

Despite careful physical examination, the best radiographic studies of each antral wall, including computed tomography, and inspection through the palatal defect, the volume of interest is difficult to define. Detailed roentgenographs of this area, that is, Caldwell's and Water's views, submental-vertex view, tomographs in two planes, and a lateral view, along with a computerized axial tomogram, define bone destruction. However, soft tissue infiltration, which often will not produce any functional or radiographic manifestations, must be estimated in keeping with clinical experience. (See Tables 6-9 and 6-10). In general the dimensions of the ports are extended to include generous margins around the walls suspected of involvement. Spread into the pterygoid or ethmoid regions may be difficult to detect radiographically. For this reason these areas are frequently included in the treated volume without having evidence of their involvement. If the floor of the orbit is involved radiographically, or if the eye is displaced or partially paralyzed, the entire orbit with its contents should be irradiated at the risk of losing the eyesight (Chapter 5). We believe that involvement of even a part of the orbit demands full irradiation of the entire orbit. Attempting to shield the globe during the latter part of the irradiation is a risky procedure. Even when the floor of the orbit is radiographically normal, the anterior beam usually encompasses the infraorbital ridge. Similarly, the hard palate is encompassed even though it is not clinically or radiographically involved.

Because of the marked eccentricity of the antrum, special techniques are used to deliver a relatively homogeneous dose to the volume. Formerly, with intracavitary sources, the maximum dose was 7500 to 9500 rad in 10 days at a point 2 cm from the source. For small lesions the fact that the depth dose decreased rapidly was regarded as an advantage. As indicated previously, however, most carcinomas of the antrum are advanced when first seen. This rapid decrease in dose then becomes a limiting disadvantage (Table 6-10).

We depend primarily on external irradiation, either alone or preoperatively, in the treatment of antral carcinomas, large or small. The most homogeneous dose distribution is obtained with ipsilateral anterior and lateral megavoltage beams modified with wedge filters. When no orbital invasion is present, the lateral beam can be directed to spare the ipsilateral and contralateral eyes. However, when the ipsilateral orbit must be irradiated, the contralateral eye must be spared. This is accomplished by angling the lateral beam slightly posteriorly. An alternative is to use a wedged pair of beams—an anterior and a superior port. Whichever port arrangement is used, care must be taken to include the ethmoid sinus in the volume of high dose. This is accomplished by crossing the midline with the anterior beam. Of course, bolus is necessary when the skin is involved by cancer.

When radiation therapy is the sole treatment, a tissue dose of 6500 to 7500 rad in 6 to 9 weeks or its biologic equivalent is usually considered optimum. This degree of fractionation is necessary if necrosis is to be kept to a minimum. We believe that if doses of this magnitude cannot control the cancer, it is rather futile to increase the dose further. The type of time-dose-volume study necessary to establish optimum factors is not available.

Shortly after treatment has started, the necrotic material decreases, and the pain and sense of fullness lessen. Edema about the orbit subsides slowly as inflammation and venous obstruction diminish.

METASTASES TO CERVICAL LYMPH NODES. Metastases to cervical lymph nodes from cancer of the antrum are usually thought of as being infrequent. However, such metastases were present in ten of thirty-one patients reviewed by Bataini and Ennuyer, eleven of fifty reviewed by Cheng and Wang, forty-eight of 224 patients reviewed by Kurohara and associates, and thirteen of sixty-three patients reviewed by Pezner and associates. These and other series indicate that the incidence of metastases to cervical nodes varies from 20% to 30%. Distant metastases are infrequent. Radical neck dissection was previously recommended for cervical lymphadenopathy in these patients. Recently, radiations have been administered to such nodes with moderate success. (See Chapter 4.) We believe that irradiation of the entire cervical chain is the treatment of choice for clinically positive metastases (Chapter 4). When nodes are enlarged on admission, the change of cure is slight, that is, 15% (Dalley, 1959; Bataini and Ennuyer).

Prophylactic irradiation of the lymph node chains when no lymphadenopathy is present cannot be justified on the basis of existing data (Pezner and associates). Of forty-seven patients who were initially assessed as having no metastasis, eight subsequently developed adenopathy. Metastases in the cervical lymph nodes was the sole cause of failure in only one of these eight.

PROGNOSIS AND RESULTS. Our present methods of treatment, whether radical surgery, irradiation, or a combination of the two, are of limited curative value in the advanced cases. Since a high proportion of the patients come initially with far-advanced carcinoma, cure rates are low. Surgery alone has been applied only to selected patients, and it is impossible to compare survival rates obtained by radical surgery with those obtained by irradiation. Survival rates obtained by irradiation alone or irradiation associated with minor surgical procedures have been reported by several large treatment centers. These will usually contain a fairly representative group of cases. Published data are presented in Table 6-11. Although some of these data are old, the scarcity of much recent data makes them of value. When radiation therapy is the sole treatment, the 5-year tumor-free survival rate of patients seen in the usual large general hospital should average above 30%. With selection of patients for surgery, higher rates can be expected. Rarely will a patient treated with positive lymph node metastases survive 5 years free of disease. Table 6-9 relates survival to the various types of extension. Carefully planned external irradiation with wedge filters, as described previously, apparently gives results superior to those obtained by predominantly intracavitary radioactive materials (Stewart, 1960). As might be expected, local control rates vary with cell type. Cantril and associates found the order to be transitional cell carcinoma, lymphoepithelioma, undifferentiated carcinoma, plasmacytoma, malignant lymphoma, and, last, squamous cell and muco-epidermoid carcinoma.

Beale and Molony selected fifty-five of their ninety-nine patients for combined preoperative irradiation and surgery. Among those patients whose resected specimens revealed no evidence of residual cancer, 48% were disease-free at 5 years. When residual cancer was found in the resected specimen, 33.5% of the patients were disease-free at 5 years. Obviously, patient selection has a major influence on survival rates obtained by this combination.

Cheng and Wang reported that seven of twelve patients treated with preoperative irradiation (6000 rad in 6 weeks) followed by radical surgery were living and

Table 6-11. Results of treatment for carcinoma of maxillary antrum (treatment usually consisted of irradiation alone or irradiation with minor surgery)

Author	Years included	Number treated	5-year survival
Hunt	1952	87	30 (34%)
Boone	1954-1963	70	(35%)
Bataini	1959-1965	19	6 (31%)
TOTAL		176	(34%)

well at 3 years (clinical stages not defined). After using the same techniques Harrison reported five of six patients with T1 lesions and nineteen of thirty-one patients with T2 lesions were free of cancer at 3 years. Very poor control rates (only three of forty) were obtained for patients with more advanced lesions.

For many anatomic sites the advantages to be found in postoperative as compared to preoperative irradiation are related to two facts: the surgical specimen may assist in defining the specific site of local residual cancer and wound healing can proceed normally. However, postoperative irradiation of the antral area is associated with serious healing problems. Large surgical defects in this area do not tolerate radiations well, and information gained from the operative specimen has not been particularly helpful. Thus preoperative irradiation is preferred.

Irradiation provides worthwhile palliation to some of the patients with locally incurable lesions. However, perhaps 20% of our patients have shown little improvement and have continued a downhill course to death.

The adenocarcinomas arise from the glandular cells of the antral mucosa. They are the same general types of cancer as occur in the major salivary glands, and for this reason they should be treated by radical surgery when possible (Roth). The cell types that have been described are cylindroma, malignant mixed tumors, adenocarcinomas, mucoepidermoid tumors, and anaplastic tumors (Rafla-Demetrious). However, irradiation may be successful. Of nineteen patients treated by combined surgery and irradiation, two were living without recurrence at 5 years (Tod). Of twenty-five treated patients with cylindromatous types of adenocarcinoma of the paranasal sinuses, nine were well after 5 years, and of ten patients with adenocarcinomas of other types, two were well after 5 years (Larsson and Martensson). Similar results were reported by Rafla-Demetrious. Of twelve treated by radiotherapy alone, one was living cancer-free at 5 years. Ten died with cancer, and one died without cancer. With combined radiotherapy and surgery, five of fifteen were living and well at 5 years. Results reported by Gamez-Araujo and associates confirm the continued poor prognosis of patients with adenocarcinoma of the paranasal sinuses. He reported two of fourteen living without disease after 5 years, two living less than 5 years, and one dead of unrelated causes at 1 month. It must be remembered, however, that these tumors may recur 10 to 15 years after treatment, and for this reason a 5-year survival rate is not the same as the permanent control rate.

Malignant lymphomas of the maxillary antrum are just as radiosensitive as malignant lymphomas elsewhere. The clinical stage of the lymphoma must be established just as described for lymphomas of the nasopharynx. A generous margin around the tumor can be included in the treated volume. Minimum doses of 5000 rad in 4 to 6 weeks are usually possible and advisable. If confined to the antral area, prognosis is good. Of eighteen patients treated by Tod (many undoubtedly understaged by current standards) nine were living without evidence of disease after 5 years. When no cervical lymphadenopathy was present, Wang and associates reported 71% were living without disease at 3 years. When lymphadenopathy was present, at least four of nine were living without evidence of disease at 3 years.

Carcinomas of the nasal fossa and ethmoid sinuses require special consideration. They present initially either as a swelling of the bridge of the nose and the medial canthi, or they produce nasal obstruction as a nasal polyp. Their central, anterior location makes direct lateral ports of limited value, since they would usually entail irradiation of the eyes if the entire volume of interest were to be encompassed. To bring these ports posteriorly and then angle them anteriorly means the exit beam will strike the opposite eye. A single anterior ^{60}Co beam may be sufficient for markedly anterior lesions. For the more extensive lesions the posterior zone of low dose should be irradiated with lateral ports. Small wedges for the lateral beams will increase the homogeneity. Common causes of failure are the same as tabulated in Table 6-10.

SUMMARY. Carcinoma of the maxillary antrum is usually squamous cell in type, but adenocarcinoma may occasionally occur. Advanced bone destruction with infiltration of adjacent soft tissues is the rule. To be effective in these advanced stages, treatment must include eradication of disease in or near tissues of importance both functionally and cosmetically. The effectiveness of radiotherapy in controlling *limited* cancers compares favorably with that of surgery. The fact that deformity with radiotherapy is less makes it preferable. On the other hand, neither radiotherapy alone nor surgery alone controls as many advanced cancers as does combined radiotherapy and surgery.

MIDLINE GRANULOMA

Midline granuloma is a progressive destructive necrosis of the upper air passages, which, if untreated, is always lethal. Bone, cartilage, and soft tissues are destroyed as it progresses (Fig. 6-11, *A*). Death occurs from infections such as meningitis, from hemorrhage, or from malnutrition. The histologic picture is one of chronic inflammation, necrosis, granulomas, small vessel vasculitis, and endarteritis.

This disease has often been confused with Wegener's granulomatosis, which is distinguishable from midline granuloma on histopathologic examination (Fauci and associates) and which is clinically different, as shown in Table 6-12. The distinction between these two diseases is critical in selecting the optimum treatment, since midline granuloma is greatly benefited by irradiation (Fig. 6-11, *B*), and Wegener's granulomatosis is best treated with systemic chemotherapy (usually cyclophosphamide). The few patients available for treatment and analysis do not enable us to sharply define the optimum radiation treatment factors. Experience suggests that wide margins of apparently normal tissue should be encompassed in the treated volume. The dose must be substantial (5000 rad or more in daily fractions of 180 to 200 rad). Fauci and associates controlled eight of ten patients irradiated with this dose. However, two patients had serious CNS sequelae either from the treatment or from the disease.

It is now clear that irradiation can provide these patients excellent long-term control. Treatment volumes are generally large, and doses required are substantial, so daily doses should probably be modest.

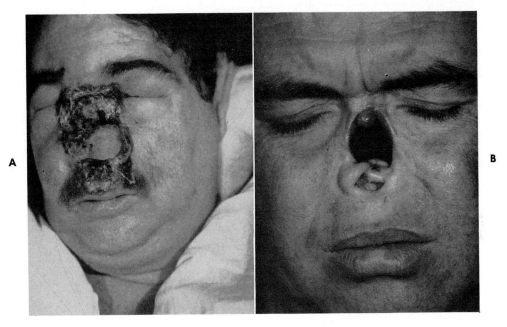

Fig. 6-11. A, Extensive lethal midline granuloma that has progressed over 6 months while patient was being treated with steroids and antibiotics. **B,** Same patient 8 months after irradiation. Patient remains well over 5 years after irradiation.

Table 6-12. Clinicopathologic criteria that distinguish midline granuloma from Wegener's granulomatosis*

Midline granuloma	Wegener's granulomatosis
Destructive upper airway lesions with characteristic extension through palate	Inflammatory upper airway disease predominantly of sinuses and nasal mucosa. Rarely, if ever, erodes through palate and face
Lungs not involved	Characteristic pulmonary infiltrates. Histopathology shows necrotizing granulomatous vasculitis
Kidneys not involved	Characteristic early focal glomerulitis, progressing to fulminant glomerulonephritis
Disseminated vasculitis very rarely, if ever, occurs	Characteristic disseminated small vessel vasculitis

*Modified from Fauci, A. S., Johnson, R. E., and Wolff, S. M.: Ann. Intern. Med. **84:**140-147, 1976.

REFERENCES

Adams, W. S., and Morrison, R.: On primary carcinoma of the middle ear and mastoid, J. Laryngol. **69**:115-131, 1955.

American Joint Committee for Cancer Staging and End Results Reporting, Manual for staging of cancer, Chicago, 1978, Whiting Press.

Arthur, K.: Radiotherapy in carcinoma of the middle ear and auditory canal, J. Laryngol. Otol. **90**:753-762, 1976.

Bataini, J. P., and Ennuyer, A.: Advanced carcinoma of the maxillary antrum treated by cobalt teletherapy and electron beam irradiation, Radiology **102**:737, 1972.

Beale, F. A., and Molony, T. J.: The role of radiotherapy in benign and malignant disease of the maxillary antrum, Otolaryngol. Clin. North Am. **9**:269-289, 1976.

Boden, G.: Radiation myelitis of the brain stem, J. Fac. Radiologists **2**:79-94, 1950.

Boland, J., and Paterson, R.: Cancer of the middle ear and external auditory meatus, J. Laryngol. **69**:468-478, 1955.

Boone, M. L., Harle, T. S., Higholt, H. W., and Fletcher, G. H.: Malignant disease of the paranasal sinuses and nasal cavity, Am. J. Roentgenol. **102**:627-636, 1968.

Borsanyi, S. J., and Blanchard, C. L.: Ionizing radiation and the ear, J.A.M.A. **181**:958-961, 1962.

Bradley, W. H., and Maxwell, J. H.: Neoplasms of the middle ear and mastoid, Laryngoscope **64**: 533-556, 1954.

Bradshaw, J. D.: Radiotherapy in glomus jugulare tumors, Clin. Radiol. **12**:227-234, 1961.

Cantril, S. T., Parker, R. G., and Lund, P. K.: Malignant tumors of the maxillary sinus, Acta Radiol. **58**:105-128, 1962.

Capps, F. C. W.: Glomus jugulare tumours of middle ear, J. Laryngol. **66**:302-314, 1952.

Chen, K. Y., and Fletcher, G. H.: Malignant tumors of the nasopharynx, Radiology **99**:165-171, 1971.

Cheng, V. S. T., and Wang, C. C.: Carcinomas of the paranasal sinuses, Cancer **40**:3038-3041, 1977.

Chiang, T. C., and Jung, P. F.: The nasopharyngoscope, and camera examination of the primary carcinoma of nasopharynx, Cancer **40**:2353-2364, 1977.

Collins, V. P., and Pool, J. L.: Treatment of antral cancer by combined surgery and radium therapy, Radiology **55**:41-45, 1950.

Dalley, V. M.: Cancer of the middle ear, J. Fac. Radiol. **4**:193-196, 1953.

Dalley, V. M.: Malignant disease of the antrum, Br. J. Radiol.**32**:378-385, 1959.

Dalley, V. M.: Radiation therapy in relation to malignant tumors of the temporal bone. In Buschke, F.: Progress in radiation therapy, vol. 3, New York, 1965, Grune & Stratton, Inc.

del Regato, J. A.: Roentgenotherapy in epitheliomas of the maxillary sinus, Surg. Gynecol. Obstet. **65**:657-665, 1937.

del Regato, J. A.: Cancer of the respiratory system and upper digestive tract. In del Regato, J. A., and Spjut, H. J.: Ackerman and del Regato's Cancer: diagnosis, treatment, and prognosis, ed. 5, St. Louis, 1977, The C. V. Mosby Co.

deSchryver, A., Wachtmeister, L., and Baryd, I.: Ophthalmologic observations on long-term survivors after radiotherapy for nasopharyngeal tumours, Acta Radiol. [Ther.] **10**:193-209, 1971.

Dias, A.: Effects on the hearing of patients treated by irradiation in the head and neck area, J. Laryngol. **80**:276-287, 1966.

Fauci, A. S., Johnson, R. E., and Wolff, S. M.: Radiation therapy of midline granuloma, Ann. Intern. Med. **84**:140-147, 1976.

Fletcher, G. H., and Million, R. R.: Malignant tumors of the nasopharynx, Am. J. Roentgenol. **93**: 44-55, 1965.

Fu, K., Newman, H., and Phillips, T. L.: Treatment of locally recurrent carcinoma of the nasopharynx, Radiology **117**:425-431, 1975.

Fuller, A. M., Brown, H. A., Harrison, E. G., and Siekert, R. G.: Chemodectomas of the glomus jugulare tumors, Laryngoscope **77**:218-238, 1967.

Gamble, J. E., Peterson, E. A., and Chandler, J. R.: Radiation effects on the inner ear, Arch. Otolaryngol. **88**:64-69, 1968.

Gamez-Araujo, J. J., Ayala, A. G., and Guillamondegui, O.: Mucinous adenocarcinomas of nose and paranasal sinuses, Cancer **36**:1100-1105, 1975.

Girden, E.: Effect of roentgen rays upon hearing in dogs, J. Comp. Physiol. Psychol. **20**:263-290, 1935.

Godtfredsen, E.: Ophthalmologic and neurologic symptoms of malignant nasopharyngeal tumours, Acta psychiat. et neurol., suppl. 34, pp. 1-323, 1944.

Grubb, W. B., and Lampe, I.: The role of radiation therapy in the treatment of chemodectomas of the glomus jugulare, Laryngoscope **75**:1861-1871, 1965.

Hanks, G. E., Bagshaw, M. A., and Kaplan, H. S.:

The management of cervical lymph node metastasis, Am. J. Roentgenol. **105**:74-83, 1969.

Harrison, D. F. N.: The management of malignant tumors affecting the maxillary and ethmoidal sinuses, J. Laryngol. Otol. **87**:749-772, 1973.

Hatfield, P. M., James, A. E., and Schulz, M. D.: Chemodectomas of the glomus jugulare, Cancer **30**:1164-1168, 1972.

Holsti, L. R., and Rinne, R.: Treatment of malignant tumours of paranasal sinuses, Acta Radiol. **6**:337-350, 1967.

Hoppe, R. T., Goffinet, D. R., and Bagshaw, M.: Carcinoma of the nasopharynx, Cancer **37**:2605-2612, 1976.

Hoppe, R. T., Williams, J., Warnke, R., Goffinet, D. R., and Bagshaw, M. A.: Carcinoma of the nasopharynx—the significance of histology, Int. J. Radiat. Oncol. **4**:199-205, 1978.

Hudgins, P. T.: Radiotherapy for extensive glomus jugulare tumors, Radiology **103**:427-429, 1972.

Hunt, A. H.: Discussion on treatment of malignant disease of the upper jaw, Proc. R. Soc. Med. **48**:75-78, 1955.

Kelemen, G.: Experimental defects in the ear and the upper airways induced by radiation, Arch. Otolaryngol. **61**:405-418, 1955.

Kurohara, S. S., Webster, J. H., Ellis, F., Fitzgerald, J. P., Shedd, D. P., and Badib, A. O.: Role of radiation therapy and of surgery in the management of localized epidermoid carcinoma of the maxillary sinus, Am. J. Roentgenol. **114**:35-42, 1972.

Larsson, L. G., and Martensson, G.: Carcinoma of the paranasal sinuses and nasal cavities, Acta Radiol. **42**:149-172, 1954.

Lederman, M.: Cancer of the nasopharynx, Springfield, Ill., 1961, Charles C Thomas, Publisher.

Lindahl, J. W. S.: Carcinoma of the middle ear and meatus, J. Laryngol. **69**:457-467, 1955.

Maruyama, Y., Gold, L. H., and Kieffer, S. A.: Radioactive cobalt treatment of glomus jugulare tumors, Acta Radiol. **10**:239-247, 1971.

Meyer, J. E., and Wang, C. C.: Carcinoma of the nasopharynx—factors influencing results of therapy, Radiology **100**:385-388, 1971.

Miller, J. R.: Results of treatment in glomus jugulare tumors with emphasis on radiotherapy, Radiology **79**:430-434, 1962.

Million, R. R., Fletcher, G. H., and Jesse, R. H.: Evaluation of elective irradiation of the neck for squamous cell carcinoma of the nasopharynx, tonsillar fossa, and base of tongue, Radiology **80**:973-988, 1963.

Moench, H. C., and Phillips, T. L.: Carcinoma of the nasopharynx: review of 146 patients with emphasis on radiation dose and time factors, Am. J. Surg. **124**:515-518, 1972.

Moskovskaya, N. V.: Effect of ionizing radiation on function of vestibular analyzer, Vestn. Otorinolaringol. **22**:43-49, 1960.

Newman, H., Rowe, J. F., and Phillips, T. L.: Radiation therapy of glomus jugulare tumor, Am. J. Roentgenol. **118**:663-669, 1973.

Palacios, E.: Chemodectomas of the head and neck, Am. J. Roentgenol. **110**:129-140, 1970.

Perez, C. A., Ackerman, L. V., Mill, W. B., Ogura, J. H., and Powers, W. E.: Cancer of the nasopharynx, Cancer **24**:1-17, 1969.

Pezner, R. D., Moss, W. T., Tong, D., Blasko, J. C. and Griffin, T. W.: Cervical lymph node metastases in patients with squamous cell carcinoma of the maxillary antrum (submitted for publication).

Rafla-Demetrious, S.: Mucous and salivary gland tumors, Springfield, Ill., 1970, Charles C Thomas, Publisher.

Raines, D., and James, A. G.: Management of cancer of maxillary antrum, Surg. Gynecol. Obstet. **101**:395-400, 1955.

Rosenwasser, H.: Glomus jugulare tumors, Arch. Otolaryngol. **83**:3-40, 1968.

Roth, M.: Adenoid cystic carcinoma of the oral cavity, paranasal sinuses, and upper respiratory tract, Am. J. Roentgenol. **78**:790-803, 1957.

Scanlon, P. W., Rhodes, R. E., Woolner, L. B., Devine, K. D., and McBean, J. B.: Cancer of the nasopharynx, Am. J. Roentgenol. **99**:314-325, 1967.

Shukovsky, L. J., and Fletcher, G. H.: Retinal and optic nerve complications in a high dose irradiation technique of ethmoid sinus and nasal cavity, Radiology **104**:629-634, 1972.

Simko, T. G., Griffin, T. W., Gerdes, A. J., Parker, R. G., Tesh, D. W., Taylor, W., and Blasko, J. C.: The role of radiation therapy in the treatment of glomus jugulare tumors, Cancer **42**:104-106, 1978.

Sinha, P. P., and Aziz, H. I.: Treatment of carcinoma of the middle ear, Radiology **126**:485-487, 1978.

Stewart, J. G.: A wedge filter approach with 4 mV radiation to the treatment of carcinoma of the alveolus and antrum, Proc. R. Soc. Med. **53**:239-242, 1960.

Tidwell, T. J., and Montague, E. D.: Chemodectomas involving the temporal bone, Radiology **116**:147-149, 1975.

Tod, M. C.: The treatment of cancer of the maxillary antrum by radium, Br. J. Radiol. **21**:270-275, 1948.

Wang, C. C., Little, J. B., and Schulz, M. D.: Cancer of the nasopharynx: its clinical and radio-therapeutic considerations, Cancer 15:921-926, 1962.

Wang, C. C.: Radiation therapy in the management of carcinoma of the external auditory canal, middle ear, and mastoid, Radiology 116:713-715, 1975.

Wang, C. C., and Doppke, K.: Osteoradionecrosis of the temporal bone—consideration of Nominal Standard Dose, Int. J. Radiat. Oncol. Biol. Phys. 1:881-883, 1976.

Wille, C.: Malign tumors in the nose and its accessory sinuses, Acta Otolaryngol., suppl. 65, pp. 1-58, 1947.

Williams, I. G.: Carcinoma of the antrum, Proc. R. Soc. Med. 43:671-674, 1950.

Williams, I. G.: Radiotherapy of tumors of glomus jugulare, J. Fac. Radiol. 8:335-338, 1957.

7
The endolarynx and hypopharynx

The justification of radiotherapy for carcinoma of the larynx and hypopharynx lies in its ability to cure and yet preserve function. No sacrifice of cure rates is warranted. Cure can be accomplished by irradiation alone in a high proportion of selected patients with limited cancers. Should radiotherapy fail, curative surgery may still be possible. When applicable, this sequence enables the radiation oncologist to preserve function without sacrificing cure rates.

Preservation of function in these valuable tissues demands respect for tissue tolerances, yet carcinomas of these areas demand high doses that usually provoke severe reactions. These parameters will be discussed on p. 219. However, the need to balance these factors should be kept in mind during the following discussion. Between 95% and 98% of all carcinomas of the larynx and hypopharynx are microscopically diagnosed as squamous cell in type. It is a remarkable fact that despite this apparent microscopic similarity, the clinical courses of laryngeal and hypopharyngeal lesions are different. Regardless of the methods of treatment, lesions of the piriform sinus are less curable than those of the aryepiglottic fold. Those of the aryepiglottic fold are less curable than those of the false cord, and those of the false cord are less curable than those of the true cord. Partial explanation of this variation in curability lies in the unequal invasive and metastasizing characteristics. Extensive invasion and metastases with hypopharyngeal lesions are to be expected, but with true cord lesions we expect limited invasion and rare metastases.

Inseparably associated with the location of these lesions and their invasive and metastasizing characteristics are other factors affecting response to irradiation. Tumors that infiltrate epiglottic or thyroid cartilage or striated muscle are less frequently eradicated locally by irradiation than those that do not. The muscle planes of the neck and perineural lymphatics provide the pathways of extension (Ballantyne). Spread from hypopharyngeal or advanced laryngeal lesions may extend upward almost to the skull. Retropharyngeal extension from lesions of the piriform sinus may be clinically imperceptible but may be identified in the surgical specimen. One must be aware of these aspects of the natural history and tailor ports to fit the anticipated spread of the cancer.

203

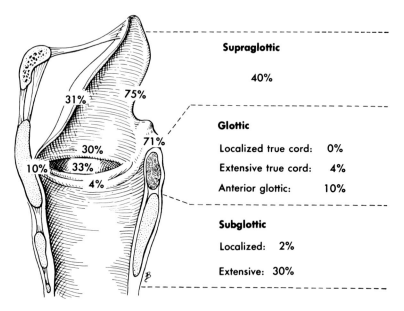

Supraglottic

40%

Glottic

Localized true cord: 0%

Extensive true cord: 4%

Anterior glottic: 10%

Subglottic

Localized: 2%

Extensive: 30%

Fig. 7-1. Incidence of lymph node metastases according to anatomic site of primary lesion. (Modified from Baclesse, F.: Br. J. Radiol., suppl. 3, 1949, and Kuhn, A. J., Devine, K. D., and McDonald, J. R.: Laryngoscope **67:**169-190, 1957.)

Infection, particularly if long-standing, produces fibrosis with vascular changes and may seriously decrease the radioresponsiveness of cancer cells. Such infection is usually associated with invasion of cartilage by tumor and is the most significant etiologic factor in the development of postirradiation cartilage necrosis.

At this point the influence of lymph node metastases on radiocurability will not be discussed. However, as has been noted in other sites, the presence of lymph node metastases signifies a particularly malignant cell type and warrants a worse prognosis (Fig. 7-1).

From the previous discussion, it is obvious that the wide differences in radiosensitivity and radiocurability justify a clinical classification, and many have been suggested. We have insisted that a simple description of the structures clinically involved is the minimum requirement for any classification. Beyond this, lesions may be grouped as endolaryngeal and hypopharyngeal. The endolaryngeal lesions are subdivided into glottic, subglottic, and supraglottic lesions. Variations in prognosis have been described among these lesions occurring in the hypopharynx (Baclesse; Lederman, 1967), and this classification will be reviewed later.

CARCINOMA OF THE ENDOLARYNX

Carcinoma of the endolarynx includes carcinoma arising from all anatomic structures of the interior of the larynx from the aryepiglottic fold to the first tracheal cartilage. The wide range of behavior of these lesions has been recognized for many years and has been emphasized in the large series reported by Baclesse, Kuhn and associates, McGavran and associates, and Micheau and associates (Fig. 7-1). These lesions are clinically separated into cancer of the glottis, subglottis, and supraglottis. The American Joint Committee on Cancer Staging and End Results Reporting developed the following revised (1978) classification of carcinoma of the larynx.

TNM CLASSIFICATION*

T— Primary tumor

TX	Tumor that cannot be assessed by rules
T0	No evidence of primary tumor

Supraglottis

TIS	Carcinoma in situ
T1	Tumor confined to region of origin with normal mobility
T2	Tumor involving adjacent supraglottic site(s) or glottis without fixation
T3	Tumor limited to larynx with fixation and/or extension to involve postcricoid area, medial wall of pyriform sinus, or pre-epiglottic space
T4	Massive tumor extending beyond the larynx to involve oropharynx, soft tissues of neck, or destruction of thyroid cartilage

Glottis

TIS	Carcinoma in situ
T1	Tumor confined to vocal cord(s) with normal mobility (including involvement of anterior or posterior commissures)
T2	Supraglottic and/or subglottic extension of tumor with normal or impaired cord mobility
T3	Tumor confined to the larynx with cord fixation
T4	Massive tumor with thyroid cartilage destruction and/or extension beyond the confines of the larynx

Subglottis

TIS	Carcinoma in situ
T1	Tumor confined to the subglottic region
T2	Tumor extension to vocal cords with normal or impaired cord mobility
T3	Tumor confined to larynx with cord fixation
T4	Massive tumor with cartilage destruction or extension beyond the confines of the larynx, or both

N—Nodal involvement

NX	Nodes cannot be assessed
N0	No clinically positive node
N1	Single clinically positive homolateral node 3 cm or less in diameter
N2	Single clinically positive homolateral node more than 3 but no more than 6 cm in diameter or multiple clinically positive homolateral nodes, none more than 6 cm in diameter
N2a	Single clinically positive homolateral node, more than 3 but no more than 6 cm in diameter
N2b	Multiple clinically positive homolateral nodes, none over 6 cm in diameter
N3	Massive homolateral node(s), bilateral nodes, or contralateral node(s)
N3a	Clinically positive homolateral node(s), one more than 6 cm in diameter
N3b	Bilateral clinically positive nodes (in this situation, each side of the neck should be staged separately; that is, N3b: right, N2a; left, N1)
N3c	Contralateral clinically positive node(s) only

M—Distant metastasis

MX	Not assessed
M0	No (known) distant metastasis
M1	Distant metastasis present

---

*From the American Joint Committee for Cancer Staging and End Results Reporting: Manual for staging of cancer, Chicago, 1978, Whiting Press.

HISTOPATHOLOGY

Predominant cancer is squamous cell carcinoma of undifferentiated carcinoma—also adenocarcinoma and others

GRADE

Well-differentiated, moderately well-differentiated, poorly to very poorly differentiated, or numbers 1, 2, 3-4

STAGE GROUPING

Stage I	T1	N0	M0
Stage II	T2	N0	M0
Stage III	T3	N0	M0
	T1 or T2 or T3, N1, M0		
Stage IV	T4, N0 or N1, M0		
	Any T, N2 or N3, M0		
	Any T, Any N, M1		

The stage of the primary tumor is determined not only by its mucosal extent but also by the presence or absence of fixation.

GLOTTIS. Glottic cancers are those arising from the true vocal cord or anterior commissure. They produce progressive hoarseness early in their development and are therefore usually diagnosed when still limited. These cancers may appear on the superior or inferior surface of the cord or may develop on its free margin. Most cord lesions are well differentiated and, apparently because of the scanty lymphatic drainage from the cord, rarely metastasize until there has been infiltration beyond the cord. The staging of carcinoma of the true cord is relatively simple and is closely related to prognosis. The status of the mobility of the vocal cords and the extent of the lesion on the mucosal surface are also the major clinical factors bearing on prognosis, since metastases are rare from this primary site.

Clinical staging and treatment require an accurate definition of tumor extent. Direct and indirect laryngeal examination are essential. Soft tissue films of the area in question, tomograms, laryngograms, and computed tomographs (Mancuso and associates) will provide additional valuable details of extent. Cancer extension into any of the normal recesses, the depth and location of neoplastic ulcerations, and fixed or enlarged normal structures may be defined by these highly useful radiographic studies.

Infiltration into the muscle underlying the cord decreases cord mobility, and in advanced cases the cord may be entirely fixed. The presence or absence of cord fixation is a good clinical index of the degree of infiltration and has been found closely related to curability by radiotherapeutic measures. McGavran and associates (1959) found on microscopic study that the muscle was always invaded when cord fixation was present. They also found the muscle invaded in half of those cases in which no fixation had been described clinically. The extent as defined on careful histologic sectioning of the resected glottis will vary from the clinically determined extent in 16% to 31%. Underestimation of extent comprises about two thirds of these variances, and overestimation of extent comprises about one third (Micheau and associates). In glottic lesions in which the cord is normally movable (Stage I and some

Table 7-1. Results of radiotherapy for limited carcinoma of the true cord*

Author	Number of patients	Well at 5 years (%)
Hibbs	27	91
Perez	47	86
Robbins	19	80
Sheline	30	80
Wang	107	73

*Carcinomas were limited to the vocal cords. Vocal cords were movable. Patients lost to follow-up were usually counted as dying of cancer.

Table 7-2. Results of laryngectomy for radiation failures*

Anatomic site	Mobility	5-year, disease-free survival
Part or all of cord involved	Normally mobile	33/41 (80%)
One or both cords or with extension above or below cords	Impaired mobility	12/16 (75%)
Locally advanced	Fixed	12/27 (44%)

*Modified from Wang, C. C.: Am. J. Roentgenol. **120:**157-163, 1974.

Stage II), the radiocurability will average better than 80%, whereas with radio-therapy for glottic lesions producing cord fixation (Stages III and IV), the 5-year control rate will be about 30% (Wang). The site of the cord lesion may also alter prognosis. Lesions located anteriorly are less likely to metastasize and more readily controlled by irradiation than those situated in the posterior one half of the cord or the arytenoid area. Extent of infiltration is highly significant. Radiographic evidence of destruction of the thyroid cartilage by tumor greatly increases the risk of postirradiation cartilaginous necrosis and decreases the chances of cure, even though some such cases can be controlled by irradiation. If a tracheostomy is required before or during treatment, the prognosis is decidedly worse. The necessity for a tracheostomy is just one manifestation of advanced cancer, and this alone probably accounts for the worse prognosis.

It has been shown in many clinics that limited cancers of the anterior two thirds of the cords are equally curable either by irradiation or surgery (Table 7-1). Certainly any cancer suitable for cordectomy is equally suited for irradiation. However, laryngofissure, even when applied with skill, may be accompanied by a significant recurrence rate of 43% (McGavran and associates, 1959). It is certain that skillfully applied radiotherapy leaves a better voice than cordectomy. Furthermore, if regrowth should develop after radiotherapy of a limited cord lesion, salvage laryngectomy is possible. The 5-year disease-free survival rate obtained from laryngectomy of radiation failures is high (Table 7-2).

Advanced carcinomas of the endolarynx involving both the true and false cords have been termed *transglottic lesions* and deserve special mention (McGavran and associates, 1961). Half of these patients present initially with ipsilateral lymph node metastases. Half of those patients presenting with ipsilateral metastases have already

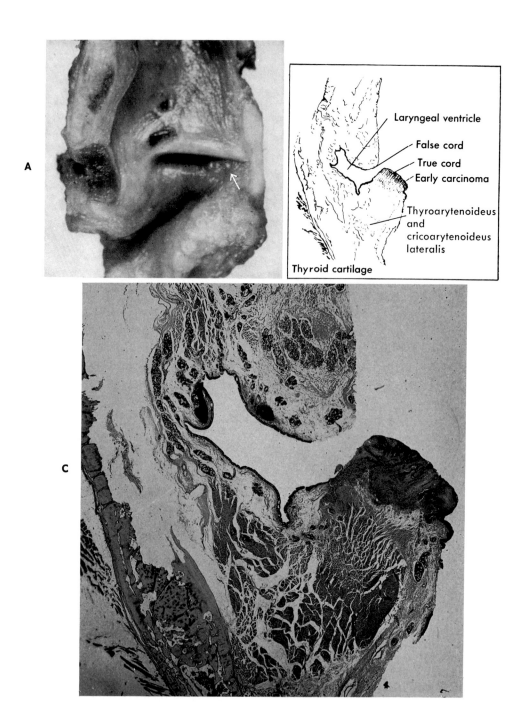

Fig. 7-2. Stage I carcinoma of the larynx. See text. (From Ackerman, L. V., and Rosai, J.: Surgical pathology, ed. 5, St. Louis, 1974, The C. V. Mosby Co.)

developed contralateral lymph node metastases. Most of the metastases are found along the upper half of the jugular chain, but the lower anterior node groups are also occasionally involved. These data demand that for transglottic lesions one should routinely include management of the lymph node chains in the plan of initial treatment.

Advanced lesions fixing the cord, invading the cartilage, or invading the arytenoid region can undoubtedly be controlled in a higher percentage of patients by

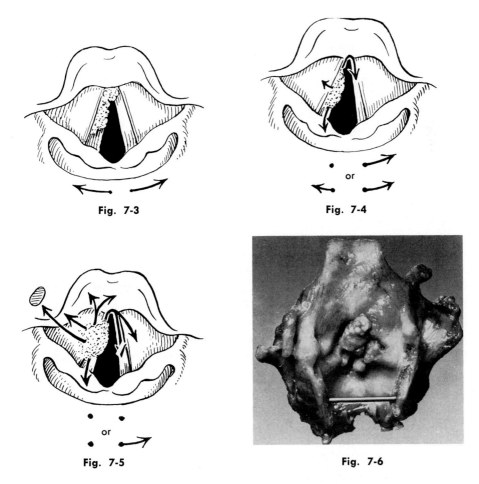

Fig. 7-3

Fig. 7-4

Fig. 7-5

Fig. 7-6

Fig. 7-3. Stage II carcinoma of the larynx. This is the same as Stage I with the addition of involvement of the anterior commissure.

Fig. 7-4. Stage III carcinoma of the larynx. As indicated by the arrows, extension is beyond the cord but not beyond the endolarynx. One cord is at least partially fixed. There are no palpable nodes.

Fig. 7-5. Stage IV carcinoma of the larynx. The cancer has spread beyond the glottis in the form of direct extension, lymph node metastasis, or both.

Fig. 7-6. Gross specimen of Stage IV carcinoma of the larynx. Cancer has infiltrated both cords and supraglottic and infraglottic regions and has extended anteriorly into the cartilage. Both cords were fixed. (W. U. neg. 55-4731; courtesy Dr. L. V. Ackerman.)

total laryngectomy alone than by radiotherapy alone. However, there continue to be reports that support the view that no fewer patients are cured when such patients are given a trial of radiotherapy, with laryngectomy being reserved for those with postirradiation persistent cancer (Jorgensen). It has been our experience that the massive glottic lesions, including transglottic lesions, should be treated by laryngectomy. A trial of radiotherapy is justified for the American Joint Committee Stage II and a limited Stage III with the realization that about one third of the patients with Stage II lesions and over one half of the patients with Stage III lesions will subsequently require laryngectomy. In this way more voices will be spared even if the 5-year tumor-free survival rate is unchanged. Although it has been more or less accepted that of such a selected group of patients, half will be cured by the trial of radiotherapy and half the radiotherapy failures will be cured by subsequent laryngectomy, the degree of selection for radiation therapy and the timing of the laryngectomy are critical. Careless application of this concept to the more advanced glottic cancers will lead to decreased cure rates.

SUBGLOTTIC REGION. Carcinoma originating in the subglottic region is not common. Much more frequently we see true cord lesions with subglottic extension. Whether the lesion of the subglottis is primary or secondary, its extent may be difficult to visualize directly or indirectly. Films of the soft tissues of the neck, laryngograms, and laminograms in both planes are essential. Even so, occult mucosal and submucosal extensions are common and lead to persistent cancer at the stoma (Figs. 7-7 and 7-8). The patient will frequently develop laryngeal obstruction and will require a tracheostomy before the diagnosis is made.

Primary lesions of the subglottic region are usually moderately well differentiated and, in comparison to supraglottic lesions, they metastasize infrequently (Fig. 7-1). These characteristics, together with the rather superficial location of these lesions, should make them amenable to irradiation. However, they have frequently been regarded as relatively radioresistant and have therefore been resected. It has become increasingly clear that radiotherapy can control some of these lesions. This fact, coupled with the realization that postsurgical stomal recurrences are common, now makes radiotherapy at least as promising as resection. We no longer hesitate to recommend irradiation for the earlier subglottic lesions. True cord lesions that have extended into the subglottic region should be classified as advanced glottic carcinomas and are best treated as other advanced cord lesions.

SUPRAGLOTTIC REGION. Lesions of the supraglottic region as a group are the most malignant of the endolaryngeal carcinomas. They are usually anaplastic microscopically, infiltrate widely, and metastasize frequently. Specific symptoms appear late, and the majority of patients present with advanced disease. Fifty-five percent of the patients present with adenopathy on admission, and metastases are bilateral or fixed in 19% (Lindberg and Jesse). Wang (1973) reported metastases present in 51% on admission. These clinical characteristics make many of the lesions difficult to control either by irradiation or surgery. Included in this group are lesions of the false cords, the laryngeal surface of the arytenoids, the infrahyoid portion of the epiglottis, and the suprahyoid portion of the epiglottis.

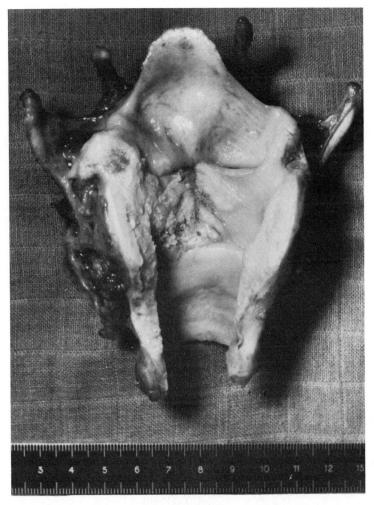

Fig. 7-7. Squamous cell carcinoma of the subglottic area extending down to the first tracheal ring. The left vocal cord is fixed. (From Micheau, C., Luboinski, B., Sancho, H., and Cachin, Y.: Cancer **38:**316-360, 1976.)

Just as for carcinomas of the glottis, limited lesions of the supraglottic area are controlled in a high percentage of patients by radiation therapy alone. Advanced cancers infiltrating deeply into the lateral walls or arytenoid areas or producing extensive edema are seldom controlled by radiation therapy alone and require surgery with or without irradiation. Surgery should usually consist of radical excision and appropriate neck dissection. Wang (1973) reported that 80% to 90% of the T1 N0 and T2 N0 lesions were controlled by radiotherapy alone, but only 10% of the T3 N1 and T4 N1 lesions were controlled by radiotherapy.

Several additional factors have been found to affect prognosis. Lesions that have perforated or even invaded the inferior two thirds of the epiglottic cartilage are difficult to cure by irradiation and should be approached surgically (McGavran and

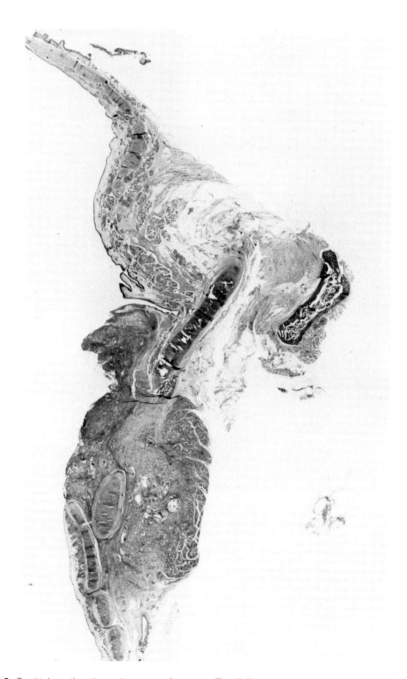

Fig. 7-8. Sagittal section through center of cancer (Fig. 7-7) showing extension up to the ventricle, down to the trachea, and through the cricothyroid membrane. (From Micheau, C., Luboinski, B., Sancho, H., and Cachin, Y.: Cancer **38:**316-360, 1976.)

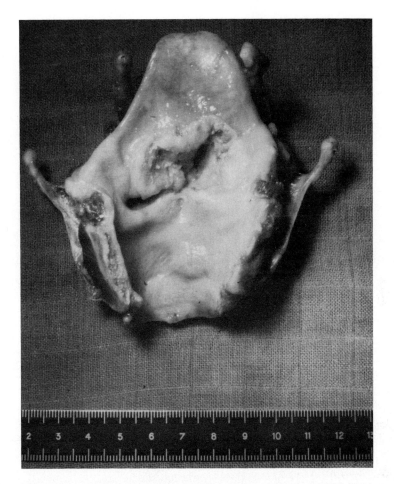

Fig. 7-9. Squamous cell carcinoma of the supraglottic area (base of the epiglottis). The true cords are involved in about one third of such cancers. (From Micheau, C., Luboinski, B., Sancho, H., and Cachin, Y.: Cancer **38**:316-360, 1976.)

associates, 1961) (Figs. 7-9 and 7-10). Lesions of the free part of the epiglottis do well even though cartilage is invaded. Lindberg and Jesse reported twenty-two of thirty-four (64%) such patients free of cancer 2 years after radiotherapy. However, if the base of the tongue or pharyngoepiglottic folds are invaded, the prognosis is very poor. A small proportion of local failures are attributable to technical defects, that is, geographic miss, inadequate dosimetry, and the like. A similar proportion are considered to fail locally because of large hypoxic components of tumor or distant metastases. Finally, patients with these cancers tend to have second primary cancers, emphysema, arteriosclerosis, and cirrhosis (Niederer and associates). Many advocate preoperative irradiation for these more advanced lesions of the supraglottic region. Thus Wang and associates (1972) reported the value of using 4500 rad in 4 weeks as a preoperative measure. However, clinical trials defining its value are still in progress.

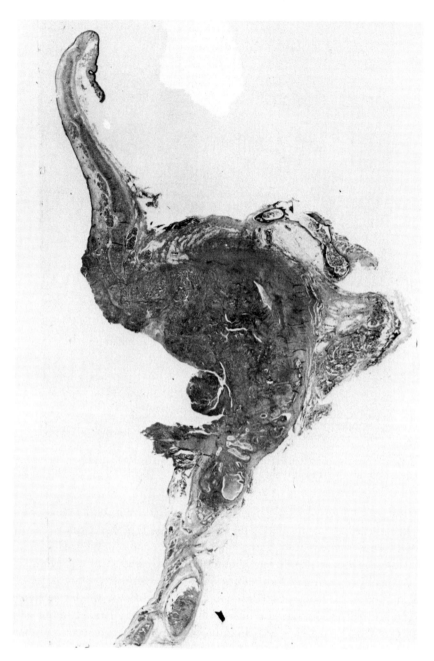

Fig. 7-10. Midsagittal section through the epiglottis shown in Fig. 7-9. The cancer has perforated the epiglottis, extended into the preepiglottic space, and destroyed the thyroid cartilage. (From Micheau, C., Luboinski, B., Sancho, H., and Cachin, Y.: Cancer **38:**316-360, 1976.)

As mentioned before, metastases to nodes develop frequently and early. A high proportion of such nodes can be controlled radiotherapeutically.

Irradiation will control 95% of the mobile nodes when the primary lesion is controlled (Bataini and associates). This statement is supported by the report of Schneider and associates who found that a dose of 6500 rad or more given at a rate of 1000 rad per week controlled nodal disease in ten of thirteen patients with nodes 3 cm or less. Two of the three failures were salvaged by surgery.

Cancers of the aryepiglottic fold are rarely diagnosed early but when diagnosed early are readily controlled by irradiation. Cancers of this site are usually advanced and have infiltrated inferiorly into the piriform sinus or laryngeal vestibule. These advanced lesions are rarely radiocurable and should be considered for radical surgery.

Cancers of the false cords spread early into the ventricle, the cartilage of the epiglottis, and the thyroid cartilage. Baclesse pointed out that extension inferiorly to the true cord is infrequent. Any of these extensions greatly reduces the chance of cure by radiotherapy. Thus, except for the T1 or T2 lesions such cancers are given 4500 to 5000 rad in 4½ to 5 weeks, then surgery is performed.

TECHNIQUE OF IRRADIATING CARCINOMA OF THE LARYNX. Endolaryngeal lesions are usually squamous cell in type, and they demand high doses. On the other hand, postirradiation laryngeal edema and necrosis are serious and may be fatal, and even a limited edema of the vocal cord is symptomatic. These sequelae definitely increase with increasing dose. They will occasionally appear with the dose levels recommended and may develop in spite of the expert use of our clinical guides.

The structures composing the larynx show striking differences in sensitivity from patient to patient, yet the same patterns of response are common. Ciliated epithelium ceases to function early in the treatment (Alexander). Secretions decrease, the mucosa becomes dry and irritated, and if the dose has been sufficiently great, edema of all mucosa develops later. This edema may be especially marked over the arytenoids after the recommended doses. These tissues show a disruption of submucosal structures, hyalinization, and scattered debris. Muscles of the larynx show no significant change. Blood vessels show the same changes as elsewhere. Cartilage shows no acute response. However, months after high doses, the perichondrium shows no further mitotic activity. Nuclei degenerate, and the cartilage also starts its degeneration, progressing in the worst circumstance to aseptic necrosis or, if an ulcer is present, to sloughing of the cartilage. Although these changes are present to some degree in all cases, most patients treated with small ports and moderate fractionation of dose retain excellent function with no significant discomfort. When larger ports are used for ulcerated lesions directly overlying cartilage, additional risks must be accepted. In small children the irradiation of these structures may result in diminished growth of the diameter of the airiway and stricture (Bonte and associates). Fortunately, the need for laryngeal irradiation is rare in this young group.

Optimum dose-time-volume relationships are of extreme importance in irradiating carcinoma of the larynx. Studies have been made for both the glottic and supraglottic cancers. Coutard emphasized the use of clinical guides and laid the foundation of modern radiotherapy for carcinoma of the larynx. Baclesse's review of the dose-time-volume factors summarizes the pioneering work of Coutard and is highly significant here because it represents a broad spectrum of dose-time relationships. The data Baclesse obtained by plotting cures, failures, and high-dose sequelae graphically according to tissue dose and fractionation suggest that, within limits, cancer control rates are not decreased by increased fractionation. However, the undesirable sequelae are definitely reduced by avoiding severe acute reactions by using the more fractionated techniques. These are the same findings that prompted earlier radiologists to extend the overall treatment period from 1 day to 2 weeks, then to 6 weeks, and now to 8 weeks and longer. Severe cartilage and soft tissue reactions after limited fractionation are strikingly reduced by greater fractionation.

The often-accepted narrow limits of doses allowed in the irradiation of carcinoma of the larynx have been emphasized many times and have been used to justify increased precision in radiotherapy technique (Herring and Compton; Kim and associates). Three concepts are important in considering doses to the larynx:

1. The justification for radiotherapy rests not only on controlling cancer, but also on preservation of the voice.

2. One cannot justify serious high-dose effects with the argument that a higher proportion of laryngeal cancers are thus controlled. Laryngectomy is available for radiation failures.

3. The optimum dose-time-volume factors are those that produce the maximum number of cured patients with good or acceptable voices.

These concepts are obviously different from those for clinical situations in which radiation therapy is the only modality for cure or when the high-dose sequelae carry less morbidity.

The technique of irradiating limited lesions of the true cord can be easily accomplished by using lateral parallel opposing portals measuring 4 × 5 or 5 × 5 cm. Precise centering of the beam is assured by using external landmarks and by taking localization films. Extension of the cancer to the anterior commissure should be encompassed by allowing the anterior border of the beam to extend 1 cm beyond the anterior edge of the thyroid cartilage. Since limited glottic cancers rarely metastasize to cervical lymph nodes, and since the more advanced glottic cancers are resected, the cervical lymph node chains are rarely irradiated during treatment of lesions of the vocal cord. The small ports previously mentioned are adequate.

With the average size and shape of the anterior portion of the neck an unwedged parallel opposed pair of beams will produce a 12% to 15% variation in dose. This variation in dose can be diminished and a sharper falloff of dose posteriorly can be achieved by combining beam angulation with wedges (Wang).

DOSE-TIME RELATIONSHIPS IN THE IRRADIATION OF CANCERS OF THE VOCAL CORD. Many attempts have been made to define the optimum dose-time relationships for carcinoma of the larynx (Baclesse; Morrison and Deeley; Fletcher and Klein; Stewart; Vaeth and associates; Horiot and associates; Aristizabal and Caldwell; Marks and associates; Wang; Kim and associates). With few exceptions the more superficial cancers of the cord are given 6000 rad in 6 weeks delivered at the rate of 200 rad five times each week. For small exophytic cancers Horiot and associates recommended 6500 rad in 6 weeks, and for the more bulky advanced glottic lesions 7000 rad in 6½ weeks. Wang recommended a dose of 6500 rad in 6½ weeks. In contrast, Morrison and Deeley found that with megavoltage beams 7000 rad in 6 weeks was well tolerated if ports did not exceed 25 cm², but 6400 rad in 6 weeks was the limit of tolerance for larger ports. This variation in optimum dose from center to center does little to support Herring's conclusion that with ±5% variations in dose there are clinically detectable increases in high-dose effects or persistence of cancer in the supraglottic region. Furthermore, the data of Horiot and associates for limited cancer of the glottis fail to show a decreased rate of persistence with increasing NSD from 1700 to 2000 rets (a variation not acceptable to Caldwell). Finally, they found there was less than 100 rets difference in the average dose given to those patients developing high-dose effects and those showing persistent cancer. Marks and associates found an almost identical "flattening" of the dose-response curve in the analysis of their data. This search for an optimum dose-fractionation pattern for the cure of limited cancer of the vocal cord has confirmed that small, superficial cancers are readily controlled by modest doses, that the dose ranges considered by Horiot and associates and by Marks and associates are on an almost flat part of the dose-response curve, and that this range of doses is usually well below the dose producing frequent serious sequelae. These limits in fractionation and dose must not be applied to any except Stage I cancers because, as the cancer enlarges, the dose required increases, the irradiated volume must be enlarged, and the incidence of sequelae quickly increases. (See the following discussion on the supraglottis.) In any case, our experience supports the findings of Horiot and associates, and we recommend their dosage schedule, that is, 6000 rad in 6 weeks for superficial cancers of the cord, 6500 rad in 6 weeks for small exophytic cancers, and 7000 rad in 6½ weeks for bulky, more advanced cancers.

Both Jorgensen and Sell, Horiot and associates, and Niederer and associates discussed other factors related to failure and high-dose effects, that is, cell type, clinical stage, anatomic site, geographic miss, etc. By far the greatest proportion of failures are from persistent cancer within the irradiated volume. There will be an occasional geographic miss, and they are most common from unrecognized cancer or cancer in situ extending subglottically.

The technique of setting up the patients for irradiation can be simple. When no special lead shielding is required and the patient is cooperative, we prefer to treat the patient in the face-up position. A comfortable rigid head rest is necessary. The external landmarks of glottic structures should be determined by patient examination, roentgenograms, and study of autopsy specimens. The relative positions of the glottic and hypopharyngeal structures with regard to external landmarks is illustrated in Fig. 7-11. A knowledge of the relationships is essential for proper beam directioning. The diameter of the usual cobalt source produces a penumbra that is

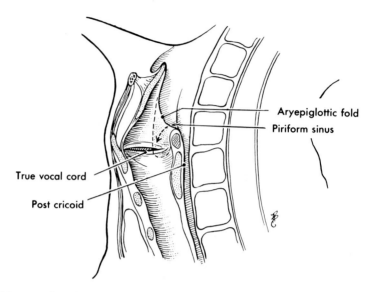

True vocal cord

Post cricoid

Aryepiglottic fold

Piriform sinus

Fig. 7-11. Diagram of the laryngeal and hypopharyngeal structures as related to the anterior portion of thyroid cartilage. The position of ports is usually determined by the relationship of the cartilages to the structures involved.

significant when using these small beams. Beam trimmers or a secondary beam-shaping technique should be used to diminish such unnecessary radiations. Among these patients with Stage I cancers of the vocal cord who are irradiated with mega-voltage beams at the dosage rates described, the limiting tissue is not the laryngeal cartilage, but the tissues of the arytenoid region. For this reason, when the size of the cancer will permit, the port should be reduced after a dose of 5000 to 5500 rad is delivered.

TECHNIQUE FOR IRRADIATING CARCINOMA OF THE SUPRAGLOTTIC REGION. The ports for treating cancers of the supraglottic area are generally larger than for those of the glottis. Cancers of this region tend to invade the aryepiglottic folds, the lateral walls of the pharynx, the vallecula, and the preepiglottic tissues. Extension inferiorly across the laryngeal ventricle occurs with advanced cancers. However, the conus elasticus limits downward extension below the upper margin of the cricoid cartilage (Micheau and associates). Furthermore, metastases to lymph nodes are present in a high proportion (55%). Adenopathy will seldom develop in patients who present no adenopathy on admission if the primary port arrangement encompasses the midjugular and subdigastric areas (Fletcher, 1970). Thus occasionally ports may be as small as 6 × 8 cm, but will generally be 8 × 10 cm or larger. Should total doses greater than 6000 rad in 6 weeks be necessary, the primary ports should be reduced if at all possible. Bilateral anterior tangential ports for lower cervical nodes are necessary if adenopathy is present on admission.

Radiation therapy should be tried as the curative treatment of choice when the cancer is not extensive (T1 N0 and T2 N0). When postirradiation persistent cancer can be diagnosed, a cure by laryngectomy should be attempted. Thus the larynx will be spared when possible, but not at the expense of lowered cure rate.

Once the cancer has become locally advanced with fixation of the larynx, subglottic extension, or destruction of cartilage, control by irradiation alone is unlikely. For these we have favored a combination of preoperative irradiation (5000 rad in 5 weeks) with radical surgery. Local control rates with this combination are good, and, with care, complications are no greater than following surgery alone (Chang and associates).

DOSE-TIME RELATIONSHIP IN THE IRRADIATION OF CANCERS OF THE SUPRAGLOTTIC REGION. The best dose-time data are those given by Shukovsky (1970). He showed that there is a sharp increase in the probability of control as the NSD increases from 1700 to 2100 rets. Limited cancers are frequently cured by 5800 to 6150 rad in 6 weeks (NSD's of 1700 to 1800 rets). More extensive cancers require doses of 6850 to 7200 rad (NSD's up to 2100 rets). A dose of 1900 rets seems to be optimal if one were to specify a single dose level. Wang and Bataini and associates concur that this range of doses seems optimal.

HIGH DOSE EFFECTS. With the type of patient selection recommended previously and with appropriate attention to beam quality, size, and fractionation, the incidence of high-dose complications is greatly reduced. The pathogenesis of radiation necrosis of laryngeal cartilage may vary, but the factors responsible for its onset are the same as those responsible for necrosis of the mandible. Normal cartilage covered by normal mucosa can withstand high doses of radiations as long as infection or trauma does not supervene. Either infection or trauma may trigger a response in irradiated cartilage, resulting in sequestration of the entire irradiated tissue. Aside from the technical factors of irradiation that affect onset of necrosis, necrosis is more likely to occur if the initial laryngeal lesion shows extensive ulceration or if surgery such as partial laryngectomy preceded irradiation. Each of these impairs the viability of the tissues in the irradiated volume.

Necrosis will be most frequent after irradiation of extensive true cord lesions and lesions of the inferior portion of the epiglottis. The exact site of necrosis is often difficult to ascertain. With two parallel opposing lateral ports, the point of highest dose is in the anterior border of the thyroid cartilage. However, in the development of cartilage necrosis, the location of the malignant lesion is more important than the point of highest dose.

As may be expected, the higher the dose within a given treatment period, or the shorter the treatment period for a given dose, the higher the incidence of necrosis. A tissue dose of 200 rad per day or 1000 rad per week for 6 weeks is probably as rapidly as one can treat without seriously increasing the incidence of necrosis.

Anyone who treats laryngeal carcinoma with curative doses of radiations will encounter some cases of high-dose effects. The following precautions will decrease their frequency.

1. The irradiation of large, deeply ulcerating, endolaryngeal lesions is almost certain to be followed by edema or cartilaginous necrosis. This fact, together with the

low radiocurability of such large lesions, has convinced us that total laryngectomy is preferable in this group of advanced cancers.

2. Small irradiated volumes always heal better than large ones. The treated volume should be as small as the margins of the lesion will permit.

3. Low daily doses (in the region of 180 rad per day) to the required total dose are associated with fewer high-dose complications than larger daily fractions in shorter overall treatment times (Baclesse).

4. If partial laryngectomy has proved inadequate, more radical surgery is preferable to irradiation. If such patients are irradiated, the chances of edema or cartilage necrosis are high and must be accepted.

5. Reirradiation even with palliative doses is hazardous. Surgery offers the best hope of control in postirradiation recurrent cases.

We have not had radiation necrosis develop in any patient given curative megavoltage irradiation for limited carcinoma of the vocal cord. We have had permanent or intermittent edema of the arytenoids in about 15% of these patients.

The symptoms of cartilage necrosis resemble those of persistent cancer. Since the treatment of persistent disease should be surgical and that of necrosis is often non-surgical, the differential diagnosis is of more than academic interest. The confusion is made worse when necrosis is initiated by recurrent growth of the cancer. Direct and indirect examinations are not usually helpful. A biopsy of the superficial tissue may not be representative of the etiologic agent. Biopsy of the deeper tissues is seldom accomplished and may trigger a more extensive necrosis. Consequently, the management of these patients is extremely difficult. To subject all such patients to a prolonged period of observation will generally mean that areas of persistent disease are allowed to become hopelessly nonresectable.

Our policy has been to biopsy the lesions immediately. If no cancer is found, the patients are given antibiotics, are placed on high-protein, high-caloric diets with associated supportive care, and are closely observed for one month. If at that time there is no improvement, a laryngectomy is considered even in the absence of a positive biopsy. This policy will mean that some noncancerous larynges will be removed, but they will be the more severe necroses. The voice that would eventually be obtained in such patients would be poor, and the chance of aspiration pneumonia is high. Thus surgery is the treatment of choice for patients with advanced edema or necrosis as well as for those with obvious postirradiation recurrence of disease. A similar policy has been recommended by Lederman and by Kagan and associates.

CARCINOMA IN SITU. The diagnosis of carcinoma in situ of the endolarynx signifies the presence of a diffuse mucosal change and the real probability of multiple foci of malignant degeneration (Stout). With a diagnosis of carcinoma in situ, several important questions need to be answered.

1. Is this the periphery of an unrecognized invasive carcinoma of the larynx? Of invasive squamous cell carcinomas of the larynx, 75% have an adjacent area of carcinoma in situ (Bauer and McGavran). Furthermore, except on the vocal cord, carcinoma in situ almost never occurs in the larynx without an associated invasive squamous cell cancer.

Table 7-3. Incidence of metastases to lymph nodes in patients with carcinoma of the supraglottis*

Stage†	N0	N1	N2	N3	Total with nodes	
T1	19	3	—	1	4/23	17%
T2	24	10	2		12/36	33%
T3	19	9	3	5	17/36	47%
T4	28	37	10	14	61/89	69%
TOTAL	90	59	15	20	94/184	51%

*Modified from Wang, C. C.: Am. J. Roentgenol. **120:**157-163, 1974.
†Clinical staging of the American Joint Committee, 1972.

2. If carcinoma in situ is on the vocal cord, did the biopsy or stripping procedure remove the entire lesion? Stripping may remove all carcinoma in situ in a proportion of carefully selected patients (Norris and Peale). However, this procedure has not been widely adopted. Although a diagnosis of carcinoma in situ does not justify radical surgery, it is so often unrepresentative of the true malignant process present that vigorous radiotherapy is frequently indicated (Stout). Under such circumstances the entire endolarynx should be given cancerocidal doses of 6000 rad in 6 weeks or its equivalent.

IRRADIATION OF METASTASES TO REGIONAL LYMPH NODES. The incidence of obvious metastases from carcinoma of the supraglottic region to regional lymph nodes is shown in Table 7-3. A proportion of the remaining patients have occult metastases to cervical nodes. This high incidence requires us to consider nodal treatment in the management of these patients. The primary lymph drainage is into nodes that are usually included in the beams directed to the primary lesion. The lower cervical and supraclavicular areas can be encompassed by using anterior beams that permit the option of shielding midline structures. However, we have often used the large parallel opposing beams encompassing the primary lesion and nodes described by Bataini and associates. With either technique the dose to the primary lesion and nodes can be tailored to the requirements for the volume of cancer in question.

The dose required to control nodal metastases varies according to the volume of the tumor. For occult foci 5000 rad in 5 weeks is uniformly adequate. For adenopathy that is barely palpable up to nodes 2.5 to 3 cm in diameter, 6500 rad in 6½ weeks to 7000 rad in 7 weeks is highly effective, that is, giving 90% to 100% control. For adenopathy 3 cm or larger, control diminishes as the tumor volume increases. Doses up to 9500 rad (1000 rad/week) given through gradually reduced ports have been used (Bataini and associates; Schneider and associates).

PROGNOSIS AND RESULTS. Factors affecting prognosis have been reviewed previously. Because of the selection of patients presented in most series, it is impossible to quote survival statistics that cannot be criticized. However, in several institutions where radiotherapy is the principal form of treatment, the possibilities of this modality can be fairly accurately evaluated. The excellent results obtained by radiotherapy of limited carcinomas of the true cord are shown in Table 7-1 and Fig. 7-12. No series reports less than 70% living and well after 5 years. Ninety percent of

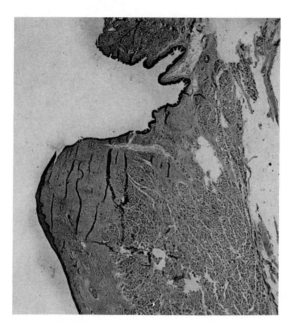

Fig. 7-12. Section through a larynx previously irradiated for squamous cell carcinoma of the true cord (5500 rad in 5 weeks). Patient died 2 years later of a coronary artery disease. There is minimal edema, and the epithelium is intact.

these patients are living and well after 5 years according to several series. When the cancer has spread beyond the true cord to the anterior commissure, the prognosis is but slightly worse. Superficial involvement of the anterior commissure and the opposite vocal cord with normal motion of both cords is still quite well controlled by irradiation (Perez and associates; Wang). However, infiltration of the deeper structures or fixation of the vocal cord reduces radiocurability sharply. When extension is beyond the larynx or when no more than ipsilateral lymphadenopathy can be found, the control rate rarely exceeds 30%. If lymphadenopathy is bilateral or if there are distant metastases, no cure by irradiation can be hoped for.

The cure rate of carcinoma of the supraglottic region is the lowest of the three subdivisions. However, one must not overlook the high radiocurability of limited supraglottic lesions. Seventy percent to 80% of the patients with early lesions will be free of cancer for at least 5 years. Shukovsky reported that forty-one of fifty-two patients (79%) with limited T1 and T2 supraglottic cancers were living and well at 2 years. Wang obtained an 89% control at 3 years with T1 lesions, 66% with T2 lesions, 21% with T3 lesions, and 23% with T4 lesions. When metastases were present, the control rate decreased, so that T3 N1 and T4 N1 were controlled in 10%. Bataini and associates reported the results obtained by ^{60}Co irradiation of 218 cancers of the supraglottic region. Results were particularly favorable in the earlier stages.

Much less information is available for subglottic lesions. Lesions arising on the true cords may extend subglottically. The prognosis is made slightly worse by such extension (Perez and associates). Distinct from this condition are the true subglottic cancers. Lampe reported no cures in five patients, and Baclesse reported one cure in ten patients. Lederman (1961) reported 36% of forty-two patients living and well at 5 years. His report, together with an appreciation of the high incidence of post-surgical stomal recurrences, has prompted us to recommend irradiation for limited subglottic lesions.

MANAGEMENT OF POSTIRRADIATION PERSISTENT CARCINOMA. One of the arguments for primary irradiation of selected carcinomas of the endolarynx is that it provides a reasonable chance for preserving the voice without decreasing the chance of control. Radical excision of a postirradiation persistence can be accomplished with acceptable risk of complications. Selection of patients for postirradiation laryngectomy was discussed previously and is summarized in the following paragraphs.

If persistent cancer is suspected, the lesion is biopsied immediately. If no cancer is found, the patient is given broad-spectrum antibiotics and adequate nutrition, and he is followed for 1 month. If after that period there is no improvement, laryngectomy is considered even in the absence of a positive biopsy. Some noncancerous larynges will be removed, but they will be the more severely damaged ones—the ones in which the voice would be very poor in any case. This sequence of management must not be confused with the planned preoperative irradiation described in the following section. The less radical procedure of partial laryngectomy with sparing of the voice can be applied to selected patients (Ballantyne and Fletcher).

The results of laryngectomy performed on postirradiation persistent carcinomas are summarized in Table 7-2. The value of careful follow-up examinations and prompt surgery is obvious.

PREOPERATIVE IRRADIATION OF CARCINOMA OF THE LARYNX. Planned combinations of irradiation and surgery are of special value in the management of advanced carcinomas of the endolarynx. The general aims of preoperative irradiation are discussed in Chapter 2. In regard to extensive lesions of the larynx and laryngopharynx, surgery fails because of occult "fingers" of cancer extending beyond the excision and because of occult foci in unresected lymph nodes. Primary irradiation apparently fails in the more advanced cancers from regrowth of the more resistant central nidus of large cancerous masses. The aim of preoperative irradiation is to eradicate the "fingers" and occult foci prior to excision of the centrally located bulky persistence. Regardless of whether this is the responsible mechanism, control rates of the more advanced lesions are improved by the combination.

The strong advocates for preoperative irradiation have been Silverstone and associates, Biller and Ogura, Levitt and associates, and Wang and associates. In view of the rationale of preoperative irradiation presented in Chapter 2 and the accumulated arguments for the use of medium- to high-dose preoperative irradiation for advanced carcinomas of the larynx and hypopharynx, we have administered such therapy frequently and recommend its use in T3 and T4 cancers of the supraglottis.

For planned preoperative irradiation, doses of 5500 rad in 5 weeks followed in 3 to 6 weeks by radical surgery have been used by Silverstone and Goldman. For combined procedures this is certainly the upper limit of dose, and 3 weeks is a minimum interval. Doses of 2000 to 3600 rad in 10 to 20 days have been recommended by Hendrickson but have been condemned by Reddi and Mercado and by Marks and associates. We do not believe such low doses will frequently eradicate occult foci at or beyond the margin of excision. We recommend a preoperative dose of 4500 to 5000 rad in 4 weeks as described by Wang and associates.

COMPLICATIONS OF COMBINED MODALITIES. There is uniform agreement that anything more than minor combinations of irradiation and surgery, regardless of the sequence, increases problems related to healing. Radical surgery increases the incidence of postirradiation sequelae just as previous high-dose irradiation increases the incidence of postoperative complications. Minor complications developed in about a fourth of the cases reported by Ditchek and Lampe. Spontaneously healing fistulas or small sloughs developed in 12%, whereas severe complications (permanent fistula, slough requiring graft, or rupture of the carotid) developed in 10%. In contrast to this experience, Chung and associates could find no difference in the number or severity of complications for any of three modalities: surgery alone, planned preoperative irradiation of 5000 rad in 5 weeks, or rescue surgery for recurrence after attempted cure by radiation therapy.

Most surgeons operating after medium to high doses report an increase in problems related to healing. However, when the alternatives are considered, the additional risks are usually accepted by both the patient and the physician, if there is a resonable possibility of cure.

SUMMARY. When irradiation and surgery are equally capable of controlling cancer of the larynx, radiotherapy is the treatment of choice, since it leaves the patient with a much better voice and often with much better deglutition. For these same reasons, irradiation is the treatment of choice for glottic lesions when the cord remains movable or partially movable, for early subglottic lesions, and for early supraglottic lesions. Advanced subglottic lesions and most of the advanced glottic lesions should probably be treated by laryngectomy. Just as in other sites, the radiosensitivity of the carcinoma determines the dose required, whereas the tolerance of the cartilage and adjacent normal soft tissues limits the dose. Because of the important functions of the larynx and hypopharynx, excessive doses may produce relatively small changes that assume great importance. However, with carefully applied radiations these sequelae are sufficiently infrequent to warrant the risk of their appearance. Carelessly applied radiations can do as much harm as unskilled surgery. The complications of overdosage (necrosis and edema) and of underdosage (persistence) demand an appreciation of the radiation tolerance of the larynx, experience with fractionated low daily dose techniques, and a continuing careful appraisal of the dose-time-volume relationships.

CARCINOMA OF THE HYPOPHARYNX

The term *hypopharynx* is anatomically well defined, but in the radiotherapeutic and surgical literature it has been given numerous meanings. The hypopharynx extends superiorly to a horizontal plane through the hyoid bone and inferiorly to a horizontal plane through the lower border of the cricoid cartilage. Classifications of hypopharyngeal cancers are simple. Three anatomic sites are included—cancers of the piriform sinus, postcricoid area, and posterior pharyngeal wall. We included cancers of the aryepiglottic folds with those of the supraglottic larynx inasmuch as they behave more like supraglottic cancers.

The hypopharynx is divided into two parts—the upper or membranous part, which extends from the pharyngo-epiglottic fold down to the arytenoid and includes the posterolateral surface of the aryepiglottic fold, and the corresponding lateral and posterior walls of the pharynx. Inferior to this is the osteocartilaginous part of the hypopharynx, which extends to the lower border of the cricoid cartilage. As the name implies, the posterior portions of the thyroid lamina and cricoid cartilage form its walls. Lesions of the piriform sinus, posterior surface of the arytenoid and cricoid cartilages, and the mouth of the esophagus are included.

Lesions of the membranous portion of the hypopharynx are definitely more curable than those of the lower portion. It has been suggested that the reason for this is that more fungating lesions occur in the upper portion, whereas more flat, ulcerating lesions occur in the lower portion. The latter tend to infiltrate more widely and metastasize earlier (Fig. 7-16). Direct and mirror examinations are the most certain ways of defining tumor extent, but roentgenograms with and without contrast media frequently assist in defining their inferior extent.

TUMOR SPREAD. Early spread to adjacent soft tissues and cartilage is the rule.

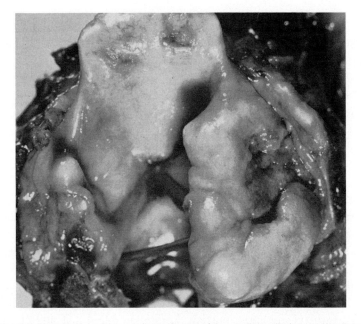

Fig. 7-13. Deeply ulcerating squamous cell carcinoma of the medial wall of the piriform sinus. Note the typical edema of the aryepiglottic fold and the arytenoid region. (W. U. neg. 55-4470; courtesy Dr. L. V. Ackerman.)

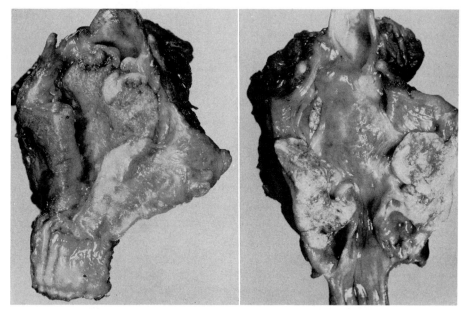

Fig. 7-14   **Fig. 7-15**

Fig. 7-14. Squamous cell carcinoma of the postcricoid region. Note the extension into the arytenoids and laterally into the piriform sinuses. (W. U. neg. 49-5584; courtesy Dr. L. V. Ackerman.)
Fig. 7-15. Fungating, infiltrating squamous cell carcinoma of the posterior wall of the hypopharynx or of the epiesophagus of Lederman. (W. U. neg. 50-3302; courtesy Dr. L. V. Ackerman.)

Lesions arising in the postcricoid region or on the medial wall of the piriform sinus invade laryngeal structures (Fig. 7-13) and may extend inferiorly to involve the upper portion of the cervical esophagus. Lesions of the lateral wall of the piriform sinus are only 1 or 2 mm from the thyroid cartilage, and they invade it early. The disease may even perforate the cartilage. The position of these lesions assures the symptoms of dysphagia or aspiration of fluids. Later, symptoms of laryngeal involvement develop. Intense radiation reaction in this region may further impair swallowing and may have fatal consequences.

The incidence of lymph node involvement will depend on the type of practice reviewed. In the average general hospital, 50% to 60% of patients with lesions of the hypopharynx will present with metastases (Fig. 7-16). Of 860 patients with carcinoma of the hypopharynx, 460 had adenopathy when first seen (Lederman). However, in our experience in a charity hospital, it was rare to see a carcinoma of the piriform sinus that had not already metastasized. The involved nodes are usually near the midcervical region and at times may be difficult to distinguish from direct extension. Lesions of the lower or osteocartilaginous portion metastasize more frequently than those of the upper portion. Lederman found that metastasis occurred in 81% of ninety-four patients with lesions in the lower part of the piriform sinus,

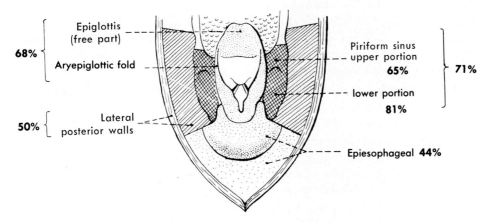

Fig. 7-16. Incidence of cervical lymph node metastases from carcinoma of the various portions of the hypopharynx. (Modified from Lederman, M.: J. Laryngol. **68:**333-369, 1954.)

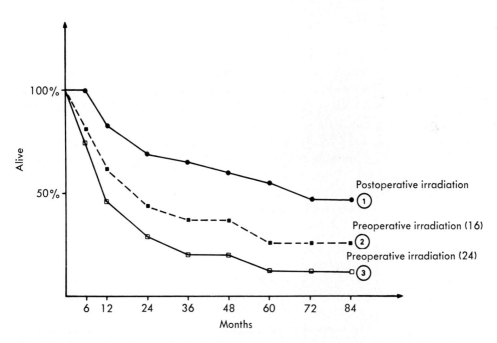

Fig. 7-17. Comparison in a randomized clinical trial between *(1)* postoperative irradiation, that is, 5500 rad given in 5½ weeks starting about 4 weeks postoperatively; *(2)* preoperative irradiation, that is, 5500 rad given in 5½ weeks ending 2 weeks prior to surgery; and *(3)* "radiation failures" prior to surgery. (From Vandenbrouck, C., Sancho, H., Le Fur, R., Richard, J. M., and Cachin, Y.: Cancer **39:** 1445-1449, 1977.)

whereas it occurred in 65% of fifty-eight patients with lesions in the upper part of the piriform sinus. About 60% of patients with lesions of the aryepiglottic folds and arytenoids will show metastases, and about 50% of those with lesions of the posterior and lateral walls will show metastases. In fifty-two patients selected for radical surgery, 84% had microscopically proved ipsilateral lymph node metastases (McGavran and associates). It is clear from these data that any treatment policy must include plans for treating regional lymph node chains.

By the time the diagnosis of cancer of the hypopharynx is made, the disease has usually reached an advanced clinical stage. Limited disease (T1 and T2) is infrequently diagnosed, and while the value of irradiation is thought to be great, this value is in fact poorly defined. In contrast, locally advanced lesions of the hypopharynx respond poorly to irradiation alone (10% to 15% are controlled). Clinical trials have shown that for T3 and some T4 lesions the highest control rates are obtained by radical laryngopharyngectomy followed by vigorous postoperative irradiation (Vandenbrouck and associates) (Fig. 7-17).

TECHNIQUE. For limited lesions we use the same guides for irradiation discussed previously for endolaryngeal lesions. The same limitations to daily dose rate and to total dose exist for the hypopharynx. The volume requiring treatment is usually great, and the ports are usually large. Parallel opposing lateral ports remain the most practical arrangement. The spinal cord and more anterior endolaryngeal structures should be spared irradiation if at all possible. If nodes are more posterior, the limited tolerance of the spinal cord must be respected. Boosting doses in this area with the electron beam or sharply angled photon beams should be developed.

If, for medical or technical reasons, irradiation is to be the sole treatment for a patient with a T3 or T4 lesions, the technique is similar to that described for an advanced lesion of the supraglottic region. Port arrangement is difficult if the lesion or its metastasis extends inferiorly a distance that requires irradiation of the upper mediastinal tissues. A double-wedge filter technique is satisfactory, and Stevens has described the use of lateral beams that seem to have some advantages should such extension be present.

The primary treatment beams should routinely include subdigastric and mid-jugular nodes when there is no adenopathy and bilateral irradiation of both jugular chains when any nodal involvement is suspected. This can be done by using large direct lateral ports. After the primary lesion has been given a dose of 6500 to 7500 rad in 7 to 8 weeks, the dose to still palpable or large cervical lymph nodes can be raised by supplementary anterior and posterior tangential beams for boosting doses to reduced ports. Additional doses of 500 to 1000 rad can be given. Lalanne and associates recommended doses of 6500 to 7500 rad given in 7 to 8 weeks (Chapter 4).

Combinations of radiotherapy and surgery. The overall cure rates obtained by radiotherapy alone or by surgery alone have been so poor that combinations of radiation and surgery are now recommended for almost every patient with technically operable primary lesions and regional nodes. Independent studies in several centers have verified that the greatest proportion of tumor-free survivals are obtained by combining radical resection with postoperative irradiation (Fletcher and Evers;

Jesse and Lindberg; Vandenbrouck and associates) (Fig. 7-17). Fletcher and Evers administered doses of 5500 to 6000 rad to ten patients when the margins of surgical excision were considered inadequate. Eight of these patients were well 1 to 6 years later. By contrast, only sixteen of 147 were well 1 to 6 years later if irradiation was delayed until the persistent cancer was obvious.

While combined irradiation and surgery are widely accepted as the treatment of choice for patients with T3 and selected T4 lesions, there is debate as to whether the irradiation should be preoperative or postoperative. Preoperative doses of 3000 rad in 3 weeks are of no value (Marks and associates). Chung and associates found that doses of 5000 rad in 5 weeks produced similar morbidity or mortality regardless of the sequence (21% major complications following surgery alone, 16% following preoperative irradiation and surgery, and 21% following salvage surgery). Thus the morbidity and mortality need not be a major factor in determining the sequence. However, Vandenbrouck and associates reported the results of a small randomized trial and found postoperative irradiation (5500 rad in 5½ weeks) produced a higher disease-free survival rate than the same dose given preoperatively (Fig. 7-17). For this anatomic site we have favored the use of postoperative irradiation for most T3 and selected T4 lesions. Obviously, in those circumstances in which the tumor seems to be fixed or the lesion is borderline resectable, we have favored preoperative irradiation with reevaluation after the 5500 rad dose.

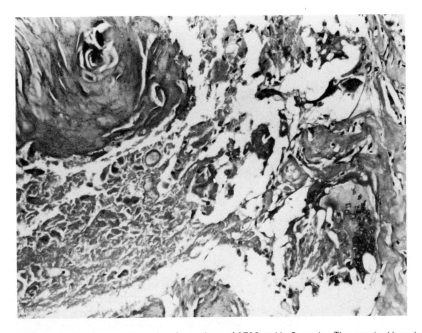

Fig. 7-18. Microscopic changes 6 weeks after a dose of 6700 rad in 8 weeks. The cervical lymph node had biopsy-proved metastasis of squamous cell carcinoma prior to irradiation. The mass, originally 10 cm in diameter, shrank to 3 cm diameter. No viable cancer remains. Keratin, dead cells, and multi-nucleated foreign body giant cells are typical findings.

Table 7-4. Results of radiotherapy of carcinoma of the hypopharynx (clinical material not selected)

Author	Number of cases	5-year cures (%)
Rennaes (1952)	84	6
Hultberg (1953)	165	14.5
Lederman (1967)	673	11
Lalanne (1971)	290	11

SUMMARY. The results obtained by radiotherapy of hypopharyngeal cancers are poor (Table 7-4). Except for the limited cancers of the hypopharynx, lesions of this area are not sufficiently radiosensitive to be frequently radiocurable. Most curable among these lesions are those of the posterior wall, those on or very near the aryepiglottic fold, small lesions, and those of the upper part of the piriform sinus. The prognosis in patients with these more favorable T1 and T2 lesions will depend on the presence or absence of cervical lymph node metastases. To be curative, irradiation must be vigorous, sparing if possible the endolaryngeal structures anteriorly and the spinal cord posteriorly. Combinations of radical resection followed by postoperative irradiation yield the highest disease-free survival rates for patients with primary T3 and T4 cancers.

REFERENCES

Ackerman, L. V., and Rosai, J.: Surgical pathology, ed. 5, St. Louis, 1974, The C. V. Mosby Co.

Alexander, F. W.: 306 laryngeal carcinomas: staging and end results, Arch. Otolaryngol. **83**:602-606, 1966.

American Joint Committee for Cancer Staging and End Results Reporting: Manual for staging of cancer, Chicago, 1978, Whiting Press.

Aristizabal, S. A., and Caldwell, W. L.: Radiation tolerance of the normal tissues of the larynx, Radiology **103**:419-422, 1972.

Baclesse, F.: Carcinoma of the larynx, Br. J. Radiol, suppl. 3, 1949.

Ballantyne, A. J.: Principles of surgical management of cancer of the pharyngeal walls, Cancer **20**:663-667, 1967.

Ballantyne, A. J., and Fletcher, G. H.: Preservation of the larynx in the surgical treatment of cancer recurrent after radiation therapy, Am. J. Roentgenol. **99**:336-338, 1967.

Bataini, J. P., Ennuyer, A., Pocet, P., and Ghossein, N. A.: Treatment of supraglottic cancer by radical high dose radiotherapy, Cancer **33**:1253-1262, 1974.

Bauer, W. G., Edwards, D. L., and McGavran, M. H.: A critical analysis of laryngectomy in the treatment of epidermoid carcinoma of the larynx, Cancer **15**:263-270, 1962.

Bauer, W. G., and McGavran, M. H.: Carcinoma in-situ and evaluation of epithelial changes in laryngopharyngeal biopsies, J.A.M.A. **221**:72-74, 1972.

Biller, H. F., and Ogura, J. H.: Planned preoperative irradiation for laryngeal and laryngopharyngeal carcinoma. In Vaeth, J. M., editor: The interrelationship of surgery and radiation therapy in the treatment of cancer, Baltimore, 1970, University Park Press.

Bonte, F. J., Stembridge, V. L., and Reef, J. D.: Effects of ionizing radiation upon the immature rabbit larynx. Am. J. Roentgenol. **105**:791-794, 1969.

Chang, T. C., Sagerman, R. H., King, G. A., Yu, W. S., Johnson, J. T., and Cummings, C. W.: Complications of high dose preoperative irradiation for advanced laryngeal-hypopharyngeal cancer, Radiology **128**:467-470, 1978.

Coutard, H.: Roentgen therapy of epitheliomas of tonsillar region, hypopharynx and larynx from 1920 to 1926, Am. J. Roentgenol. **28**:313-331, 1932.

Ditchek, T., and Lampe, I.: Radical surgery after

intensive high-energy irradiation, Arch. Surg. 86:534-539, 1963.

Fletcher, G. H., and Klein, R.: Dose-time-volume relationships in squamous cell carcinoma of the larynx, Radiology 82:1032-1042, 1964.

Fletcher, G. H., and Evers, W. T.: Radiotherapeutic management of surgical recurrences and postoperative residuals in tumors of the head and neck, Radiology, 95:185-188, 1970.

Fletcher, G. H., Jesse, R. H., Lindberg, R. D., and Koons, C. R.: The place of radiotherapy in the management of the squamous cell carcinoma of the supraglottic larynx, Radiology 108:19-26, 1970.

Fletcher, G. H., and Hamberger, A. D.: Causes of failure in irradiation of squamous cell carcinoma of the supraglottic larynx, Radiology 111: 697-700, 1974.

Ghossein, N. A., Bataini, J. P., Ennuyer, A., Stacey, P., and Krishnaswamy, V.: Local control and site of failure in radically irradiated supraglottic laryngeal cancer, Radiology 112:187-192, 1974.

Hendrickson, F. R.: The results of low dose preoperative radiotherapy for advanced carcinoma of the larynx. In Vaeth, J. M., editor: The interrelationship of surgery and radiation therapy in the treatment of cancer, Baltimore, 1970, University Park Press.

Herring, D. F., and Compton, D. M.: The degree of precision required in the radiation dose in cancer radiotherapy, Enviromed, Inc., Report No. EMI-216.

Horiot, J., Fletcher, G. H., Ballantyne, A. J., and Lindberg, R.: Analysis of failures of early vocal cord tumors, Radiology 103:663-665, 1972.

Hudson, W. R., and Cavanaugh, P. J.: Combined surgical and radiation management of carcinoma of the laryngopharynx, Trans. Am. Laryngol. Rhinol. Otol. Soc., pp. 254-270, 1965.

Jesse, R. H., and Lindberg, R. D.: The efficacy of combining radiation therapy with a surgical procedure in patients with cervical metastasis from squamous cell cancer of the oropharynx and hypopharynx, Cancer 35:1163-1166, 1975.

Jorgensen, K.: Carcinoma of the larynx. I. Treatment mainly by primary irradiation. Acta Radiol. (Ther.) 9:401-419, 1970.

Jorgensen, K., and Sell, A.: Carcinoma of the larynx. II. Treatment by ^{60}Co supervoltage irradiation, Acta Radiol. [Ther.] (Stockh.) 10: 161-173, 1971.

Kagan, A. R., Calcaterra, T., Ward, P., and Chan, P.: Significance of edema of the endolarynx following curative irradiation for carcinoma, Am. J. Roentgenol. 120:169-172, 1974.

Kim, J. C., Elkin, D., and Hendrickson, F. R.: Carcinoma of the vocal cord, Cancer 42:1114-1119, 1978.

Kuhn, A. J., Devine, K. D., and McDonald, J. R.: Cervical metastases from squamous cell carcinoma of the larynx, Laryngoscope 67:169-190, 1957.

Lalanne, G. M., Cachin, T., Juillard, G., and Lefur, R.: Telecobalt therapy for carcinoma of the laryngopharynx, Am. J. Roentgenol. 111: 78-84, 1971.

Lampe, I.: Radiotherapy of carcinoma of the larynx, Proceedings of the Third National Cancer Conference, Philadelphia, 1957, J. B. Lippincott Co.

Lederman, M.: Cancer of the laryngopharynx, J. Laryngol. 68:333-369, 1954.

Lederman, M.: Epi-oesophageal cancer with special reference to tumors of the post cricoid region, Br. J. Radiol. 28:173-183, 1955.

Lederman, M.: Place of radiotherapy in treatment of cancer of the larynx, Br. Med. J. 1:1639-1646, 1961.

Lederman, M.: Cancer of the pharynx, J. Laryngol. 81:151-172, 1967.

Levitt, S. H., Beachley, M. C., Zimberg, Y., Pastore, P. N., DeGiorgi, L. S., and King, E. R.: Combination of preoperative irradiation and surgery in the treatment of cancer of the oropharynx, hypopharynx, and larynx, Cancer 27: 759-767, 1971.

Lindberg, R. D., and Jesse, R. H.: Integrated approach to management of cancers of the larynx and hypopharynx. In Oncology 1970, Proceedings of the Tenth International Cancer Congress, Chicago, 1971, Year Book Medical Publishers, Inc.

McGavran, M. H., Spjub, H. J., and Ogura, J. H.: Laryngofissure in the treatment of laryngeal carcinoma, Laryngoscope 69:44-53, 1959.

McGavran, M. H., Bauer, W. C., and Ogura, J. H.: The incidence of cervical lymph node metastases from epidermoid carcinoma of the larynx and their relationship to certain characteristics of the primary tumor, Cancer 14:55-66, 1961.

Mancuso, A. A., Hanafee, W. N., Juillard, G. J. F., Winter, J., Jr., and Calcaterra, T. C.: The role of computed tomography in the management of cancer of the larynx, Radiology 124:243-244, 1977.

Marks, J. E., Lowry, L. D., Lerch, I., and Griem, M. L.: Glottic cancer; an analysis of recurrence as related to dose, time, and fractionation, Am. J. Roentgenol. 117:540-547, 1973.

Marks, J. E., Kurnik, B., Powers, W. E., and

Ogura, J. H.: Carcinoma of the pyriform sinus, Cancer **41**:1008-1015, 1978.

Marks, J. E., Freeman, R. B., Lee, F., and Ogura, J. H.: Carcinoma of the supraglottic larynx, Am. J. Roentgenol. Radium Ther. Nucl. Med. **132**: 255-260, 1979.

Markson, J. L., and Flatman, G. E.: Myxoedema after deep x-ray therapy to the neck, Br. Med. J. **1**:1228-1230, 1965.

Micheau, C., Luboinski, B., Sancho, H., and Cachin, Y.: Modes of invasion of cancer of the larynx, Cancer **38**:316-360, 1976.

Morrison, R., and Deeley, T. J.: The treatment of carcinoma of the larynx by supervoltage radiotherapy, Clin. Radiol. **13**:145-148, 1962.

Nass, J. M., Brady, L. W., Glassburn, J. R., Prasasvinichai, S., and Schatanoff, D.: Radiation therapy of glottic carcinoma. Int. J. Radiat. Oncol. Biol. Phys. **1**:867-872, 1976.

Niederer, J., Hawkins, N. V., Rider, W. D., and Till, J. E.: Failure analysis of radical radiation therapy of supraglottic laryngeal carcinoma. Int. J. Radiat. Oncol. Biol. Phys. **2**:621-629, 1977.

Norris, C. M., and Peale, A. R.: "Untreated" carcinoma of the larynx. Ann. Otol. Rhinol. Laryngol. **77**:468-476, 1968.

Paterson, R.: Treatment of malignant disease by radiotherapy, ed. 2, Baltimore, 1963, The Williams & Wilkins Co.

Perez, C. A., Holtz, S., Ogura, J. H., Dedo, H. H., and Powers, W. E.: Radiation therapy of early carcinoma of the true vocal cords, Cancer **21**:764-771, 1968.

Reddi, R. P., and Mercado, R.: Low dose preoperative radiation therapy in carcinoma of the supraglottic larynx, Radiology **130**:469-471, 1979.

Schneider, J. J., Fletcher, G. H., and Barkley, H. T.: Control by irradiation alone of non-fixed clinically positive lymph nodes from squamous cell carcinoma of the oral cavity, oropharynx, supraglottic larynx, and hypopharynx. Am. J. Roentgenol. **123**:42-48, 1975.

Shukovsky, L. J.: Dose, time, volume relationships in squamous cell carcinoma of the supraglottic larynx, Radiology **108**:27-29, 1970.

Silverstone, S. M., and Goldman, J. L.: Combined therapy, irradiation and surgery, for advanced cancer of the laryngopharynx, Am. J. Roentgenol. **90**:1023-1031, 1963.

Silverstone, S. M., Goldman, J. L., and Ryan, J. R.: Combined high dose radiation therapy and surgery of advanced cancer of the laryngopharynx. In Vaeth, J. M., editor: The interrelationship of surgery and radiation therapy in the treatment of cancer, Baltimore, 1970, University Park Press.

Stevens, K. R., Fry, R. F., and Stone, V. C.: A new technique for irradiating thoracic inlet tumors. In press.

Stewart, J. G.: Late effects of radiation—the radiotherapists' problem, Br. J. Radiol. **42**:797-798, 1969.

Stout, A. P.: Intramucosal epithelioma of the larynx, Am. J. Roentgenol. **69**:1-13, 1953.

Vandenbrouck, C., Sancho, H., Le Fur, R., Richard, J. M., and Cachin, Y.: Results of a randomized clinical trial of preoperative irradiation versus postoperative in treatment of tumors of the hypopharynx, Cancer **30**:1445-1449, 1977.

Vaeth, J. M., Green, J. P., and Schroeder, A. F.: Radiation therapy of cancer of the vocal cord and NSD implications, Am. J. Roentgenol. **114**: 63-64, 1972.

Wang, C. C.: Laryngopharyngeal cancer: five-year results after x-ray therapy, N. Engl. J. Med. **255**:1033-1035, 1956.

Wang, C. C.: Megavoltage radiation therapy for supraglottic carcinoma result of treatment, Radiology **109**:183-186, 1973.

Wang, C. C., Schulz, M. D., and Miller, D.: Combined radiation therapy and surgery for carcinoma of the supraglottic and pyriform sinus, Am. J. Surg. **124**:551-554, 1972.

8

The thyroid

The ablation of normal thyroid function with ^{131}I is a well-established, simple procedure, and basically the effect does not differ from externally administered radiations. Early injury of small blood vessels, acute inflammatory response in the epithelial cells of the follicle, necrosis, and hemorrhage follow in sequence. Regeneration may be partial. The most obvious late damage is seen in the blood vessel changes. The turnover time of the follicular cells is several months. It requires months and even years for radiation-induced hypothyroidism to develop in some patients.

Less appreciated is the fact that external irradiation of the normal thyroid gland in the process of treating patients for carcinoma of the larynx or pharynx, breast, or lymphoma also decreases thyroid function. Ten years after vigorous irradiation, Einhorn and Wikholm found three of forty-one patients hypothyroid, whereas the remaining thirty-eight showed decreased thyroid reserve. Microscopic changes include impairment of cellular reproduction as manifested by an inhibition of goitrogenic hyperplasia. Similar changes were reported by Markson and Flatman. Radiation-induced destruction of thyroid tissue stimulates an increase in thyroid antibodies. These antibodies in turn suppress thyroid function (Jonsson and associates). The precise contribution of this change to the late injury of the gland and suppression of thyroid function is still speculative (Einhorn and Einhorn). For the relationship of thyroid injury to cardiac changes and the possible increased sensitivity of the gland after lymphangiogram, see p. 244.

CARCINOMA OF THE THYROID GLAND

Carcinoma of the thyroid gland exhibits a variety of cell types with widely differing growth characteristics. A single staging system for thyroid cancer as proposed by the American Joint Committee has not been widely accepted because of the lack of correlation of the differentiated types with size (T) and involvement of lymph nodes (N). In the case of papillary adenocarcinomas several reports suggest that prognosis improves with increasing number of involved lymph nodes. We would agree, however, that fixed nodes (N2) carry a poor prognosis. Lymph node metastases in medullary carcinomas also worsen prognosis. For the sake of discussion we choose to accept the pathologic classification and prognostic factors proposed by Woolner. The rela-

233

Table 8-1. Classification of thyroid carcinoma in 1181 cases into relative incidences of various types of thyroid carcinoma*

Histologic type	Percent
Papillary	62.3
Follicular	17.6
Medullary	6.5
Anaplastic	13.6

*Modified from Woolner, L. B.: Semin. Nucl. Med. **1:**481-502, 1971.

Table 8-2. Prognostic features of thyroid cancers by type*

Type	Percent incidence	Percent survival (actuarial)		
		5 years	10 years	20 years
Papillary adenocarcinoma				
Occult (less than 1.5 cm)	37	100	100	100
Intrathyroid (larger than 1.5 cm)	53	99	98	98
Extrathyroid (locally invasive)	10	83	63	52
Follicular adenocarcinoma				
Vascular invasion, slight	50	100	97	100
Vascular invasion, moderate to marked	50	68	41	26
Medullary carcinoma				
Negative lymph nodes	48	95	100	—
Positive lymph nodes	52	70	49	—
Anaplastic carcinoma	—	1	—	—

*Prognostic classification of thyroid carcinoma proposed by Woolner. Note that for both papillary and follicular adenocarcinoma the presence or absence of lymph node metastases is not considered. In the case of follicular adenocarcinoma those patients with lymph node metastases generally have the more aggressive vascular invasive pattern. (Modified from Woolner, L. B.: Semin. Nucl. Med. **1:**481-502, 1971.)

tive incidences for the various histologic types of thyroid carcinoma are shown in Table 8-1. Prognostic factors for each histologic type, particularly in the differentiated thyroid carcinomas as described by Woolner, are shown in Table 8-2. In this classification *papillary adenocarcinoma* of the thyroid includes those tumors that have some degree of follicle formation admixed with a papillary tumor. *Follicular adenocarcinomas* have no element of papillary differentiation apparent on multiple section examination. *Medullary carcinoma*, first described by Hazard, exhibits a varying degree of amyloid stroma in what might otherwise be classified as a poorly differentiated carcinoma of the thyroid. Further subclassification of anaplastic or undifferentiated thyroid carcinomas does not appear to have any particular advantage in therapeutic decisions.

Differentiated cell types

PAPILLARY ADENOCARCINOMA. Papillary adenocarcinoma is by far the most common neoplasm of the thyroid gland. Characteristically this type of tumor is well differentiated and slow growing. Psammoma bodies are not uncommonly seen in

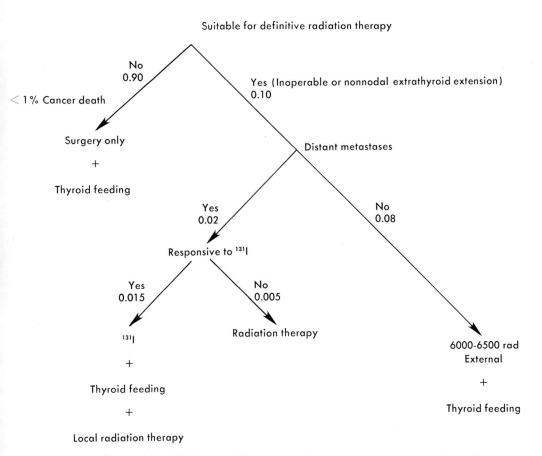

Suitable for definitive radiation therapy

No
0.90

Yes (Inoperable or nonnodal extrathyroid extension)
0.10

< 1% Cancer death

Surgery only

+

Thyroid feeding

Distant metastases

Yes
0.02

No
0.08

Responsive to ¹³¹I

Yes
0.015

No
0.005

Radiation therapy

¹³¹I

+

Thyroid feeding

+

Local radiation therapy

6000-6500 rad
External

+

Thyroid feeding

Fig. 8-1. A decision tree for papillary adenocarcinoma of the thyroid. No more than 10% of patients will be candidates for local irradiation or ¹³¹I therapy for distant metastasis. Of those patients with metastasis, three fourths can be expected to respond to therapeutic doses of ¹³¹I. For patients with nonnodal residual disease or extension into adjacent tissues, postoperative irradiation can be expected to reduce the incidence of local recurrence.

histologic preparation. Metastases to regional lymph nodes, even in the absence of a palpable primary tumor, are not uncommon. Hematogenous metastases are infrequent, but when they do occur the organs involved are lung, bone, liver, and brain. Multicentric foci of tumor within the thyroid gland are common but seem to bear no relationship to prognosis. Invasion of adjacent muscle or thyroid cartilage represents the only bad prognostic feature found in this tumor with the exception of the discovery of distant metastases. At the time of surgical intervention only about 2% of patients will be found to have distant metastases, and approximately 8% will be found to have locally invasive tumor, making eradication by surgery impossible (Fig. 8-1).

FOLLICULAR ADENOCARCINOMA. By definition papillary elements are not present within these tumors. At least half of these tumors exhibit vascular invasion, which illustrates the aggressiveness of the primary tumor and clearly sets it apart

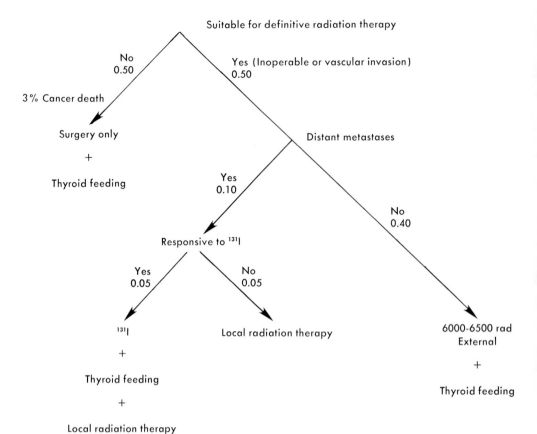

Fig. 8-2. A decision tree for follicular adenocarcinoma of the thyroid. Half of the patients with this disease are successfully managed by surgery alone. For the remainder, one in five will have evidence of distant metastasis, and half of this group will be responsive to ^{131}I therapy. For the remainder who are inoperable or likely to have local recurrences following surgery alone, irradiation can contribute significantly to local control.

from papillary adenocarcinoma. Lymph node metastases are not common, but when present usually indicate a worse prognosis than the similar situation seen in papillary adenocarcinoma. In the more aggressive lesions hematogenous metastases to lung and bone may be the presenting complaint. About 10% of these patients or less than 2% of all patients with thyroid carcinoma may present with symptoms of metastases (Fig. 8-2). Hürthle cell carcinoma of the thyroid is a variant of follicular adenocarcinoma.

MEDULLARY CARCINOMA. In 1959 Hazard and associates described this variant of undifferentiated carcinoma with characteristic amyloid formation. It comprises 6% to 8% of all thyroid carcinomas. This tumor may be familial in origin and associated with pheochromocytomas, parathyroid adenomas, multiple mucosal neuromas, and calcitonin production. Approximately one half of these tumors will metastasize to lymph nodes. The possibility of monitoring calcitonin levels in family members is intriguing, but there is no clear evidence that early thyroidectomy will result in cure or an improved survival of the patients with this neoplasm.

Graze and associates reported on their experience with a large kindred with familial medullary carcinoma. In the initial screening with calcium infusion, twelve patients were identified with abnormal provocative tests; all twelve at surgery were found to have bilateral carcinomas, and seven had metastases to lymph nodes. Subsequent screenings with provocative tests (calcium infusion or pentagastrin stimulations test) detected sixteen additional patients with elevated calcitonin levels. At surgery none of the second series of patients had lymph node metastases, and only two had bilateral tumors. In the second series the patients with carcinoma were considerably younger, and the tumors were much smaller. Since the presence or absence of cervical lymph node metastases is the most significant prognostic factor in this tumor, programs to identify familial medullary carcinoma and efforts at early detection are clearly justified.

Undifferentiated cell types

Anaplastic carcinoma of the thyroid occurs in less than 15% of patients and is a highly malignant form of neoplasia. The median survival with this disease is approximately 6 months. In comparison to papillary adenocarcinoma of the thyroid these tumors tend to appear approximately three decades later in life. Tumor growth is rapid and the outcome invariably fatal.

Treatment

The treatment of choice for operable carcinoma of the thyroid gland is surgery. However, there is rather vigorous debate about the optimum extent of the surgery. We believe that for most differentiated carcinomas surgery should include the lobe of involvement and isthmus with any contiguous lymph nodes. There is no clear indication for radical neck dissection in the treatment of differentiated thyroid carcinoma. The fact that thyroid carcinoma may involve both lobes in a multicentric occult form does in itself not justify total thyroidectomy for these patients. This is especially true for papillary carcinoma in which lobectomy with limited dissection of accessible nodes provides excellent local control and cure (Crile). Both local recurrence and distant metastases are more frequent in follicular carcinoma, and this pattern is not altered by more radical surgical procedures. There is no place for prophylactic neck dissection in the treatment of either type of differentiated thyroid carcinoma (Cady and associates). Medullary carcinomas frequently present with features that make the primary tumor inoperable, particularly when lymph node metastases are present. For the undifferentiated carcinomas palliation may be substantial, but there is no evidence that any form of local therapy influences the ultimate fatal outcome.

We do not believe that a palpable, nonfunctioning thyroid nodule should be treated primarily by thyroid feeding and observation for regression. Proper treatment plans can only be formulated after the histologic nature of the nodule is determined. In those patients with undifferentiated carcinomas delay in diagnosis while a trial of thyroid feeding is undertaken may result in less successful palliative procedures. The morbidity and mortality of thyroid surgery are extremely low, and the information provided by such a surgical procedure will result in more appropriate therapeutic decisions.

Other than surgery, irradiation holds the only real hope for cure of carcinoma of the thyroid. For this reason external irradiation is the unquestioned treatment of choice for the inoperable but still apparently localized carcinoma. This is true regardless of cell type. One should not wait for known persistent carcinoma to produce symptoms before irradiating. The literature does not offer ready documentation of the role of external irradiation in the treatment of thyroid cancers; however, the published results of small series of inoperable cases of differentiated thyroid carcinoma by Sheline and associates and Smedal and associates, as well as results of treating undifferentiated carcinomas by Smedal and Meissner give some indication of the value of local irradiation when complete surgical removal is not possible. Our approach to the selection of patients for definitive irradiation of differentiated cell types is shown in Figs. 8-1 and 8-2. It is clear that only a relatively small number of patients who present with papillary carcinoma would be appropriate candidates for postoperative irradiation. A slightly larger proportion of patients with follicular adenocarcinoma will be at risk with local recurrence as the only manifestation of failure, and they should be included in the group to receive vigorous local irradiation. For patients with medullary carcinoma local irradiation should be considered for all inoperable lesions and for those patients with cervical lymph node metastases. For the undifferentiated carcinomas local irradiation should be considered a palliative procedure only.

We do not believe that routine ablation of the remaining thyroid gland following definitive surgical treatment is indicated. For the majority of patients with differentiated thyroid cancer this procedure would not be expected to offer any significant benefit, since survival rates are high with surgery alone. The use of ^{131}I should be restricted to treatment of distant metastases only. Pochin has shown that approximately three fourths of those patients with papillary carcinomas and half of those with follicular carcinomas will be responsive to some degree to therapeutic doses of ^{131}I. This is not the case for undifferentiated cell types or medullary carcinoma of the thyroid. A determination of the degree of function of the metastases is difficult to make in the presence of a normally functioning thyroid gland. The thyroid gland acts as an iodine trap, and the uptake of the metastases, which at best is less than a normal gland, will have less ^{131}I available for uptake. In addition, the presence of a normal functioning gland usually implies normal TSH levels. In the absence of a normal functioning thyroid gland endogenous TSH increases dramatically to stimulate function of some cancers of the thyroid. For these two reasons we believe the first step in the evaluation of patients with metastases is to totally ablate the remaining functional thyroid gland with a single dose of 100 mCi of ^{131}I. After such a dose thyroid function should be reduced to near zero in about 2 months, and TSH will have had the opportunity to stimulate the differentiated metastatic lesions. At that time a second dose of ^{131}I can be given to evaluate concentration of the ^{131}I in the metastatic lesions. If uptake is demonstrated, Pochin recommends doses of 150 mCi of ^{131}I at 2-month intervals. Two days after this therapeutic dose the patient resumes thyroid feeding and continues on medication until 4 weeks before the next dose is planned. The interval between subsequent doses is expanded. In successfully treated cases an average of just over five doses of 150 mCi in a mean time of 3½ years was used by Pochin.

Many believe that those cancers responding to ^{131}I therapy are usually the same tumors that respond to TSH suppression therapy. Desiccated thyroid effectively suppresses TSH production, and in so doing it may suppress cancer growth. This virtually blocks any possibility of effective ^{131}I therapy for 1 to 2 months. Triiodothyronine produces the same physiologic effect as desiccated thyroid, but after its withdrawal the return of function to normal is more rapid (8 days) than after thyroid withdrawal (1 to 2 months). For this reason triiodothyronine is the suppressing agent of choice when one anticipates alternating ^{131}I therapy with TSH suppression therapy. It is our belief that these two methods of therapy should be alternated in most patients with functioning metastases. At the same time one can justifiably add local external irradiation to lesions of weight-bearing bones and large soft tissue masses producing pressure on vital structures.

It is far more difficult to evaluate the role of TSH suppression by thyroid feeding in patients with surgically treated lesions and no evidence of dissemination. Clark and associates observed that multiple foci of origin or residual occult local cancer was found after limited surgical procedures in 123 of 218 patients (56.4%). This would certainly speak against the observed successful outcome of the majority of patients with papillary adenocarcinoma of the thyroid being treated surgically, unless TSH suppression were achieved in nearly all patients or the existence of untreated occult cancer had no clinical significance. Cady and associates in a review of 792 patients with differentiated thyroid carcinomas noted that less than half of their patients maintained thyroid feeding. As they point out, patients with less than subtotal thyroidectomy would be able to avoid the myxedema associated with thyroid deficiency, and thus the group with the greatest likelihood of persistent foci of carcinoma could neglect therapeutic thyroid medication. Despite this possible bias their review indicated a significant reduction in mortality for those patients who continued taking exogenous thyroid. This protective effect, however, was not noted in patients with follicular carcinoma. Until such time as a precise method of determining the value of thyroid feeding is available, we recommend such therapy for all patients with differentiated thyroid cancers.

EXTERNAL IRRADIATION. In patients with residual disease following surgery or those with inoperable primary tumors all known cancer should be irradiated vigorously with a curative aim. Since midline blocking cannot be employed, the usual dose-limiting structure is the spinal cord (Figs. 8-3 and 8-4). A tumor dose of about 6500 rad in 7 weeks should be given for differentiated thyroid carcinomas and slightly less dose for medullary carcinomas. This dose can usually be delivered through a single anterior portal with minimal risk of spinal cord, tracheal, or esophageal damage.

Once the disease has spread beyond the neck, curative dose levels are no longer

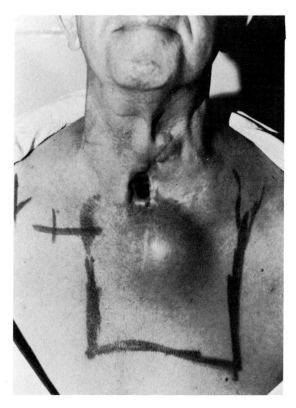

Fig. 8-3. Postoperative recurrent Hürthle cell carcinoma of the thyroid. Patient had his larynx removed at the time of thyroidectomy. The cancer has recurred both above and below the stoma. Disease in both areas was controlled by irradiation for 7 years.

justified. If such a widespread carcinoma is functioning, palliative therapy should consist of external irradiation combined with ^{131}I therapy or with thyroid feeding. Palliative external irradiation alone is the only treatment for nonfunctioning carcinomas.

RESULTS. Carcinoma of the thyroid is not a common disease. Furthermore, the differentiated histologic types have excellent survival times, and any claims for the superiority of one technique or another are difficult to substantiate. On the other hand, the undifferentiated histologic types are usually nonresectable and usually kill rather quickly. Patients with papillary or follicular carcinomas may live for years with their cancer, regardless of the clinical stage. Results of irradiation are therefore difficult to evaluate. However, there is no longer any question but that vigorous irradiation of local differentiated cancer does produce beneficial, long-lasting, and often permanent control. With irradiation alone, Smedal and associates reported an 85% 5-year survival in surgically nonresectable lesions—a survival equal to their results of radical surgery plus irradiation in the more limited stages. Similarly, Sheline and associates reported that of nine patients with nonresectable papillary carcinomas, five were tumor-free at 5 years after irradiation. Of eight

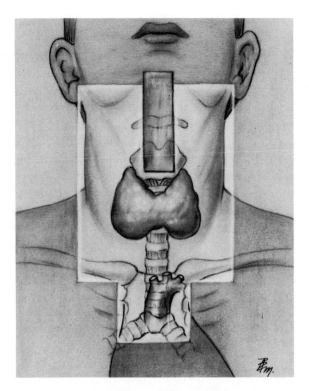

Fig. 8-4. Volume of interest in the irradiation of locally advanced carcinoma of the thyroid gland. The glottis should be shielded if at all possible. The superior mediastinum should usually be included in the high-dose volume.

patients with nonresectable follicular carcinoma, six were tumor-free at 5 years.

Tubiana and Lacour reported 5-year survivals in twenty of twenty-nine inoperable patients with papillary carcinomas and six of sixteen patients with follicular carcinomas. Unfortunately, it is difficult to define the role of radiation therapy in most published series of the treatment of thyroid cancer. This is true both because this is an uncommon neoplasm and because the histologic features and prognostic criteria are not uniformly defined in all series. We do believe, however, that the guidelines for selection of patients for definitive irradiation shown in Figs. 8-1 and 8-2 form a rational basis for approaching the management of this disease. Most series contain a large proportion of surgically treated patients, with radiotherapy being reserved for the surgical failures. This limits our evaluation of radiotherapy alone in the management of this cancer.

Radiation-induced thyroid carcinoma

There is no longer any doubt that irradiation of benign disease about the head and neck has resulted in an increased probability of development of thyroid cancer. Almost all these malignancies are of the well-differentiated type, and most are papillary adenocarcinomas (Favus and associates). Recognition of this problem has led to "recall" of many patients who received thymic or tonsillar irradiation as children. Careful studies with thyroid imaging procedures have resulted in detection of extremely small areas of nonuptake of isotope in the thyroid gland. Although surgery in such patients without palpable nodules has resulted in the discovery of thyroid carcinoma in the earliest stage, we do not believe that scanning or lobectomy is appropriate unless a palpable nodule is present. The approach by Swelstad and associates seems more appropriate. Patients with a history of head and neck irradiation are given physical examinations. If no nodule is palpated, a thyroid scan is not performed. For those patients with a palpable nodule and an abnormal thyroid scan surgery is recommended. Unfortunately, the patient at risk for developing thyroid carcinoma following low-dose irradiation about the head and neck area has a cumulative risk that is not mitigated by a single examination that shows no evidence of disease. The best approach would be an annual physical examination of the thyroid gland of patients at risk and appropriate studies if a definite nodule develops.

REFERENCES

Cady, B., Sedgwick, C. E., Meissner, W. A., Bookwalter, J. R., Romagosa, V., and Werber, J.: Changing clinical, pathologic, therapeutic, and survival patterns in differentiated thyroid carcinoma, Ann. Surg. 184:541-553, 1976.

Clark, R. L., Ibanez, M. L., and White, E. C.: What constitutes an adequate operation for carcinoma of the thyroid, Arch. Surg. 92:23-26, 1966.

Crile, G.: Changing end results in patients with papillary carcinoma of the thyroid, Surg. Gynecol. Obstet. 132:460-468, 1971.

Einhorn, J., and Wikholm, G.: Hypothyroidism after external irradiation to the thyroid region, Radiology 88:326-328, 1967.

Einhorn, J., and Einhorn, N.: Effects of irradiation of the endocrine glands. In Vaeth, J. M., editor: Radiation effect and tolerance, normal tissue, Baltimore, 1972, University Park Press.

Favus, M. J., Schneider, A. B., Stachura, M. E., Arnold, J. E., Yun Ryo, U., Pinsky, S. M., Colman, M., Arnold, M. J., and Frohman, L. A.: Thyroid cancer occurring as a late consequence of head-and-neck irradiation, N. Engl. J. Med. 294:1019-1025, 1976.

Greze, K., Spiler, I. J., Tashjian, A. H., Melvin, K. E., et al.: Natural history of familial medullary thyroid carcinoma, N. Engl. J. Med. 299:980-985, 1978.

Hazard, J. B., Hawk, W. A., and Crile, G., Jr.: Medullary (solid) carcinoma of the thyroid: a clinicopathological entity, J. Clin. Endocrinol. 19:152-161, 1959.

Jonsson, J., Einhorn, N., Fagraeus, A., and Einhorn, J.: Organ antibodies after local irradiation, Radiology 90:536-540, 1968.

Markson, J. L., and Flatman, G. E.: Myxoedema after deep x-ray therapy to the neck, Br. Med. J. 1:1228-1230, 1965.

Pochin, E. E.: Radioiodine therapy of thyroid cancer, Semin. Nucl. Med. 1:503-515, 1971.

Sheline, G. E., Galante, M., and Lindsay, S.: Radiation therapy in the control of persistent thyroid cancer, Am. J. Roentgenol. 97:923-930, 1966.

Smedal, M. I., and Meissner, W. A.: The results of x-ray treatment in undifferentiated carcinoma of the thyroid, Radiology 76:927-935, 1961.

Smedal, M. I., Salzman, F. A., and Meissner, W. A.: The value of 2 MV roentgen-ray therapy in differentiated thyroid carcinoma, Am. J. Roentgenol. 99:352-364, 1967.

Swelstad, J., Scanlon, E. F., Murphy, E. D., Garces, R., and Khandekar, J. D.: Thyroid disease following irradiation for benign conditions, Arch. Surg. 112:380-383, 1977.

Tubiana, M., Lacour, J.: External radiotherapy and radioiodine in the treatment of 359 patients of thyroid cancer, Br. J. Radiol. 48:894-907, 1975.

Woolner, L. B.: Thyroid carcinoma: Pathologic classification with data on prognosis, Semin. Nucl. Med. 1:481-502, 1971.

9

The heart and blood vessels

THE HEART

Portions of the heart are given substantial doses during the irradiation of internal mammary lymph nodes and cancers of the lungs and mediastinum. Accumulated data show that functional and microscopic changes are occasionally produced by commonly used techniques. As in other anatomic sites, changes apparently depend on dose, volume, and fractionation.

Cardiac damage

Damage may be to the pericardium, directly on the myocardium, or to the blood vessels. A combination of these tissues may be damaged in a given situation.

INCIDENCE. The incidence of cardiac damage after the various irradiation techniques is impossible to establish. Occasional case reports, coupled with reports from several centers, comprise our data (Cohn and associates; Jones and Wedgwood; Catteral; Vaeth and associates; Stewart and Fajardo). The administration of 5000 to 6000 rad to the internal mammary nodes was found to produce cardiac damage in 3% to 4% in one department (Stewart and associates). However, many other therapists have delivered similar doses with slightly different fields and beams without producing clinical manifestations of heart disease. Cohn and associates reported an incidence of 6% in patients irradiated for Hodgkin's disease. The fractionation scheme and portal size were shown to be important in the production of cardiac damage.

PERICARDIUM. The pericardium is a relatively avascular, double-layered mesothelial sheath. It must retain its thin, highly flexible qualities if it is to minimize damping of the cardiac contractions. The two layers are normally lubricated and glide over one another without rubbing. Radiations damage these qualities of the pericardium in several ways.

Acute pericarditis. Radiation-induced acute pericarditis may appear a few weeks to several years after irradiation. It is diagnosed by the development of fever, tachycardia, substernal pain, and pericardial friction rub. Pericardial effusion is frequent, and cardiac tamponade may develop. The cardiac silhouette is widened. As might be expected, the ECG shows inversion and flattening of T waves, elevation of the ST segment, and decrease of the QRS segment.

243

The course of acute pericarditis is variable, being self-limiting in about half the patients. The remainder show recurrence or develop chronic constrictive pericarditis.

The dose-time-volume relationships for acute pericarditis have been clarified by Stewart and Fajardo. Most patients will have had at least 4000 rad in 4 weeks to a major portion of the heart. Yet the disease is not common even after 5000 to 6000 rad in 5 to 6 weeks. This has led to inquiries into the possibility of associated factors. Mediastinal tumors may invade or become attached to the pericardium. It is conceivable, although unlikely, that radiations compound the pericardial injury initiated by tumor invasion. Rapid radiation-induced tumor regression of a thymoma or Hodgkin's disease at times creates a necrotic mass adjacent to the pericardium. This could conceivably trigger the acute reaction. It has been suggested that in selected patients this might contribute to the development of pericarditis. However, it is not a factor in most cases (Stewart and Fajardo).

A surprising proportion of the patients who develop postirradiation pericardial effusion will do so after they have developed myxedema. Rogoway and associates suggested that the prolonged high iodide level after lymphangiogram provokes thyroid hyperplasia and thus increases the radiovulnerability of the thyroid gland. He also suggests that the irradiated gland may not be able to compensate with hyperplasia for an iodide-induced defect. Obviously, thyroid function must be evaluated in these patients before concluding that the damage is directly on the pericardium and not indirectly through the thyroid gland. The study of these changes in man and rabbit confirms that most of the changes are a result of direct cellular damage to the pericardium, myocardium, and blood vessels and not to the various indirect mechanisms.

Chronic pericarditis. Chronic pericarditis is usually manifested by chronic constrictive changes associated with myocardial or endocardial fibrosis or with varying degrees of effusion. The latent period from irradiation to onset of chronic pericarditis varies from 6 months to several years. It may or may not be preceded by acute pericarditis. Symptoms and signs are dyspnea, varying severity of chest pain, venous distention, and pleural effusion. Paradoxic pulse and fever may be present. ECG may show a decreased QRS voltage, flat or inverted T wave, and elevation of the S-T segment. The cardiac silhouette is enlarged.

The morphologic changes are not specific for radiation damage. The pericardium is thickened due to deposition of collagen. The two layers are frequently fused or adherent to each other by a fibrinous exudate. The pericardium may be adherent to the heart and pleura. The blood vessels in the pericardium show the characteristic subendothelial connective tissue proliferation. Usually the underlying myocardium appears normal on gross examination.

The etiologic factors resulting in chronic constrictive pericarditis are apparently the same as those for acute pericarditis. Less than half the patients showing chronic constrictive pericarditis will give a clinical history of previous acute pericarditis. The treatment of chronic constrictive pericarditis depends on its severity—that is, antipyretics for fever, pericardiocentesis for tamponade, and pericardectomy for severe constrictive symptoms.

MYOCARDIUM. Excluding the blood vessels and connective tissues, the myocardium is composed of a stable cell population. This lack of mitotic activity in cardiac muscle makes the myocardium one of the more radioresistant tissues. However, doses of a clinical level produce a variety of subcellular changes in the muscle fibers that appear distinct from those secondary to radiation-induced vascular damage (Burch and associates). We believe, however, that most changes seen in heavily irradiated myocardium can be accounted for by radiation-induced vascular damage. Direct radiation injury of the muscle fiber is a minor factor, but fibrosis between muscle bundles is present on microscopic examination. This is diffuse in distribution and does not resemble changes seen in an infarct. Whether such fibrosis is secondary to small vessel occlusion or parallel with it is not known. Direct damage to the conducting mechanism has not been demonstrated after clinically employed doses but may occur after high single doses.

CARDIAC BLOOD VESSELS. Blood vessels of the heart show the same response to radiations as blood vessels elsewhere. (These changes, which are occlusive in nature, are described in detail in the following discussion.) However, injury of cardiac vessels is more serious than radiation-vascular injury in most other sites. It is therefore worthy of special attention. No specific vessels are more affected than others. The consequences of radiation-induced vessel occlusion are the same as those from other causes. A high single dose of radiations is used as a nonoperative technique for producing myocardial infarction in experimental animals (Stone and associates). The incidence of infarction from clinically used doses is unknown. This is especially difficult to determine, since many of the patients are beyond middle age and those infarctions produced by the radiations are impossible to identify. Treatment is the same as that for myocardial infarction from other causes.

In an excellent study, Stewart and Fajardo defined some of the risks of *carditis* (clinical manifestations of pericardial or myocardial damage) as related to the rad and ret doses, fractionation, and proportion of the heart in the high-dose volume. When at least half the heart must be included in the highly dosed volume, as is the case for selected patients with Hodgkin's disease, a ret dose of 1500 (about 4400 rad in 4 to 5 weeks) will produce mild carditis in about 5%. When high-dose *reirradiation* of the mediastinum is necessary and the heart is included in the irradiated volume, the risk of carditis is much greater, that is, 40%. By contrast, when the volume is smaller, as is used in the treatment of the internal mammary nodes, a ret dose of 1850 is required to produce mild carditis in 5%. Changes in shielding and fractionation will modify the volume and the ret dose and thus influence the incidence of heart damage.

Stewart and Fajardo have likewise emphasized the importance of differentiating between radiation-induced carditis and persistence of cancer. The treatment is obviously different. Most patients with carditis are treated conservatively, since the lesions will clear spontaneously. However, the occasional more acute and progressive tamponade may be mistaken for mediastinal compression by cancer and the patient allowed to go untreated or mistreated.

Prednisone is often administered as part of a multidrug chemotherapy regimen for Stages III and IV Hodgkin's disease. When mediastinal irradiation is followed by intermittent withdrawal of prednisone (as is commonly done between cycles of MOPP [a combination consisting of vincristine, nitrogen mustard, procarbazine, and prednisone] therapy), latent "radiation injury" of the heart sometimes develops (Castellino and associates). These changes diminish when prednisone is reinstituted. When such steroids are omitted from the MOPP regimen from the start of therapy, the "withdrawal" changes do not develop. Fortunately, the elimination of prednisone from the MOPP regimen does not seem to diminish its effectiveness.

Adriamycin-induced myocardial damage is a widely recognized toxic response. The incidence of this response, along with the incidence of pericardial effusions and fibrosis, are increased when adriamycin is combined with cardiac irradiation (Eltringham and associates). We have made every effort to avoid the simultaneous use of these two agents and to use caution, even if they are used separately as long as 2 to 3 weeks apart.

BLOOD VESSELS

The fact that cellular viability and organ function in every anatomic site depend on the integrity of blood vessels makes a knowledge of vessel radiation response important. The acute reactions in highly radiosensitive tissues such as hemopoietic tissue and gut are initiated before radiation-induced vascular changes are apparent. By contrast, the late reactions in the brain and myocardium are almost entirely secondary to radiation-induced vascular changes. An impaired blood supply quickly leads to local changes in nutrition, electrolytes, and tissue oxygenation. This decreases the ability of tissues to respond to injury. No other single system is so significant in regulating cellular radiosensitivity. Radiations damage blood vessels of all sizes, and the damage is in the direction of impairing normal circulation. A circulation already impaired by a cancerous mass may improve rapidly as the mass shrinks.

Just as for other tissues, the radiation-induced effects are acute and chronic and depend on vessel size, location, associated vascular disease, dose-time-volume factors, and, finally, the stresses to which the irradiated volume may be subjected.

ACUTE VASCULAR CHANGES. The first and most noticeable gross postirradiation vascular change is the cutaneous or mucosal erythema. The intensity of the erythema is greater when the dose is higher and the area is larger. Erythema of the skin appears in waves—the first day, the second to third week, and at the end of the first month. The mechanisms of these erythemas are not known, but the first erythema is thought to be a vascular response to local extracapillary cell injury, whereas the later erythemas are presumed to be due to direct capillary damage. The erythema is not a result of nerve injury. It has been suggested that a histamine-like substance is produced by the injury and that this diffuses through tissues to produce erythema slightly beyond the margins of the irradiation. However, the erythema is not decreased by antihistamines. At this time the vessels maintain their ability to respond to a scratch test by vasoconstriction. Wheal formation is not produced by histamine. Skin temperature rises several degrees with onset of erythema, suggesting that vasodilation and not merely vasocongestion occurs. Although the responses of vasoconstriction and vasodilation are reduced, they still occur with the local administration of epinephrine or acetylcholine (Moss and Gold). Direct observation of arterioles and capillaries in the bat's wing, frog's web, nail fold, and through transparent windows confirms that acute radiation-induced small blood vessel damage is nonspecific.

During this acute phase, damage of the vessel endothelium is not striking. With doses used clinically, however, some endothelial cells are killed and mural thrombi may form to narrow or obliterate the vessel lumen. The functions of small blood vessels have been defined in terms of their ability to deliver metabolic needs to cells and carry waste products from cells. These types of functions depend not only on blood flow rates but also on transmission and transport of nutrients and waste products through the capillary wall. Both layers of the capillary wall—the endothelium and the basement membrane—must be considered in studies of capillary wall permeability. However, data are scanty and the relative contribution of each remains uncertain. A few hours to a few weeks after moderate doses of radiations there is an increased permeability of the capillary wall.

As might be expected, the rapidly proliferating endothelial cells of newly devel-

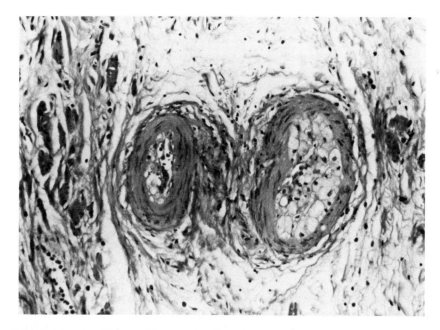

Fig. 9-1. Arteries from a 34-year-old woman irradiated 5 months previously with 6500 rad for carcinoma of the cervix. Fatty deposits in the intima have caused great narrowing of the lumina.

oping capillaries are more sensitive to radiations than endothelial cells in older capillaries (Gillette and associates). This fact is of use in timing radiation therapy for neovascularization of the cornea and in explaining some of the inhibitory effects of early irradiation on wound healing.

One of the most constant early alterations seen in the capillaries and prearterioles after irradiation is dilatation of the vessel. This can be accompanied by endothelial cell swelling, degeneration and necrosis, and cellular inflammatory infiltrate. Increased vascular permeability with resulting tissue edema is a common early manifestation (Fig. 9-1). The pathogenesis of this increased vascular permeability is not clear, since endothelial cell damage may appear minimal or absent, although edema can be severe. It is possible that irradiation interferes at least temporarily, with vasomotor regulatory mechanisms, with resulting hemodynamic alterations conducive to tissue edema.

We recognize increased capillary permeability as local edema, and it may be seen after doses of 500 rad or more. Various substances such as labeled plasma, erythrocytes, Evans blue dye, and colloidal gold permeate the capillary walls more rapidly after irradiation. The peak change develops 2 weeks after a single exposure. The contribution of the thrombi and vasodilation to the increased permeability is unknown. At this point the capillaries exhibit increased fragility. Bleeding occurs more readily even though the clotting mechanism is normal. These composite responses to radiation-induced injury resemble an inflammatory response (Reinhold). Like an inflammatory response, they subside as the chronic vascular changes become manifest.

CHRONIC VASCULAR CHANGES. After the acute reaction subsides and before major narrowing of the lumen develops, diffusion of material through the capillary wall decreases. The vessel wall may not appear seriously damaged. However, the ultrafiltration properties of the endothelial lining are decreased (Reinhold). Furthermore, the basement membrane of the capillary wall is thickened, and it is presumed to contribute to decreased capillary permeability during the chronic phase. The connective tissue barrier between the capillaries and the dependent tissues is increased due to extracapillary fibrosis. The cause of this extracapillary fibrosis is unknown, although Rubin and Casaret related this to a connective tissue reaction after the "leakage" of plasma constituents from the capillary.

Still later the number of small vessels is decreased through the process of vessel occlusion (Fig. 9-2). Arteriolar capillary intimal hyalinosis proceeds as a discontinuous process. Radiations in cancerocidal doses inhibit capillary sprouting and vascular remodeling (van den Brenk). This probably contributes to postirradiation delays of wound healing. However, vascular endothelium appears to recover rapidly, and there is a possibility that migrating unirradiated endothelial cells account for this apparent rapid recovery. This aspect of small vessel injury needs to be clarified.

The most frequent changes in vessels of medium and small caliber, particularly arteries, occur in the intima. These are manifested by swelling and vacuolation of the endothelial cells. Later, proliferation of endothelial cells and lipid deposits may

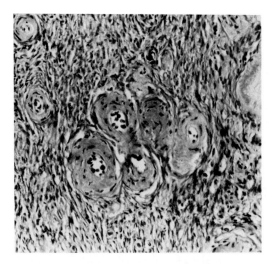

Fig. 9-2. Small blood vessels 5 months after irradiation with 6500 rad in 7 weeks. Walls are strikingly thickened and lumen is narrowed.

occur. These lesions resemble atheromatous plaques but differ in their location, since atheromatous plaques rarely occur spontaneously in small arteries. These lesions are not specific for radiation, since any physical or chemical damage to the vessel, especially the adventitia, will result in similar lesions. This is particularly true in experimental situations in which animals are rendered hyperlipemic by dietary means. In man there is no evidence of a relationship between serum cholesterol levels and development of the foamy lesions in the intima after irradiation. These lesions can be seen a few days after radiation and they can persist for many years. Concomitant with these intimal changes, vacuolation and degeneration of the smooth muscle cells of the media may occur. Repair with fibrosis of the media is seen in chronic lesions. Narrowing of the lumen occurs as a result of concentric fibrosis and loss of vascular elasticity, but thrombosis and intimal proliferation also play important roles.

In the superficial part of the cutis extensive dilatation of capillaries, recognized as telangiectasia, is seen. The telangiectatic vessels arise from existing capillaries and are presumed to be a result of greater flow through the few remaining damaged small blood vessels.

The sequelae of small blood vessel obliteration vary with the organ in question. Vasculoconnective tissue of the skin can tolerate extensive damage before necrosis is produced. On the other hand, rather minor defects in the vasculature of the brain, myocardium, kidney, or lungs may result in seriously limited function.

In addition to these direct radiation-induced changes in small blood vessels, there are changes secondary to tumor shrinkage. Thus quantitative studies show improved vascular filling following irradiation. Also, vessels in large tumors revert in appearance to those seen in small tumors (Hilmas and Gillette; Reinhold). This is fundamental to the process of radiation-induced reoxygenation of the tumor.

The popularity of a dose of 6000 rad in 6 weeks is a recognition of the tolerance of most normal vasculoconnective tissues. The incidence of necrosis of normal tissues increases rather rapidly when doses higher than 6000 rad in 6 weeks are delivered to large volumes. A wide variety of factors modifies the response of small vessels—tissue oxygen, associated inflammatory reactions, sclerotic changes in the aged patient, hypertension, associated trauma such as surgery, fractionation scheme, and so forth. The recognition of these factors and the exploitation of fractionation is the basis for individualization of technique.

LARGE BLOOD VESSELS. High doses of radiations produce little recognizable acute change in large blood vessels. The changes affecting large, elastic arteries occur usually as a late manifestation. Although a direct effect of radiation on the cellular elements of the media cannot be excluded, the changes seen are similar to those observed after damaging the adventitial vessels nourishing most of the vascular wall. These can be produced experimentally by burning or freezing the adventitia. Extensive dissection around the vessels with stripping of their blood supply is likely to be a predisposing factor, although this is by no means a prerequisite for such a radiation-induced change. The changes basically consist of degeneration of muscular cells of the media. This can be a patchy, localized process or present itself as a wide zone of cystic medial necrosis. Weakening of the walls of the vessel may lead to rupture. More often a process of fibrosis of the media is observed. The intima overlying the areas of media degeneration usually develops changes indistinguishable from those of ordinary atherosclerosis (Lindsay and associates). Again, these changes can be produced experimentally by damaging the vessel adventitia by chemical or physical means. The pathogenesis of these experimental lesions appears to be interference with the nutrition of the arterial wall by damage of the adventitial vasa vasorum. It seems likely that a similar mechanism operates in radiation-induced damage to large arteries, that is, it is mediated through narrowing and occlusion of the vasa vasorum by the radiation. In clinical situations, one has also to consider the added factors of the presence of tumor cells and the tissue reactions they may elicit as contributing to the vessels' decreased blood supply. Already mentioned is the important factor of extensive surgical dissection of the vessel adventitia. This decreased strength of the vessel wall attains unusual importance when radical neck dissection is performed after high doses have been given to the carotid arteries (Roscher and associates). Rupture may occur.

Changes within the lumen are more obvious. Single large doses of 1500 to 2000 rad produce arteriosclerosis and atherosclerosis in 30 to 40 weeks. This sclerosis is confined to the irradiated zone (Lindsay and associates). Fractionated doses of 3000 to 5000 rad seem to produce less severe changes than the large single doses.

Asscher found that radiations sensitize blood vessels to hypersensitive changes. Hypertension from any cause produces early profound hypertensive vascular damage in irradiated blood vessels. Unirradiated blood vessels subjected to the same hypertension may appear relatively normal for months. When hypertension develops years after high-dose irradiation, the patient can, because of the hypertension, develop a localized vascular insufficiency leading to necrosis of the irradiated volume.

Silverberg and associates compared a variety of parameters in nine patients with atherosclerotic carotid artery disease associated with neck irradiation with forty unirradiated control patients. The nine irradiated patients with occlusive carotid artery disease were younger than the controls, had less peripheral vascular and less coronary artery disease, and had less frequent hyperlipemia and hypercholesterolemia. These findings support the recognition of radiation-induced carotid artery disease as a clinical entity. Reconstructive carotid surgery on these patients should be approached as if radiation were not a factor, even though there may be some periarterial fibrosis and increased difficulty in separating the plaques from the vascular media (Silverberg and associates).

In childhood, the aorta and other large vessels grow in proportion to increasing body surface area and not in relation to chronologic age (Taber and associates). Doses of 2500 to 2800 rad in 2 to 3 weeks to large vessels arrest growth in vessel diameter (Colguhoun). The significance of this effect is greatest in infancy and diminishes in adolescence.

REFERENCES

Asscher, A. W.: The delayed effects of renal irradiation, Clin. Radiol. 15:320-325, 1964.

Burch, G. E., Sohal, R. S., Sun, S. C., Miller, G. C., and Colcolough, H. L.: Effects of radiation on the human heart, Arch. Intern. Med. 12: 230-234, 1968.

Castellino, R. A., Glatstein, E., Turbow, M. M., Rosenberg, S., and Kaplan, H. S.: Latent radiation injury of lungs or heart activated by steroid withdrawal, Ann. Intern. Med. 80:593-599, 1974.

Catterall, M.: The effect of radiation upon the heart, Br. J. Radiol. 33:159-164, 1960.

Cohn, K. E., Stewart, J. R., Fajardo, L. F., and Hancock, E. W.: Heart disease following radiation, Medicine 46:281-298, 1967.

Colguhoun, J.: Hypoplasia of the abdominal aorta following therapeutic irradiation in infancy, Radiology 86:454-456, 1966.

Eltringham, J. R., Fajardo, L. J., and Stewart, J. R.: Adriamycin cardiomyopathy: enhanced cardiac damage in rabbits with combined drug and cardiac irradiation, Radiology 115:471-472, 1975.

Gillette, E. L., Maurer, G. D., and Severin, G. A.: Endothelial repair of radiation damage following beta irradiation, Radiology 116:175-177, 1975.

Hilmas, D. E., and Gillette, E. L.: Tumor microvasculature following fractionated x irradiation, Radiology 116:165-169, 1975.

Jones, A., and Wedgwood, J.: Effects of radiations on the heart, Br. J. Radiol. 33:138-158, 1960.

Lindsay, S., Kohn, H. I., Dakin, R. L., and Jew, J.: Arteriosclerosis due to roentgen radiation, Circ. Res. 10:51-60, 1962.

Moss, W. T., and Gold, S.: The acute effects of radiations on the physiology of small blood vessels, Radiology 90:294-299, 1963.

Pierce, R. H., Hafermann, M. D., Kagan, A. R.: Changes in the transverse cardiac diameter following mediastinal irradiation for Hodgkin's disease, Radiology 93:619-624, 1969.

Reinhold, H. S.: Radiations and the neurocirculation. In Vaeth, J. M., editor: Radiation effect and tolerance, human tissue, Baltimore, 1972, University Park Press.

Rogoway, W. M., Finkelstein, S., Rosenberg, S. A., and Kriss, J. P.: Myxedema developing after lymphangiography and neck irradiation, Clin. Res. 14:133, 1966.

Roscher, A. A., Steele, B. C., and Woodward, J. S.: Carotid artery rupture after irradiation of the larynx, Arch. Otolaryngol. 83:472-476, 1966.

Rubin, P., and Casaret, G. W.: Clinical radiation pathology, Philadelphia, 1968, W. B. Saunders Co.

Silverberg, G. D., Britt, R. H., and Goffinet, D. R.: Radiation-induced carotid artery disease, Cancer 41:130-137, 1978.

Stewart, J. R., Cohn, K. E., Fajardo, L. F., Hancock, E. W., and Kaplan, H. S.: Radiation-induced heart disease, Radiology 89:302-310, 1967.

Stewart, R., and Fajardo, L. F.: Dose response in human and experimental radiation-induced heart disease, Radiology 99:403-408, 1971.

Stewart, R., and Fajardo, L. F.: Radiation induced heart disease. In Vaeth, J. M., editor: Radiation effect and tolerance, human tissue, Baltimore, 1972, University Park Press.

Stone, H. L., Bishop, V. S., and Guyton, A. C.: Progressive changes in cardiovascular function after unilateral heart irradiation, Am. J. Physiol. 206:289-293, 1964.

Taber, P., Kosobkin, M. T., Gooding, L. T., Palubinskas, A. J., and Neuhanser, E. B. D.: Growth of the abdominal aorta and renal arteries in childhood, Radiology 102:129-134, 1972.

Vaeth, J. M., Feigenbaum, L. Z., and Merill, M. D.: Effects of intensive radiation on the human heart, Radiology 76:755-762, 1961.

10

The lung and thymus

RESPONSE OF NORMAL LUNG TO IRRADIATION

The trachea and lungs are composed of many types of tissues, most of which tolerate moderate doses of radiations well. The airway is lined with ciliated columnar epithelium that is shed only with high doses. This was emphasized by Lacassagne when a beam sufficient to produce a loss of esophageal epithelium was directed to the rabbit's mediastinum and no noticeable early change in the tracheal lining was produced. However, striking cytologic changes do appear later. The tracheal and bronchial epithelia thicken, and the proportion of goblet cells increases (Engelstadt; Bergmann and Graham). Although the ciliated epithelium may appear relatively normal after doses of 5000 to 6000 rad in 5 to 6 weeks, the cilia cease to function early. Mucus-secreting glands cease to function, and dry, irritated mucosa results. Bronchoscopic examination of patients with typical clinical and radiographic findings of radiation pneumonitis reveals an edematous, red, vascular bronchial mucosa. Bronchial narrowing results from the edema. Secretions are thick and sticky and tend to accumulate. These gross changes persist for months, even though later the chest film may show only a slight haziness. Although such airway changes cannot explain the parenchymal and pleural alterations to be described, they may explain some of the transient radiographic changes resulting from ventilatory disturbances, that is, atelectasis with mediastinal shifting. Transient benefit may be obtained from agents that shrink the mucosa or decrease secretions. The airway may be unusually dry because of the damage to mucous glands. A nonproductive cough from such a cause may be benefited by a humidifier. Months later, in an extreme case of radiation pulmonary fibrosis, the accumulation of secretions with secondary infection may lead to sloughing of bronchial epithelium and a necrotizing bronchitis. This reaction should not be confused with the early bronchial radiation epithelitis. Four classic phases are recognized in the development of radiation-induced pneumonitis (Engelstadt).

1. Beginning 2 hours after a vigorous irradiation and lasting 24 to 48 hours, lymph follicles degenerate, and the bronchial mucosa becomes hyperemic, with increased transudate and moderate leukocytic infiltration. Dose-dependent edema of the mucosa is not ordinarily of any clinical significance provided that daily doses are kept

253

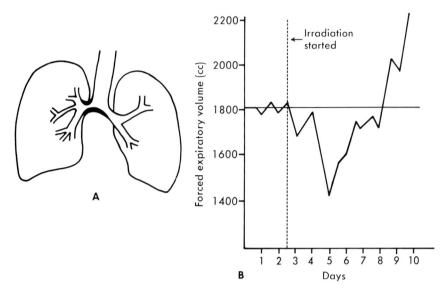

Fig. 10-1. A, Critically situated carcinoma of the right mainstem bronchus with marked bronchial narrowing. **B,** Graph of forced respiratory volume before and 1 week after high daily bronchial doses of 250 to 330 rad. Whether decrease in expiratory volume is related to continued cancer growth, infection, or radiation-induced edema is speculative. Striking functional improvement occurred beginning the sixth day. (Modified from Cameron, S. J., Grant, I. W. B., Lutz, W., and Pearson, J. G.: Clin. Radiol. **20:** 12-18, 1969.)

within conventional ranges. However, if the airway is already seriously narrowed by tumor, ventilatory function studies have shown that significant swelling may follow two or three daily bronchial doses of 250 to 300 rad (Cameron and associates) (Fig. 10-1). We have never seen this type of swelling show clinical manifestations.

2. A latent stage of relatively normal function lasts for 2 to 3 weeks.

3. The degenerative stage begins from 1 to 3 weeks up to 6 months after a single large dose and several weeks after the usual fractionated course. This stage corresponds to a clinical decrease in pulmonary function and is often termed acute radiation pneumonitis. The endothelial cells of small vessels swell, may slough, and leave a surface favorable for thrombus formation. Through these damaged vascular walls plasma passes to accumulate in the interstitial tissues. Also, there are changes in the proliferating alveolar lining cells. They swell, slough, and are enmeshed in exudate, which escapes through the septal walls. This exudate is compressed during inspiration and forms the hyaline membrane so characteristic of this stage of radiation pneumonitis.

If the dose has not been too high, septal cells proliferate, migrate into the alveolus, scavenge the cellular debris, and assist in clearing the alveolus. The interstitial and alveolar exudates are absorbed, and the hyaline membrane is lysed as the process of repair is initiated.

4. The last stage, that of regeneration, is marked by reepithelization of the alveoli

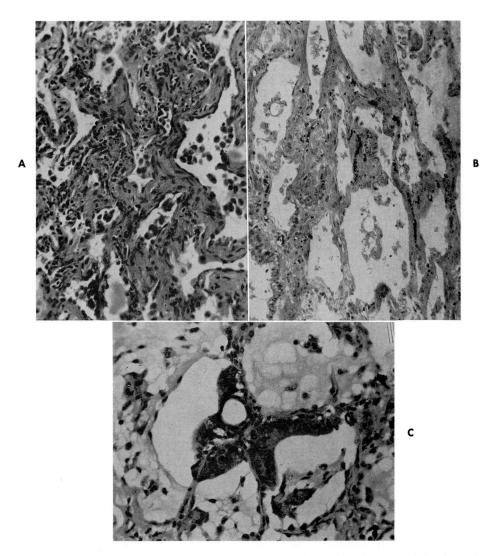

Fig. 10-2. Radiation-induced changes in the lung. **A,** Marked fibrosis and edema of alveolar walls typical of late radiation-induced pulmonary fibrosis. **B,** Low-power photomicrograph showing extensive debris in alveoli and changes described in **A. C,** Metaplasia of epithelial lining occurring in the course of radiation-induced pulmonary fibrosis. (W. U. negs. 50-6003 and 50-6001; courtesy Dr. L. V. Ackerman.)

and the airway, and reestablishment of the microvasculature. In addition, after doses of 4500 rad or higher (1000 rad per week), there will be residual interstitial fibrosis in all tissues, progressive vascular sclerosis, and permanent decrease in all functions. Bone production is not unusual (Fig. 10-2).

CLINICAL CHANGES. Clinically, only a degenerative phase early and a regenerative phase late can be recognized. During the degenerative phase, dyspnea and a

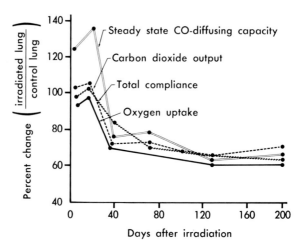

Fig. 10-3. Radiation-induced changes in pulmonary function in dogs. The irradiated lung was given 4500 rad (correct for increased transmission) in 20 to 25 fractions in 23 to 27 days, 200 kv. The irradiated lung was compared to the nonirradiated lung to obtain percent change. (Modified from Teates, C. D.: J. Appl. Physiol. **20:**628-636, 1965.)

cough occasionally productive of a thick white sputum may develop, particularly if the field has been large and the dose has been high. Fever and night sweats may be present. Usually these symptoms will subside in 2 to 3 months, and no further symptoms will be noticed despite positive radiographic findings. If the volume of irradiation has been large and the dose has been high, the clinical signs and symptoms of acute radiation pneumonitis appear in 3 to 6 weeks. The patient becomes progressively more dyspneic, coughs up thick white sputum, is cyanotic, and develops fever and severe sweats. Capilloalveolar block is the most disabling physiologic change (Fig. 10-3).

When both lungs are encompassed as in hemibody irradiation with a single dose of 1000 rad, the incidence of pneumonitis is 84%, whereas with a dose of 800 rad it is 29% (Fryer and associates). About 6 months may be required for patients to develop symptoms.

If lung destruction has been extensive, symptom-producing permanent fibrosis develops during the regenerative phase. Despite its usual unilateral distribution, this late fibrosis may completely disable the patient. Cough, as well as hemoptysis, dyspnea, orthopnea, and clubbing of the fingers, may be severe. Multiple abscess formation and secondary infection with the resulting chills, fever, and night sweats develop in the extreme cases. Death may result from infection. Right heart failure secondary to progressive decrease of the pulmonary capillary bed has been reported (Whitfield and associates; Stone and associates). However, this condition is unlikely unless extremely large fields are employed (Fig. 10-10). Pneumonectomy has proved beneficial in some of the most severe cases (Bergmann and Graham). Radiation pulmonary fibrosis can be severely disabling or even fatal, but such a case would be

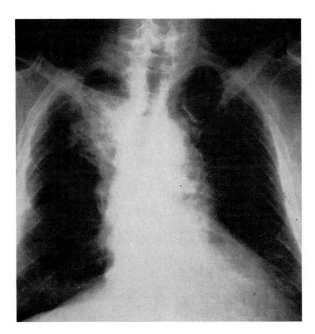

Fig. 10-4. Pulmonary fibrosis 10 months after irradiation for carcinoma of the esophagus. Patient was given a calculated dose of 5500 rad in 39 days through a cylindrical volume measuring 7 × 20 cm centered at the middle third of the esophagus (1000 kv; hvl, 3 mm Pb).

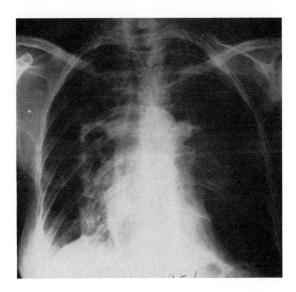

Fig. 10-5. Radiation pneumonitis after 24 mev betatron therapy. A calculated 4900 rad in 32 days was delivered to the midchest through a 12 × 15 cm anterior port. Note the sharp outline of the irradiated volume, which appeared 6 months later. (W. U. neg. 55-4001; courtesy Dr. W. E. Powers.)

considered rare. The incidence and severity can be diminished by carefully avoiding irradiation of large volumes of normal lung tissue to high doses.

RADIOGRAPHIC CHANGES. In early stages, several months after a relatively high dose, the film may reveal only a haziness of the irradiated lung field (Widmann; Bate and Guttmann). In later stages, this becomes a patchy consolidation of the irradiated volume. Finally, the patches coalesce. In late, severe stages, when fibrosis is complete, the normal architecture of the lung may not be visible. The pattern of reaction may follow the configuration of field applied (Figs. 10-4 to 10-6). Atelectasis, with

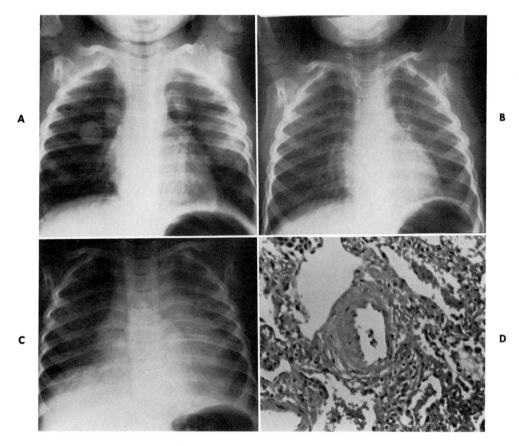

Fig. 10-6. Radiation reaction in child's lung. **A,** Bilateral pulmonary metastases from Wilms' tumor. Patient was given 1200 rad midchest (uncorrected) with parallel opposing anterior and posterior ports. Patient was also given actinomycin D. Two months later, a thoracotomy was done for persistent densities. Multiple small foci of Wilms' tumor were scattered throughout the lung. The same radiation therapy and chemotherapy were then repeated. **B,** Two months after the second course of therapy. All densities have disappeared but patient had clinical symptoms of radiation pneumonitis. **C,** One year after **A.** Patient has pulmonary hypertension with cardiac enlargement. Patient died 1 year later from pulmonary hypertension. **D,** Microscopic slide of patient's lung taken at autopsy. Pulmonary arteriole shows marked intimal proliferation. This proliferation could result either from irradiation directly, or secondarily due to the increased pulmonary blood pressure accompanying pulmonary fibrosis (H & E; × 137). (Courtesy Dr. Harvey White.)

mediastinal shifting, pleural and pericardial adhesions, pleural thickening, and calcified plaques, may be present. Bate and Guttmann were able to show that with tissue doses of 3000 to 5000 rad in 3 to 5 weeks to limited volumes, thirty-five of fifty patients showed radiographic evidence of radiation fibrosis. The picture was frequently reversible. Only seven of the thirty-five presented symptoms. Libshitz and Southard found that radiographic changes are rare with doses of less than 3000 rad in 3 weeks but are usually manifested after doses of 4000 rad in 4 weeks. They anticipate that radiation pneumonitis will appear 1 week earlier for each 1000 rad increment over 4000 rad. This is in keeping with the report of Salazar and associates who found radiation-induced pulmonary fibrosis in more than half of the patients given an equivalent of 5000 rad in 5 weeks through commonly used portals and in 100% of those given the equivalent of 6000 rad in 6 weeks. Radiation pneumonitis (extent and severity not specified) was much less frequent but developed as expected to some degree in nearly all patients given an equivalent of 6000 rad in 6 weeks.

Other than in children total thoracic irradiation is seldom justified. However, when it is judged necessary in adults, a midchest dose of 2500 rad delivered at a rate of 150 rad each day should not be exceeded (Newton; Newton and Spittle). For young children a total dose of 1400 to 1500 rad given with daily fractions of 150 rad is near the limit of tolerance. However, even with this dose there are indications that the subsequent size and mechanical properties of the chest are affected. It is not known whether this is caused directly by irradiation or indirectly from the presence of a lung with "stunted" growth during a period of chest wall growth (Wohl and associates).

PATHOLOGIC PHYSIOLOGY. The pathologic physiology of the irradiated lung is related to both vascular and airway injury. However, it is often difficult to define how much of a given functional change is attributable to vascular pathology and how much is attributable to airway pathology. Radiation-induced changes in some of the more common functions are shown in Fig. 10-3. Carbon monoxide diffusing capacity decreases strikingly as one would expect with hyaline membrane formation, interstitial fibrosis of septa, and thrombosis or progressive vascular sclerosis. Compliance is seriously decreased by the interstitial sclerosis (Sweany and associates; Moss and associates). It follows that lung volumes are diminished. Poor ventilation of the irradiated segment and incomplete oxygenation of the blood contributes to the patient's disability in proportion to the ratio of damage to normal lung.

The functional changes produced in clinical practice were studied by Brady and associates. Doses delivered to carcinomas of the lung and adjacent normal lung varied from 6000 rad in 40 days to 2000 rad in 11 days. Pulmonary mechanics, ventilation, volumes, and blood gas tensions showed few significant changes that could be attributed to radiation therapy delivered through the usual, carefully tailored portals. Breath-holding pulmonary diffusing capacity decreased markedly with high doses given through large ports. Brady's study confirmed the relative "safety" of giving effective doses to modest volumes and the hazards of giving high doses to large volumes.

In evaluating the postirradiation clinical findings it must be remembered that

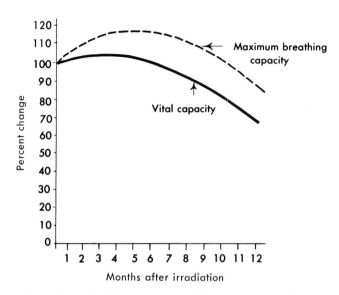

Fig. 10-7. Change in maximum breathing capacity and vital capacity after irradiation of the lung for bronchogenic carcinoma. Maximum breathing capacity improves dramatically up to the sixth month, then decreases slowly, probably when the cancer begins to enlarge. Vital capacity improves initially, but also decreases. The contribution of the radiations to the decreased functions is usually masked by the regrowth of the cancer. (Modified from Deeley, T. J.: Clin. Radiol. **11**:33-39, 1960.)

sites of metastases can easily mask the contribution of irradiation to lung changes. Furthermore, high and particularly destructive doses are justified only for small cancers in limited volumes. Under such circumstances only a fraction of the total lung volume is destroyed. These destroyed areas may not be clinically significant if the remainder of the lung compensates. Perhaps the major reason for the wide variation in clinical radiation response is the wide individual variation in preirradiation pulmonary reserve.

Radiation pulmonary fibrosis requires from 6 months to several years to develop fully. It therefore need be anticipated only in those irradiated patients surviving this developmental period. Because of their frequent long-term survival, it will appear most frequently in patients irradiated subsequent to radical mastectomy and in patients after mediastinal irradiation for Hodgkin's disease. Although such pulmonary fibrosis is not uncommon, symptom-producing fibrosis is relatively infrequent, and severely disabling fibrosis is rare. No attempt should be made to minimize the frequency and dangers of pulmonary fibrosis, but one should never withhold vigorous treatment of smaller malignant lesions of the mediastinum, lungs, or chest wall solely from the fear of its appearance. If fields are kept as small as is clinically permissible and if tangential ports are employed when possible, the frequency of radiation pulmonary fibrosis will be kept at a minimum (Chapters 11, 12, and 20).

TREATMENT OF RADIATION PNEUMONITIS. As long as cancer of the breast,

Hodgkin's disease, or cancers within the thorax are irradiated, radiation pneumonitis will be produced. In the great majority of patients, radiographic manifestations of the changes will be the first and indeed the only evidence of radiation pneumonitis. Usually the opacity will decrease or disappear with no symptoms or treatment. The defects can be identified and quantitated by pulmonary function studies. When the early symptoms are sufficiently severe to justify treatment, steroids may be of help. About half the patients will have early marked relief (Whitfield and associates; Moss and associates). When the fibrosis is well established, steroids are of no value. In severe cases, oxygen may be necessary. Antibiotics do not seem to help unless there is secondary infection (Moss and associates). Sedatives can be used to allay the cough. Still later, if the disease is unilateral and if the patient's condition justifies major surgery, pneumonectomy may help (Bergmann and Graham).

Prophylactic administration of cortisone to animals given whole chest irradiation will decrease the incidence of serious acute reactions (Moss and associates). However, prophylactic administration of cortisone to patients receiving lung irradiation is not indicated. The best prophylaxis is carefully directed beams, keeping the volume of high dose radiation as small as possible.

The cessation of cortisone administration to patients who have previously had lung irradiation (as might occur with cyclic MOPP therapy) may activate a latent radiation pneumonitis (Castellino and associates). Fear of this has often led to eliminating prednisone from the MOPP combination.

RADIOTHERAPY OF CARCINOMA OF THE LUNG

The high incidence of carcinoma of the lung, coupled with the relative ineffectiveness of the best methods of treatment, has made carcinoma of the lung one of the radiation oncologist's most formidable problems. Pneumonectomy can be performed in a fraction of these patients (35%), but 75% of these patients with resectable carcinoma die from metastases undetected at the time of surgery. Radiotherapy fails not only for this same reason, but also from frequent nonsterilization of the primary lesion. Care for this large group of patients will continue to be primarily palliative. However, occasionally a patient is cured by irradiation or by surgery. These few curable patients must not be lost because of a pessimistic approach to the treatment of carcinoma of the lung.

We have adopted a modified version of the World Health Organization's classification of lung cancer as follows:

1. Squamous cell carcinoma
2. Undifferentiated large cell carcinoma
3. Undifferentiated small cell carcinoma (includes oat cell carcinoma)
4. Adenocarcinoma
5. Bronchiolalveolar carcinoma
6. Miscellaneous and rare types (includes giant cell carcinoma, clear cell carcinoma, carcinosarcoma, carcinoids, and others)

Squamous cell carcinoma comprises the majority of the bronchogenic carcinomas seen at our institution (about 60%). Histologic grading is based primarily on their degree of keratinization.

Undifferentiated large cell carcinoma is a heterogeneous group comprising dedifferentiated squamous cell carcinoma, adenocarcinoma, and some mixed types as disclosed by electron microscopic studies.

Undifferentiated small cell carcinoma includes small round, lymphocytic-like types as well as the so-called oat cell carcinoma. In recent years evidence has accumulated that this tumor derives from Kultchitsky-like cells present in the bronchial epithelium and presumably of neural crest origin. About one third of lung cases seen at autopsy at our hospitals are of this type.

Adenocarcinoma and bronchiolalveolar carcinoma are closely related entities, the latter having a characteristic growth pattern. Both may be scar-related. These tumors account for between 10% and 15% of our bronchogenic carcinomas and, like squamous cell carcinoma, are amenable to histologic grading.

A review of the pathogenesis of carcinoma of the lung contributes little that cannot be correctly surmised from the reasons for failure previously presented. It is likely that most bronchogenic carcinomas are preceded by the superficial intra-epithelial changes of carcinomas in situ (Black and Ackerman). At this stage there are no physical signs or symptoms and no radiographic evidence of the disease. Study of the bronchial cells in the sputum may suggest the diagnosis if the diagnosis is

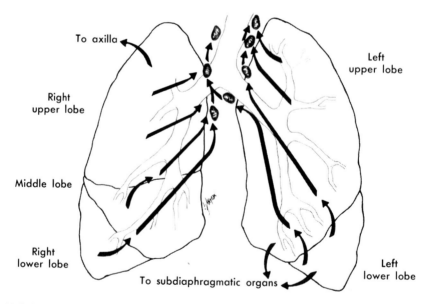

Fig. 10-8. Lymphatic drainage of various lobes of the lungs. Note the crossover from lingula of left upper lobe and upper portion of left lower lobe to right paratracheal nodes. Also, there are direct routes to the abdominal organs and axillae once the pleura is crossed. Lymph drainage does not parallel arteries or veins, nor does it remain distinct for each lobe. (Modified from Nohl, H. C.: Thorax **11:**172-185, 1956.)

suspected. Otherwise it is necessary to wait for the signs and symptoms of advanced carcinoma or its recognition on the radiograph. Distant metastases frequently produce the initial signs or symptoms.

Three fourths of all bronchogenic carcinomas arise in the hilar regions from major bronchi. About one fourth of the lesions will arise from peripheral bronchi. Direct extension of the cancer occurs along the bronchi, thus reaching and invading the pericardium, the vagus, phrenic and recurrent laryngeal nerves, the esophagus, the trachea, and major vessels. Peripherally, the cancer may cross the pleural space to the chest wall, brachial plexus, ribs, and diaphragm.

The lymphatic drainage of the lungs is shown in Fig. 10-8. On autopsy examination, cancer of the lung has spread to hilar lymph nodes in over 90% of the patients. However, carcinoma of the lung does not spread in a predictable stepwise fashion. The principles of regional node dissection proved valuable in many other anatomic sites are of limited value in treating carcinoma of the lung. Mediastinal lymph nodes as well as blood vessels are usually involved by the time the diagnosis is established. The highly vascular composition of the lung with its dual circulation of bronchial and pulmonary vessels provides ready anatomic opportunities for blood vessel invasion. It is not surprising that radiation oncologists fail to cure 90% of the cancers of the lung because of obvious or occult hematogenous spread at the time of the original diagnosis. Pretreatment evaluation of intrathoracic tumor extent depends heavily on radiographic findings and on mediastinoscopy and bronchoscopy. An assessment of mediastinal spread by mediastinoscopy is shown in Table 10-1. Bronchoscopy serves not only as a means for tumor biopsy but also to assess proximity of the cancer to the carina, the probable presence of subcarinal nodes, and the appearance of the endobronchial component. A search for extrathoracic metastases with brain, liver, and bone scans and a skeletal series will be justified for selected patients.

Although autopsy findings are not entirely applicable to the clinical situation (Table 10-2), they assist in defining the metastasizing potential of the various histologic types. A proportion of patients have no spread beyond the thorax at the time of autopsy (Table 10-2). Such data argue strongly for more aggressive combinations of surgery and postoperative irradiation.

Table 10-1. Distribution of positive mediastinal biopsies (mediastinoscopy) according to the site of the primary cancer

Lobe	Percent with positive medi- astinal nodes*	Percent of positive mediastinal nodes in each region†		
		Right paratracheal	Left paratracheal	Subcarinal
Right upper lobe	60	64	4	32
Right lower lobe	36	42	12	46
Left upper lobe	42	16	42	42
Left lower lobe	25	21	29	50

*Based on data from Goldberg, E. M., Glickman, A. S., and Kahn, F. R.: Cancer **25**:347-353, 1970.
†Based on data from Carlens, F.: Chest **65**:442-445, 1974.

Table 10-2. Distribution of lung cancer as found at autopsy in patients dying within 1 month of lung resection that, at the time, was presumed to be curative*

Histologic type of cancer	Number of patients	Number with persistent disease	Number with distant metastases	Sites of distant metastases
Squamous cell	131	44 (33%)	22 (17%)	Distant nodes, 6; adrenal gland, 5; liver, 5; other lung and kidney, 3
Small cell	19	13 (70%)	12 (63%)	Liver, 7; nodes, 6; adrenal gland, 4; brain and kidney, 2
Adenocarcinoma	30	13 (43%)	12 (40%)	Adrenal gland, 7; brain, 5; lymph nodes, 4; vertebrae, 3
Large cell	22	3 (17%)	3 (14%)	Kidney, 3; adrenal gland, liver, and other lung, 3
TOTAL	202	73 (35%)	49 (24%)	Adrenal gland, 18; lymph nodes, 17; liver, 16; kidney and other lung, 6

*Modified from Mathews, M. J., Kanhouwa, S., and Pickern, J.: Cancer Chemother. Rep. III. **4**:63-67, 1973.

Clinical staging of cancer of the lung has never been popular primarily because the surgeon's needs are met by the separation of operable from inoperable and resectable from nonresectable cases. However, the American Joint Committee has proposed the stage classification on p. 226. It is being used more and more in national protocols.

INDICATIONS FOR RADIOTHERAPY. The treatment of cancer of the lung must take into account three aspects of spread of this disease.

1. Local intrapulmonary spread of the primary lesion (Table 10-4)
2. Patterns and incidences of spread to regional nodes—hilar, mediastinal, supraclavicular, and axillary (Table 10-1)
3. Patterns and incidences of spread to more distant structures (Tables 10-2 and 10-3)

Our limitations in defining spread to each of these three areas obviously limit our ability to tailor treatment in keeping with the true extent of the disease. Recognition of this has strongly influenced us to use chemotherapy and to systematically irradiate large apparently normal volumes that, on a statistical basis, account for frequent failure. Surgery is the treatment of choice for all apparently localized, resectable squamous cell carcinomas and adenocarcinomas of the lung. However, surgery has been unable to cope satisfactorily with 95% of these lesions. Smart questioned surgery as the primary treatment for limited cancers and irradiated forty operable lesions. Nine patients (22.5%) survived 5 years. Morrison and associates reported the results of a clinical trial comparing surgery and megavoltage radiotherapy in apparently resectable cancers. Fifty-eight patients were in the study. Twenty-eight were selected at random for radiotherapy and thirty for surgery. Irradiated patients were given 4500 rad in 4 weeks to a volume encompassing the radiographic

Table 10-3. Distribution of metastasis from bronchial carcinoma (all histologic types)*

Cell type	Liver	Adrenal	Bone	Brain	Other
Epidermoid	30.5	27.4	24.4	13.7	
Small cell	61.9	39.2	37.5	30.5	Abdominal lymph nodes 56.6%
Adenocarcinoma	44.8	42.9	39.9	25.4	
Large cell	39.6	36.4	28.9	29.4	Abdominal lymph nodes 36.0%

*From Muggia, F. M., Hansen, H. H., and Chervu, L. R.: Diagnosis in metastatic sites. In Straus, M. J., editor: Lung cancer clinical diagnosis and treatment, New York, 1977, Grune & Stratton, Inc., by permission.

Table 10-4. Roentgenographic findings according to histologic type of lung cancer*

Radiographic finding	163 Squamous cell carcinomas (%)†	126 Adeno-carcinomas (%)‡	114 Small cell undifferentiated carcinomas (%)§	97 Large cell undifferentiated carcinomas (%)‖
Peripheral lesion	31	74	32	65
Atelectasis	37	10	18	13
Consolidation	20	15	24	25
Hilar/perihilar abnormality	40	18	78	32
Mediastinal abnormality	2	3	13	10
Pleural effusion	4	5	5	2
No abnormality	3	1	0	0
Single abnormality	64	70	38	58

*From Green, R. F.: Lungs and mediastinum. In Steckel, R. J., and Kagan, A. R., editors: Diagnosis and staging of cancer, Philadelphia, 1976, W. B. Saunders Co.
†Data from Byrd, R. B., Miller, W. E., Carr, D. T., et al.: The roentgenographic appearance of squamous cell carcinoma of the bronchus, Mayo Clin. Proc. **43:**327, 1968.
‡Data from Lehar, T. J., Carr, D. T., Miller, W. E., et al.: Roentgenographic appearance of bronchogenic adenocarcinoma, Am. Rev. Resp. Dis. **96:**245, 1967.
§Data from Byrd, R. B., Miller, W. E., Carr, D. T., et al.: The roentgenographic appearance of small cell carcinoma of the bronchus, Mayo Clin. Proc. **43:**337, 1968.
‖Data from Byrd, R. B., Miller, W. E., Carr, D. T., et al.: The roentgenographic appearance of large cell carcinoma of the bronchus, Mayo Clin. Proc. **43:**333, 1968.

abnormality plus a 2 cm margin. At 1 year 64% of the irradiated patients were living and 43% of the resected patients were living. However, at 4 years only 7% of the irradiated patients were living and 23% of the resected patients were living. Although one might argue that the doses of radiations were low and the margins of apparently normal lung were narrow, we believe this study supports the superiority of surgery for resectable squamous cell carcinoma of the lung. Although both modalities of treatment will probably fail if metastases are present, surgery is definitely more likely to succeed in controlling the primary lesion of squamous cell type. The same is true for adenocarcinoma of the lung.

TNM CLASSIFICATION*

T—Primary tumor

TX   Tumor proven by the presence of malignant cells in bronchopulmonary secretions but not visualized roentgenographically or bronchoscopically, or any tumor that cannot be assessed

T0   No evidence of primary tumor

TIS   Carcinoma in situ

T1   Tumor 3.0 cm or less in greatest diameter, surrounded by lung or visceral pleura, and without evidence of invasion proximal to a lobar bronchus at bronchoscopy

T2   Tumor more than 3.0 cm in greatest diameter, or a tumor of any size that either invades the visceral pleura or has associated atelectasis or obstructive pneumonitis extending to the hilar region. At bronchoscopy, the proximal extent of demonstrable tumor must be within a lobar bronchus or at least 2.0 cm distal to the carina. Any associated atelectasis or obstructive pneumonitis must involve less than an entire lung, and there must be no pleural effusion

T3   Tumor of any size with direct extension into an adjacent structure such as the parietal pleura or the chest wall, the diaphragm, or the mediastinum and its contents; or a tumor demonstrable bronchoscopically to involve a main bronchus less than 2.0 cm distal to the carina; or any tumor associated with atelectasis or obstructive pneumonitis of an entire lung or pleural effusion

N—Nodal involvement

N0   No demonstrable metastasis to regional lymph nodes

N1   Metastasis to lymph nodes in the peribronchial or the ipsilateral hilar region, or both, including direct extension

N2   Metastasis to lymph nodes in the mediastinum

M—Distant metastasis

MX   Not assessed

M0   No (known) distant metastasis

M1   Distant metastasis present

HISTOPATHOLOGY

Squamous cell carcinoma, adenocarcinoma, undifferentiated large cell, undifferentiated small cell (oat cell cancer)

GRADE

Well-differentiated, moderately well-differentiated, poorly to very differentiated, or numbers 1, 2, 3-4

STAGE GROUPING

Occult stage	TX N0 M0		Occult carcinoma with bronchopulmonary secretions containing malignant cells but without other evidence of the primary tumor or evidence of metastasis to the regional lymph nodes or distant metastasis
Stage I	TIS N0 M0		Carcinoma in situ
	T1 N0 M0 ⎫		Tumor that can be classified T1 without any metastasis or
	T1 N1 M0 ⎬		with metastasis to the lymph nodes in the peribronchial
	T2 N0 M0 ⎭		and/or ipsilateral hilar region only, or a tumor that can be classified T2 without any metastasis to nodes or distant metastasis†
Stage II	T2 N1 M0		Tumor classified as T2 with metastasis to the lymph nodes in the peribronchial and/or ipsilateral hilar region only

---

*From the American Joint Committee for Cancer Staging and End Results Reporting: Manual for staging of cancer, Chicago, 1978, Whiting Press.

†TX N1 M0 and T0 N1 M0 are also theoretically possible, but such a clinical diagnosis would be difficult if not impossible to make. If such a diagnosis is made, it should be included under Stage I.

Stage III   T3 with any N or M⎱   Any tumor more extensive than T2, or any tumor with me-
                    N2 with any T or M⎰   tastasis to the lymph nodes in the mediastinum, or any
                    M1 with any T or N   tumor with distant metastasis

In contrast to the conclusion that primary surgery is preferable for the squamous cell type, this is not true for small cell carcinoma. Thus, in a clinical trial randomizing patients between surgery and irradiation, the mean survival of seventy-one surgically treated patients was 199 days, whereas that of seventy-three irradiated patients was 284 days (Medical Research Council). A few were cured. However, it is now clear from many series that for small cell carcinoma local irradiation combined with multidrug chemotherapy can produce survival rates superior to any single modality. Even so, the overall results remain unsatisfactory, with death most often from widespread metastases.

Squamous cell carcinoma and adenocarcinoma

The criteria of inoperability employed by the thoracic surgeon determine which patients with squamous cell carcinoma and adenocarcinoma are to be evaluated for irradiation as the initial form of therapy. (As yet various combinations of chemotherapy have failed to improve survival of patients with these cell types.) Briefly, lesions are generally nonresectable when tumor is found to have destroyed bone, invaded the pericardium, involved the sympathetic chain, brachial plexus, or recurrent laryngeal or phrenic nerves, produced bloody pleural effusion that contains cancer cells, extended on the mucosa to within 2 cm of the trachea, extended to the esophagus, or metastasized to the scalene nodes or distantly or extensively to local nodes. Heroic attempts to cure some patients in this group by radical resection have been disheartening. In addition, there will be a small number of patients judged nonresectable because of their inability to tolerate any radical surgical procedure and those already disabled because of pulmonary insufficiency. The patients with squamous cell carcinoma and well-differentiated adenocarcinoma judged nonresectable must be separated into at least three major subdivisions.

1. A small number of patients will be judged nonresectable because critically located limited lesions have involved nonresectable vital organs (tracheal wall or carina, major blood vessels, and others). In our experience this group of patients is small. To this group should be added those patients who, although operable in a technical sense, are inoperable because of other physical reasons and those apparently operable patients who refuse surgery. Patients in these three categories with squamous cell carcinomas should be given vigorous irradiation with a curative aim, provided their general physical condition permits. It should be emphasized that patients found to have limited but nonresectable cancers at thoracotomy are not necessarily incurable by radiotherapy. Long-term survivals have been obtained even when the mediastinum was involved or when the aorta or the vena cava were involved (Guttmann; Bloedorn). It is now obvious that one should not delay irradiation of the surgically incurable patient until symptoms appear. Rather, treatment should begin immediately and should be vigorous if tumor extent warrants.

2. Patients in this group have been judged nonresectable because of locally

advanced squamous cell carcinoma with or without thoracotomy. This is a large pro-portion of the patients, and the clinical extent of the cancer varies widely. Small, critically located cancers were previously discussed. Any primary bronchogenic car-cinoma not enclosed by a 10 × 15 cm port should not be treated to a high-dose level, that is, over 4500 rad in 4 to 5 weeks. This type of clinical staging is arbitrary, but as treated volumes are enlarged to encompass larger cancers, normal lung tolerance becomes an increasingly serious dose-limiting factor. Such patients should be treated with a palliative aim only if they have symptoms amenable to radiotherapy. Cough, hemoptysis, dyspnea, superior vena caval obstruction, esophageal obstruction, and pain are frequently temporarily relieved by such irradiation. In treating this group of patients it is not necessary (in fact, it may be harmful) to routinely attempt in-clusion of all known cancer. Only those areas suspected of producing symptoms, or likely to produce symptoms, are irradiated. Rarely are tumor doses exceeding 3000 to 4500 rad in 3 to 4 weeks necessary for maximum palliation in this group. In a clinical trial Deeley found that 3000 rad in 3 weeks gave longer survival and less sequelae than the higher dose of 4000 rad in 4 weeks. A point of diminishing returns is reached as the dose is increased and the volume becomes larger. When the pri-mary tumor is no longer encompassed by a 10 × 15 cm beam, high doses often do more harm than good.

3. Once the squamous cell carcinoma or adenocarcinoma has spread beyond the hemithorax and mediastinum, the radiation oncologist must concern himself with the distant metastasis as well as the primary lesion. Indeed, the distant metastasis may justify his major efforts. In this group the irradiation is planned with a view of pallia-tion, although the fact is appreciated that life will not be measurably prolonged. There is no limit to the manifestations of metastasis. Thus treatment must be tailored to fit a wide spectrum of clinical findings.

TECHNIQUE OF EXTERNAL IRRADIATION. The relatively great skin-tumor dis-tances associated with radiotherapy of most pulmonary malignancies demand multi-portal irradiation techniques developed with simulation and repeated portal veri-fication films.

Before selecting the optimum field arrangement, the size, shape, and position of the volume to be irradiated must be determined. In this, the radiation oncologist is limited by his frequent inability to radiographically differentiate tumor from inflam-matory reaction or atelectasis. Large lesions near the hilum are usually associated with these changes, whereas the extent of peripheral lesions and smaller hilar lesions may be truly represented on the film. Computed tomograms, bronchograms, bronchoscopy, esophagrams, and, of course, thoracotomy give additional useful information. However, there is no way to precisely ascertain tumor extent in every patient, and large errors in tumor localization are unavoidable (Figs. 10-9 and 10-10). How much of a given radiographic abnormality is cancer? Should all areas of in-creased density be encompassed by the beams just to be safe? Overholt and Rumel emphasized the problem when they found tumor to correspond with suggested radiographic extent in only 17% of all lesions. Most of this 17% was composed of

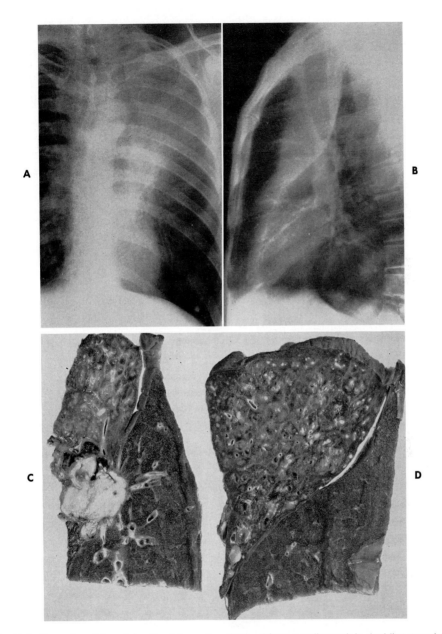

Fig. 10-9. Illustration of the misleading information obtained from a radiograph in deciding on volume to be irradiated. **A** and **B,** Posteroanterior and lateral roentgenograms of a patient with biopsy-proved bronchogenic carcinoma in left upper lobe of bronchus. The films do not permit one to define volume of involvement and suggest a much more extensive lesion than is obvious in gross specimens shown in **C** and **D.** Note relatively small tumor that is capable of producing extensive obstructive atelectasis. Such a lesion should be treated by a relatively small port over the hilum rather than by irradiation of entire left upper lung field. (W. U. negs. 55-730, 55-731, and 55-786; from Ackerman, L. V.: Acta Radiol. Interamericana **5:**28-36, 1955.)

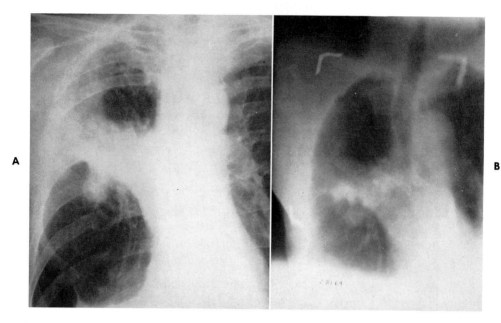

Fig. 10-10. A, Routine chest film showing infiltration of a proved bronchogenic carcinoma. Compare with **B. B,** Same lesion as shown in **A,** but film is taken in treatment position with telecobalt beam. Often, in taking such localization films, additional information can be obtained relative to extent of disease.

peripheral lesions. Thus, in ignorance, excessive field margins may be allowed in one direction whereas inadequate ones may be taken in another. Also within the lung, the sites of origin and patterns of metastases vary with histologic type (Table 10-4). These characteristics, along with those illustrated in Tables 10-1, 10-2, and 10-3 and the uncertainties illustrated in Fig. 10-9, impact heavily on the radiation techniques.

Certain assumptions have proved justifiable:

1. If an entire lung or lobe is atelectatic, only the region of the blocked bronchial orifice and mediastinum need be treated. This can be done with a small field. The bronchus will often reopen, and the atelectasis will be relieved, thus assisting in defining the real limits of the cancer (Fig. 10-11).

2. In the treatment of hilar lesions or lesions near the hilum, the adjacent mediastinum can and should be routinely included in the treatment field (Table 10-1).

3. The spinal cord and the uninvolved lung need not be irradiated to a dose carrying a high risk of injury. Simple reduced ports and angulation of beams are recommended if the doses to the spinal cord would otherwise be excessive (Chapter 22).

4. Although undifferentiated and oat cell carcinomas are more radiosensitive than other bronchogenic carcinomas, their frequently early metastases diminish the chances of cure. With these lesions we are justified in using more generous ports and somewhat lower tissue doses. Planned prophylactic irradiation of the brain and chemotherapy in patients with small or oat cell carcinoma are discussed on the following pages.

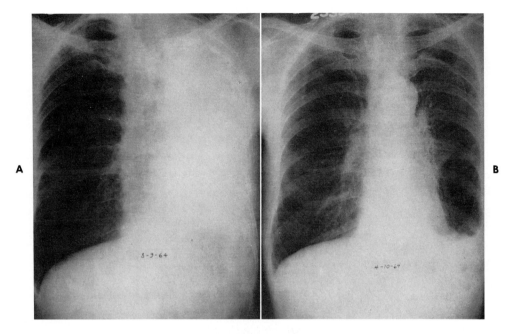

Fig. 10-11. A, Pretreatment film showing complete atelectasis of left lung due to cancer plugging left mainstem bronchus. **B,** Same patient 4 weeks later after onset of therapy. Treatment was given with 10 × 10 cm anterior and posterior telecobalt beams centered over obstructed bronchus. A total dose of 3500 rad had been given to the midchest tissues. This film was taken at completion of therapy. This is an expected response if atelectasis has not persisted more than 8 to 10 days.

Regardless of these limitations in defining the involved volume, the radiation oncologist must make an estimate of tumor extent before proceeding with irradiation. When treatment can be given with a curative aim, a generous 3 cm margin of normal tissue should be included in the treatment field in both the anteroposterior and lateral projections. Simulation and films confirming the beam directioning and correct field shape and size are essential. Peripheral small tumors may move significantly on inspiration and expiration. This should be evaluated fluoroscopically. Obviously, beams should be shaped to spare as much normal lung as possible. The following three arrangements are available:

1. Tumors of the apex may be treated with a parallel pair of opposed anterior and posterior beams encompassing the primary site, hilum, mediastinum at and above the carina, ipsilateral axillary, and supraclavicular area. If there is concern that the brachial plexus is involved, the ports should be enlarged to encompass at least the lower one half of the cervical segment of the spinal cord as well. Cancers in this region may be regarded as peripheral tumors. They respond well, can be given high doses, and can be locally controlled. The severe shoulder and arm pain that develops in many of these patients signals nerve invasion. The need for including the lower cervical cord and adjacent nerve plexus is clear but often overlooked.

2. High doses to small hilar lesions can be delivered in part with simple anterior

and posterior ports using megavoltage radiations. In many cases the use of parallel opposing ports will be superior to that of rotational techniques (Guttmann). The spinal cord dose should not exceed 4500 rad in 4 weeks. Oblique anterior and posterior or lateral portals are easily arranged if a boosting lung dose is to be given.

3. Small, markedly eccentric peripheral lesions may be better treated by sharply angled crossfiring ports centered around the point nearest the tumor. However, the proportion of such cancers referred for irradiation will be small. The hilum and mediastinum should also be irradiated in this group.

The question of the optimum dose-time relationship for squamous cell carcinomas and adenocarcinomas of the lung remains controversial. As indicated previously, our experience suggests that tissue doses of 5000 to 6000 rad in 6 weeks are tolerated if ports, exclusive of the mediastinum, are no larger than 10 × 10 cm. However, the fact that this dose is tolerated does not necessarily indicate that it should be given.

There is no single "optimum" dose for squamous cell carcinoma of the lung. The dose required to consistently eradicate squamous cell carcinoma of the lung will vary according to the size of the cancerous mass as well as numerous biologic factors. In addition, eradication of the lesion in the lung does not routinely increase survival rate. Failure to recognize the difference between the end points of local control and survival has resulted in much confusion concerning the recommended doses for patients with squamous cell carcinoma of the lung.

However, in developing our efforts to increase survival, we need a definition of the dose-time factors that will commonly eradicate *local* tumor. Local control is seldom achieved with doses below 1450 ret (4500 rad in 4 to 5 weeks) (Eisert and associates, 1976). Although these workers failed to find further increased local control with higher doses, Salazar and associates (1976) reported increased shrinkage of tumor mass with an increased dose of up to 6000 rad in 6 or more weeks. It would be a major radiobiologic inconsistency if local control of squamous cell carcinoma and adenocarcinoma of the lung was not dose-related between 4500 and 6500 rad. The experience to date indicates that about 50% of squamous cell carcinomas of the lung will be locally controlled by doses of 6000 rad in 6 weeks. Small tumor masses, as in lymph nodes, will be controlled 90% of the time.

The frequency of widespread metastases from squamous cell carcinoma and adenocarcinoma of the lung seriously limits the impact that local control of the primary lesion has on long-term survival. The relationship of survival rates to doses is shown in Fig. 10-12. There is no more than a suggestion that at 3 years survival is increased with higher doses.

When fields no larger than 10 × 10 cm, exclusive of the mediastinal port, are sufficient, a daily dose of 170 to 180 rad to the center of the tumor for 5 days each week to a total of 5000 to 6000 rad is tolerated. Tumor-skin distances are least for apical lesions. Also, cross firing beams damage less normal lung before and after passing through tumors of this site. For these reasons higher tumor doses in the apex are more easily delivered and better tolerated. If the size of the tumor in the lung requires a portal much larger than 10 × 10 cm, the total dose should be reduced (4500 rad in 5 weeks), or after this dose, port size should be reduced.

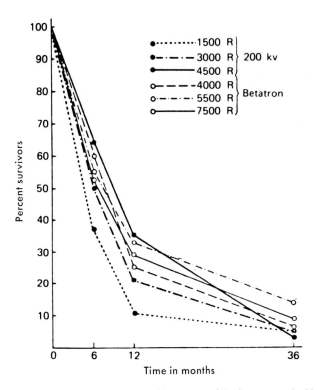

Fig. 10-12. Survival rates of patients with inoperable cancer of the lung treated with various doses of radiations. Little, if any, difference in long-term survival can be shown between these groups of patients with advanced disease. (From Pierquin, D., Gravis, P., and Gelle, X.: J. Radiol. Electrol. **46:** 201-216, 1965.)

In the search for improved survival and for a less demanding therapy, a variety of atypical patterns of fractionation and doses have been tested.

One of the most popular variations from standard fractionation patterns is the split-course technique (Levitt; Abramson and Cavanaugh; Guthrie and associates; Salazar and associates; Aristizabal and Caldwell; Lee and associates; Scruggs and associates). This technique calls for the administration of about two thirds of the dose (3000 to 3500 rad midchest in 3 weeks). Then, after a 2- to 3-week interval of no irradiation, a chest film is taken for reevaluation. Often the atelectasis will have diminished, and the infection will have cleared. A beam of reduced size can then be used to complete treatment. In these patients with chronic obstructive pulmonary disease even a small reduction in beam size may be critical. In addition, the reevaluation provides a special opportunity to select those patients most likely to benefit from intensive local irradiation. Thus, even though the split-course technique for cancer of the lung may not cure more patients, it has special merits. Since some of the patients treated by this technique will survive for many years, spinal cord tolerance *must* be respected.

Normally ventilated lung transmits more ionizing radiations than a comparable volume of fat, muscle, or bone. Emphysematous lung transmits still more radiations, and atelectatic lung less. A solid tumor separated from the skin portal by normal lung would naturally receive a higher dose of radiations than a similar tumor embedded in an equal volume of muscle. The magnitude of this difference depends on the thickness of intervening normal lungs, ribs, vertebrae, pleural effusion, and the quality of the beam. Normal lung immediately beyond the mass may alter backscatter to the mass slightly. The complexity of this problem increases still further as one encounters different thicknesses of these tissues for each of several directed beams. For beams passing through the mediastinum, the dose to the tumor may be truly represented by standard depth dose tables, whereas for beams passing through large thicknesses of expanded lung, large correction factors should be added.

Our own measurements indicate that with a ^{60}Co beam no correction is necessary for straight anterior or posterior mediastinal beams. In contrast, about 30% should be added to the calculated midline dose from a straight lateral beam traversing normal lung. The use of computed tomograms to assess the effective densities of these intervening tissues will likely increase precision in dose delivery.

At present we must accept a greater variation in dose in the treatment of cancers of the lung than in any other tissue. Lung tolerance has been established with lung doses calculated from standard isodose curves. The actual doses to the lung and the tumor are higher than this calculated value.

EXTRATHORACIC METASTASES FROM SQUAMOUS CELL CARCINOMA. Metastases to bone have usually been given doses of 4000 to 4500 rad in 4 to 5 weeks. They respond well to this dose level. If substantial longevity is anticipated, such doses are warranted. Efforts to shorten the overall treatment time by using high daily fractions have been effective in relieving pain for a limited period. We do not recommend this technique if survival is expected to exceed 3 to 4 months or if a bone is in danger of fracture.

Metastases to the brain respond to doses of 4000 to 4500 rad in 4 to 5 weeks. The whole brain should be included in the port.

CLINICAL CARE. Patients with nonresectable squamous cell carcinoma or adenocarcinoma being irradiated will require general supportive care as well as specific medication directed toward relieving signs and symptoms. The major therapeutic effort will be directed to maintenance of the patients' nutrition and control of obstructive pneumonitis. Proper treatment planning will minimize radiation-induced anorexia, but it cannot be entirely eliminated. For this reason, too, diet is important.

A large proportion of these patients will show clinical and radiographic improvement of obstructive pneumonitis on antibiotic therapy alone. Such infections should be treated aggressively. By such means, fever, sweats, cough, and dyspnea may be relieved prior to an actual radiation-induced tumor regression.

The possibility of reducing radiation reactions in normal lung by chemical means has interested many serious workers in this field. This is of particular importance, since the reaction in normal lung adds considerably to the hazards of vigorous irradiation. No clinically useful chemical agent has been found. ACTH and cortisone have been used with the aim of reducing the severity of the acute reaction and of reducing already developed pulmonary fibrosis (Cosgriff and Kligerman; Whitfield and associates; Moss and associates). Adrenocorticoid therapy reduces the symptoms and produces objective improvement in function and in the roentgenographic findings during the acute phase of radiation pneumonitis. However, it is questionable if any decrease in the incidence or severity of late change will occur (Rubin and associates). Adrenocorticoid therapy should not be used during irradiation with the hope of reducing lung damage.

Superior vena caval obstruction

Clinical symptoms suggestive of superior vena caval obstruction will develop in 5% of all patients with cancer of the lung. The primary cancer producing these symptoms will be in the right upper lobe 80% of the time. On the other hand, 15% to 20% of the cancers of the right upper lobe will eventually produce superior vena caval obstruction. Of all patients in which carcinoma of the lung is the cause of this syndrome, 31% will have squamous cell carcinoma, 34% small or oat cell carcinoma, 20% undifferentiated or anaplastic carcinoma, 6% adenocarcinoma, and 6% unclassified carcinoma (Polackwich and Straus). Lymphomas and metastases from extrapulmonary primary carcinomas will comprise a small proportion (6% and 7%, respectively). The anatomy of the venous network affected in superior vena caval obstruction is discussed by Okay and Bryk. The edema and venous back pressure resulting from the obstruction may make bronchoscopy, mediastinoscopy, and biopsy hazardous. In this situation, if the clinical and radiographic diagnoses are straightforward and histologic verification is impossible or inadvisable, radiotherapy without a cellular diagnosis is not only justified but is mandatory. Of course one must consider the differential diagnosis, that is, the benign processes of aortic aneurysm or constrictive fibrosis.

Venous compression is caused most often by direct invasion (68%) and less frequently by metastases. Of those patients who come to autopsy with superior vena caval obstruction, 70% also have pericardial or cardiac invasion. Thus the minimum volume considered for irradiation should include the mediastinum along with the radiographically obvious disease. If the cancer is also a producer of inappropriate antidiuretic hormone, the head and neck and brain edema can be made even worse. In such a case, radiations serve the double function of relieving obstruction and reducing the abnormal hormone.

The immediate need of these patients is for relief of the brain and airway edema. Dexamethasone (Decadron) hastens the decrease of intracranial edema. It is not indicated otherwise. Eighty percent of the patients show a prolonged reduction in obstructive symptoms after doses of 4000 to 4500 rad in 4 to 5 weeks. Cure has been rarely reported (Watson), but cure is not a realistic aim for patients with superior vena caval obstruction. Should obstructive symptoms recur, a second dose of 3500 rad in 3 to 4 weeks can be given. Whether initial large daily fractions as advocated by Rubin, that is, 400 rad per day or more to the cancer, are superior to the more conventional daily fractions of 180 to 200 rad is not settled (Cameron and associates). Certainly those patients presenting with critical embarrassment of respiration justify emergency irradiation together with supportive care. However, in his enthusiasm to relieve the patients, the radiation oncologist should not overlook the need for proved dose-time relationships. The concept that a critically ill patient demands large daily fractions should be applied with care.

Small cell and oat cell carcinoma of the lung

As illustrated in Fig. 10-13, small cell and oat cell carcinomas metastasize earlier and kill more frequently and rapidly than squamous cell carcinomas or adenocarcinomas. An occasional patient with this disease has been cured with irradiation, and life is prolonged with irradiation (Medical Research Council). Even so, the post-irradiation survival rates at all intervals are poor.

Although the initial response is often dramatic with rather low doses, recurrence is common unless doses are carried to substantial levels or chemotherapy is added. Thus, when radiation alone was used, the Medical Research Council recommended doses in the range of 4000 rad in at least 4 weeks. A dose-control plot by Choi and Carey confirms the need for this dose level (Fig. 10-14). Finally, Holoye and associates gave 6000 rad by a split-course technique in addition to administering chemotherapy. They verified that this dose was adequate but did not verify that a dose of this magnitude was necessary.

Optimum combinations of drugs and dose of radiations are yet to be defined. However, the combination of irradiation of the bulky tumor mass (usually the primary lesion and mediastinal nodes) and brain irradiation with systemic chemotherapy is the treatment of choice for small cell carcinoma of the lung.

The incidence of metastases to the brain varies widely from one series to another and according to the histologic type (Tables 10-2 and 10-3). However, several factors are important in assessing the potential of "prophylactic" brain irradiation.

1. Of 149 patients who died of bronchial carcinoma and had complete autopsies, 130 had microscopic evidence of metastases. Cancer was found as a single metastasis in eighty-eight, and in thirteen the brain was the only organ involved (Luomanen and Watson).

2. Several autopsy series report an overall incidence of metastases in the brain of over 40% (Line and Deeley; Luomanen and Watson).

3. Whether treatment was local irradiation or chemotherapy, the brain was the anatomic site of first metastasis in 26% (8/30) (Chan and associates) and 20% (8/39) (Holoye and associates).

Such data as these and the fact that many of the currently used chemotherapeutic agents are not effective against metastases to the brain have encouraged trials of "prophylactic" irradiation of the brain regardless of the associated modalities of treatment (Kent and associates; Cox and associates; Choi and Carey; Moore and associates). In a randomized study Cox and associates found doses of 2000 rad in 2

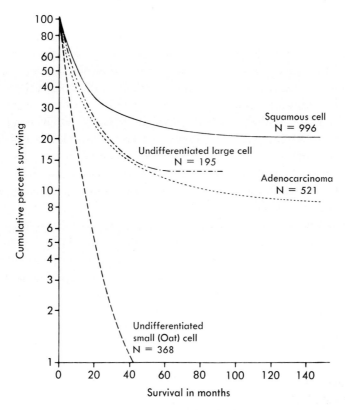

Fig. 10-13. Cumulative survivals of patients with cancer of the lung according to histologic diagnosis. (From Mountain, C. F., Carr, D. T., and Anderson, W. A. D.: Am. J. Roentgenol. **120:**130-138, 1974.)

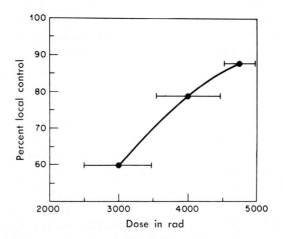

Fig. 10-14. Local control for small cell and oat cell carcinoma of the lung with various doses of radiations. (From Choi, C. H., and Carey, R. W.: Cancer **37:**2651-2657, 1976.)

weeks to be relatively ineffective in prolonging the lives of patients with this cell type. Choi and Carey in a nonrandomized study judged it effective. There is no longer major disagreement as to the effectiveness of "prophylactic" irradiation of the brain in decreasing the subsequent clinical manifestations of intracranial metastases. Three hundred ninety patients with small cell cancer of the lung and with no clinical or brain scan evidence of intracranial metastases were given "prophylactic" brain irradiation (3000 rad using 10 daily fractions combined with a multidrug chemotherapy regimen) (Moore and associates). Only six of 152 patients with advanced disease and six of 88 patients with limited disease developed intracranial metastases. Patients are thus spared the neurologic complication of metastases by a well-tolerated irradiation. Whether or not this irradiation prolongs life is yet to be clarified (Cox and associates).

PROGNOSIS AND RESULTS. Irradiated patients will have been judged incurable by surgery. This group will consist of patients with localized lesions in nonresectable sites, poor-risk patients with otherwise resectable lesions, and patients with widespread advanced carcinoma. One can hardly imagine a group of patients in greater need. In the early use of radiations, the failure to obtain any long-term survivors in this group of irradiated patients led many radiation oncologists and surgeons to doubt the value of vigorous irradiation, or of any irradiation at all. Some believed it worse than useless (Shorvon). Nothing could be further from the truth. As the indications for radiotherapy have become well-recognized and the techniques of administering it have become more precise, good results have increased and harmful sequelae have decreased.

Under favorable circumstances, the primary lung lesion, whether adenocarcinoma, squamous cell carcinoma, or small cell carcinoma, can be eradicated with irradiation. On postmortem microscopic examination, Churchill-Davidson found no residual primary tumor in four of ten patients selected for vigorous irradiation (minimum tumor dose of 5000 rad in 7 weeks). Bloedorn and associates found no residual cancer in seventeen patients after a dose of 4000 rad in 4 weeks. Similarly, Brooks and associates found no cancer in the irradiated volume in four patients at autopsy (more than 4000 rad in 5 to 6 weeks). They did not suggest how frequently this could be accomplished. Roswit and associates reported that preoperative administration of 4000 to 5000 rad in 6 weeks destroyed all microscopic evidence in a group of mixed histologic types of cancer in twenty-one of 136 patients. A higher dose should be given if the volume is small. With such a dose, a significant number of 5-year survivors can be obtained by irradiation alone. The reports of Smart, of Hilton and Pilcher, and of Morrison and associates have been cited previously. One further study helps in deciding care for the inoperable patient. Guttmann administered vigorous irradiation (5000 to 6000 rad in 5 to 6 weeks) to ninety-five patients proved nonresectable at thoracotomy. Fifty-eight percent of the patients were living at 1 year, 27% at 2 years, and 7.4% at 5 years. In contrast, survival was very poor after similar doses were administered to the known residual cancer after incomplete cancer resection. It is now clear that the patient found to be non-

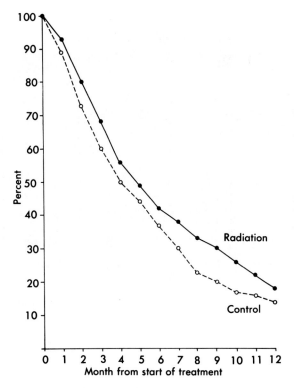

Fig. 10-15. Percentage of patients with nonresectable carcinoma of the lung surviving to indicated month. (From Roswit, B., Patno, M. P., Rapp, R., Veinbergs, A., Stuhlborg, J., and Reid, C. B.: Radiology **90:**688-697, 1968.)

resectable at thoracotomy should not have a so-called palliative resection. Instead, a biopsy should be taken, and the chest should be closed. If the disease is apparently still localized, curative irradiation is fully justified. Radical radiotherapy was given to 132 patients with nonresectable cancer (Hellman and associates). After 6 months 62% were living, after 1 year 33% were living, and after 2 years 11% were living. Only five patients had clinically significant fibrosis. In a nationwide prospective randomized study, the comparative value of radiotherapy and placebo was studied (Roswit and associates). Irradiation produced a greater proportion of survivals at each interval (Fig. 10-15). However, the difference was not great. Such results are not encouraging, but they settle once and for all any question of the value of irradiation for the silent but nonresectable cancer. Some of these patients are curable; in others, radiotherapy blocks the development of irreversible symptoms. For those patients who have already developed symptoms, radiotherapy holds a major promise of relief.

PALLIATION. How frequently palliation follows irradiation depends on the criteria for irradiation and technique. Brown employed criteria similar to those given previously. He reported that 46% of the treated patients showed improvement,

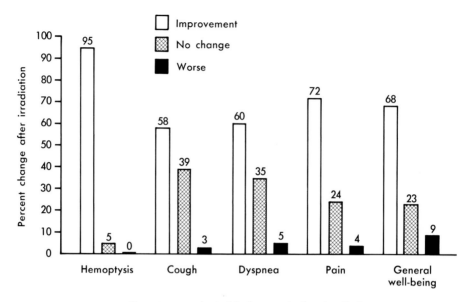

Fig. 10-16. Graphic illustration of extent of palliation offered by radiotherapy in inoperable carcinoma of the lung. (Based on data from Line, D., and Deeley, T. J. In Deeley, T. J., editor: Carcinoma of the bronchus, New York, 1972, Appleton-Century-Crofts.)

whereas 23% became worse. The fate of the remainder was unknown. Hustu and Nickson produced symptomatic improvement of 113 of 186 patients. Some symptoms are more frequently relieved than others.

Hemoptysis will be suppressed almost routinely but may occasionally recur (Fig. 10-16). Superior vena caval obstruction will occur in about 5% of all patients with bronchogenic carcinoma. Of 107 patients presenting this complication, eighty-five had right lung lesions, usually in the upper lobe or the main bronchus (Szur and Bromley). Four thousand to 4500 rad tissue dose in 3 to 4 weeks produced improvement in 69% of their patients; 79% showed no further recurrence of obstruction. Obstructive pneumonitis and atelectasis will be relieved in about 20% of the treated patients presenting this symptom (Mayer and Roswit) (Fig. 10-11). Cough is nearly always decreased and often eliminated entirely. Pain due to pleural involvement or nerve invasion is seldom relieved, but the chest discomfort associated with bronchial obstruction and infection is frequently relieved (Fig. 10-16). Patients with pleural effusion seem to derive little benefit from irradiation (Brooks and associates). Pain from distant osseous metastases is frequently relieved by irradiation (Fig. 10-16). Fever, sweats, pulmonary hypertrophic osteoarthropathy, loss of appetite, and dysphagia are relieved with varying frequency, but we rarely see a paralyzed nerve regain its function. The extent of palliation is shown graphically in Fig. 10-16.

The age of the patient does not seem to affect prognosis, although the Karnofsky performance index is closely correlated with outcome. The histologic type has the same significance as it does elsewhere in the body. Patients with the more malignant oat cell and undifferentiated lesions show a better immediate response to irradiation, but their subsequent life is shorter and the ultimate prognosis remains worse. Patients with upper lobe lesions appear to have a better prognosis and respond more satisfactorily to irradiation than do those with lower lobe lesions (Brown; Haas and Harvey; Haas and associates). The reason for this has not been defined, although it may be a consequence of shorter distances and better depth doses near the apex. Also, it is not unlikely that lesions of the apex produce symptoms at an earlier stage than those of the base. They may be grouped with other peripheral lung lesions.

Radiographic improvement does not necessarily coincide with clinical improvement, particularly if the disease is widely disseminated. However, significant radiographic improvement will be observed in about 50% of the treated patients (Roswit and associates). This will be most striking in those with peripherally located lesions or in those in whom the obstruction of a major bronchus is relieved. Bone may reform when a superior sulcus tumor is treated vigorously.

POSTOPERATIVE IRRADIATION. Combinations of irradiation and surgery have been considered with a view toward improving the results of surgery alone or irradiation alone. Just how often transected or residual neighboring cancer is the cause of failure is not known. However, mediastinal lymph node metastases and mediastinal infiltration are commonly suspected as the cause of failure of pneumonectomy and lobectomy. Paterson and Russell reported the 3-year survival rate was 4% when metastases to the mediastinum had occurred but 41% when the mediastinum was negative. It follows that postpneumonectomy mediastinal irradiation should be evaluated. In a carefully randomized prospective study, Paterson and Russell compared pneumonectomy alone with pneumonectomy followed by mediastinal irradiation. By a three-field technique, 4500 rad was delivered to the mediastinum in 3 to 4 weeks. At 3 years, 36% of ninety-nine patients having only surgery were living. Thirty-three percent of 103 patients having postoperative mediastinal irradiation were living. This study failed to show that there was any benefit from routine postpneumonectomy irradiation of the mediastinum. However, in a more recent study Green and associates found that postpneumonectomy or postlobectomy irradiation of the mediastinum improved survival among patients with metastases to hilar or mediastinal nodes but not among patients without metastases (Table 10-5). All histologic types seemed to benefit equally. These results, along with the distribution of local recurrences as described by Spjut and Mateo and the data in Table 1, have prompted us to reconsider postoperative irradiation. Once the lung is removed, the emptied hemithorax tolerates high doses well. The entire mediastinum plus the hemithorax are logical volumes to include in the irradiation of postpneumonectomy patients.

PREOPERATIVE IRRADIATION. The former popularity of preoperative irradiation for carcinoma of the lung was not so much a measure of its success as it was a manifestation of the desperate search for an improved method of treatment. To be rational, preoperative irradiation should be directed toward the causes of surgical failure.

Table 10-5. Comparison of 5-year survival rates for carcinoma of the lung with and without postoperative irradiation*

Histological type	Treatment	
	Surgery alone	Surgery plus irradiation
Patients without node metastases		
Squamous-cell carcinoma	10/37 (27%)	12/43 (28%)
Adenocarcinoma	3/16 (19%)	2/8 (25%)
Anaplastic carcinoma	1/11 (9%)	2/8 (25%)
TOTAL	14/64 (22%)	16/59 (27%)
Patients with node metastases		
Squamous-cell carcinoma	1/16 (6%)	6/28 (21%)
Adenocarcinoma	0/6 (0%)	10/16 (62%)
Anaplastic carcinoma	0/8 (0%)	7/22 (32%)
TOTAL	1/30 (3%)	23/66 (35%)
FINAL TOTAL	15/94 (16%)	39/125 (31%)

*From Green, N., Kurohara, S. S., George, F. W., and Crews, Q. E.: Radiology **116**:405-407, 1975.

However, the causes of operative failure are poorly documented. At postmortem examination regional lymph node metastases are still present in over half the failures, whereas 42% of the failures have recurrence in the bronchial stump, chest wall, parietal pleura, or residual ipsilateral lung (Spjut and Mateo). In addition, we see in Table 10-2 that at least in one study of patients whose resection was recent, 35% still had residual local disease and 24% already had distant metastases. The logical areas for attack by preoperative irradiation are the mediastinum and ipsilateral hemithorax. It is difficult to imagine long-term benefit from less than full cancerocidal doses to cancer spread to these areas.

The general principles of preoperative irradiation along with the possible modes of action are discussed in Chapter 2. Preoperative irradiation would most likely make its greatest contribution in patients with minimal and perhaps even occult strands of cancer cells extending across the lines of excision. It is conceivable, although unlikely, that residual but still locally confined regional lymph node metastases could be rendered resectable by low-dose preoperative irradiation. However, for carcinoma of the lung, it is remote that either of these extensions is the sole cause of surgical failure. Several studies are noteworthy.

1. Mallams and associates and Paulson gave preoperative doses of 3000 rad in 10 to 12 days to cancers of the lung apex. Four weeks later pneumonectomy was performed. Of forty-six patients suitable for 3-year follow-up, nine were living. This is a higher survival rate than has been obtained with either resection or irradiation alone. These good results were not obtained by others who reproduced the combination. There is little enthusiasm for it.

2. Mediastinal lymph nodes can often be cleared of all microscopic evidence of metastases. Bloedorn found that of seventeen patients explored before and after

irradiation, nine showed disappearance of metastases. He even had an occasional patient survive 5 years after vigorous irradiation of a mediastinum previously proved to contain metastases.

3. Metastases to lymph nodes seem more radiocurable than the primary cancer. At the time of postirradiation thoracotomy, proved lymph node metastases were sterilized 77% of the time; the primary lesion, given the same dose, was sterilized in 35% of the cases (Bloedorn).

4. Of 109 initially nonresectable cancers (judged nonresectable without thoracotomy in forty-six and at thoracotomy in sixty), 75% were judged resectable after irradiation. Of the 109 patients, 12% lived 1 year (Bloedorn).

Two nationwide randomized clinical trials testing the value of preoperative irradiation have been reported. The trial conducted by the Veterans Administration was reported by Shields and associates and showed preoperative irradiation to be of no value. Similarly, the Collaborative National Study confirmed the uselessness of routine preoperative irradiation for bronchogenic carcinoma. A somewhat higher preoperative dose used by Crowley and associates (5500 to 6000 rad in 5½ to 6 weeks to larger volumes) produced a major increase in postoperative complications without increasing cure rates.

Summary

Bronchogenic carcinoma rarely produces alarming symptoms while still limited to the lung. Spread beyond the lung is almost impossible to eradicate by radical surgery, vigorous irradiation, or chemotherapy; but surgery is more effective in controlling the localized disease. Less than 10% of patients with carcinoma of the lung are curable. External irradiation holds the greatest promise for significant palliation of patients with inoperable squamous cell carcinoma. In this group, if all known disease can be included in a 10 × 15 cm port and if the patient can tolerate vigorous irradiation, an attempt should be made to cure the patient. Although failure to cure will follow in all but a few patients, maximum palliation will have been provided. In the patient with nonresectable squamous cell carcinoma irradiation should not be withheld until symptoms or signs develop. For although some of the sequelae of extensive mediastinal invasion are reversible with irradiation, others are not. Such irreversible sequelae can be prevented from developing by early irradiation.

Small cell or oat cell carcinomas are quite radioresponsive, but their early wide dissemination limits the value of local irradiation. Local irradiation to the bulk of the tumor mass combined with multimodal chemotherapy holds promise of extending palliation.

THE THYMUS

Although the functions of the thymus are still poorly understood, it is recognized as critical to the development of the thymic-dependent or cellular immunity. The thymus and the circulating small lymphocytes assist in distinguishing self-antigens from foreign antigens. They also produce cell-mediated immune reactions. It might be expected that early in life a disturbance in this system would lead to the development of an immunologic deficient state. Surgical removal of the thymus in the newborn may produce alterations in immunity, but thymectomy in older children and adults does not produce immunologically related problems, even though there may be a decrease in lymphocytes. Similarly, irradiation of the adult thymus may produce a decrease in lymphocytes, but no resulting immunologically related problems have been proved (p. 313). The normal thymus is unavoidably irradiated in the treatment of Hodgkin's disease and carcinoma of the esophagus, lung, and breast. Although several workers have speculated that irradiation of the thymus accelerates the development of metastases, this point remains to be proved.

THYMOMAS. Tumors of the thymus occur at all ages but are most common during middle age. Thymoma is the most common primary tumor of the anterior mediastinum. Ten percent of thymomas are simple benign cysts, and 30% are judged to be invasive (the gross finding necessary to categorize a thymic neoplasm as malignant). Ten to fifteen percent of all patients with myasthenia gravis will have a thymoma, whereas 15% to 50% of all patients with thymoma will have myasthenia gravis.

Recent electron microscopic studies by several authors have clarified the histogenesis of thymoma. Basically all thymomas are of epithelial origin with a variable amount of nonneoplastic lymphocytic component. The epithelial cells may be polygonal or spindle shaped. Although subtypes of thymoma can be produced by the predominance of one or another cellular component, this does not materially affect the prognosis. Any of these types may or may not be invasive.

The borderline between benign and malignant thymoma is vague. Unlike most cancers for which the pathologist has a histologic means for distinguishing benign from malignant neoplasms, this is not usually possible with thymomas. With thymoma the status of the capsule and the presence or absence of active invasion are the decisive criteria. With gross signs of invasion there is no question; superior vena caval obstruction, nerve paralysis, and seeding on the pleura are obvious signs of malignant change. However, the less obvious types of invasion require that the entire capsule be removed and that a diagnosis of capsular or pericapsular invasion be made only after a careful inspection. Batata and associates observed that the benign lesions were usually in older females, asymptomatic, noninvasive, and completely encapsulated. A poor prognosis was warranted if the tumor was in a younger male patient, had a low lymphocyte count, was predominantly right-sided, and if symptoms of pressure were present. The similarity of the clinical evolution of this tumor and Hodgkin's disease in some patients has been recognized by Pons and associates. It is obviously important to exclude thymic lymphoma from the group of thymomas.

TREATMENT. Radiotherapy should be given for those tumors showing invasion, that is, about 30% of all thymomas. When the thymoma was malignant, Batata reported that no patients were cured by surgery alone. Whether or not radiotherapy should also be given to the apparently totally excised noninvasive thymomas is unsettled. If such a noninvasive thymoma is not enmeshed in important mediastinal structures and is removed cleanly, we have advised against routine postoperative irradiation. However, for large lesions enmeshed in important structures or for thymomas that are only partially resected, we have advised that postoperative irradiation be given even though there may be no gross invasion. Such a decision may seem quite arbitrary, but in the absence of a histologic guide it is the best we can do.

The supraclavicular areas should be encompassed in the irradiated volume when adenopathy is present. Prophylactic irradiation of these areas has been recommended and we believe it is appropriate, but its contribution to survival remains to be measured.

No conclusive time-dose studies have been reported for the irradiation of these tumors. Marks and associates reported local control in all of their nine patients who were given doses from 3000 rad in 10 fractions to 4800 rad in 24 fractions. They recommend a minimum dose of 4000 rad in 20 fractions for occult residual disease to at least 4500 rad in 5 to 6 weeks for larger masses. We have given tissue doses of 4500 to 5000 rad in 5 to 6 weeks to the entire mediastinum, using parallel opposing anterior and posterior megavoltage beams. After a spinal cord dose of 3500 to 4000 rad, two oblique posterior ports sparing the cord can be used. If the mass is large or if there is a persistent mass after 4500 to 5000 rad and a 2- to 3-week break in treatment, we suggest a boosting dose of 1000 to 1500 rad in 1 to 2 weeks through reduced oblique or lateral ports. Care must be taken to avoid the spinal cord, but the risk of heart, lung, or esophageal damage must be accepted with the higher dose.

RESULTS. An evaluation of the role of radiotherapy in the management of malignant thymomas is difficult because of the infrequency of this neoplasm. Of twenty-four patients reported by Batata, five (21%) were alive and well 5 years after irradiation, seven (29%) were alive with disease, and twelve (50%) were dead with disease. No patient who had surgery alone for a malignant thymoma was cured. Bernatz and associates reported that only 17% of those patients with malignant thymoma survived 10 years after treatment. There were no 20-year survivors (Payne and Clagett). Pons and associates reported control in four of fourteen patients, and Ariaratnam and associates reported control in six of eleven patients. Thus it is important to define the invasive thymomas early and to proceed with irradiation without waiting for clinical manifestations of persistence. Cell type should not influence dose and has little effect on ease of control.

REFERENCES

Abramson, N., and Cavanaugh, P.: Short course radiation therapy in carcinoma of the lung, Radiology 96:627-630, 1970.

Ackerman, L. V.: Changing concepts in the pathology of cancer of the lung, Acta Radiol. Interamericana 5:28-36, 1955.

Ariaratnam, L. S., Kalnicki, S., Mincer, F., and Botstein, C.: The management of malignant thymoma with radiation therapy, Int. J. Radiat. Oncol. Biol. Phys. 5:77-80, 1979.

Aristizabal, S. A., and Caldwell, W. L.: Radical ir-

radiation with the split course technique in carcinoma of the lung, Cancer 37:2630-2635, 1976.

Baker, N. H., Cowley, R. A., and Linberg, E.: A follow-up in patients with bronchogenic carcinoma "locally cured" by preoperative irradiation, J. Thorac. Cardiovasc. Surg. 44:298-302, 1963.

Batata, M. A., Aguilar, R. I., Huvos, A. G., Beattie, E. J.: Current concepts of thymomas, Phoenix, Ariz., Nov., 1972, American Society of Therapeutic Radiologists.

Bate, D., and Guttmann, R. J.: Changes in lung

and pleura following two-million-volt therapy for carcinoma of the breast, Radiology **69:**372-383, 1957.

Bergmann, M., and Graham, E. A.: Pneumonectomy for severe irradiation damage, J. Thorac. Surg. **22:**549-564, 1951.

Bernatz, P. E., Harrison, E. G., and Clagett, O. T.: Thymoma: a clinicopathologic study, J. Thorac. Cardiovasc. Surg. **42:**424-444, 1961.

Black, H., and Ackerman, L. V.: The importance of epidermoid carcinoma in situ in the histogenesis of carcinoma of the lung, Ann. Surg. **136:**44-55, 1952.

Bloedorn, F. G.: Rationale and benefit of preoperative irradiation in lung cancer, J.A.M.A. **196:** 340-341, 1966.

Brady, L. W., Germon, P. A., and Cander, L.: The effects of radiation therapy on pulmonary function in carcinoma of the lung, Radiology **85:**130-134, 1965.

Brooks, W. D. W., Davidson, M., Thomas, C. P., Robson, K., and Smithers, D. W.: Carcinoma of the bronchus, Thorax **6:**1-16, 1951.

Brown, D. E. M.: X-ray therapy and carcinoma of the bronchus, Br. J. Radiol. **25:**472-475, 1953.

Byrd, R. B., Miller, W. E., Carr, D. T., et al.: The roentgenographic appearance of squamous cell carcinoma of the bronchus, Mayo Clin. Proc. **43:** 327, 1968.

Cameron, S. J., Grant, I. W. B., Lutz, W., and Pearson, J. G.: The early effects of irradiation on ventilatory function in bronchial carcinoma, Clin. Radiol. **20:**12-18, Jan., 1969.

Castellino, R. A., Glatstein, E., Turbow, M. M., Rosenberg, S., and Kaplan, H. S.: Latent radiation injury of lungs or heart activated by steroid withdrawal, Ann. Intern. Med. **80:**593-599, 1974.

Chan, P. Y., Byfield, J. E., Kagan, A. R., and Aronstam, E. M.: Unresectable squamous cell carcinoma of the lung and its management by combined bleomycin and radiotherapy, Cancer **37:**2671-2676, 1976.

Choi, C. H., and Carey, R. W.: Small cell anaplastic carcinoma of lung, Cancer **37:**2651-2657, 1976.

Churchill-Davidson, I.: A technique of simulated rotation therapy for the treatment of carcinoma of the bronchus, Proc. R. Soc. Med. **46:**463-464, 1953.

Collaborative National Study: Preoperative irradiation of cancer of the lung, Cancer **23:**419-429, 1969.

Cosgriff, S. W., and Kligerman, M. M.: The use of ACTH and cortisone in the treatment of postirradiation pulmonary reaction, Radiology **57:**537-540, 1951.

Cox, J. D., Petrovich, Z., Paig, C., and Stanley, K.: Prophylactic cranial irradiation in patients with inoperable carcinoma of the lung, Cancer **42:**1135-1140, 1978.

Crowley, R. A., Wizenberg, M. J., and Linberg, E. J.: Role of radiation therapy and surgery in treatment of bronchogenic carcinoma, Ann. Thorac. Surg. **8:**229-236, 1969.

Deeley, T. J.: The effects of radiation on the lungs in the treatment of carcinoma of the bronchus, Clin. Radiol. **11:**33-39, 1960.

Deeley, T. J.: A clinical trial to compare two different tumour dose levels in the treatment of advanced carcinoma of the bronchus, Clin. Radiol. **17:**299-301, 1966.

Deeley, T. J.: The treatment of carcinoma of the bronchus, Br. J. Radiol. **40:**801-822, 1967.

Eisert, D. R., Cox, J. D., and Komaki, R.: Irradiation for bronchial carcinoma: reasons for failure, Cancer **37:**2665-2670, 1976.

Engelstadt, R. B.: Pulmonary lesions after roentgen and radium irradiation, Am. J. Roentgenol. **43:**676-681, 1940.

Fryer, C. J., Fitzpatrick, P. J., and Rider, W. D.: Radiation pneumonitis: experience following a large single dose of radiation, Int. J. Radiat. Oncol. Biol. Phys. **4:**931-936, 1978.

Green, N., Kurohara, S. S., George, F. W., and Crews, Q. E.: Postresection irradiation for primary lung cancer, Radiology **116:**405-407, 1975.

Greene, R. F.: Lung and mediastinum. In Steckel, R. J., and Kagan, A. R.: Diagnosis and staging of cancer, Philadelphia, 1976, W. B. Saunders Co.

Guthrie, R. T., Ptacek, J. J., and Hass, A. C.: Comparative analysis of two regimens of split course radiation in carcinoma of the lung, Am. J. Roentgenol. **117:**605-608, 1973.

Guttmann, R. J.: Results of radiation therapy in patients with inoperable carcinoma of the lung whose status was established at exploratory thoracotomy, Am. J. Roentgenol. **93:**99-103, 1965.

Haas, L. L., and Harvey, R. A.: Radiation management of otherwise hopeless thoracic neoplasms, J.A.M.A. **154:**323-326, 1954.

Haas, L. L., Harvey, R. A., and Melchor, C. F.: Radiation management of apical lung tumors, J. Thorac. Surg. **33:**496-525, 1957.

Hellman, S., Kligerman, M. M., Von Essen, C. F., and Scibetta, M. P.: Sequelae of radical radiotherapy of carcinoma of the lung, Radiology **82:**1055-1061, 1964.

Hilton, G., and Pilcher, R. S.: Carcinoma of the bronchus. In Carling, E. R., Windeyer, B. W., and Smithers, D. W., editors: Practice in radiotherapy, St. Louis, 1955, The C. V. Mosby Co.

Holoye, P. Y., Samuels, M. L., Lanzotti, V. C., Smith, T., and Barkley, H. T.: Combination chemotherapy and radiation therapy for small cell carcinoma, J.A.M.A. **237**:1221-1224, 1977.

Hustu, H. O., and Nickson, J. J.: Carcinoma of the lung: results of radiological treatment, Am. J. Roentgenol. **91**:95-104, 1964.

Jacobson, L. E., and Knauer, I. S.: Correction of factors for tumor dose in chest cavity due to diminished absorption and scatter in lung tissue, Radiology **67**:863-876, 1956.

Johnson, P. M., Sagerman, R. H., and Jacox, H. W.: Changes in pulmonary arterial perfusion due to intrathoracic neoplasm and irradiation of the lung, Am. J. Roentgenol. **102**:637-644, 1968.

Kent, C. H., Brereton, H. D., and Johnson, R. E.: "Total" therapy for oat cell carcinoma of the lung, Int. J. Radiat. Oncol. Biol. Phys. **2**:427-432, 1977.

Killen, D. A., Yukoski, C. F., and Gobbel, W. G.: Combination 5-fluorouracil and x-radiation therapy for nonresectable bronchogenic carcinoma, J. Thorac. Cardiovasc. Surg. **54**:299-303, 1967.

Komaki, R., Cox, J. D., and Eisert, D. R.: Irradiation of bronchial carcinoma. II. Int. J. Radiat. Oncol. Biol. Phys. **2**:441-446, 1977.

Kornelsen, R. O.: Tumor dose in the chest cavity, Br. J. Radiol. **27**:289-293, 1954.

Lacassagne, A.: Action des rayons du radium sur les muqueuses de l'oesophage et de la trachée chez le lapin, Compt. Rend. Soc. Biol. **84**:26-27, 1921.

Lee. R. E., Carr, D. T., and Childs, D. S.: Comparison of split-course radiation therapy and continuous radiation therapy for unresectable bronchogenic carcinoma: 5 year results, Am. J. Roentgenol. **126**:116-122, 1976.

Levitt, S.: Split-dose approach in radiation therapy, Radiol. Clin. North Am. **7**:293-299, 1969.

Libshitz, H. I., and Southard, M. E.: Complications of radiation therapy: the thorax, Semin. Radiol. **9**:41-49, 1974.

Line, D. H., and Deeley, T. J.: The necropsy findings in carcinoma of the bronchus, Br. J. Dis. Chest **65**:238-242, 1971.

Luomanen, R. K. J., and Watson, W. L.: Autopsy findings. In Watson, W. L., editor: Lung cancer—a study of five thousand Memorial Hospital cases, St. Louis, 1968, The C. V. Mosby Co.

Mallams, J. T., Paulson, D. L., Collier, R. E., and Shaw, R. R.: Presurgical irradiation in bronchogenic carcinoma, superior sulcus type, Radiology **82**:1052-1054, 1964.

Marks, R. D., Wallace, K. M., and Pettit, H. S.: Radiation therapy control of nine patients with malignant thymoma, Cancer **41**:117-119, 1978.

Medical Research Council: Five year follow-up of medical research council comparative trial of surgery and radiotherapy for primary treatment of

small celled or oat celled carcinoma of the bronchus, Lancet **2**:501-505, 1969.

Moore, T. N., Livingston, R., Heilbrun, L., Elteringham, J., Skinner, O., White, J., and Tesh, D.: The effectiveness of prophylactic brain irradiation in small cell carcinoma of the lung, Cancer **41**:2149-2153, 1978.

Morrison, R., Deeley, T. J., and Cleland, W. P.: The treatment of carcinoma of the bronchus, Lancet **1**:683-684, 1963.

Moss, W. T., and Haddy, F. J.: The relationship between oxygen tension of inhaled gas and severity of acute radiation pneumonitis, Radiology **75**:55-58, 1960.

Moss, W. T., Haddy, F. J., and Sweany, S. K.: Some factors altering the severity of acute radiation pneumonitis: variation with cortisone, heparin, and antibiotics, Radiology **75**:50-54, 1960.

Muggia, F. M., Hansen, H. H., and Chervu, L. R.: Diagnosis in metastatic sites, lung cancer clinical diagnosis and treatment, New York, 1977, Grune & Stratton, Inc.

Newton, K. A.: Total thoracic irradiation combined with intravenous injection of autogenous marrow, Clin. Radiol. **11**:14-21, 1960.

Newton, K. A., and Spittle, M. F.: Analysis of 40 cases treated by total thoracic irradiation, Clin. Radiol. **20**:19-22, 1969.

Okay, N., and Bryk, D.: Collateral pathways in occlusion of the superior vena cava and its tributaries, Radiology **92**:1493-1498, 1969.

Overholt, R. H., and Rumel, W. R.: Clinical studies of primary carcinoma of the lung, J.A.M.A. **114**:735-742, 1940.

Paterson, R., and Russell, M. H.: Lung cancer, value of postoperative radiotherapy, Clin. Radiol. **13**:141-144, 1962.

Paulson, D. L.: The survival rate in superior sulcus tumors treated by presurgical irradiation, J.A.M.A. **196**:342, 1966.

Payne, W. S., and Clagett, O. T.: Surgery of the thymus gland. In Shields, T. W., editor: General thoracic surgery, Philadelphia, 1972, Lea & Febiger.

Perez, C. A.: Radiation therapy in the management of carcinoma of the lung, Cancer **39**:901-916, 1977.

Petrovich, Z., Ohanian, M., Cox, J.: Clinical research on the treatment of locally advanced lung cancer, Cancer **42**:1129-1134, 1978.

Polackwich, R. J., and Straus, M. J.: Superior vena caval syndrome. In Straus, M. J., editor: Lung cancer, New York, 1977, Grune & Stratton, Inc.

Pons, A., Armand, J. P., Voigt, J. J., and Combes, P. F.: Évaluation des resultats de la radiothérapie dans 14 cas de thymomes malins, Bull. Cancer **64**:79-92, 1977.

Roswit, B.: Palliation by chemotherapy, J.A.M.A. **196:**848-849, 1966.

Roswit, B., Patno, M. P., Rapp, R., Veinbergs, A., Stuhlborg, J., and Reid, C. B.: The survival of patients with inoperable lung cancer: a large-scale randomized study of radiation therapy versus placebo, Radiology **90:**688-697, 1968.

Roswit, B., and White, D. C.: Severe radiation injuries of the lung, Am. J. Roentgenol. Radium Ther. Nucl. Med. **129:**127-136, 1977.

Rubin, P., Andrews, J. R., Paton, R., and Flick, A.: Response of radiation pneumonitis to adrenocorticoids, Am. J. Roentgenol. **79:**453-464, 1958.

Rubin, P., Green, J., Holzwasser, G., and Gerle, R.: Superior vena caval syndrome, Radiology **81:**388-401, 1963.

Salazar, O. M., Rubin, P., Brown, J. C., Feldstein, M. L., and Keller, B. E.: Predictors of radiation response in lung cancer, Cancer **37:**2636-2650, 1976.

Salazar, O. M., Rubin, P., Brown, J. C., Feldstein, M. L., and Keller, B. E.: The assessment of tumor response to irradiation of lung cancer: continuous versus split-course regimens, Int. J. Radiat. Oncol. Biol. Phys. **1:**1107-1118, 1976.

Scruggs, H., El-Mahdi, A., Marks, R. D., and Constable, W. C.: The results of split-course radiation therapy in cancer of the lung, Am. J. Roentgenol. **121:**754-760, 1974.

Shields, T. W., Higgins, G. A., Lawton, R., et al.: Preoperative x-ray therapy as an adjuvant in the treatment of bronchogenic carcinoma, J. Thorac. Cardiovasc. Surg. **59:**49-61, 1970.

Shorvon, L. M.: Carcinoma of the bronchus with special reference to its treatment by radiotherapy, Br. J. Radiol. **20:**443-449, 1947.

Smart, J.: Can cancer of the lung be cured by irradiation alone? J.A.M.A. **195:**1034-1035, 1966.

Spjut, H. J., and Mateo, L. E.: Recurrent and metastatic carcinoma of lung, Cancer **18:**1462-1468, 1965.

Stone, D. J., Schwarz, M. J., and Green, R. A.: Fatal pulmonary insufficiency due to radiation effect upon the lung, Am. J. Med. **21:**211-226, 1956.

Sweany, S. K., Moss, W. T., and Haddy, F. J.: The effects of chest irradiation on pulmonary function, J. Clin. Invest. **38:**587-593, 1959.

Teates, C. D.: The effects of unilateral thoracic irradiation on pulmonary blood flow, Am. J. Roentgenol. **102:**875-882, 1968.

van den Brenk, H. A. S.: Radiation effects on the pulmonary system. In Berdjis, C. C., editor: Pathology of irradiation, Baltimore, 1971, Williams & Wilkins Co.

Watson, W. L.: Oat cell lung cancer. In Watson, W. L., editor: Lung Cancer. A study of five thousand Memorial Hospital Cases, St. Louis, 1968, The C. V. Mosby Co.

Whitfield, A. G. W., Bond, W. H., and Melville, W.: Pulmonary irradiation effects and their treatment with cortisone and ACTH, J. Fac. Radiol. **6:**12-22, 1954.

Whitfield, A. G. W., Bond, W. H., and Kunkler, P. B.: Radiation damage to thoracic tissues, Thorax **18:**371-380, 1963.

Wohl, M. E. B., Griscom, N. T., Traggis, D. G., and Jaffee, J.: Effects of therapeutic irradiation delivered in early childhood upon subsequent lung function. Pediatrics **4:**507-516, 1975.

11

The breast

RESPONSE OF THE NORMAL BREAST TO IRRADIATION

The duct system of the female breast is the result of a progressive invagination of embryonal ectoderm. This process begins as an ectodermal thickening about the sixth week of development and at birth has produced the fifteen to twenty primary milk ducts in addition to sparse acini. From the standpoint of development at least, the breast can be regarded as a highly specialized sweat gland of the apocrine type.

This specialization of embryonal ectoderm is accompanied by alterations in resistance of the invaginated epithelium to radiations. Before considering the radio-responsiveness of the normal mammary gland, it should be recalled that the quantity and function of both the ductal and alveolar epithelium are determined by endocrine activity.

Endocrine secretions, and consequently growth activity, within the breast vary with age, phase of menstrual cycle, stage of pregnancy, and activity of nursing. In general, growth activity is closely related to radioresponsiveness. In fact, in rabbits, such growth rate changes in the breast have been shown to alter radioresponsiveness of the mammae. Turner and Gomez reported the details of these alterations. They found that the rudimentary duct epithelium, before the growth stimulus of the estrogenic hormone had become effective, was relatively resistant to roentgen rays—660 rad (skin) in one dose produced a slight depression of subsequent growth; 2640 rad (skin) in one dose, marked depression; and 3980 rad, total inhibition (140 kv, unfiltered; target-skin distance, 30.5 cm; 144 rad per minute). After estrogen stimulation of the prepubertal breast, the radioresponsiveness of the duct epithelium was increased from 30% to 50%. However, when growth of the duct system was complete (that is, after the rapid growth of puberty), 3300 rad (skin) in one dose was necessary to completely inhibit subsequent lobuloalveolar growth. After 6 days of pseudo-pregnancy, the radioresponsiveness of the cells had increased, for only 2640 rad (skin) was necessary to inhibit further growth. Epithelial cells lining the lobuloalveolar system and developing at the end of pseudopregnancy or the middle of pregnancy are extremely radioresponsive; 720 rad (skin) in one dose was sufficient to inhibit their subsequent ability to secrete milk. However, at all other stages of lactation 2640 rad (skin) was necessary to completely inhibit the secretion of milk.

289

Whenever the exposure to roentgen rays was sufficient to temporarily inhibit either subsequent growth or lactation, the irradiated gland regressed to a duct system. Subsequent pregnancies or pseudopregnancies failed to stimulate the growth of the lobuloalveolar system or lactation.

It has been difficult to demonstrate variations in radioresponsiveness subsequent to fluctuations in endocrine activity in the human female breast. A few results in children who were irradiated for mammary hemangiomas have been recorded (Fig. 11-1). Doses of 300 rad or less to the infant's breast produced no clinically detectable deformity in later life (Kolar and associates). However, doses above this level may produce hypoplasia of the breast if the port is sufficiently large to encompass the infant breast bud, areola, or even adjacent soft tissues. The skin may appear normal even in the presence of marked suppression of growth. In such patients, pregnancy will not usually stimulate growth of the tuboalveolar system, so that lactation will not occur. Doses currently being given to the whole chest for metastatic Wilms' tumor (1200 rad in less than 2 weeks) may be sufficient to produce suppression of growth of

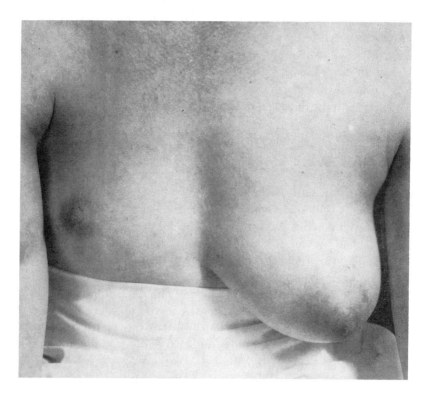

Fig. 11-1. Effect of irradiation on the infant breast. The patient was treated for a large cystic hygroma when she was less than 1 year of age. She was given 1900 rad (air) through a 15 × 15 cm port directed to the chest wall, including the breast (200 kv; filter, 0.5 mm Cu plus 1 mm Al; TSD, 50). This photograph was taken 20 years later. Skin changes are minimal, but marked underdevelopment of right breast is obvious. There is also shortening of the right clavicle. The patient has not been pregnant, so that status of lactation is unknown. (From Martin, J. A.: Tex. J. Med. **50:**220, 1954.)

the breasts, but we have not observed such growth suppression. During the prepubertal period, when the breast consists principally of a slowly expanding duct system, 1500 to 2000 rad (skin) through a single port directly over the breast in 8 days will strikingly impair development, whereas 3000 to 4000 rad (skin) in 30 days will not only permanently arrest growth of glandular epithelium but will also produce an associated severe fibrosis and shrinkage of the breast. Irradiation of the male breast

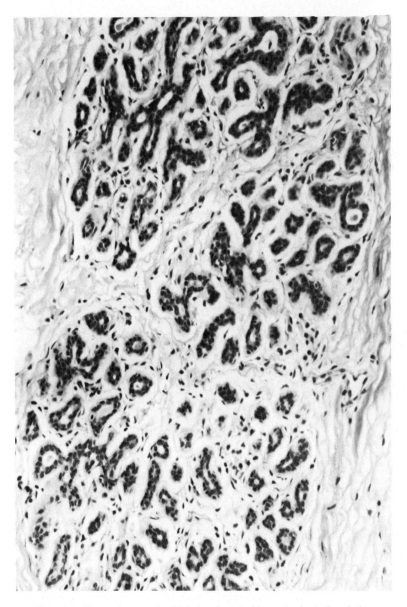

Fig. 11-2. Photomicrograph of lobule of normal breast prior to irradiation.

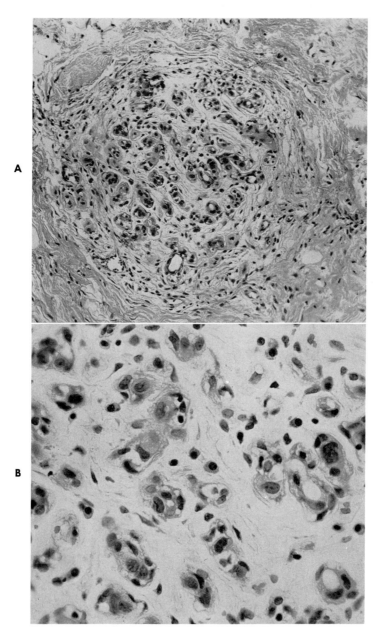

Fig. 11-3. Effect of radiations on normal adult breast. In 3 weeks the patient received 2100 R (air) through a medial tangential port and 2100 R (air) through a lateral tangential port. Ports were 10 × 20 cm (400 kv; hvl, 3.5 mm Cu; TSD, 70). Two and one-half months later the breast was removed. **A,** Radiation effect on normal lobule. **B,** High-power magnification of the same lobule showing abnormal cells with vacuolation of the cytoplasm and distortion of nuclei. (W. U. negs. 56-5106 and 56-5107; from Ackerman, L. V.: Proceedings of the Twenty-Second Seminar of the American Society of Clinical Pathologists, 1957, American Society of Clinical Pathologists.)

with a dose of 1500 rad given at the rate of 500 rad per day for 3 successive days will prevent subsequent estrogen-induced proliferation of breast tissue. Use is made of this effect prior to the administration of estrogen in the treatment of carcinoma of the prostate.

The morphologic effects of radiations on normal adult breast parenchyma have been studied after preoperative irradiation and on tissue obtained at autopsy. The commonly administered midbreast dose of 5000 rad in 5 weeks delivered through medial and lateral tangential beams produces massive destruction of lobules. The ducts shrink, and the cells lining the ducts show pyknotic nuclei and condensation of cytoplasm (Figs. 11-2 to 11-4). Periductal stroma proliferates and shows a striking lamellated appearance with many wide tissue spaces. These changes are not entirely specific for radiation effect, but except as a result of radiation, they are rarely seen in the breast.

In practice, it is customary to administer such irradiation over a period of weeks or even months. Short-term variations in sensitivity such as might occur during the menstrual cycle have gone undetected. It does not seem unreasonable to assume, however, that variations similar to those appearing in the rabbit may also occur in the human being.

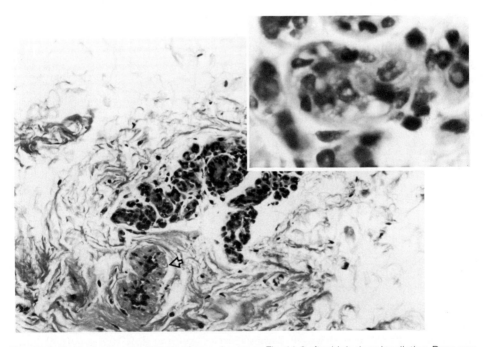

Fig. 11-4. Photomicrograph of lobule of same breast as Fig. 11-2 after high-dose irradiation. Dose was 6000 rad in 7 weeks given 7 years before this section. There is marked atrophy of lobule and perilobar and periductal fibrosis (arrow). Inset shows marked nuclear pleomorphism, vacuolization of nuclei, and cytoplasm.

Irradiation of the human lactating breast is seldom carried out, and the dose required to alter lactation has not been established. Here, again, the response of the human breast will probably be in the same direction as that described previously for the rabbit by Turner and Gomez.

The natural and artificially produced fluctuation in radioresponsiveness of the normal rabbit's breast has stimulated some workers to investigate the effects of sex hormones on the radiosensitivity of breast cancer. Microscopic studies do not suggest that a similar proliferation of breast cancer can frequently be produced by estrogens (Emerson and associates), although augmentation of growth has been reported (Macdonald). Huseby and Thomas observed an estrogen-induced cancer regression in the presence of estrogen-induced breast tissue proliferation. Such changes in "normal" breasts of women advanced in age are infrequent. The idea of increasing the radiosensitivity of carcinoma of the breast by estrogen administration has not yet been realized.

CARCINOMA OF THE BREAST

The role of radiotherapy in the management of adenocarcinoma of the breast varies widely, depending on the clinical stage, pathologist's findings in the resected specimen, the general clinical status of the patient, and the patient's requests. In the more limited stages, radiotherapy is often combined with surgery, whereas in the more advanced stages radiotherapy is usually combined with hormonal therapy, ablative procedures, or chemotherapy. The great value of radiotherapy as a palliative agent in advanced cancer of the breast is uniformly agreed on. The same cannot be said for the use of radiation therapy as a curative modality either postoperatively or alone.

Many investigators have shown by a variety of analyses that cancer of the breast is present, growing, and metastasizing years before the primary lesion is clinically detectable (McKinnon; Park and Lees; Bond). This becomes increasingly clear as one analyzes late results and finds deaths from cancer occurring as long as follow-up is maintained.

This fact has led to the widespread misconception that cancer of the breast has so often metastasized beyond the regional nodes that the great majority of patients should be treated as if they had hematogenous metastases. However, this concern for occult distant metastases must not lead to an "undertreatment" of the primary mass and its regional metastases to lymph nodes. This would not only promote the self-fulfilling prophecy that loco-regional treatment does little to increase survival but would also ensure that an increased proportion of these patients, whatever their eventual outcome, would be plagued with otherwise preventable loco-regional recurrence. A conservative estimate is that 60% of the women have hematogenous metastasis at the time of original therapy (Bross). Another 25% of the patients have no regional metastasis or hematogenous metastases. This leaves a bare 15% of all breast cancer patients whose outcome might be modified by treatment of regional nodes. A portion of this 15% may be controlled by axillary dissection. Not counting the problem of cancer regrowth on the chest wall or internal mammary nodes, this leaves a small proportion of the original group of patients on which the value of radio-therapy can be tested. It is not surprising that many surgeons, radiation oncologists, and chemotherapists have lost their enthusiasm for radical mastectomy and questioned the value of radiotherapy.

Whatever the combination of surgery and radiotherapy, we are convinced that control of the primary cancer and its regional spread should be a major aim for those patients with no proved distant disease. Should there be no occult hematogenous metastasis, loco-regional treatment provides a good chance for cure. Should there be occult hematogenous metastasis, the patient still may remain symptom-free for many years. The absence of local pain, ulceration, vascular obstruction, nerve compression, and source for additional metastasis may provide the patient with years of near-normal life. Finally, loco-regional control provides the maximum opportunity for chemotherapy to be used in a true adjuvant sequence.

Factors affecting treatment decisions and end results

Although we recognize that a variety of clinical and histologic factors influence therapeutic decisions and end results, we also recognize that the behavior of cancer of the breast is often capricious and frustrating. Clinico-pathologic characteristics that warrant special consideration in assessing the indications for treatment are the following:

More favorable	Less favorable
1. Small primary tumor	1. Large primary tumor
2. No metastases to regional nodes	2. Metastases to regional nodes
3. No vascular or lymphatic invasion	3. Invasion of vessels or lymphatics
4. Low invasive potential, that is, "pushing" border; increased lymphocytic infiltration; solitary primary lesion	4. High invasive potential, that is, infiltrating border; no increased lymphocytic infiltration; multiple foci of origin
5. Outer quadrants	5. Inner quadrants

Selected clinicopathologic features warrant special attention because of their bearing on clinical staging, treatment, and results.

1. *Size of the primary breast lesion.* The larger the primary breast cancer the greater the chances of regional and distant metastases (Fig. 11-5). Lane found that cancers up to 1.5 cm in diameter had metastasized to regional nodes in 38% of the patients. Cancers over 4.5 cm in diameter had metastasized to regional nodes in 70% of the patients. Also the larger the primary cancer the greater the chances of skin, muscle, and chest wall invasion with the associated worsening of prognosis (Fig. 11-6). The "T" categories of the TNM stage classification recognize this correlation between size of the primary lesion and the incidence of local and distant spread. The T1 category includes primary lesions less than 2 cm, T2 category includes primary lesions from 2 cm to 5 cm in diameter, and T3 category includes primary lesions greater than 5 cm in diameter.

2. *Status of regional lymph nodes.* The most important single local factor in determining prognosis is the presence or absence of metastases to regional lymph nodes. The distribution, number, and size of the metastases are also important (Fig.

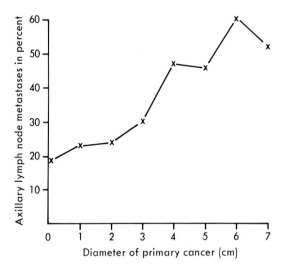

Fig. 11-5. Percent of patients who had metastases to axillary lymph nodes as related to size of the primary lesion. (Based on data from Haagensen, C. D., et al.: The lymphatics in cancer, Philadelphia, 1972, W. B. Saunders Co.)

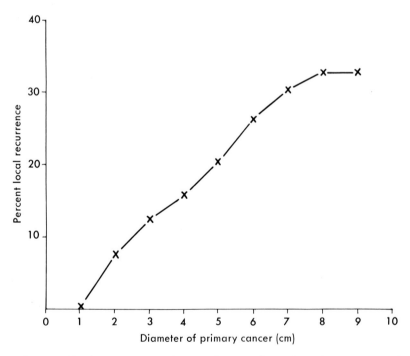

Fig. 11-6. Percent of local recurrence as related to diameter of the primary breast cancer. (Based on data from Donegan, W. L.: Local and regional recurrence. In Spratt, J. S., and Donegan, W. L., editors: Cancer of the breast, Philadelphia, 1967, W. B. Saunders Co.)

11-7). If the metastases are confined to the low axillary lymph nodes or if they are clinically occult, the prognosis is still good.

Generally, involvement of axillary nodes is orderly and stepwise with the sequence of involvement being the lowest nodes (inferior to the lower border of the pectoralis muscles) first and the highest nodes (superior to the upper border of the pectoralis muscles) last. Not only are the lowest nodes involved first, but they are also involved in greater numbers than nodes at other levels. However, disease-free survival rates are more closely correlated with the *total* number of axillary nodes involved rather than the specific level of involvement (Smith and associates). The likelihood that the patient will be disease-free within a period of 5 years is greatly diminished when the number of involved nodes exceeds four (Table 11-1). The

Table 11-1. Disease-free survival rate correlated with the number of involved axillary lymph nodes*

Histologic status of axillary nodes	Patients disease-free at 5 years	
	Number	Percent
No metastases	206	81
1-3 positive nodes	90	33
>4 positive nodes	97	19

*Modified from Fisher, B.: Surgical approaches in treatment of primary breast cancer. In Castro, J. R., ed. Current concepts in breast cancer and tumor immunology, New York, 1974, Medical Examination Publishing Co., Inc.

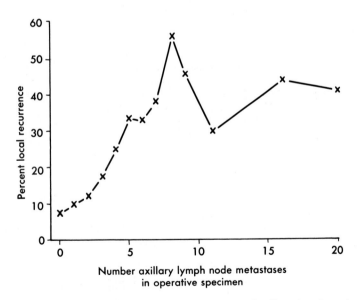

Fig. 11-7. Percent of local recurrence as related to number of axillary lymph nodes containing metastases. (Based on data from Donegan, W. L.: Local and regional recurrence. In Spratt, J. S., and Donegan, W. L., editors: Cancer of the breast, Philadelphia, 1967, W. B. Saunders Co.)

10-year survival rate is similarly correlated with the number of involved axillary nodes. Thus, when four or less nodes were positive, the 10-year determinate survival rate was 45% (fifty-seven of 126), and when five or more nodes were involved, it was 13% (ten of seventy-five) (Smith and associates). If the palpable axillary node is greater than 2.0 cm or is fixed, the prognosis is poor. The incidence and distribution of metastases to lymph nodes vary with the location of the primary lesion (Table 11-8).

3. *Status of blood vessels.* The finding of cancer invading blood vessels is particularly ominous if the lymph nodes also contain cancer (Kister and associates). The presence of skin edema, especially if more than one third of the skin of the breast is involved, is a particularly ominous finding.

4. *Histologic type and cellular growth pattern.* The histologic classification of cancer of the breast according to invasiveness and metastasizing capabilities has considerable prognostic value. Furthermore, it is a highly useful guide for the radiation oncologist in selecting patients most likely to benefit from postoperative irradiation.

The following histologic classification of carcinoma of the breast lists the recognized microscopic patterns in order of decreasing metastasizing potential. Inflammatory carcinoma is not regarded as a distinct histologic type. It is a breast cancer with extensive lymphatic permeation and is included here because of its clinical significance. The prognosis of Paget's disease depends largely on whether it is associated with in situ or infiltrating duct carcinoma.

HISTOLOGIC CLASSIFICATION

		Histologic type	Approximate percent of total group of cancers of breast
Infiltrating and metastasizing	Ductal in origin	1. Inflammatory carcinoma	>1
		2. Scirrhous carcinoma	80
		3. Medullary carcinoma	4
		4. Colloid (mucinous) carcinoma	3
		5. Tubular (well differentiated) carcinoma	>1
		6. Infiltrating papillary carcinoma	1
	Lobular	1. Infiltrating lobular carcinoma	7
Noninfiltrating and nonmetastasizing		1. Duct carcinoma in situ { Papillary / Solid (comedo)	2
		2. Lobular carcinoma in situ	2
Paget's disease of nipple		1. With in situ duct carcinoma	
		2. With invasive duct carcinoma	

The presence of lymphocytic and/or plasmacytic infiltrate in and around breast cancers has been interpreted as a host immune reaction to the presence of the tumors, is more frequently found in tumors of higher nuclear grade, and correlates with improved survival (Black, McDivitt).

These immunomorphologic changes tend to be more marked in the smaller and presumably "earlier" tumors and are rarely observed in large tumors. It is not clearly established whether the duration of the tumor, the immune response, or both are responsible for the improved survival (Zimmerman and associates).

Similarly, it is widely accepted that a sharply circumscribed (pushing) tumor border is a favorable prognostic sign in breast cancer. However, if medullary and colloid carcinomas are excluded, this might not be the case (Silverberg and associates).

Standardized forms of examining and reporting of breast specimens and lymph nodes, such as those recommended by the National Cancer Institute Breast Cancer Task Force and the World Health Organization (Cottier), if generally adopted will provide a substantial uniform data base to help solve the many remaining questions on these clinicomorphologic correlations.

When considering any modality of local treatment, one must take into account the well-documented multicentricity of breast cancer. Gallager and Martin, using whole organ sections, found duct carcinoma in situ or severe atypia away from the primary site in over 75% of 157 breasts, whereas more than half had additional primary sites or multiple sites of invasion.

On the other hand, little is known about the latency of such atypias and intraductal neoplasias. In the case of lobular carcinomas in situ for instance, a trend to a more conservative approach in management appears to be taking place. Recent publications indicate that the risk of developing infiltrating carcinoma is not high enough to justify mastectomy in all breasts harboring lobular carcinoma in situ (Wheeler and associates; Ackerman and Katzenstein; Haagensen and associates).

This conservatism cannot be extended to intraductal carcinoma, since axillary node metastasis is a well-known complication of seemingly in situ duct cancers. Here, undetected microinvasiveness is the most likely explanation.

The criteria for selecting patients for postoperative irradiation are discussed later. The selection is based on the probability of residual local cancer either in the primary site or regional lymph nodes. After mastectomy duct and lobular carcinoma in situ are unlikely to recur locally; when their rare metastases do occur, they are usually confined to the low axillary lymph nodes. Surgery cures these types in a very high proportion. Postoperative irradiation is not routinely justified for these types. Unfortunately, these two types comprise less than 5% of all carcinomas of the breast. By contrast, inflammatory and scirrhous carcinoma account for most local recurrences and metastasize commonly to regional lymph node groups.

Clinical staging of cancer of the breast

Haagensen and Cooley have grouped the factors of the original Haagensen and Stout criteria of inoperability to form four clinical stages.

Stage A   No clinically involved lymph nodes and none of the grave signs listed under Stage C
Stage B   Clinically involved axillary nodes less than 2.5 cm in diameter and none of the grave signs listed under Stage C
Stage C   The presence of any one of five grave signs:
1. Edema of the skin limited in extent (less than a third of the skin involved)
2. Ulceration of skin
3. Solid fixation of the primary tumor to the chest wall
4. Axillary lymph nodes 2.5 cm or more in diameter
5. Fixation of the axillary lymph nodes to the surrounding tissues
Stage D   All more advanced cancers

This classification makes no use of the size of the primary lesion except that the large cancer may produce skin changes or become fixed to deep structures. It does use the size of axillary lymph node metastasis. The definitions of inflammatory carcinoma, clinically involved nodes, fixation to the chest wall, and fixation of axillary nodes require special attention in this and other staging procudures.

The American Joint Committee on Cancer Staging and End Result Reporting has used the TNM (T—primary tumor; N—regional lymph nodes; M—distant metastasis) system and recommends the following stage classification (1978 revision).

TNM CLASSIFICATION*

T— Primary tumor
Clinical-diagnostic classification
TX   Tumor cannot be assessed
T0   No evidence of primary tumor
TIS   Paget's disease of the nipple with no demonstrable tumor†
T1*   Tumor 2 cm or less in greatest dimension
    T1a   No fixation to underlying pectoral fascia or muscle
    T1b   Fixation to underlying pectoral fascia and/or muscle
T2*   Tumor more than 2 cm but not more than 5 cm in its greatest dimension
    T2a   No fixation to underlying pectoral fascia and/or muscle
    T2b   Fixation to underlying pectoral fascia and/or muscle
T3*   Tumor more than 5 cm in its greatest dimension
    T3a   No fixation to underlying pectoral fascia and/or muscle
    T3b   Fixation to underlying pectoral fascia and/or muscle
T4   Tumor of any size with direct extension to chest wall or skin‡
    T4a   Fixation to chest wall
    T4b   Edema (including peau d'orange), ulceration of the skin of the breast, or satellite nodules confined to the same breast
    T4c   Both of above
    T4d   Inflammatory carcinoma
Postsurgical treatment–pathologic classification
TX   Tumor cannot be assessed
T0   No evidence of primary tumor

---

*From the American Joint Committee on Cancer Staging and End Results Reporting: Manual for staging of cancer, Chicago, 1978, Whiting Press.
† Paget's disease with a demonstrable tumor is classified according to size of the tumor.
‡ Chest wall includes ribs, intercostal muscles, and serratus anterior muscle, but not pectoral muscle.

TIS		Preinvasive carcinoma (carcinoma in situ), noninfiltrating intraductal carcinoma, or Paget's disease of nipple
T1	**T1a**	Same as clinical-diagnostic classification*
	T1b	**i:** tumor <0.5 cm
		ii: tumor 0.5-0.9 cm
		iii: tumor 1.0-1.9 cm
T2	**T2a** **T2b**	Same as clinical-diagnostic classification
T3	**T3a** **T3b**	Same as clinical-diagnostic classification
T4	**T4a** **T4b** **T4c** **T4d**	Same as clinical-diagnostic classification

N—Nodal involvement
Clinical-diagnostic classification

NX	Regional lymph nodes cannot be assessed clinically
N0	No palpable homolateral axillary nodes
N1	Movable homolateral axillary nodes
N1a	Nodes not considered to contain growth
N1b	Nodes considered to contain growth
N2	Homolateral axillary nodes considered to contain growth and fixed to one another or to other structures
N3	Homolateral supraclavicular or infraclavicular nodes considered to contain growth or edema of the arm

M—Distant metastasis

MX	Not assessed
M0	No (known) distant metastasis
M1	Distant metastasis present
	Specify _____

GRADE

Well-differentiated, moderately well-differentiated, poorly to very poorly differentiated, or numbers 1, 2, 3-4

STAGE GROUPING

Stage I	T1a	N0 or N1a	
	T1b	N0 or N1a	M0
Stage II	T0	N1b	
	T2a	N0 or N1a or N1b	
	T2b	N0 or N1a or N1b	M0
Stage III	Any T3	N1 or N2	M0
Stage IV	T4	Any N	Any M
	Any T	N3	Any M
	Any T	Any N	M1

R—Residual tumor

R0	No residual
R1	Microscopic residual tumor
R2	Macroscopic residual tumor
	Specify _____

---

*Dimpling of the skin, nipple retraction, or any other skin changes except those in T4b may occur in T1, T2, or T3 without the classification.

Cancers of the breast are, at least in one sense, favorably situated because no vital structures need limit the dose that can be given. Skin, ribs, and the intervening connective tissues are the limiting organs. This absence of vital structures has encouraged radiation oncologists to treat carcinoma of the breast with high doses.

Radiation-induced microscopic changes in breast cancer

High doses of radiations produce characteristic microscopic changes both in normal connective tissues and in cancer cells. If the dose is high, the tumor may be completely replaced by fibrosis. Postirradiation changes in the unsterilized tumor consist of the development of abnormal mitosis, atypical nuclei, and even giant cells. These changes do not indicate increased dedifferentiation of the tumor cells but more likely are indicative of cellular obsolescence. In addition to the obvious cyto-lethal effects manifested by a decrease in tumor size, sublethal injuries to remaining cancer cells and radiation-induced hyaline degeneration of connective tissues may produce a beneficial growth restraint. The cancer cells are often encased by the dense fibrous tissue and may remain in a quiescent state for months or years.

It is an extremely difficult problem for the pathologist to assign predictive value to histologic changes in tumor after irradiation. This is particularly true for carcinoma of the breast. The presence of mitosis, at times apparently increased over that seen in preirradiation biopsies, is often considered by pathologists as evidence of radio-resistance. Yet this interpretation is not uncommonly belied by the patient's subsequent clinical course. The dilemma stems, at least in part, from the pathologist's attempt to make projections of a dynamic process from a static source, a histologic preparation. It must be remembered that a relatively increased number of mitoses may be seen as a result of delay or arrest in the mitotic cycle as well as by true increase in cellular division. Furthermore, one cannot predict from a histologic preparation the reproductive potential of cells arising from such mitotic divisions.

These effects of radiations on the viability and reproducibility of cancer cells must be remembered not only when radiotherapy is the sole treatment but also in evaluating preoperative irradiation. Studies of the recently irradiated breast led early workers to conclude that this cancer was almost invariably radioresistant (Lenz). The highly fractionated technique of Baclesse (1965) proved capable of arresting clinical evidences of local growth for 5 years or more in at least a third of all patients treated for cure and in at least half of all patients presenting with no palpable axillary adenopathy. About a fourth of 101 advanced primary lesions were histologically sterilized by this technique. Finally, Pierquin and associates used combinations of external megavoltage beams with interstitial implants of radioactive sources to raise the combined dose in the primary breast mass to 9000 to 10,000 rad. Cancerous masses of various sizes are usually controlled by doses of this level (Table 11-2). The need for doses of this magnitude has been and will likely continue to be a deterrent to widespread use of radiations to treat the unresected breast mass. It is also a strong argument for lumpectomy when radiation therapy is to be used to treat the otherwise intact breast. The dose required for eradication of metastases of various sizes in regional lymph nodes is discussed on p. 310.

Table 11-2. Control of primary breast masses by combined doses of 9000 to 10,000 rad*

Diameter of breast mass	Recurrent growth within 5 years
0-2 cm	0 in 13
2-5 cm	0 in 21
>5 cm	2 in 14

*From Pierquin, B., Baillet, F., and Wilson, J. F.: Am. J. Roentgenol. Radium Ther. Nucl. Med. **127:**645-648, 1976.

Table 11-3. Incidence of metastases found in axillary lymph nodes 6 weeks after preoperative irradiation (4500 rad tissue dose given with daily fractions of 175 rad)*

	Positive axillary nodes	Extranodal disease
Surgery only	39% (76/196)	40/76
Preoperative irradiation	21% (21/99)	4/21

*Modified from Schryver, A. D.: Int. J. Radiat. Oncol. Biol. Phys. **1:**601-609, 1976.

Preoperative irradiation

The general aims, principles, and possibilities of preoperative irradiation have been discussed in Chapter 2. All that has been discussed there is particularly applicable in the treatment of carcinoma of the breast. Interest in preoperative irradiation of the breast was prompted by the feeling that results could not be improved further by surgery alone. Serious attempts to evaluate preoperative irradiation in carcinoma of the breast have been sparse. However, clinical trials have encouraged continued evaluation of this sequence. Baclesse (1965) reported the operative findings in 101 patients who had been given high doses. Sixty-three percent were initially judged inoperable but were later operated on. No viable tumor was found in a fourth. Forty-one percent were free of cancer at 5 years, and 35% were free of cancer at 10 years. White and associates were likewise impressed with the capability of radiotherapy to convert borderline inoperable lesions to operable lesions. Their impression was that local recurrences were fewer and the 5-year survival rate was increased. A preoperative dose of 3500 to 5000 rad was given with a ^{60}Co beam.

A randomized clinical trial comparing surgery alone with preoperative and post-operative irradiation was reported by Wallgren and associates. Nine hundred sixty patients were entered into the study. As might be expected, during the first several years of the study there was no significant difference in survival. However, the incidence of loco-regional failure was reduced from 17% to 5% by preoperative and postoperative therapy. Doses of 4500 rad in 175 rad fractions were delivered to the volume at risk. This preoperative irradiation produced a notable decrease in the incidence of positive nodes and in the incidence of extranodal spread found in the resected specimen (Table 11-3). Although follow-up is still somewhat limited, Wallgren and associates obtained a significant increase in survival by using pre-operative irradiation.

In summarizing the information given in Chapter 2 as it applies to operable carcinoma of the breast, we can speculate that, as a result of preoperative irradiation,
the growth rate and transplantability of breast cancer will be decreased, the tumor
bed will be less susceptible for implant take and growth, loco-regional recurrences
are diminished, but eradication of the primary cancer will only rarely be achieved
with the preoperative doses recommended. Will these changes increase the cure
rate? Will preoperative irradiation be superior to postoperative irradiation, especially when postoperative irradiation can be applied with the additional understanding
gained from study of the resected specimen? Wallgren and associates have shown
that the cure rate is increased by preoperative irradiation, and preoperative irradiation is more effective in this regard than postoperative irradiation.

Radiotherapy alone after simple excision of the palpable mass or after lumpectomy

The unusually high dose necessary to control a substantial proportion of unresected primary breast cancers was cited on p. 310. On the other hand, if the palpable

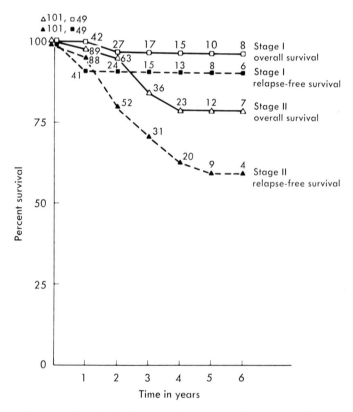

Fig. 11-8. Cumulative overall survival and relapse-free survival of Stages I and II patients treated with
radiation therapy alone after excision biopsy. (From Prosnitz, L. R., Goldenberg, I. S., Packard, R. A.,
et al.: Cancer **39**:917-923, 1977.)

tumor is excised (lumpectomy) but the breast is otherwise left intact, vigorous but well-tolerated doses of radiations control the local disease with remarkable consistency.

The aims of lumpectomy followed by irradiation are to preserve the breasts, the muscles, and the nerves of the chest wall without decreasing the rate of control. To be completely successful in these aims, the primary tumor mass must be sufficiently small for excision without serious deformity to the breast. This depends on the relative sizes of the breast and the mass. Seldom will masses suitable for this sequence be as large as 5 cm, and most have been about 3 cm or less in diameter. Axillary lymphadenopathy has often been present in patients selected for this sequence, but adenopathy should seldom be larger than 2 cm. This selects a more favorable local lesion for this sequence of management. Peters and, more recently, Prosnitz and associates recommend that it be used for selected patients with clinical Stages I and II lesions.

Simple excision of the palpable mass in Stages I and II will leave cancer in the breast in at least 25% of the patients (Peters). Therefore doses of radiations must be

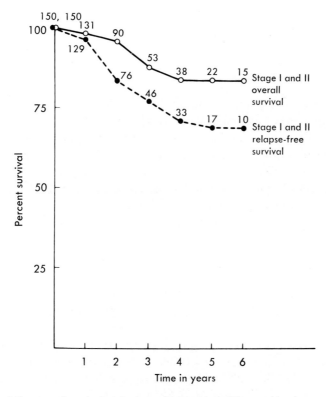

Fig. 11-9. Cumulative overall survival and relapse-free survival of the combined group of Stages I and II patients treated primarily with radiation therapy only after excision biopsy. (From Prosnitz, L. R., Goldenberg, I. S., Packard, R. A., et al.: Cancer **39**:917-923, 1977.)

of a high level. The entire breast and regional nodes are given a minimum of 5000 rad through a combination of tangential and direct portals (p. 316). Boosting doses of 1000 to 1500 rad through small portals should be directed to the lumpectomy site and to the initially suspicious lymphadenopathy. Some have preferred to deliver the boosting dose with interstitial techniques. When doses lower than those mentioned before have been used, local persistence rates have been considerable (Atkins and associates).

The postirradiation appearance of the breast depends on the selection of patients, the relative magnitude of the surgery, fractionation of the radiation therapy, and other details of technique. A carefully fractionated technique is essential if the hard fibrotic changes are to be minimized.

In many of the small published series there were no local recurrences with this technique. In a collection of 150 patients from four institutions there were ten recurrences, five of which were permanently controlled by subsequent mastectomy (Prosnitz and associates). These overall survival and disease-free survival rates shown in Figs. 11-8 and 11-9 are competitive with those obtained by other modalities. In addition, the breast and axilla remain intact. Ten and 15-year follow-up data on large numbers of patients treated by lumpectomy plus irradiation are not available. However, 5 years and longer follow-up data are available and provide us with sufficient optimism for us to continue to recommend the procedure on a selective basis.

Postoperative irradiation of the chest wall and regional lymph nodes

Despite radical attempts to remove the primary breast cancer and its metastases in axillary lymph nodes, loco-regional disease is unavoidably left behind in a substantial proportion of patients. This varies widely, depending on the factors mentioned earlier. Recurrence of the cancer on the chest wall and in the regional lymph nodes is a major catastrophe in the eyes of the patient. A bleeding necrotic ulcer, obstruction of regional vessels, or invasion of the brachial plexus contribute major problems over long periods of time during the patient's last months or years of survival. Systematic steps for preventing or diminishing such problems are therefore extremely important.

In addition we now have reason to believe that postoperative irradiation will, in selected patients, increase the 5-year disease-free survival rates. This will be detailed below, but the promise of increased local control and possibly increasing disease-free survival emphasize the need to identify patients at high risk for postoperative loco-regional recurrences.

By using the original Haagensen and Stout criteria to select operable cases and by skillfully performing the radical mastectomy, local persistence and skin metastases will appear in no more than 15% of the operable cases within the first 5 years. However, these recurrences will continue to develop, and the incidence may reach 20% by the tenth postoperative year (Spratt). Chest wall recurrence will be more frequent when axillary lymphadenopathy is found (Fig. 11-7) and when the breast mass is large or involves the skin by attachment or edema (Fig. 11-6). Dao and Nemoto found recurrence in eleven of forty patients whose operative specimen showed fifteen or more positive axillary nodes or a primary lesion 5 cm or larger. If a large number of axillary lymph nodes is involved, the local recurrence rate may reach 45% (Spratt). Of fifty-five patients whose operative specimen showed no axillary metastases, none developed local recurrence, although four of the fifty-five died of disseminated metastases (Dao and Nemoto). Patients with primary lesions 1 cm or less in diameter rarely develop chest wall recurrence. Patients with lesions 8 cm or more in diameter develop local recurrence 33% of the time (Spratt).

In our experience most recurrences appear initially within 3 cm of the operative scar or deep to or near the edges of the skin graft. The mechanism of local recurrences is unknown, but one should consider the following:

1. Transection of the peripheral extensions of the primary lesion
2. Wound implantation from cut vessels that ooze blood or lymph containing viable tumor emboli
3. Retrograde movement of tumor cells to the edges of the operative wound as described by Gricouroff

It seems likely that all of these mechanisms are at one time or another responsible for local recurrences.

Whatever the precise mechanisms for recurrences on the chest wall, we can identify patients at high risk for such recurrences as those with the following:

1. Large primary lesion (The recurrence rate is considerable with lesions larger than 3 cm [Fig. 11-6].)
2. Fixation of the primary lesion to the skin, skin edema, or ulceration
3. At least four or at least 20% of the resected axillary lymph nodes involved with metastases (Fig. 11-7)
4. Inflammatory carcinoma
5. Multiple invasive primary lesions

There are a variety of randomized studies all indicating that postoperative irradiation of the chest wall diminishes the incidence of recurrences on the chest wall (Paterson and Russell; Wallgren and associates; Fisher and associates). The incidence of recurrence on the chest wall in the unirradiated controls varies with patient selec-

Table 11-4. Effect of various doses of radiations on the control of clinically occult metastases in the supraclavicular region (axilla was positive in the surgical specimen)*

Dose	Percent developing nodes in supraclavicular region within 5 years
No irradiation	20-26
3500 rad in 3 weeks	11-13
4500-5000 rad in 5 weeks	1.5
5000-5500 rad in 7 weeks	1.2

*Modified from Fletcher, G. H., and Shukovsky, L. J.: J. Radiol. Electrol. **56**:383-400, 1975.

Table 11-5. The value of radiation therapy on loco-regional control rates in patients with cancer of the breast*

Anatomic site	Incidence of clinical recurrence in specified patient group after mastectomy only (%)	Incidence of clinical recurrence in specified patient group with post-operative radiation therapy (%)
Supraclavicular nodes (if axilla was positive in resected specimen)	20-26	1.5
Parasternal nodes (if axilla was positive in resected specimen or lesion was central or in medial half of breast)	Clinically obvious 9 Histologically 53	0
Chest wall	33 to 45 (if axilla was extensively involved or primary lesion was 6 to 7 cm in diameter)	10 (if more than 20% of the axillary nodes were positive or locally advanced disease in breast)

*Modified from Fletcher, G. H.: Int. J. Radiat. Oncol. Biol. Phys. **1:**769-779, 1976. (For specific treatment factors see Table 11-7 and p. 316.)

tion, as pointed out before. The overall incidence of postoperative recurrence on the chest wall following tissue doses of 4500 to 5000 rad in 5 weeks drops to less than 5%. In patients with a high risk of recurrence, that is, those with more than four positive axillary nodes, the postoperative, postirradiation rate of recurrence on the chest wall may approach 10% (Fletcher) (Tables 11-4 and 11-5).

UNRESECTED METASTASES IN REGIONAL LYMPH NODES. There are at least three important questions that we must consider in establishing indications for postoperative irradiation of regional nodes.

1. What is the incidence of metastases to the regional chains of nodes in the various clinical circumstances?

2. Does irradiation in well-tolerated doses eradicate subclinical metastases in regional nodes?

3. Does eradication of subclinical metastases in regional nodes modify subsequent problems related to local recurrence, and does it increase disease-free survival rates?

Seldom does the surgeon resect more regional lymph nodes than those located in the axilla. Paraclavicular and internal mammary nodal chains constitute additional important lymph drainage routes, which must also be considered. Recurrences in the axilla are rare after the classic axillary dissection. On the other hand, after anything less than the classic axillary dissection we believe full irradiation of the axilla is justified. Supraclavicular nodes are rarely involved when axillary dissection yields histologically negative nodes. By contrast, of those patients whose supraclavicular area is initially normal but whose axillary nodes are histologically involved, 20% to 25% subsequently develop clinical evidence of metastases in supraclavicular nodes (Paterson and Russell; Robbins and associates). The internal mammary nodes, like the axillary nodes, constitute a primary drainage area from the breast. This is espe-

Table 11-6. Comparison of radical mastectomy alone with radical mastectomy associated with dissection of internal mammary nodes*

	Treatment	
	Radical mastectomy	Radical mastectomy with dissection of internal mammary nodes
Number of patients studied	543	506
Overall 5-year survival (%)	70	70
Patients with positive axillary nodes (%)	58	55
5-year survival rate of patients with positive axillary nodes and inner or medial quadrant T1 or T2 primaries (%)	52	71

*From Lacour, J., Bucalossi, P., Cacers, E., Jacobelli, G., Koszarowski, T., Le, M., Rumeau-Rouquelle, C., and Veronesi, U.: Cancer **37:**206-214, 1976.

cially important for cancers in the medial half of the breast and for those in the sub-areolar tissues (Table 11-8). The arguments for irradiating the internal mammary chain of nodes are precisely the same arguments the surgeon uses to justify axillary dissection. "Curative" treatment, including axillary dissection and sometimes post-operative chemotherapy, without serious consideration of treatment of the internal mammary chain is, at best, inconsistent. Until recently neither surgery (Urban) nor irradiation (Guttmann) directed toward the internal mammary nodes could be shown to increase the disease-free survival rate. However, the large randomized study of Lacour and associates did show that removal of the internal mammary chain at the time of the radical mastectomy increased the disease-free survival rate in a selected subgroup of patients (patients with T1 and T2 lesions of the medial quadrants who had histologically verified metastases in axillary nodes) (Table 11-5).

A review of the techniques used in the often-quoted randomized trials (Paterson and Russell; Kaae and Johansen; Fisher and associates) creates serious doubt that the internal mammary chain was actually encompassed or, when encompassed, was given what is now accepted as an adequate dose (Fletcher and Montague). By con-trast, the recent series of Host and Brennhovd (Figs. 11-10 and 11-11), the analysis by Lacour (Table 11-6), and the review by Fletcher and Montague (p. 312) verify that adequate irradiation of the internal mammary chain as part of the loco-regional treat-ment does indeed increase disease-free survivals.

The radiocurability of subclinical metastases in regional lymph nodes can be determined by comparing the surgically removed axillary contents with and without preoperative irradiation and by comparing the incidence of metastases developing in a regional nodal area with and without previous irradiation. Both types of studies have been done, and both confirm the ability of well-tolerated doses of radiations to eradicate and control a significant proportion of regional subclinical metastases.

1. *Studies of axillary contents after preoperative irradiation.* These types of studies are of limited significance, since they depend on the thoroughness of the

Table 11-7. Probability of tumor control—responses of masses of various volumes to various doses*

Tumor diameter	Dose (rad)	Frequency of control (%)
Subclinical	5000 (5 weeks)	>90
2.5-3 cm	7000 (7 weeks)	90
>5 cm	7000-8000 (8-9 weeks)	30
>5 cm	8000-9000 (8-10 weeks)	56
>5-15 cm	8000-10,000 (10-12 weeks)	75

*Modified from Fletcher, G. H., and Shukovsky, L. J.: J. Radiol. Electrol. **56**:383-400, 1975.

axillary dissection and the ability of the pathologist to identify and examine all axillary lymph nodes. In addition, we must remember that the full effects of the radiations are slow in becoming manifested. Furthermore, when cancer cells are found after irradiation, the pathologist cannot accurately assess their future potential for growth. Wallgren and associates reported the results of such a study and found that 6 weeks after delivering 4500 rad (175 rad per daily fraction) to the axillary nodes, the incidence of positive nodes in the dissected axilla was reduced to one half its unirradiated value (Table 11-3).

Guttmann administered a tissue dose of 5000 rad in 5 weeks to internal mammary and paraclavicular regions after biopsy proof of metastases to either or both regions. Sixty percent of 148 patients were living at 5 years. Some patients with biopsy-proved regional metastases to lymph nodes were irradiated vigorously but died with widespread metastases. Autopsy studies of twenty such patients failed to reveal residual cancer in any of the areas that were initially shown to have metastases.

2. *Studies of incidence of metastases developing in nodal areas with and without elective irradiation.* Fletcher and Shukovsky analyzed data relevant to the effectiveness of various doses of radiations in eradicating subclinical nodal disease in carcinoma of the breast (Table 11-7). It has been an almost uniform finding that elective irradiation (4500 to 5000 rad in 5 to 6 weeks) of subclinical metastases in regional lymph nodes will decrease the subsequent development of clinically obvious disease in the treated volume to about one tenth of its unirradiated incidence (Table 11-5). The degree to which this is dose-related is shown in Table 11-7.

DOES POSTOPERATIVE IRRADIATION INCREASE DISEASE-FREE SURVIVAL?
It has been the conventional wisdom that postoperative irradiation of the regional nodes and the chest wall does not increase disease-free survival rates. This conclusion seems to have been supported by the studies of Paterson and Russell, Kaae, and Fisher and associates. We now have several reasons to doubt this conclusion.

1. The work of Lacour and associates cited before indicates that removal of the internal mammary nodes at the time of mastectomy increases disease-free survival in selected patients. These results suggest that in selected patients postoperative irradiation of the internal mammary chain will likewise increase disease-free survival rates.

2. Host reported the results of a randomized study designed to measure the value

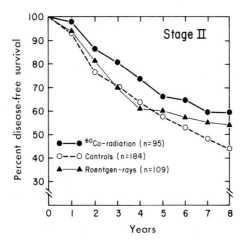

Fig. 11-10. Effect of postoperative ^{60}Co irradiation on disease-free survival rate (clinical Stage II). The difference between unirradiated patients and those patients irradiated with ^{60}Co is significant. The difference between the unirradiated patients and those patients irradiated with orthovoltage beams is not significant. (Modified from Host, H., and Brennhovd, I. O.: Int. J. Radiat. Oncol. Biol. Phys. **2:**1061-1067, 1977.)

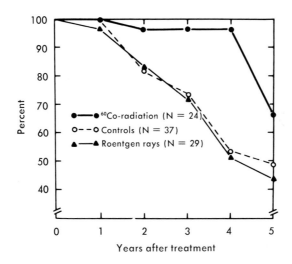

Fig. 11-11. Effect of postoperative ^{60}Co irradiation on survival of patients with four or more involved axillary lymph nodes in the resected specimen. The difference is statistically significant. (Modified from Host, H., and Brennhovd, I. O.: Int. J. Radiat. Oncol. Biol. Phys. **2:**1061-1067, 1977.)

of postirradiation of the chest wall and regional nodes following radical mastectomy. The survival curves so obtained are shown in Figs. 11-10 and 11-11. Patients with pathologically proved axillary metastases were irradiated with megavoltage beams and modern portal arrangements. The increased survival in the patients given postoperative irradiation is statistically significant and must now be taken into consideration as a major factor in our reevaluation of the role of postoperative irradiation.

3. Wallgren and associates found improved survival when preoperative irradiation was given but no improved survival when postoperative irradiation was given. This difference is unexplained.

4. Fletcher and Montague compared the survival rates at 5 and 10 years in two groups of patients. Of two hundred eighty-seven patients who had radical mastectomy *only*, 11.5% had microscopically involved axillary nodes (average of five per axilla when positive), and the 5- and 10-year survival rates were 71.7% and 54%, respectively. Of three hundred fifty-six patients who had radical mastectomy, 65.7% had microscopically involved axillary nodes (average of six per axilla when positive). They were given *postoperative irradiation* and showed 5- and 10-year survival rates of 71.3% and 56% respectively.

There can no longer be any reasonable doubt about the ability of acceptable doses of radiations to eradicate disease in these nodes nor any question but that the eradication of such disease increases survival.

In our efforts to restrict irradiation to those who benefit from it we must consider the merits and limitations of reserving postoperative irradiation for only those patients who develop clinical manifestations of loco-regional recurrence. If we wait

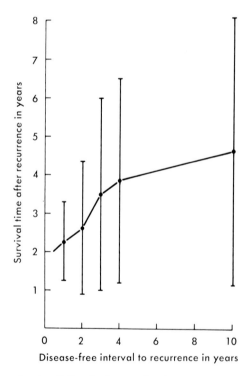

Fig. 11-12. Survival time *after* irradiation for loco-regional recurrent cancer of the breast plotted against disease-free interval measured from initial mastectomy to recurrence. The common long post-recurrent survival justifies a serious effort to control loco-regional disease. (From Chu, F. C. H., Lin, F. J., Kim, J. H., Huh, S. H., and Garmatis, C. J.: Cancer **37**:2677-2681, 1976.)

until recurrences are clinically obvious, not only are higher doses required for tumor eradication, but local control is achieved less often. A good example of the best that can be achieved has been reported by Chu and associates (Fig. 11-12). Their results are excellent, but in addition to diminished loco-regional control, there is a good possibility that some patients develop their initial distant metastases during the "waiting" period. Indeed such would have to be the case to account for the increased disease-free survival rate reported by Host.

EFFECTS OF LOCAL NODAL IRRADIATION ON SYSTEMIC IMMUNITY TO CANCER OF THE BREAST. In 1974 Stjernsward summarized carefully selected data from five diverse clinical studies (Bruce, Fisher and associates, Kaae, and two series from Paterson and Russell) to support his contention that local irradiation modified systemic immunity to cancer of the breast, resulting in increased distant metastases. His argument was supported by such changes as decreased peripheral lymphocyte count, radiation-induced reduction in the barrier function of nodes, and reduction in the ability of the nodal lymphocytes to initiate tumor immune responses. However, Perez has critically reviewed this concept and concluded that once tumor cells have reached the regional nodes, an immune response is rather quickly developed. This response then becomes a systemic response, and its presence no longer depends on the integrity of regional nodes. At this point, local irradiation of regional nodes does not appear to interfere with the immune aspects of cancer spread. Furthermore, reexamination of the data manipulations by Stjernsward has since shown that his aforementioned conclusions were not justified (Levitt and Fletcher). Finally, comparisons made in the randomized studies of Wallgren and associates and Host fail to show any increase in either the number or decrease in the time of appearance of distant metastases in irradiated patients. For these reasons, Stjernsward's arguments can no longer be used as arguments against postoperative irradiation.

From the preceding discussions it is clear that there are many parameters that have a bearing on the incidence of postoperative recurrence on the chest wall, metastases to unresected regional nodes, and distant spread. Not only is the rationale for postoperative irradiation based on these data, but also the indications for integrated hormonal manipulation and the rapidly changing potential of chemotherapy.

Considerations relative to chemotherapy

In addition to the problems related to loco-regional recurrences, about 60% of the patients treated with curative intent will eventually manifest distant metastases. At highest risk are patients who have large primary cancers and those who, on axillary dissection, have more than four nodes involved by cancer (Table 11-1). The proportion of such patients showing distant metastases continues to increase as long as follow-up is maintained. For this 60% we obviously need modalities that control or delay distant metastases. Chemotherapy provides a potential for such control for a fraction of the premenopausal patients at high risk for occult metastases. If, at the same time, such systemic chemotherapy significantly diminishes loco-regional recurrences, the vigor of conventional loco-regional treatment should be reassessed.

Table 11-8. Incidence of metastases to internal mammary lymph nodes according to primary site*

Involving medial quadrant or subareolar region	
When axillary nodes are positive, internal mammary nodes will be positive in 53%	(152) (286)
When axillary nodes are negative, internal mammary nodes will be positive in 15.8%	(52) (340)
Confined to outer quadrants, excluding subareolar region	
When axillary nodes are positive, internal mammary nodes will be positive in 42%	(11) (26)
When axillary nodes are negative, internal mammary nodes will be positive in 1 in 8	

*Urban, J. A.: Personal communication, 1968.

Such a reassessment should include consideration of both limited and radical surgery with and without radiation therapy for a variety of combinations of chemotherapeutic agents. The complexity of such a clinical study is obvious.

The premenopausal patient at high risk for occult metastases should be given postoperative adjuvant chemotherapy. The incidence of local recurrence is decreased or delayed by this chemotherapy. We do not know if this modification in loco-regional recurrence is permanent or if it duplicates the control of metastases to lymph nodes and the chest wall that is achieved by postoperative irradiation. Until we know the incidence of long-term loco-regional control following a specific surgical procedure combined with specific chemotherapy, we have continued to insist on loco-regional irradiation in this high-risk group.

INFLAMMATORY CARCINOMA OF THE BREAST. Well-fractionated high-dose irradiation (6000 rad or more plus boosting doses to the chest wall, and 5000 rad or more plus boosting doses to the axilla at 750 rad per week) sometimes followed by simple mastectomy controls loco-regional disease in about one half of the patients with inflammatory carcinoma of the breast (Barker and associates). Preirradiation and postirradiation chemotherapy (5-fluorouracil [5-FU], doxorubicin [Adriamycin], and cyclophosphamide [Cytoxan]) seem to increase loco-regional control to an even higher proportion of patients and perhaps extend survival (Blumenschein and associates). These combinations are being studied.

Very severe skin reactions may be produced by administering such agents as doxorubicin (Adriamycin) during radiation therapy. An interval of about 2 weeks between these two modalities greatly diminishes their combined local damage (Aristizabal and associates; Philips and associates). It is obvious from this discussion that close collaboration of the oncologic disciplines is essential in the care of patients at high risk for occult distant metastases.

The danger of damaging underlying lung is a constant concern during the planning of radiation therapy. Every effort is made to limit the volume of normal lung in the high-dose volume. Radiation-induced fibrosis of the lung apex is to be expected and in our experience is never symptom-producing. High doses reach the underlying pericardium and heart from the photon beam directed to the internal mammary chain. If the port is large and the cardiac dose exceeds 4500 rad in 4 weeks, a certain proportion of patients will develop electrocardiographic changes. Stewart and associates reported that of 117 patients given irradiation to the internal mammary chain, four developed heart abnormalities (Chapter 9). Guttmann had no cases in her survivors. We have not encountered this sequela in our practice. The use of a photon beam in this anatomic site has the questionable additional benefit of irradiating the mediastinal nodes. If the disadvantages of mediastinal irradiation outweigh the advantages, it is simple to reduce the dose to mediastinal structures by using an appropriate electron beam.

Finally, although the palliative value of loco-regional irradiation in the apparently locally confined but inoperable cancer of the breast is not questioned, there has remained some question of its *curative* value. However, of those patients selected as inoperable by the triple biopsy technique, 60% were living 5 years after irradiation alone (Guttmann). Fletcher and Montague used the usual clinical methods for selecting inoperable lesions. After vigorous irradiation, 27.1% were living at 5 years. The same type of clinical problem is encountered in the management of previously unirradiated patients who develop postmastectomy loco-regional recurrences. The fact that many of these patients and many of the patients who are primarily inoperable will survive for long periods emphasizes the importance of carefully planned high-dose loco-regional radiation therapy. Such irradiation does not preclude hormonal or chemotherapy management when indicated.

Summary of indications for irradiation

1. The histologic classification was given previously. Radiation therapy cannot generally be justified in noninfiltrating and nonmetastasizing cancers. (It is likely that irradiation alone will favorably modify the outcome of patients with multiple foci of noninvasive, nonmetastasizing carcinoma of the breast. Indeed, this would seem to be a strong indication for irradiation alone, providing no mass could be detected by palpation, mammography, or other means. This specific problem has not been studied in depth, and a clinical trial is necessary to define the precise role of irradiation.)

2. Preoperative irradiation in initially clearly operable patients seems to be as effective in decreasing loco-regional recurrence as postoperative irradiation (Wallgren and associates). However, the highly useful information obtainable from the resected specimen is not available preoperatively to assist in selecting patients at high risk for loco-regional recurrences and distant metastasis. In addition, there is certainly a radiation-induced increase in problems related to healing. Therefore we recommend preoperative irradiation only in the borderline *inoperable* patient with the hope that subsequent resection will be possible.

3. Patients with upper outer quadrant lesions less than 5 cm who show no microscopic evidence of axillary lymph node metastases are unlikely to develop local recurrence. They are unlikely to develop axillary or internal mammary node me-

tastases later. After radical mastectomy, we do not advocate routine postoperative irradiation for these patients.

4. Candidates for lumpectomy and irradiation were defined on p. 304.

The following criteria apply to postmenopausal and paramenopausal patients.

5. If metastases to axillary lymph nodes are found in the surgical specimen, we advocate irradiation of the internal mammary and paraclavicular node areas. The chest wall is also irradiated in these patients if four or more nodes are involved, if one fifth of all nodes removed are involved, or if any of the signs of an advanced primary lesion are present (fixation to muscle or skin, edema or erythema of skin, or primary lesion greater than 5 cm in maximum diameter).

6. If the primary lesion is located in the subareolar tissues or in the medial quadrants, irradiation of the internal mammary and paraclavicular chain is recommended, whether metastases are found in the axilla or not.

7. In patients with locally inoperable cancer but no distant disease, the chest wall, breast, and lymph node areas are irradiated vigorously. The subsequent course of such patients is highly variable. Some patients will become candidates for limited mastectomy. Some will live for years with their loco-regional disease stabilized or controlled. Most will die by 5 years, but they will have been made much more comfortable because of the vigorous loco-regional irradiation. The need for combining such irradiation with chemotherapy is clear.

PREMENOPAUSAL PATIENTS. Premenopausal patients at high risk for loco-regional recurrence require special consideration in view of the decreased incidence of local recurrences achieved with chemotherapy (see discussion on p. 313).

Technique

The patient at high risk for postoperative loco-regional recurrence and the patient who has just had a lumpectomy present quite similar problems to the radiation oncologist. In both patients the chest wall must be given a substantial dose without damaging the underlying lung. In addition, the internal mammary and paraclavicular nodes must be irradiated without damaging the heart, brachial plexus, or associated important tissues. The intention with both categories of patients is to completely eradicate suspected loco-regional residual cancer. These lymph node areas (Figs. 11-13 to 11-16) can be treated more effectively by a field arrangement separate from that best-suited for irradiation of the breast proper or the skin flaps on the chest wall (Fletcher and Montague). Medial and lateral tangential ports are simple and effective in delivering the desired dose to the breast with minimal injury to the lung (Fig. 11-17). Sufficient angulation or shifting of the medial tangential port to include the ipsilateral internal mammary lymph nodes decreases homogeneity within the breast and increases the irradiated volume of normal lung. A narrow port placed at the medial edge of the medial tangential port not only delivers a higher dose to the internal mammary nodes, but also permits better arrangement of tangential ports (Fig. 11-17). Supraclavicular, retroclavicular, and axillary lymph

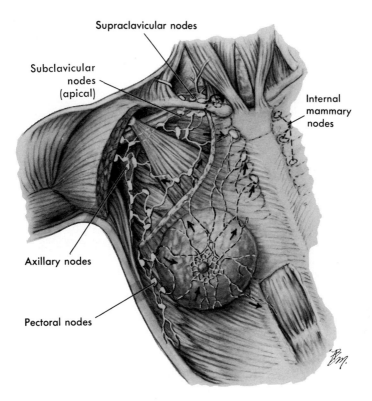

Fig. 11-13. Lymph drainage and lymph node groups of the breast. The volume requiring irradiation must usually be planned to encompass axillary, infraclavicular, supraclavicular, and internal mammary chains.

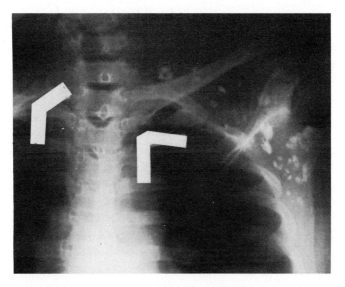

Fig. 11-14. Hand lymphangiogram showing location and distribution of axillary, infraclavicular, and supraclavicular lymph nodes. Note that it is generally possible to encompass these nodes with little irradiation of the lung.

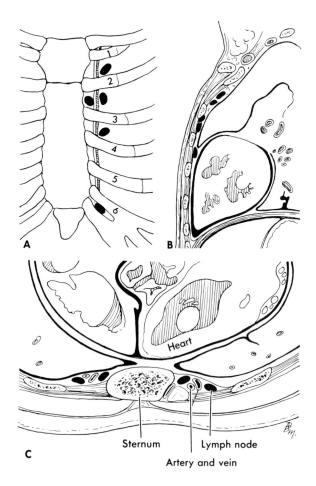

Fig. 11-15. Internal mammary chain of lymph nodes shown in three views. The chain usually extends from the first to the sixth interspaces along course of internal mammary vessels. The proximity of the heart makes irradiation of a segment of the heart unavoidable.

nodes are best treated with parallel opposing anterior and posterior ports of ^{60}Co or megavoltage beams. In practice it is usually more convenient to use a single anterior dogleg-shaped portal. Such a field is readily shaped with modified lead bricks (Fig. 11-18). Care must be taken to avoid as much lung as possible by having the patient raise her arm until it is at least at a right angle to the body. A dose of 5600 rad (maximum surface dose) in 5 fractions per week for 5 weeks is well tolerated. One may be tempted to deliver this dose in a shorter overall period. However, efforts to do this have resulted in severe fibrosis that produces a "frozen" shoulder and brachial plexus damage. In our experience, this dose is the maximum in the overall time of 5 weeks. Although this port delivers an adequate dose to the internal mammary and paraclavicular nodes, a supplementary port must be used for the axillary nodes when they have not been completely removed. A posterior port

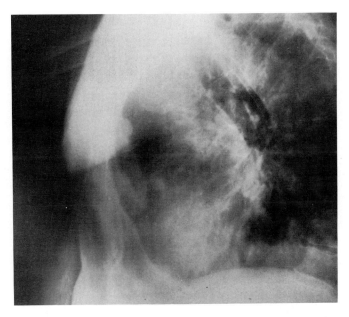

Fig. 11-16. Lateral radiograph of chest showing size and position of metastases from carcinoma of the breast to internal mammary lymph nodes. (Courtesy Dr. D. Koch.)

accomplishes this quite readily. Compensating filters should be used by those dissatisfied with the unaltered beam. The delivery of an excessively high dose in the thinner superior portion of the shoulder can be prevented by selectively shielding this volume after the desired dose has been given. No direct axillary port is necessary in patients of average anteroposterior dimensions. If available, an electron beam of suitable energy (usually about 12 to 15 mev) is excellent for irradiating the internal mammary chain.

The lateral tangential port should be brought laterally to at least the midaxillary line. The medial tangential port is brought to the lateral edge of the narrow internal mammary port. When irradiation of the chest wall or the breast is planned, such tangential beams are sufficient and are highly practical; yet they damage the lung very little. The junction of the upper border of the tangential beams with the lower border of the paraclavicular beam must be as far superior as the axilla will permit (Fig. 11-18). This reduces the volume of irradiated lung to a minimum. Homogeneity of the dose is increased if wedges (15 to 30 degree wedges with ^{60}Co or 4 mev beams) are used. Techniques employing a direct beam of electrons have been described (Chu and associates). However, these techniques are not significantly superior to the more practical and common technique of medial and lateral tangential beams.

Subcutaneous nodules are often the first manifestation of loco-regional recurrence. The characteristics of megavoltage beams, even those used tangentially, may result in a deficient dose to the skin and these subcutaneous tissues. Tangential ^{60}Co

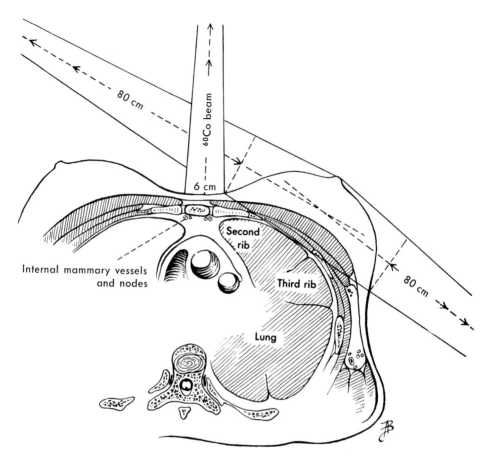

Fig. 11-17. Diagram of a cross section through the thorax at level of nipple. Fields are arranged for treatment of inoperable carcinoma of the breast or postlumpectomy. A similar arrangement is suitable for postoperative use. The narrow, straight anterior telecobalt or, preferably, an electron beam is centered over the ipsilateral internal mammary chain. The tangential beams are so angled as to encompass the chest wall to midaxillary line. Scatter to the lung is negligible. Surface dose can be increased to desired level by using a bolus for part of the treatment.

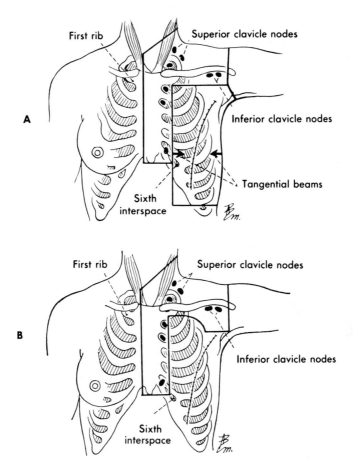

Fig. 11-18. A, Common shape for beams encompassing the internal mammary, paraclavicular, and high axillary nodes. Shaped lead bricks are simple to make for this treatment. **B,** Modification of beams as described in **A,** to permit addition of tangential beams directed to chest wall.

or megavoltage beams must be used with bolus for at least a part of the treatment. A satisfactory schedule is to use bolus on alternate days.

Skin grafting is a common necessity in the performance of mastectomy. The need for irradiating the grafted area frequently arises. Doses recommended in the following discussion will almost certainly slough a newly applied graft. Six to eight weeks should usually elapse before high doses are given to the graft. (See Chapter 3 for a discussion of this problem.)

Dose

Serious early attempts to define the optimum time-dose relationships for carcinoma of the breast were made (Green; Cohen; Friedman and Pearlman; De Moor and associates). From these studies, as well as previously mentioned reports, it was obvious that although the necessary dose was usually high, a wide variation in the dose was required to eradicate the disease. A single curve such as defined by De Moor and associates was insufficient to define this relationship. It is now accepted that a dose of 5000 rad in 5 weeks is sufficient to eradicate microscopic foci of cancer 90% of the time (Fletcher and associates, 1971). The dose required to eradicate large tumor masses of this disease is often higher than skin and subcutaneous tissue can tolerate, thus, the increasing popularity of interstitial techniques and lumpectomy. However, Table 11-7 relates the parameters of tumor volume and dose to incidence of control when external beams are used. The minimum dose recommended for palpable tumor is the highest tolerated by the normal tissues. This dosage level is much better established than is the optimum lethal dose for masses of carcinoma of the breast.

It is generally accepted that 90% of the time a dose of 5000 rad in 5 weeks is sufficient to eradicate subclinical foci left after lumpectomy (Table 11-7). However, for this situation Bataini and associates failed to find a clear-cut dose-response relationship. It is likely that such inconsistencies can be explained by examining the completeness of the lumpectomy. It has been our concern that unless the surgeon is acutely aware of the importance of removing the entire mass with a surrounding margin of grossly normal tissue, the radiation oncologist can no longer be certain he is dealing with subclinical foci. Indeed, it is this concern that has prompted our routine use of boosting doses of 1500 to 2000 rad to the lumpectomy site.

Unresected primary lesions, 2 cm or more in diameter (T2 and T3), are controlled in two thirds of the patients by doses of 8000 rad in 8½ weeks whereas less than one third are controlled by doses of 7000 rad or less (Bataini and associates).

The clinically negative axilla will, on axillary dissection, yield involved lymph nodes about 30% of the time. Doses of 6000 rad in 6 weeks to the unresected negative axilla will produce a control rate at 5 years of 85% (Bataini and associates). After this dose, salvage surgery for recurrences is well tolerated. Clinically positive axillary masses require boosting doses in keeping with total doses shown in Table 11-7.

In view of the high doses that are required to control a high proportion of masses in the breast it is not surprising that lumpectomy and interstitial irradiation have achieved widespread acceptance. When tangential ^{60}Co or megavoltage beams are used with or without bolus on alternate days or for the first half of the treatment, soft tissue doses of 5000 rad in 5 weeks are well tolerated. Each field should be treated each day. The homogeneity and magnitude of the dose in the skin and subcutaneous soft tissues depend on a variety of technical and anatomic factors, that is, compensating filters, bolus, Lucite end-plate, and presence or absence of the breast (Grant and associates; Hanson and Grant). The optimum combination of these factors used with the available ^{60}Co or megavoltage unit is often a matter of one's clinical experience and cannot be otherwise spelled out. Attempts to deliver high doses in short periods using skin-sparing radiations may produce intense fibrosis of the entire volume. Serious damage to the brachial plexus has been reported with such a technique. Furthermore, when fractions are reduced from 5 each week to 3 each week, the total dose must be reduced about 20% if a major increase in soft tissue necrosis is to be avoided (Montague).

The technique of irradiation after simple mastectomy is essentially the same as that after radical mastectomy. We routinely include the chest wall in our treated volume if a simple mastectomy only has been performed. If distant metastases are obvious, the high doses mentioned previously are probably not justified.

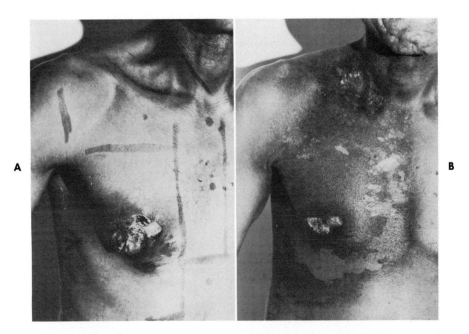

Fig. 11-19. A, Adenocarcinoma of male breast judged inoperable and treated primarily by irradiation. The same ports are used as for cancer of female breast. **B,** At the completion of irradiation (5000 rad in 22 days delivered to regional lymph nodes, ^{60}Co, SSD 80 cm, and 4300 rad in 20 days, surface of chest wall by tangential beams, 280 kv; 1.9 mm Cu hvl). Skin reaction progressed to moderate moist reaction. Patient died 11 months later of generalized metastases with no local regrowth.

On p. 316 we gave the technique for irradiating the intact breast and regional nodes after lumpectomy. This same technique is used for irradiating carcinoma of the male breast (Fig. 11-19).

Palliative irradiation

Despite the controversy regarding the curative value of radiotherapy in carcinoma of the breast, there can be no doubt about its value as a palliative agent. The large ulcerated primary breast tumor can be made to heal or shrink, and axillary or supraclavicular nodes can be eradicated or reduced in size (Fig. 11-20). Painful

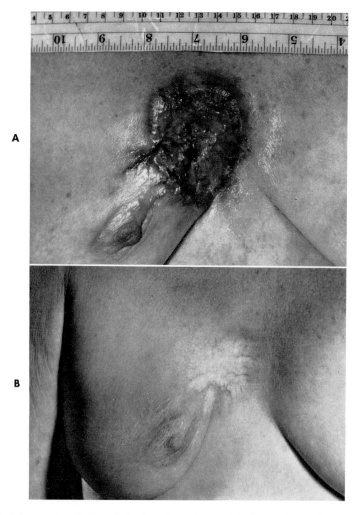

Fig. 11-20. A, Large ulcerated medially placed carcinoma of the breast. It was fixed to the underlying sternum and costal cartilages and was judged inoperable. Small axillary nodes were present. Patient was given dose previously described. **B,** Same patient 2 years later, with no evidence of recurrence either of the primary lesion or in the regional nodes.

osseous metastases respond dramatically with relief of pain in over 70% of the patients, and occasionally recalcification will occur. To arrest bone destruction and thereby decrease pain and prevent or delay pathologic fracture is certainly among the most gratifying types of palliation, both for the patient and for the physician (Figs. 11-21 and 11-22). When a patient with known generalized metastases from carcinoma of the breast complains of pain characteristic of osseous metastases, irradiation of the site of pain is indicated even in the absence of roentgenographic or bone scan evidence of disease. As long as the recognized combined effects of chemotherapy and radiation therapy on normal tissues are taken into consideration, there

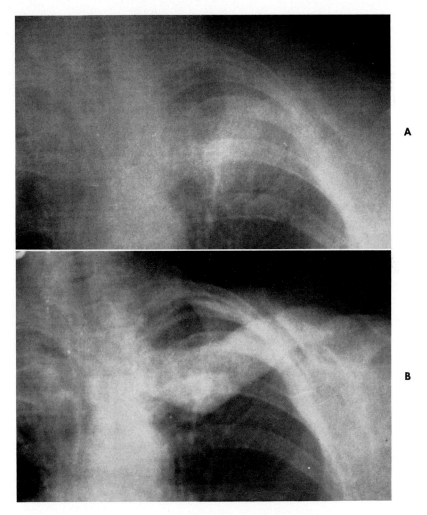

Fig. 11-21. A, Almost complete destruction of left clavicle from widespread carcinoma of the breast. **B,** Same patient 6 months after palliative irradiation of 3000 rad in 3 weeks using 1000 kv; hvl, 3 mm Pb.

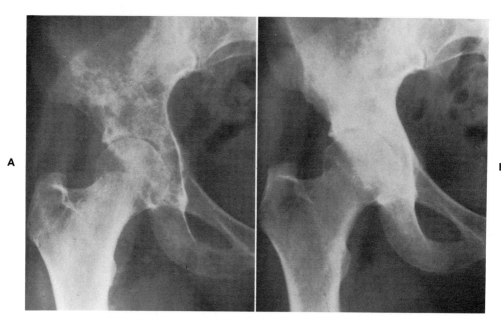

Fig. 11-22. A, Massive destruction of right acetabular area by metastatic adenocarcinoma of breast. **B,** Same patient 10 months after palliative irradiation of 2700 rad to the involved volume in 3 weeks (^{60}Co, 80 cm SSD).

are no contraindications to using these two modalities together. When high doses of radiations are required, agents such as doxorubicin (Adriamycin) should be discontinued as mentioned earlier. Agents such as cyclophosphamide (Cytoxan), bleomycin, and 5-fluorouracil (5-FU) need to be discontinued when certain organ sites are in the high-dose volume (Chapter 1).

Palliative irradiation of the primary breast lesion is not an innocuous treatment. However, some patients will live several years with known metastases. This fact should be kept in mind in planning palliative irradiation of the primary lesion. If survival of 6 months is anticipated, a full course of local irradiation should be considered. Although all areas of potential spread need not be included in the field, the area of irradiation remains large. A relatively high minimal tissue dose is required to produce significant decrease in skin ulceration, size of tumor, or reduction in pain from brachial plexus involvement. No single field arrangement is best for all these patients.

Clinically significant pain-producing osseous metastases will develop in about 50% of those patients in whom curative treatment is not attempted or attempted and failed. About 70% to 80% of those patients having pain from osseous metastases receive good relief after irradiation. About 28% will present radiographic evidence of varying degrees of recalcification (Johnson and associates) (Table 11-9). Osseous metastases are usually satisfactorily treated by single fields or by two fields if long bones of the extremities are to be irradiated. A minimal tissue dose of 2500 to 3500

Table 11-9. Efficacy of radiation therapy in treatment of carcinoma of the breast metastatic to bone*

Author	Number of patients	Subjective improvement (%)	Objective improvement
Bouchard	23	65	6 of 23
Lenz and Fried	81	70	14 of 31
Leddy and Desjardins	92	80	
Garland and associates	79	70	10 of 38
Johnson and associates	148	93	28%
TOTAL	423	72%	31%

*Modified from Chu and associates: Am. J. Roentgenol. **77:**438-447, 1957.

rad in 10 to 15 days is sufficient if medium-sized ports are used. (For a discussion of the effects of irradiation on osseous tissue, see Chapter 21.) Metastases from carcinoma of the breast to abdominal viscera, the lungs, or the brain are usually the cause of death in these patients. The specific volume of soft tissue requiring irradiation and the dose necessary to produce the desired palliation must be weighed in each case. Concurrent hormonal and chemotherapy management should always be evaluated.

Summary

The continued evaluation of therapeutic modalities available for carcinoma of the breast has not answered to the satisfaction of many oncologists the questions concerning the role of modified radical mastectomy with or without irradiation versus the role of various limited operative procedures (simple mastectomy or lumpectomy) in combination with irradiation. It is now obvious that limited masses of cancer cells in either nodes or the breast can be controlled by irradiation in a high proportion of patients. This fact can be effectively employed to increase cure rates, to prolong symptom-free survival, and to decrease the deformity of radical mastectomy without shortening survival. However, indications and techniques continue to be questioned and refined.

Whether the patient lives 1 year or 20 years, control of the cancer in the chest wall and in the regional lymph nodes is a fully justified aim. The argument that cancer of the breast is usually disseminated when the diagnosis is made should not lull radiation oncologists into doing less in patients with apparent local cancer of the breast.

Modified radical mastectomy is the operation chosen by most surgeons for patients with operable lesions. However, we have been increasingly impressed with the results of less radical procedures coupled with radiotherapy.

Our current recommendations for combining modified radical mastectomy and radiation therapy have been discussed. In patients found to be locally inoperable, but who show no distant metastases, we treat the primary lesion and the associated lymph node areas. The cancer will frequently be sufficiently radiosensitive to be locally eradicated. After simple mastectomy or lumpectomy in selected patients, we have elected to irradiate the internal mammary and paraclavicular nodes together with vigorous irradiation of the soft tissues of the chest wall.

Prophylactic systemic chemotherapy for the premenopausal patient at high risk for distant metastases looks encouraging and is justifying a reevaluation of the need for postoperative irradiation in this group. Radiation therapy is highly useful in such patients in treating specific symptoms produced by localized foci. The combinations of radiation therapy with chemotherapy require special consideration of normal tissue tolerance, depending on the drug used and the anatomic site requiring irradiation.

REFERENCES

Ackerman, L. V., and Katzenstein, A. L.: The concept of minimal breast cancer and the pathologist's role in the diagnosis of "early carcinoma," Cancer 39:2755-2763, 1977.

Andreassen, M., Dahl-Iversen, E., and Sorensen, B.: Glandular metastases in carcinoma of the breast, Lancet 1:176-178, 1954.

Aristizabal, S. A., Miller, R. C., Schlichtemeier, A. L., Jones, S. E., and Boone, M. L.: Adriamycin—irradiation cutaneous complications, Int. J. Radiat. Oncol. Biol. Phys. 2:325-332, 1977.

Atkins, H., Hayward, J. L., Klugman, D. J., and Wayte, A. B.: Treatment of early breast cancer: a report after ten years of a clinical trial, Br. Med. J. 2:423-429, 1972.

Baclesse, F.: Roentgen therapy as the sole method of treatment of cancer of the breast, Am. J. Roentgenol. 62:311-319, 1949.

Baclesse, F.: Preoperative irradiation in high and fractionated doses in the treatment of breast cancer with the exclusion of Stage I, J. Radiol. Electrol. 43:826-830, 1962.

Baclesse, F.: Five-year result in 431 breast cancers treated solely by roentgen rays, Ann. Surg. 161:103-104, 1965.

Barker, J. L., Nelson, A. J., and Montague, E. D.: Inflammatory carcinoma of the breast, Radiology 121:173-176, 1976.

Bataini, J. P., Picco, C., Martin, M., and Calle, R.: Relation between time-dose and local control of operable breast cancer treated by tumorectomy and radiotherapy or by radical radiotherapy alone, Cancer 42:2059-2065, 1978.

Black, M. M.: Immunology of breast cancer: clinical implications. Prog. Clin. Cancer 6:115-137, 1975.

Block, G. E., Lampe, I., Vial, A. B., and Coller, F. A.: Therapeutic castration for advanced mammary cancer, Surgery 47:877-884, 1960.

Blumenschein, G. R., Montague, E. D., Eckles, N. E., Hortobagyi, G. N., and Barker, J. L.: Sequential combined modality therapy for inflammatory breast cancer, Breast 2:16-20, 1976.

Bond, W. H.: The influence of various treatments on survival rates in cancer of the breast. In Jarrett, A. S., editor: treatment of carcinoma of the breast, Maidenhead, England, 1967, Syntex Pharmaceuticals.

Bonadonna, G., Brusamolino, E., Valagussa, P., et al: Combination chemotherapy as an adjuvant treatment in operable breast cancer, N. Engl. J. Med. 294:405-410, 1976.

Bouchard, J.: Skeletal metastases in cancer of breast; study of character, incidence and response to roentgen therapy, Am. J. Roentgenol. 54:156-171, 1945.

Bross, I. D., and Blumenson, L. E.: Predictive design of experiments using deep mathematical models, Cancer 28:1637-1650, 1971.

Bruce, J.: The enigma of breast cancer, Cancer 24:1314-1318, 1969.

Butcher, H. R., Seaman, W. B., Eckert, C., and Saltzstein, S.: An assessment of radical mastectomy and postoperative irradiation therapy in the treatment of mammary cancer, Cancer 17:480-485, 1963.

Chu, F. C. H., Sved, D. W., Echer, G. C., Nickson, J. J., and Phillips, R.: Management of advanced breast carcinoma, Am. J. Roentgenol. 77:438-447, 1957.

Chu, F. C., Nisce, L., and Laughlin, J. S.: Treatment of breast cancer with high energy electrons produced by 24 Mev betatron, Radiology 81:871-880, 1962.

Chu, F. C. H., Lin, F. J., Kim, J. H., et al.: Locally recurrent carcinoma of the breast, Cancer 37:2677-2681, 1976.

Clarke, K. H.: A system of dosage estimation for the tangential irradiation of breast without bolus, Br. J. Radiol. 23:593-597, 1950.

Cohen, L.: Radiotherapy in breast cancer, Br. J. Radiol. 25:636-642, 1952.

Cole, M. P.: The place of radiotherapy in the management of early breast cancer; a report of two clinical trials, Br. J. Surg. **51:**261-264, 1964.

Cottier, H., et al: A proposal for a standardized system of reporting human lymph node morphology in relation to immunological function, J. Clin. Pathol. **26:**317-331, 1973.

Crile, G.: Rationale of simple mastectomy without radiation for clinical stage I cancer of the breast, Surg. Gynecol. Obstet. **120:**975-982, 1965.

Crile, G.: The smaller the cancer the bigger the operation? J.A.M.A. **199:**736-738, 1967.

Dahl-Iversen, E., and Tobiassen, T.: Radical mastectomy with parasternal and supraclavicular dissection for mammary carcinoma, Ann. Surg. **157:**170-173, 1963.

Dao, T. L., and Nemoto, T.: The clinical significance of skin recurrence after radical mastectomy in women with cancer of the breast, Surg. Gynecol. Obstet. **117:**447-453, 1963.

DeMoor, N. G., Durbach, D., Levin, J., and Cohen, L.: Radiation therapy in breast cancer: optimal combination of technical factors; analysis of five-year results, Radiology **7:**35-52, 1961.

Diczfalusy, G., Notter, F. E., and Westman, A.: Estrogen excretion in breast cancer patients before and after ovarian irradiation oophorectomy, J. Clin. Endocrinol. **19:**1230-1244, 1959.

Emerson, W. J., Kennedy, B. J., Graham, J. N., and Nathanson, I. T.: Pathology of primary and recurrent carcinoma of the human breast after administration of steroid hormones, Cancer **6:**641-670, 1953.

Fisher, B., Carbone, P., Economou, S. G., et al: L-Phenylalanine mustard (L-PAM) in the management of primary breast cancer. A report of early findings, N. Engl. J. Med. **292:**117-122, 1975.

Fletcher, G. H.: Reflections on breast cancer, Int. J. Radiat. Oncol. Biol. Phys. **1:**769-779, 1976.

Fletcher, G. H., and Montague, E. D.: Radical irradiation of advanced breast cancer, Am. J. Roentgenol. **93:**573-584, 1965.

Fletcher, G. H., Montague, E. D., and White, E. C.: Evaluation of irradiation of the peripheral lymphatics in conjunction with radical mastectomy for cancer of the breast, Cancer **21:**791-797, 1968.

Fletcher, G. H., Montague, E. D., and White, E. C.: Radiation therapy in the definitive management of breast cancer: Oncology 1971, Proceedings of the Tenth International Cancer Congress **6:**48-54, 1971.

Fletcher, G. H., and Shukovsky, L. J., Memoires originaux: the interplay of radiocurability and tolerance in the irradiation of human cancers, J. Radiol. Electrol. **56:**383-400, 1975.

Fletcher, G. H., and Montague, E. D.: Does adequate irradiation of the internal mammary chain and supraclavicular nodes improve survival rates? Int. J. Radiat. Oncol. Biol. Phys. **4:**481-492, 1978.

Friedman, M., and Pearlman, A. W.: Time-dose relationship in irradiation of recurrent cancer of the breast, Am. J. Roentgenol. **73:**986-998, 1955.

Gallager, H. S., and Martin, J. E.: The study of mammary carcinoma by mammography and whole organ sectioning, Cancer **23:**855-873, 1969.

Gallager, H. S., and Martin, J. E.: Early phases in the development of breast cancer, Cancer **24:**1170-1178, 1969.

Garland, L. H., Baker, M., Picard, W. H., and Sisson, M. A.: Roentgen and steroid hormone therapy in mammary cancer metastic to bone, J.A.M.A. **144:**997-1004, 1950.

Garland, L. H., Hill, H. A., Mottram, M. E., and Sisson, M. A.: Cancer of the breast, Surg. Gynecol. Obstet. **98:**700-704, 1954.

Grant, W., Cundiff, J. H., and Hanson, W. F.: Use of auxiliary collimating devices in the treatment for breast cancer with ^{60}Co teletherapy units. I. Dosimetric considerations, Am. J. Roentgenol. Radium Ther. Nucl. Med. **127:**649-652, 1976.

Green, A.: In Saner, F. D.: The breast, Baltimore, 1950, Williams & Wilkins Co.

Guttmann, R.: Radiotherapy in the treatment of primary operable carcinoma of the breast with proved lymph node metastases, Am. J. Roentgenol. **89:**58-63, 1963.

Guttmann, R.: Radiotherapy in locally advanced cancer of the breast, Cancer **20:**1046-1050, 1967.

Haagensen, C. D., and Stout, A. P.: Carcinoma of the breast, results of treatment, Ann. Surg. **116:**801-815, 1942.

Haagensen, C. D., and Stout, A. P.: Carcinoma of the breast, Ann. Surg. **118:**1-32, 1943.

Haagensen, C. D., and Cooley, E.: Treatment of early mammary carcinoma, Ann. Surg. **157:**157-169, 1963.

Haagensen, C. D., Lane, N., Lattes, R., and Bodian, C.: Lobular neoplasia (so-called lobular carcinoma in situ of the breast), Cancer **42:**737-769, 1978.

Handley, R. S., and Thackray, A. C.: Invasion of internal mammary lymph nodes in carcinoma of the breast, Br. Med. J. **1:**61-63, 1954.

Hanson, W. F., and Grant, W.: Use of auxillary collimating devices in the treatment for breast cancer with ^{60}Co teletherapy units. II. Dose to the skin, Am. J. Roentgenol. Radium Ther. Nucl. Med. **127:**653-657, 1976.

Host, H.: Postoperative radiotherapy in breast

cancer, Edinburgh European Radiology Conference, Edinburgh, July, 1976.

Host, H., and Brennhovd, I. O.: The effect of postoperative radiotherapy in breast cancer, Int. J. Radiat. Oncol. Biol. Phys. 2:1061-1067, 1977.

Hultborn, K. A., and Tornberg, B.: Mammary carcinoma. The biologic character of mammary carcinoma studied in 517 cases by a new form of malignancy grading, Acta Radiol. (suppl.) 196: 1-143, 1960.

Huseby, R. A., and Thomas, L. B.: Histological and histochemical alterations in the normal breast tissues of patients with advanced breast cancer being treated with estrogenic hormones, Cancer 7:54-74, 1954.

Kaae, S., and Johansen, H.: Simple mastectomy plus postoperative irradiation by the method of McWhirter for mammary carcinoma, Ann. Surg. 157:175-179, 1963.

Kennedy, B. J.: The role of castration in breast cancer, Arch. Surg. 88:743-746, 1964.

Kister, J., Sommers, S. C., Haagensen, C. D., and Cooley, E.: Re-evaluation of blood-vessel invasion as a prognostic factor in carcinoma of the breast, Cancer 19:1213-1216, 1966.

Kolar, J., Bek, V., and Vrabec, R.: Hypoplasia of the growing breast after contact x-ray therapy for cutaneous angiomas, Arch. Dermatol. 96:427-430, 1967.

Lacour, J., Bucalossi, P., Cacers, E., et al: Radical mastectomy versus radical mastectomy plus internal mammary dissection, Cancer 37:206-314, 1976.

Lane, N., Goksel, H., Salerno, R. A., and Haagensen, C. D.: Clinico-pathologic analysis of surgical curability of breast cancers, minimum ten-year study of personal series, Ann. Surg. 153:483-498, 1961.

Leddy, E. T., and Desjardins, A. U.: Treatment of inoperable, recurrent and metastatic carcinoma of breast, Am. J. Roentgenol. 35:371-383, 1936.

Lenz, M.: Tumor dosage and results in roentgen therapy of cancer of the breast, Am. J. Roentgenol. 56:67-74, 1946.

Lenz, M., and Fried, J. R.: Metastases to skeleton, brain and spinal cord from cancer of breast; effect of radiotherapy, Ann. Surg. 93:278-293, 1931.

Levitt, S. A., McHugh, R. B., and Song, C. W.: Radiotherapy in the postoperative treatment of operable cancer of the breast, Cancer 39:933-940, 1976.

Lumb, G.: Changes in carcinoma of the breast following irradiation, Br. J. Surg. 38:82-93, 1950.

MacDonald, I.: Sex steroids for palliation of disseminated mammary carcinoma, J.A.M.A. 172: 1288-1289, 1960.

McCredie, J. A., Inch, W. R., and Sutherland, R. M.: Effect of postoperative radiotherapy on peripheral blood lymphocytes in patients with carcinoma of the breast, Cancer 29:349-356, 1972.

McDivitt, R. W.: Tumors of the breast, AFIP Atlas of Tumor Pathology. 2 series Fascicle 2 (pp. 61-62), Armed Forces Institute of Pathology, 1968.

McKinnon, N. E.: Limitations in diagnosis and treatment of breast and other cancers, Can. Med. Assoc. J. 73:614-625, 1955.

McWhirter, R.: A comparision of the radiosensitivity of primary tumours and their regional lymphatic metastases, Br. J. Radiol. 27:649-651, 1954.

McWhirter, R.: A comparison of the radiosensitivtherapy in the treatment of breast cancer, Br. J. Radiol. 28:128-139, 1955.

Meyer, K. K.: Radiation-induced lymphocyte-immune deficiency, Arch. Surg. 101:114-121, 1970.

Montague, E. D.: Experience with altered fractionation in radiation therapy of breast cancer, Radiology 90:962-966, 1968.

Nathanson, I. T.: Sex hormones and castration in advanced breast cancer, Radiology 56:535-552, 1951.

Nathanson, I. T., Rice, C., and Meigs, J. V.: Hormonal studies in artificial menopause produced by roentgen rays, Am. J. Obstet. Gynecol. 40: 936-945, 1940.

Order, S. E.: Beneficial and detrimental effects of therapy on immunity in breast cancer, Int. J. Radiat. Oncol. Biol. Phys. 2:377-380, 1977.

Pathology Working Group. Breast Cancer Task Force. National Cancer Institute: Standardized management of breast specimens, Am. J. Clin. Pathol. 60:789, 1973.

Park, W. W., and Lees, J. C.: The absolute curability of cancer of the breast, Surg. Gynecol. Obstet. 93:129-152, 1951.

Paterson, R., and Russell, M. H.: Clinical trials in malignant disease. II. Breast cancer: value of irradiation of the ovaries, J. Fac. Radiol. 10:130-133, 1959.

Paterson, R., and Russell, M. H.: Clinical trials in malignant disease. III. Breast cancer: evaluation of postoperative radiotherapy, J. Fac. Radiol. 10: 175-180, 1959.

Perez, C. A., Stewart, C. C., and Wagner, B.: Role of the regional lymph nodes in tumor immunity. Interaction of radiation and host immune defense mechanisms in malignancy, Conference, March 23-27, 1974, Greenbrier, W. Va.

Peters, M. V.: Carcinoma of the breast—wedge resection and irradiation, J.A.M.A. 200:134-135, 1967.

Phillips, T. L.: Chemical modification of radiation effects, Cancer **39**:987-999, 1977.

Pierquin, B., Baillet, F., and Wilson, J. F.: Radiation therapy in the management of primary breast cancer, Am. J. Roentgenol. Radium Ther. Nucl. Med. **127**:645-648, 1976.

Prosnitz, L. R., Goldenberg, I. S., Packard, R. A., et al: Radiation therapy as initial treatment for early stage cancer of the breast without mastectomy, Cancer **39**:917-923, 1977.

Robbins, C. G., Lucas, J. C., Fracchia, A. A., et al: An evaluation of postoperative prophylactic radiation therapy in breast cancer, Surg. Gynecol. Obstet. **122**:979-982, 1966.

Schryver, A. D.: The Stockholm breast cancer trial: preliminary report of a randomized study concerning the value of pre-operative or postoperative radiotherapy in operable disease, Int. J. Radiat. Oncol. Biol. Phys. **1**:601-609, 1976.

Silverberg, S. G., Chitale, A. R., and Levitt, S. H.: Prognostic significance of tumor margins in mammary carcinoma, Arch. Surg. **102**:450-454, 1971.

Smith, J. A., Gamez-Araujo, J. J., Gallager, H. S., et al: Carcinoma of the breast, Cancer **39**:527-532, 1977.

Spratt, J. S.: Locally recurrent cancer after radical mastectomy, Cancer **20**:1051-1053, 1967.

Stewart, J. R., Cohn, K. E., Fajardo, L. F., Hancock, E. W., and Kaplan, H. S.: Radiation-induced heart disease, Radiology **89**:302-310, 1967.

Stjernsward, J.: Decreased survival related to irradiation postoperatively in early operable breast cancer, Lancet **2**:1285-1286, 1974.

Taylor, S. G.: Endocrine ablation is disseminated mammary carcinoma, Surg. Gynecol. Obstet. **115**:443-448, 1962.

Turner, C. W., and Gomez, E. T.: The radiosensitivity of the cells of the mammary gland, Am. J. Roentgenol. **36**:79-93, 1936.

Urban, J. A.: Radical mastectomy with en bloc in continuity resection of the internal mammary lymph node chain, Proceedings of the Third National Cancer Conference, Philadelphia, 1957, J. B. Lippincott Co.

Urban, J. A.: What is the rationale for an extended radical procedure in early cases? J.A.M.A. **199**:742-743, 1967.

Wallgren, A., Arner, O., Bergstrom, J., Blomstedt, B., Granberg, P., Karnstrom, L., Raf, L., and Silfversward, C.: Preoperative radiotherapy in operable breast cancer, Cancer **42**:1120-1125, 1978.

Watson, T. A.: Cancer of the breast, Am. J. Roentgenol. **96**:547-559, 1966.

Wheeler, J., Enterline, H. T., Roseman, J. M., et al: Lobular carcinoma in situ of the breast. Long term followup, Cancer **34**:554-563, 1974.

White, W. C.: The problem of local recurrence after radical mastectomy for carcinoma, Surgery **19**:149-153, 1946.

White, E. C., Fletcher, G. H., and Clark, R. L.: Surgical experience with preoperative irradiation for carcinoma of the breast, Ann. Surg. **155**:948-956, 1962.

Williams, I. G.: The role of radiotherapy and surgery in the treatment of primary breast cancer, Proceedings of the Third National Cancer Conference, Philadelphia, 1957, J. B. Lippincott Co.

Williams, I. G., and Cunningham, G. J.: Histological changes in irradiated carcinoma of the breast, Br. J. Radiol. **24**:123-133, 1951.

Wise, L., Mason, A. Y., and Ackerman, L. V.: Local excision and irradiation: an alternative method of the treatment of early mammary cancer, Ann. Surg. **174**:392-399, 1971.

Zimmerman, K. W., Montague, E. D., and Fletcher, G. H.: Frequency, anatomical distribution and management of local recurrences after definitive therapy for breast cancer, Cancer **19**:67-74, 1966.

Zimmerman, A., et al: The problem of immunity to breast cancers. Progress in clinical and biological research. In Montague, A. C. W., editor: cancer. vol. 12. New York, 1977, Alan R. Liss, Inc.

12

The gastrointestinal tract

Carcinomas of the gastrointestinal tract including those of the esophagus, stomach, pancreas, liver, and large intestine account for a large proportion of cancer deaths each year. The histologic types vary from the predominately squamous cell carcinomas of the esophagus to the adenocarcinomas of the large bowel. The radiation oncologist is confronted with the high incidence of early distant metastases from esophageal cancers and the seriously dose-limiting characteristics of the abdominal viscera. Although much heralded, the drug 5-fluorouracil has proven a disappointment in the management of tumors of the gastrointestinal tract. This has led radiation oncologists to reappraise the role of ionizing radiations in the treatment of these tumors. Irradiation of cancers of the gallbladder, biliary tract, and pancreas is usually considered as purely palliative, but the mere fact that palliation is possible is a major step forward in the treatment of these otherwise dismal tumors. The indications for irradiation and the results of treatment vary widely with each anatomic site. Thus carcinoma of the upper two thirds of the esophagus has its greatest chance for cure and palliation with external beam irradiation, whereas carcinoma of the colon remains primarily a surgically treated disease. Except for gastrointestinal tract tumors developing in the esophagus or pelvis, there are severe dose-limiting problems that will continue to restrict the role of radiation therapy.

THE ESOPHAGUS
Response of the normal esophagus to irradiation

The esophagus is lined with stratified squamous epithelium similar to that of the buccal mucosa. This epithelium, together with the thin submucosa and muscularis mucosae, forms longitudinal folds imparting a distensible character to the esophagus. The external muscle layer consists of striated fibers in the superior portion of the esophagus and smooth muscle fibers in its lower portion. This muscle layer is thin, varying in thickness from 0.5 to 2.2 mm. Surrounding loose connective tissue separates the esophagus from other mediastinal structures. Lymph drainage of the upper third of the esophagus empties into the supraclavicular and lower cervical nodes. That of the lower third usually empties inferiorly into nodes surrounding the cardia or along the lesser curvature of the stomach. Lymph drainage of the middle third

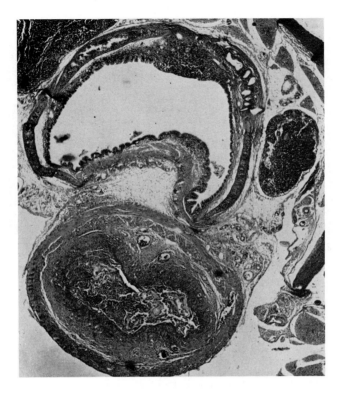

Fig. 12-1. This section was taken 12 days after single dose of 1400 rad directed to the rat's mediastinum (220 kv; hvl, 1 mm Cu; TSD, 50 cm). As noted by Lacassagne, esophageal epithelium is severely damaged, whereas tracheal epithelium is apparently normal.

may be similar to that of the upper third but more frequently simulates that of the lower third.

The epithelium of the esophagus is moderately radiosensitive, and from the meager evidence available we believe its sensitivity is similar to that of the buccal mucosa (Fig. 12-1). Reepithelization of the normal esophagus will vary with the intensity of the irradiation. A single massive dose of 3000 rad delivered to the rat's esophagus produces a complete desquamation of the epithelium in 10 days (Jennings). By the fourteenth day, reepithelization starts from the edge of the défect. In addition, islands of epithelization can be seen in the center of the defect. This probably starts from local residual resistant cells rather than seeding from other sites. In irradiating patients with bronchogenic carcinoma, the normal esophagus is frequently unavoidably included in the field. Doses of the level of 5000 to 6000 rad in 6 to 8 weeks are delivered to these segments of the esophagus. This produces a moderately severe dysphagia that will usually subside within 1 to 2 weeks after cessation of irradiation. Esophagrams taken at the height of the acute reaction will show the margins of the barium column to be serrated (Fig. 12-2). Reepithelization is rapid, and several weeks later the new epithelium may appear normal. The submuco-

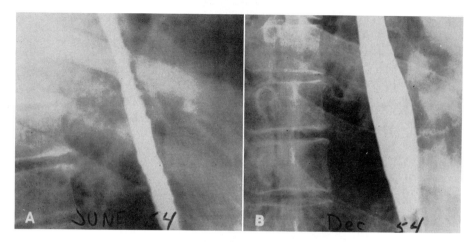

Fig. 12-2. Esophagram during acute radiation esophagitis. **A,** The serrated margins, a common finding after such irradiation, according to Seaman. **B,** Complete return to normal 6 months later. (W. U. negs. 56-558 and 56-559; from Seaman, W. B., and Ackerman, L. V.: Radiology **68:**534-541, 1957.)

sa thickens largely from edema. With excessively high doses the edema may be extreme (Fig. 12-3).

The external muscle layer tolerates radiations well, but even here excessively high doses produce striking damage. The muscle cells may show an absence of cellular delineation and a loss of nuclear detail. No symptoms have been attributed directly to the muscle damage. However, if doses have been excessive, the combined repair of all these radiation-induced lesions may produce esophageal stenosis, a tendency to ulcerate, and even esophageal perforation. In rats, muscle damage is sufficient to produce weakness of the esophageal wall. Esophageal diverticula with herniation of the mucosa through the defect are common (Jennings). This has not been reported in man. Phillips and Margolis concluded that a dose of 6300 rad in 30 fractions (1850 rets) would produce late clinically significant esophageal damage (ulceration or stenosis) in 5% of the patients. The incidence of damage is increased to 50% with 6650 rad in 30 fractions (2000 rets). However, the small number of patients makes these data very uncertain.

Radiotherapy of carcinoma of the esophagus

Progress in preoperative and postoperative care, anesthesia, and antibiotics has greatly reduced the mortality of surgery of the esophagus. However, the morbidity and mortality of esophagectomy are still high, and cure rates remain depressingly low. As will be seen later, there has also been progress in radiotherapy technique that has encouraged a more enthusiastic radiotherapeutic approach. Some increase in the number of cured patients has followed these efforts, but here also survival rates do not justify much optimism. In desperation, combinations of radiation therapy and surgery have been studied, but the cure rates remain poor.

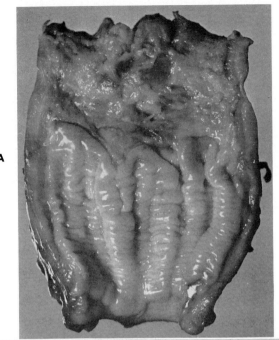

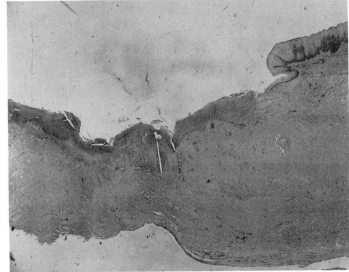

Fig. 12-3. A, Gross specimen of the esophagus from patient irradiated for carcinoma of lung. The esophagus was included in irradiated volume. Calculated dose to esophagus was 7100 rad in 48 days through 6 × 10 cm skin portals (24 mev betatron). **B,** Low-power enlargement of section taken from specimen shown in **A.** Note sharp edge separating area of necrosis from markedly edematous esophageal wall. (From Seaman, W. B., and Ackerman, L. V.: Radiology **68:**534-541, 1957.)

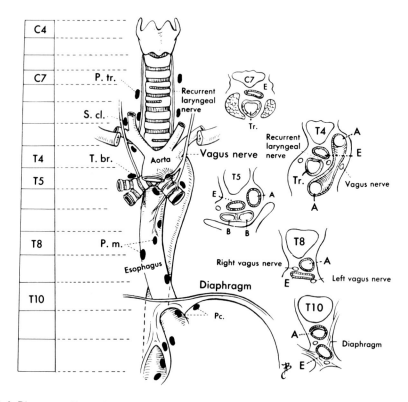

Fig. 12-4. Diagrams of important anatomic relations of the esophagus. These structures are invaded early and should be frequently included in volume of irradiation: *P. tr.,* Paratracheal; *S. cl.,* supraclavicular; *T. br.,* tracheobronchial; *P. m.,* posteromediastinal; *Pc.,* paracardial.

Like the mucosa of the oral cavity, the mucosa of the esophagus may develop leukoplakia, carcinoma in situ, or single or multiple foci of invasive squamous cell carcinoma. In the oral cavity, larynx, and cervix, squamous cell carcinomas are frequently radiocurable. Were it not for the tendency of the esophageal neoplasm to metastasize early, we might expect results similar to those obtained for histologically similar lesions elsewhere. The radiotherapeutic approach to carcinoma of the esophagus is based on the following five facts:

1. Carcinoma of the esophagus is nearly always squamous cell in type and frequently is poorly differentiated. The primary lesion is sufficiently radiosensitive to be locally radiocurable in well over half the patients treated radically.
2. The thin submucosal and muscular layers of the esophagus provide little resistance to the invasion of neighboring vital structures. These structures are rarely resectable but are easily included in the irradiated volume (Fig. 12-4).
3. Vigorous irradiation of this volume is usually well tolerated in those patients capable of swallowing liquids.
4. Evidence is now available indicating that lymph node metastases from squamous cell carcinoma of the esophagus can at least occasionally be controlled by irradiation.

5. Although improved, the mortality and morbidity of curative surgery remain high.

The following factors limit the success of irradiation:

1. Local lymph nodes are involved early. Such node metastases demand a high dose over a larger volume.
2. Distant metastases are common.
3. Nutritional deficiencies, the invasion of vital structures, and the development of fistulae leave the patient in a poor general condition.

To some extent the same factors limit the success of surgery. When nodes containing metastases are found in the operative specimen, the prognosis is extremely poor. Cancer of the esophagus is obviously unresectable in the presence of distant metastases or fixation to the trachea, bronchus, aorta, or vertebrae. Even when resection of a squamous cell carcinoma is technically possible, occult extensions beyond the limits of excision are usually present. Only 1% to 4% of all patients seen with squamous cell carcinoma are cured by surgery. Only 5% to 20% of patients selected for resection of squamous cell carcinoma are cured. With resection, adenocarcinomas of the esophagus are more frequently cured than squamous cell carcinomas. For this reason survival rates of the two cell types should be reported separately. Only in this way will the relative merits of radiation therapy for the treatment of squamous cell carcinoma of the esophagus become clear (Millburn and associates). We agree with Millburn and associates that there is a strong argument for radiation therapy of squamous cell carcinoma for all portions of the esophagus. Surgery remains the unquestioned treatment of choice for the adenocarcinomas.

The fact that 30% of the patients with squamous cell carcinoma show only a localized cancer at autopsy has kept alive the search for a more effective treatment. Bloedorn and Kasdorf have presented some interesting statistics relative to carcinoma of the esophagus. At least 30% of the patients have demonstrable distant metastasis on admission. Of 100 consecutive patients with carcinoma of the esophagus (all stages and all portions of the esophagus), seventy already have metastasis to the mediastinal lymph nodes, abdominal lymph nodes, or both. Thirty have metastasis to subdiaphragmatic nodes with or without mediastinal node involvement. If the primary lesion is in the lower half of the esophagus, abdominal lymph nodes are involved in 35%. These nodes are involved 15% of the time when the primary lesion is in the upper half of the esophagus. Of those patients selected for thoracotomy, 25% show gross local extraesophageal visceral invasion, and all of these have metastasis to lymph nodes.

When first seen, roughly 40% of the patients are clinically ineligible for radical treatment because of advanced local cancer or distant metastasis. On the other hand, surgical and autopsy data suggest that between 25% and 30% of all patients are still potentially curable by virtue of a limited (apparently resectable) primary cancer and metastasis apparently confined to regional lymph nodes.

Although such data are invaluable in developing new treatment policies, they have not directed radiation oncologists to procedures leading to an increased cure rate.

CLINICAL STAGING. A meaningful, well-accepted clinical stage classification for carcinoma of the esophagus has been slow in appearing. Following are the suggestions of The American Joint Committee (1978).

TNM CLASSIFICATION*

T—Primary tumor

T0	No demonstrable tumor in the esophagus
TIS	Carcinoma in situ
T1	A tumor 5 cm or less of esophageal length, produces no obstruction,† and has no circumferential involvement and no extraesophageal spread‡
T2	A tumor more than 5 cm in esophageal length with no extraesophageal spread‡ or a tumor of any size that produces obstruction† or that involves the entire circumference and with no extraesophageal spread
T3	Any tumor with extraesophageal spread‡

N—Nodal involvement

N0	No clinically palpable nodes
N1	Movable, unilateral, palpable nodes
N2	Movable, bilateral, palpable nodes
N3	Fixed nodes

Thoracic esophagus

NX	Regional lymph nodes for the upper, midthoracic, and lower thoracic esophagus that are not ordinarily accessible for clinical evaluation (clinical evaluation)
N0	No positive nodes (surgical evaluation)
N1	Positive nodes (surgical evaluation)

M—Distant metastasis

MX	Not assessed
M0	No (known) distant metastasis§
M1	Distant metastasis present

STAGE GROUPING

Stage I	TIS N0 M0	Carcinoma in situ
	T1 N0 M0 ⎱ T1 NX M0 ⎰	Tumor in any region of the esophagus that involves 5 cm or less of esophageal length, produces no obstruction, has no extraesophageal spread, does not involve the entire circumference, and shows no regional lymph node metastases or remote metastases

---

*From the American Joint Committee for Cancer Staging and End Results Reporting: Manual for staging of cancer, Chicago, 1978, Whiting Press.

†Roentgenographic evidence of significant impediment to the passage of liquid contrast material past the tumor or endoscopic evidence of esophageal obstruction.

‡Extension of cancer outside the esophagus is seen by clinical, roentgenographic, or endoscopic evidence of the following:

1. Recurrent laryngeal, phrenic, or sympathetic nerve involvement
2. Fistula formation
3. Involvement of the tracheal or bronchial tree
4. Vena cava or azygos vein obstruction
5. Malignant effusion—mediastinal widening itself is not evidence of extraesophogeal spread

§In the cervical esophagus any lymph node involvement other than that of cervical or supraclavicular lymph nodes is considered distant metastasis. For the thoracic esophagus any cervical, supraclavicular, scalene, or abdominal lymph nodes are considered distant metastasis.

Stage II   A tumor of any size with no extraesophageal spread and no distant metastasis

Cervical esophagus

T1	N1	M0	
T1	N2	M0	Any tumor with palpable, movable, regional nodes
T2	N1	M0	
T2	N2	M0	
T2	N0	M0	A tumor >5 cm in length with negative nodes

Thoracic esophagus

T2	NX	M0	Lymph nodes cannot be assessed (clinical-diagnostic evaluation)
T2	N0	M0	A tumor more than 5 cm in length or a tumor of any size with obstruction or circumferential involvement with no lymph node involvement (postsurgical treatment-pathologic evaluation)

Stage III   Any esophageal cancer at any level with

Any T3	Distant metastases
Any N3 (cervical)	Extraesophageal spread
Any N1 (thoracic)	Fixed lymph node metastases
Any M1	Any intrathoracic esophageal carcinoma including either upper and midthoracic region or lower thoracic region with any positive findings in regional lymph nodes

CONTROL OF THE PRIMARY LESION AND REGIONAL METASTASES. Control of the primary lesion by radiotherapy is not unusual. Watson and Brown emphasized this point when they reported the microscopic findings in four autopsies. The patients had been given vigorous mediastinal irradiation. None had persistence of the primary neoplasm. We believe these findings are common after complete irradiation. The majority of such patients will die with both local and distant lymph node metastases. However, good palliation is provided in these cases. We have given postoperative irradiation to vital mediastinal structures known to contain tumor, but at autopsy no tumor could be found in these structures. For this reason we believe that extraesophageal infiltration can be controlled in a significant proportion of patients in whom no resection is done as well as in those in whom resection is carried out.

Few data are available relative to the eradication of metastatic nodes in the irradiated volume. We know from the results of radical surgery that local nodes are rarely the only nodes involved. We have had one patient with biopsy-proved supraclavicular lymph node metastases from carcinoma of the esophagus live over 4 years after irradiation only. Others have reported 5-year survivals of such patients (Marcial and associates). We know also that lymph node metastases from carcinoma of the lung can occasionally be controlled. As a result of this knowledge, should the areas of known lymph drainage—that is, the supraclavicular and epigastric regions—be radiated routinely? We believe that the supraclavicular areas should be irradiated, but irradiation of the draining abdominal nodes has not increased the cure rate.

After irradiating all except terminal patients, Marcial and associates concluded that it was impossible at present to define the criteria for selecting patients for irradiation. The statement that once obstruction is complete, radiotherapy is not indicated should not be accepted until one is certain the obstruction is not produced by an exophytic lesion. Furthermore, symptoms related to tracheal, bronchial, or nerve involvement may be prevented or delayed by radiotherapy even though obstruction remains the major symptom.

PREOPERATIVE IRRADIATION. Poor control by either resection alone or irradiation alone has naturally led to combinations of the two modalities. The various general aspects of preoperative irradiation were discussed in Chapter 2. Just how the combination of modalities might act to improve survival in patients with carcinoma of the esophagus is not known. Many techniques are feasible, but optimum doses and intervals have not been defined. We know from the results of both surgery and radiotherapy alone that cure is infrequent. This suggests that if preoperative irradiation is to improve cure rates, it must eradicate extraesophageal cancer, that is, that disease in nodes or fascial planes. It follows that the volume requiring preoperative irradiation is large, and it is likely that the optimum dose is high.

Preoperative irradiation for carcinoma of the esophagus has been tested with a variety of dose-time factors. Nakayama and associates used doses of 2000 rad in 3 days. Small volumes encompassing the primary cancer were used, and surgery was performed 4 to 7 days later. At the other end of the dosage spectrum is the work of Doggett and associates. They irradiated large volumes, which included not only the primary cancer but also the mediastinal and upper abdominal nodes. Doses of 3500 to 4400 rad in 4 weeks were given to the total volume with boosting doses of 1500 to 2200 rad given to the primary lesion. Surgery was performed after 4 to 5 weeks. They concluded that no patients benefited from the combined therapeutic approach when the tumor was proved to involve adjacent mediastinal structures or had metastasized to upper abdominal nodes. Akakura and associates reported slightly better experience with a similar technique. Parker and Gregorie advocate preoperative doses of 4500 rad (volume unspecified). In their experience, after using surgery alone, irradiation alone, and preoperative irradiation, the best results were obtained with the combination of two modalities (12% 2-year survivors).

The large size of the esophageal mass in most patients would seem to call for much higher doses of radiations than are commonly recommended. There are no good data on this subject, but lesions 8 to 10 cm in length are common. If our experience with squamous cell carcinoma in other anatomic sites is a valid guide, we can hardly expect doses in the range of 6000 rad in 6 weeks to control a significant proportion of such large cancerous masses. Even so, Pearson concluded that about 50% of his patients developed local recurrence following such doses, and Guernsey and Knudsen found no residual cancer in seven of twenty-three patients given slightly higher doses. For these reasons combinations of irradiation and surgery might have some advantage over either one alone. Yet sporadic attempts to use preoperative or postoperative irradiation have yielded little to justify their recommendation. Nakayama and Kinoshita, Marks and associates, and Parker and Gregorie recommended combined treatment whereas Goodner and Groves and Rodriguez-Antunez failed to find it useful. Fraser and associates used preoperative doses of 5000 rad in 5 weeks to more than 6000 rad in 6 weeks and reported four of eleven patients free of disease at 5 or more years. They found no increase in cure rates with postoperative "salvage" irradiation.

The potential of combinations of irradiation and surgery as recommended by Fraser and associates must be weighed against the potential of irradiation alone as recommended by Pearson.

TECHNIQUE. In the esophagus, as elsewhere, the routes of tumor spread define the volume requiring irradiation. The longitudinal extent of spread is impossible to determine by films or by palpation (Scanlon and associates). Grossly submucosal and periesophageal lymphatic permeation is frequently undetectable. Many surgeons have been deceived by such spread and have transected the tumor. For this reason we believe it is usually advisable to irradiate generous, apparently normal, margins of the esophagus. The entire length of the esophagus should be irradiated for the longer lesions. Spread in depth is equally difficult to assess unless the tumor is far advanced, producing nerve paralyses or obvious fixation to neighboring organs. For this reason the irradiated volume should always extend laterally at least 4 cm on each side of the middle of the esophagus (Fig. 12-5). A similar margin anteroposteriorly is advisable.

The only technique by which this cylindrical volume measuring 18 to 20 cm long and 6 to 8 cm in diameter can be adequately irradiated is with external irradiation. Neither interstitial techniques nor linear sources in an esophageal catheter can possibly produce as desirable a dose distribution. With external irradiation, the volume can be irradiated homogeneously. The minimum dose to the volume should be at least 5000 rad delivered in 5 weeks (Marcial and associates; Pearson, 1977). The

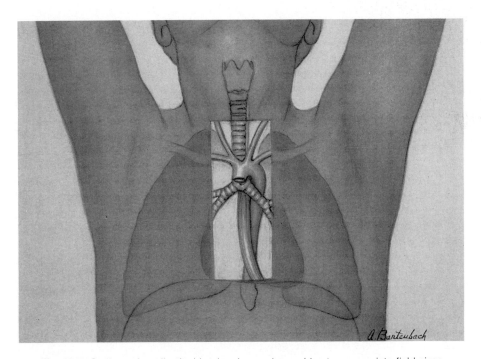

Fig. 12-5. Outlines of mediastinal landmarks used as guides to appropriate field sizes.

maximum should rarely exceed 6500 rad in 8 weeks (Phillips and Margolis). This means a daily dose of 180 to 200 rad to the volume using ^{60}Co or megavoltage beams.

We have favored irradiation of the entire esophagus and contiguous supradiaphragmatic node areas to a dose of 4500 rad at the rate of 180 rad per day through anterior and posterior opposed portals (each port treated each day). Following this the treatment portals are simulated with the patient in a prone position, using a cross-table lateral film and filling the esophagus with barium. Using this technique the esophagus usually moves from 1 to 5 cm anterior to its location in the supine position. A rotational technique with narrow beams is used to deliver an additional 2000 rad. With this technique the dose to the spinal cord is kept to a minimum. For lesions involving the posterior pharyngeal wall above the cricoid and for lesions of the upper cervical esophagus, we have favored a combination of anterior and posterior portals supplemented after the first 5000 rad by posterior oblique beams or when possible the lateral beams described by Stevens and associates. Whatever the combination of ports the dose to the spinal cord should be limited to 5000 rad given at the rate of 180 rad per day. Millburn and associates reported that one of their surviving patients developed symptoms of cord damage. Pearson (1971) had no such damage in any of his ninety-one patients.

Formerly, for patients with severe obstruction, we encouraged a preirradiation bypass procedure. With experience we have lost our enthusiasm for this procedure. The colon or stomach in the substernal location complicates the beam arrangement,

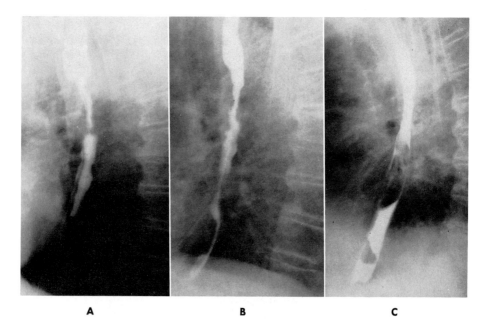

| A | B | C |

Fig. 12-6. Lateral esophagram of patient with proved squamous cell carcinoma of the middle third of the esophagus. **A,** Patient was treated by a rotational technique. **B,** Same patient at end of irradiation. **C,** Same patient 14 months after irradiation.

since they must also be avoided. Furthermore, barium in the intact esophagus is convenient, if not essential, for confirming beam alignment. In spite of arguments to the contrary, we have found gastrostomy to be the best route for maintaining nutrition of patients unable to take adequate nutrition by mouth or nasogastric tube.

PROGNOSIS AND RESULTS. Some improvement in swallowing may be noticed as early as 2 weeks after the beginning of treatment. Swallowing, although slightly painful, is frequently otherwise nearly normal by the end of irradiation. Dysphagia from the desquamation of esophageal epithelium will usually begin during the third week and reach a peak near the end of irradiation. After irradiation, reepithelization begins early and proceeds rapidly from the periphery of the desquamated surface and from islands of epithelium within the boundaries of the area. An esophagram taken near the end of therapy will usually show a widening of the stenotic defect, and on fluoroscopy the walls will appear less rigid. The film may appear normal. The

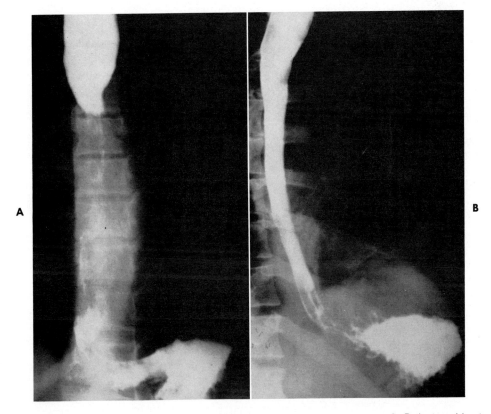

Fig. 12-7. Esophagram of patient with advanced carcinoma of the esophagus. **A,** Patient could not maintain his nutrition by mouth. Gastrostomy was performed 2 weeks before irradiation. By a rotational technique, patient was given a calculated 4900 rad in 46 days to a cylinder 6.5 × 18 cm centered on the lesion. **B,** Same patient 6 months later. The gastrostomy is closed, and the patient gained weight.

lesion will generally continue to regress for the next 3 to 4 weeks (Figs. 12-6 and 12-7).

Perforation with fatal mediastinitis is a common occurrence in the natural course of this disease (Fig. 12-8). If tumor has already destroyed the full thickness of the esophageal wall, we believe mediastinitis will soon follow regardless of whether irradiation is given. If, during treatment, a patient develops a rapid pulse with little

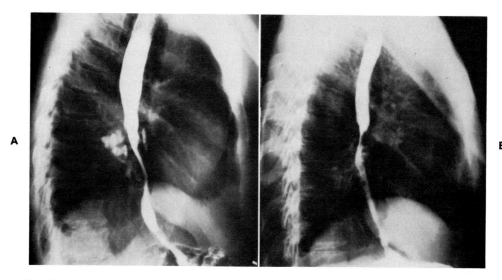

Fig. 12-8. A, Preirradiation esophagram of a patient with biopsy-proved squamous cell carcinoma of the esophagus. Perforation of esophagus has occurred. **B,** Two months after an esophageal dose of 5400 rad in 5 weeks (^{60}Co, SSD 80 cm, 6 × 15 cm portals). The perforations have closed.

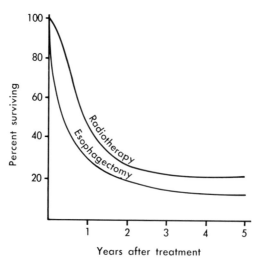

Fig. 12-9. Comparison of survival rates obtained for carcinoma of the esophagus. (Modified from Pearson, J. G.: Cancer **39:**882-890, 1977.)

or no fever and with dull substernal pain, perforation is likely to have occurred. The prognosis is very poor in such patients. Antibiotics may assist such a patient in recovering from one episode only to have another episode end fatally within a few days. Progression of the mediastinitis and extension of the cancer to the walls of major blood vessels may lead to rupture of the vessels and rapid death. Although radiotherapy has been blamed for the rupture of such arteries (Marcial-Rojas and Castro), we believe infiltrating cancer is invariably responsible. Figures indicate a larger number of cures of the middle third have been obtained by surgery. The reason for this is not that surgery is necessarily more successful but that surgery is more often applied to limited lesions of this area. We have no hesitation in recommending primary radiotherapy for limited cancers of the middle third.

The cure rates for carcinoma of the lower third of the esophagus were mentioned previously. The importance of cell type is revealed for this segment when the squamous cell carcinomas and the adenocarcinomas are considered separately (Millburn and associates). About half the surgical cures for the entire esophagus are adenocarcinomas from the lower third. Yet adenocarcinomas comprise only about 10% of all carcinomas of the esophagus. Millburn and associates have argued that all squamous cell carcinomas, including those of the lower third, should be treated by irradiation. Certainly radiation therapy should be given an adequate trial for squamous cell carcinomas of the lower third.

The results of radiation therapy in the treatment of all carcinomas of the esophagus have been reported by Dickson and by Pearson (1977). Pearson's results are shown in Table 12-1, and his total experience is illustrated graphically in Figs. 12-9 and 12-10. The results of various workers are shown in Table 12-2.

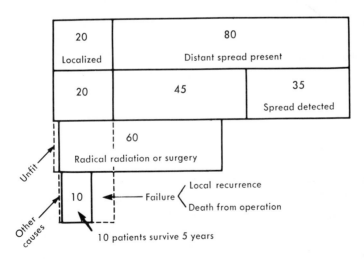

Fig. 12-10. Of any 100 typical patients as they present with esophageal cancer in the entire community of Edinburgh, 35% are demonstrably unsuitable for any radical treatment. No more than twenty are believed to have tumor truly confined to esophagus, and no more than ten of these will be alive 5 years later. Of the 60% of patients with squamous cell carcinoma selected for radical irradiation, 17% survived 5 years (48 5-year survivals from 288 radically irradiated patients). (From Pearson, J. G.: Cancer **39**:882-890, 1977.)

Table 12-1. Comparison of results of surgery and radiotherapy in the treatment of carcinoma of the esophagus*

	Surgery	Radiotherapy
Cervical esophagus	4/25 (25%)	19/76 (25%)
Upper half of thoracic esophagus	12/126 (9%)	17/109 (16%)
Lower half of thoracic esophagus	32/281 (11%)	12/103 (12%)
TOTAL	48/432 (11%)	48/288 (17%)

*From Pearson, J. G.: Cancer **39**:882-890, 1977.

Table 12-2. Comparison of survival rates obtained for squamous cell carcinoma of the esophagus*†

Author	Number of patients	5-year survival (%)
Radiation therapy only		
Krishnamurthi (1965)	100	4
Marcial and associates (1966)	145	6
Pearson (1977)	228	17
Pierquin and associates (1966)	115	3
Nakayama and associates (1965)	100	6
Millburn and associates (1968)	64	9
Surgery only		
Shedd and associates (1955)	134	0
Postlethwait and associates (1957)	121	4
Vander Vennert (1965)	150	1
Loeb (1965)	111	1

*Modified from Millburn, L., Hendrickson, F. R., and Faber, P.: Am. J. Roentgenol. **103**:291-299, 1968.
†Treatment by irradiation and surgery are tabulated separately, but percent survival is based on all patients seen. Survival rates in many series are based on the number treated, which may give an apparent superior cure rate.

The palliative value of irradiation of carcinoma of the esophagus cannot be measured adequately in terms of longevity. Tumor regression, with disappearance of the stenosis and improvement in swallowing, is worth all the demands of vigorous irradiation. With this comes an increase in weight and a notable improvement in the patient's outlook. When all patients are accepted for irradiation and a complete course of radiation therapy is given, dysphagia will improve in 75% to 80%. Obstructing symptoms will recur in a significant number.

Pain due to the local irritation of ulceration and stenosis is frequently relieved before treatment is completed. Radiation-induced esophagitis may persist for 2 to 3 weeks. Posterior extension of the cancer into nerve roots, producing back pain and referred pain, is a sign of advanced disease.

Summary

A successful method of treating carcinoma of the esophagus remains a challenge to both the surgeon and the radiation oncologist. Despite numerous ingenious techniques in both specialties, the problem is essentially unsolved. This disease is not controlled more often because of spread beyond the mediastinum before the diagnosis is made (Fig. 12-10). Our present radiotherapeutic efforts are of considerable palliative value and are fully justified on this basis alone. An occasional cure will be obtained if treatment is planned with this possibility in mind.

STOMACH
Response of the normal stomach to irradiation

With the exception of its mucosa, the human stomach tolerates high doses of radiations. The mucosa, with its variety of cells, exemplifies the selective effects of radiations both morphologically and functionally. A mucus-secreting columnar epithelium covers the surface of the stomach and the gastric pits. The pits open into the gastric glands proper, which contain four types of cells. At the necks of the gastric glands, the mucous neck cells are prominent. These proliferate rapidly and in so doing represent the source of cells of the gastric pits and some of the cells of the gastric glands. Deeper in the glands, parietal cells that produce the precursor of hydrochloric acid and the zymogenic or chief cells that produce pepsin are found. Argentaffin cells are scattered between the zymogenic cells and the basement membrane. These four cell types vary in their proportions from one section of the stomach to another.

Gastric secretions are controlled by a complex neurohumoral mechanism. Radiations alter gastric secretions by injuring mucosal cells directly and by altering both the neural and blood-borne stimuli that regulate gastric secretions. The picture is even more complex when one remembers that various regions of the stomach have different functions. To define radiation-induced changes in gastric function, several types of studies are necessary—local irradiation of gastric mucosa, local irradiation with gastric shielding, and total body irradiation. The concern here is with those situations likely to be encountered clinically.

Dawson vividly described the radiation-induced histologic changes in the dog, and Palmer and Templeton believe similar changes occur in man. With more voluminous patient material, Goldgraber and associates attempted to correlate microscopic and physiologic changes in patients given gastric irradiation as a part of treatment for peptic ulcers. Their detailed report forms the basis for the discussion to follow.

The changes to be described occur after a dose of 1600 rad delivered to the fundus of the stomach in 10 days (250 kvp; hvl, 1.5 mm Cu; target-skin distance, 50 cm). A radiation gastritis begins in about 1 week and may persist in a diminishing degree for a month or more. Hyperemia, edema, microscopic hemorrhages, and exudation are typical, but no symptoms accompany the radiation gastritis. The first detectable microscopic changes are found in the glandular tubules. Cell death begins in the depths of the glands and proceeds toward the neck cells. Their epithelia slough, and, as a result, the gastric mucosa is thinned while presenting an edematous inflammatory reaction (Fig. 12-11).

The gastric glands show interesting and apparently paradoxic responses to irradiation. Within them, the zymogenic pepsin-secreting chief cells appear more easily

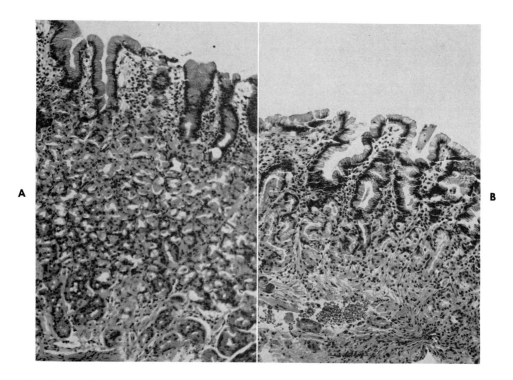

A B

Fig. 12-11. A, Normal gastric mucosa (magnification × 110). **B,** Gastroscopic biopsy showing thinning of the gastric mucosa 3 weeks after delivering a calculated 1500 rad to the mucosa in 10 days (magnification × 100) (250 kv; hvl, 1.5 mm Cu; TSD, 50 cm). (From Goldgraber, M. B., Rubin, C. E., Palmer, W. L., Dobson, R. L., and Massey, B. W.: Gastroenterology **27:**1-20, 1954.)

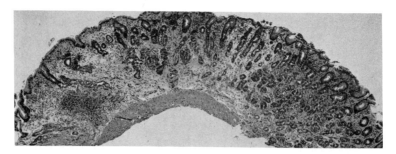

Fig. 12-12. Low-power magnification of gastric mucosa after dose described in Fig. 12-11, *B.* Note the patchiness of the glandular atrophy. (From Goldgraber, M. B., Rubin, C. E., Palmer, W. L., Dobson, R. L., and Massey, B. W.: Gastroenterology **27:**1-20, 1954.)

destroyed than the parietal acid-producing cells. Not in keeping with this constant microscopic finding is the observation that a decrease in free hydrochloric acid precedes the more gradual diminution in pepsin secretion. Goldgraber and associates noted this apparent discrepancy but found that both of these alterations in gastric secretions may begin prior to any histologic changes. They thought all cells in the depth of the glands were equally damaged by irradiation. This point remains to be clarified. Reepithelization of the glands is accomplished by downward proliferation of the mitotically active yet relatively resistant cells of the neck region.

Soon after the onset of radiation-induced glandular changes, the gastric pits deepen. The surface epithelium together with the epithelium of the pits becomes flattened, loses its mucus, and, if the dose is high, may exfoliate. After doses mentioned previously, the surface epithelium generally remains intact. The volume of mucus secreted is sharply reduced.

The destructive and regenerative changes described do not appear evenly over the stomach wall but are reported to be patchy (Fig. 12-12). Secretions are depressed for variable periods from a few weeks to several years despite earlier and apparently complete morphologic recovery of the glands. Individual variation seems to be great in this regard.

We now irradiate the stomach often in the course of treating Hodgkin's disease. Doses of 4000 rad delivered to the pylorus and antral regions of the stomach through beams 8 to 10 cm wide rarely produce any lasting symptoms, although we have seen several asthenic young adults develop ulcers within the midline following the use of extended mantle fields. These lesions have healed in every case with conservative management.

More intense local irradiation of the stomach may produce serious or even fatal necrosis of the stomach wall. Such ulceration appeared in forty-four of 256 patients with vigorous irradiation of the retroperitoneal lymph node area for carcinoma of the testicle (Roswitt and associates; Bowers and Brick; Hamilton). Gastric perforation occurred in eleven patients. All of the ulcers appeared in the irradiated volume. In a study made several months after irradiation of a part of the stomach, gastric secretions did not seem markedly affected (Brick). Since only the distal part of the stomach was irradiated, the findings in these patients are certainly not to be compared with those observed in patients treated for peptic ulcer. The patients developing radiation-induced ulcers had received about 4500 rad or even more at the level of the eleventh dorsal vertebra in 32 to 55 days (1000 kvp; target-skin distance, 70 to 100 cm; hvl, 3 mm Pb). Perforation of ten of the ulcers occurred within 6 months of the completion of irradiation (Brick). Still higher doses have been given using centrally fixed intragastric radioactive sources in the dog (Fox and associates; Littman and associates). Early death within several weeks or even days follows massive destruction of the stomach wall.

Doses of radiations that are delivered to the stomach by the moving strip technique are generally about 2500 rad in 8 to 12 days (NSD of 1100 rets). We have never observed significant immediate or late sequelae other than the common postirradiation nausea.

Carcinoma of the stomach

Most carcinomas of the stomach are adenocarcinomas. They arise from the mucus-producing cells, which, as mentioned previously, are the most radioresistant cells of the normal gastric epithelium. Adenocarcinomas arising from parietal or chief cells are rare.

The radiation tolerance of the normal stomach wall has been discussed before. Doses of the order of 5000 rad in 5 to 8 weeks are followed by frequent mucosal ulcerations and occasional perforations. It is not unreasonable to expect that eradication of gastric adenocarcinoma requires a dose of this level or even higher. In addition to this limiting tolerance of the stomach wall, the tolerance of the kidneys and of adjacent small bowel must be kept in mind. With such limitations, the curative possibilities of radiotherapy in the treatment of even early adenocarcinomas of the stomach are remote. The disease usually produces relatively minor symptoms early, and it is not frequently diagnosed until late. This, coupled with the relative radioresistant characteristics of the tumor, makes it radioincurable and, when possible, makes radical resection the treatment of choice. Resection with a curative aim is possible in only a percentage of all patients (44% of the group referred to the Mayo Clinic [Berkson and associates]) and is successful in a still smaller fraction (14%). Unfortunately, the causes for surgical failure (extensive infiltration of neighboring structures and peritoneal, liver, and lymph node metastases) are not significantly influenced by irradiation. Irradiation of advanced gastric carcinomas has been tried repeatedly. Irradiation alone or in combination with chemotherapy has been disappointing. True palliation from irradiation alone is uncommon.

Malignant lymphoma of the stomach

Primary malignant lymphoma of the stomach, in contrast to the frequently seen generalized malignant lymphoma, is a rare and occasionally curable disease (Chapter 20). It comprises only 1.5% to 5.2% of all gastric malignancies. Up to the time of Redd's summary, 847 cases had been reported. Therefore no single clinician has had an extensive personal experience with the disease.

Several reviews of the clinical, histologic, and therapeutic aspects of this disease have been published (Redd; Friedman; Wolferth and associates; Fraser and associates). The distribution of primary malignant lymphoma of the gastrointestinal tract is shown in Table 12-3. Proper evaluation to exclude a generalized malignant lymphoma should follow the diagnosis of gastric involvement. Care should be exercised to rule out some exuberant lymphoid infiltrates around peptic ulcers, the so-called pseudolymphomas. Some long-term "cures" of gastric lymphoma are due to this misdiagnosis. The great majority of non-Hodgkin's lymphomas of the gastrointestinal tract show a diffuse histologic pattern.

The clinical and radiographic manifestations of gastric malignant lymphoma

Table 12-3. Primary site of involvement in 83 patients with malignant lymphoma of the gastrointestinal tract*

Primary site	Number of patients
Esophagus	1
Stomach	40
Small bowel	25
Ileal cecal	8
Large bowel	5
Rectum	4

*Modified from Bush, R. S., and Ash, C. L.: Radiology **92**:1349-1354, 1969.

overlap those of adenocarcinoma to such an extent that laparotomy or gastroscopy with biopsy and brushings is always necessary to differentiate the two. At the time of laparotomy, gastric resection is indicated if it is technically possible. This decreases the chances of subsequent hemorrhage and perforation. Berger and associates reported that three of their patients developed gastric perforation during irradiation. Complete removal of the tumor is infrequent, however, and the clinical impressions of local extent and node involvement are frequently inaccurate even at laparotomy (Crile and associates). When gastrectomy is inadvisable or when resection is thought to be incomplete, postoperative irradiation is indicated. Even advanced lesions may be cured by irradiation (Jenkinson and associates; Redd). Irradiation will be indicated in all but a few cases. Lymph nodes will be involved in about 80% of the patients. It is for this reason that generally the whole abdomen should be encompassed and carried to a midabdominal dose of 3000 rad in 6 to 8 weeks or more (Fraser and associates). When more limited ports are used, adjuvant chemotherapy should be considered.

TECHNIQUE OF IRRADIATION. A dose sufficient to eradicate most primary malignant lymphomas of the stomach can be given even though epigastric ports must be large. However, nodal spread is unpredictable, and the use of limited tailored ports is frequently followed by regional recurrence (Fraser and associates). It is for this reason that total abdominal irradiation with appropriate kidney and liver shielding is now preferred.

The optimum total dose has not been established. A wide variation in dosage has been used in reported cases. Despite this uncertainty we recommend a dose to the primary tumor of 3500 to 4500 rad, depending on the residual tumor present, or if resection has not been performed, a dose of 4000 to 5000 rad. The dose to the remainder of the abdomen depends on tolerance and can rarely exceed 3000 rad in 6 to 8 weeks.

PROGNOSIS AND RESULTS. Of the 474 cases collected and reviewed by Snoddy and generally treated by local or regional port irradiation, only fifty (10%) of the patients survived 5 years or longer. Thirteen of the survivors were treated with irradiation only, twenty-five with surgery only, and twelve with combined surgery and irradiation. Redd reported a total of fifty-five survivors in the 847 cases recorded in the world literature. Apparently localized and completely resectable lesions yielded a 5-year survival rate of 58% (Allen and associates). These figures cannot be used to prove the relative superiority of surgery, since patients with early malignant lymphoma were selected for resection alone. Generally, in those with the advanced disease, partial resection and subsequent irradiation or irradiation after biopsy is given with adjuvant chemotherapy.

SUMMARY. Primary malignant lymphoma of the stomach is a rare, occasionally curable disease. Laparotomy is usually necessary before the diagnosis is made, but good cytologic preparations obtained by brushing and multiple biopsies may provide a preoperative diagnosis. Resection at the time of laparotomy is probably indicated if technically possible and if the patient can tolerate the procedure. Irradiation will be indicated in those patients with persistent disease and in the inoperable patients. Even those with advanced disease have been cured by such irradiation, so that every effort should be made to adequately irradiate the volume of known involvement. When the volume of irradiation is limited to the primary tumor, post-irradiation adjuvant chemotherapy should be considered.

SMALL INTESTINES

Various interesting morphologic and functional changes are produced by small bowel irradiation. There are changes in gastrointestinal motility manifested as anorexia, vomiting, gastric retention, and diarrhea. The etiology of some of these changes is known, but little is known about the causes of others.

Epithelium of the small bowel is highly radiosensitive, and histologic changes are striking. Within 24 hours of single doses of 500 to 1000 rad, mitotically active cells of the crypts show a maximum destruction. Reepithelization is extensive within 96 hours (Montagna and Wilson). However, the tips of the villi show a maximum cellular destruction in 96 hours, and complete reepithelization is microscopically complete several days later. It should be recalled here that cells on the tips of the villi originate as daughter cells from those of the crypts, and reepithelization of the tips depends on mitotically normal crypt epithelium. Therefore repair of the tips of the villi is rapidly completed once the source of cells from the crypts is reestablished. The tissues deep to the epithelium show edema, capillary congestion with occasional small hemorrhages, and degeneration of lymphoid tissue.

The late gross and microscopic changes consist of progressive fibrosis associated with marked edema (Figs. 12-13 and 12-14). The mucosa may ulcerate, and small bowel stricture and obstruction may follow. The process is locally progressive, and surgery may be required (Fig. 12-15).

The physiologic changes subsequent to small bowel irradiation are both local and remote. As in irradiation of various other tissues of the body, irradiation of the small bowel produces a prolongation of gastric emptying. Gastric emptying returns to normal 1 to 2 weeks after cessation of irradiation. The mechanism of this remote effect of localized irradiation is unknown, but it is suspected of being a consequence of radiation-induced cellular breakdown products liberated into the circulation.

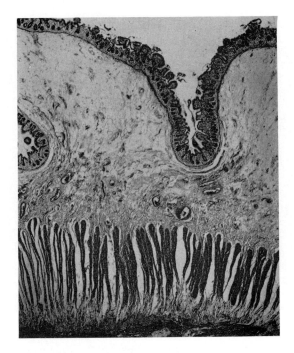

Fig. 12-13. Changes in small bowel 1 year after 4000 to 5600 rad in 5 weeks (1000 kv; hvl, 3 mm Pb; TSD, 70 cm). Note absence of lymphoid tissue and striking submucosal edema.

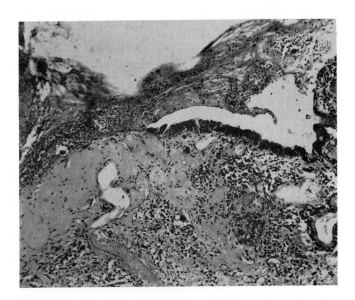

Fig. 12-14. Radiation-induced ulceration of small bowel following 4000 to 5000 rad in 5 weeks (1000 kv; hvl, 3 mm Pb; TSD, 70 cm).

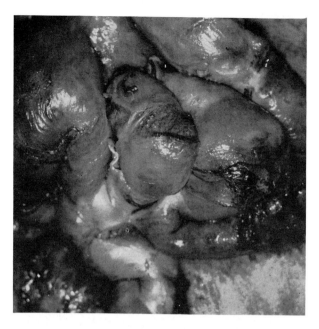

Fig. 12-15. Radiation-induced small bowel obstruction after vigorous whole pelvis irradiation for carcinoma of the bladder. Minimum dose to the pelvis exceeded 4900 rad in 5 weeks. After surgical relief of obstruction, patient lived 3 years before dying of carcinomatosis. Bowel wall was leathery and edematous. Changes above pelvis were result of chronic obstruction.

After a single dose of as low as 700 rad, there is a sudden decrease in the rate of diffusion of sugars through the mucous membrane. The recovery of bowel function follows rather closely the morphologic recovery described previously. These effects on absorption should be kept in mind in supplementing the nutrition of patients receiving abdominal irradiation.

Although there is variation in the severity with which absorption is decreased, there is generally a progressive decrease in local biochemical and physicochemical processes in the villi. The precise roles of other changes are unknown—changes in vessel permeability, motility changes, nerve plexus, and mucosal damage.

Small bowel injury should be a concern in any patient receiving abdominal or pelvic irradiation.

After a given dose of radiations, the proximal small bowel shows greater response than do the distal segments (Baker and Mitchell). This is true of all functions and of histologic changes. Severe injury to the intestinal epithelium may appear when irradiation of the upper abdomen is given in conjunction with systemic actinomycin D. These two agents are frequently used in the treatment of Wilms' tumor and testicular neoplasms. Gastrointestinal symptoms in such patients deserve special attention, and daily doses should be reduced. Concannon and associates irradiated the upper abdomen of dogs given 50 mg actinomycin D/kg. With daily midplane doses of

125 rad × 12 the dogs survived, but when 158 rad were given daily, four of six dogs died.

The great radiosensitivity of the small bowel, especially the epithelial lining, accounts for the "gastrointestinal death" after total body irradiation. The widespread destruction of this epithelium results in serious loss of fluids and electrolytes. The area also serves as a portal for septicemia, especially with the associated loss of immune responses.

Primary cancer of the small bowel

Once the clinical diagnosis of primary malignant tumor of the small bowel is made, laparotomy is necessary for confirmation. At that time surgical treatment should be carried out if at all possible. A localized malignant lymphoma of the small bowel can conceivably be irradiated with a curative aim. Regardless of whether the lymphoma is truly localized or associated with lymph node involvement, we prefer whole abdominal irradiation. The dose-time equivalence is similar to that usually recommended for non-Hodgkin's lymphoma. Cox has recommended a midabdominal dose of 2500 rad in 6 weeks and has recommended chemotherapy for patients with Stages III and IV lesions but not for those with Stages I and II lesions. The rare carcinomas of the small bowel should be treated surgically. However, carcinoid of the small bowel, even when advanced, may show remarkable regression after total abdominal irradiation with doses of 2500 rad in 6 weeks (Gaitan-Gaitan and associates). We have not had an opportunity to verify this.

CARCINOMA OF THE PANCREAS

White reviewed the radiation histopathology of the pancreas and made the following conclusions:

1. Acinar and islet cells are radioresistant in the usual range of therapeutic doses.
2. Cellular changes can be identified after very high doses of irradiation.
3. Very little is known about the effects of ionizing radiation of the pancreas.

It is very likely that the dose-limiting features of the gut of the upper abdomen preclude detailed analysis of the effects of high-dose irradiation on the normal pancreas. It is conceivable that some of the late histopathologic effects of irradiation of this organ may be determined from evaluation of the autopsied pancreas of patients who died long after total nodal irradiation for Hodgkin's disease. For the present we have little useful information to guide us in determining the tolerance of this organ.

Carcinoma of the pancreas is almost always fatal. Cure by surgical treatment is generally less than 10% for patients with resectable lesions. In our own institution median survival during a representative 5-year period was 2.9 months. The adjuvant or therapeutic use of 5-fluorouracil has been disappointing. The same can be said for multidrug combinations (Schein and associates). Early detection is difficult, and despite the use of computed tomographic scans of the abdomen, actual tumor localization is often uncertain.

Green and associates reported the value of irradiation as a palliative modality for inoperable carcinoma of the pancreas. In seventeen of twenty-two patients referred to them because of pain, they achieved excellent palliation with average doses of 1440 rad in 14 days. Haslam and associates reported the results of treatment in twenty-nine patients with nonresectable adenocarcinoma of the pancreas seen in a 10-year period. Doses as high as 6000 rad were employed using a triple split-course technique. The crude survival for these selected patients was 25% at 2½ years following diagnosis. Such results indicating a palliative response and the possibility of a prolongation of survival have encouraged us to continue to recommend irradiation for inoperable or nonresectable carcinoma of the pancreas. Tepper and associates reached the same conclusion following a review of 145 patients with carcinoma of the pancreas in a 10-year period. They suggest that irradiation following surgical resection of carcinoma of the pancreas may improve results and that preoperative irradiation in patients known to have carcinoma of the pancreas (proven by aspiration biopsy) may improve survival. A dose of approximately 5000 rad is recommended in either instance.

CARCINOMA OF THE GALLBLADDER AND BILIARY TRACT

The results of surgical treatment of carcinoma of the gallbladder and biliary tract are poor. Five-year survival rates are less than 5%. Carcinomas of this area are resectable less than 20% of the time. Radiation therapy may play a role in treatment of tumors in these sites. Our own experience has been reviewed by Smoron. For patients given at least 4000 rad the median survival following completion of treatment was 15 months, and in the group receiving less than that dose the median survival was 2.5 months. The usual reason for delivery of less than 4000 rad was patient debilitation. With the availability of techniques for aspiration and cytologic diagnosis of lesions in the region of the pancreas and gallbladder, the radiation oncologist can now proceed with palliative treatment of patients deemed inoperable without the need for laparotomy to establish the diagnosis. For the present we recommend irradiation of inoperable lesions to a dose of 5000 rad in 5½ weeks.

It is clear that we do not know the ultimate results of such irradiation. It is also clear that surgical results are extremely poor and chemotherapeutic agents are usually of questionable benefit.

LARGE INTESTINE

The effects of irradiation on the large intestine and rectum are discussed in detail in Chapter 17.

Carcinoma of the colon

Carcinoma of the colon is the second leading cause of cancer deaths in the United States. At least half the carcinomas of the large intestine are located within the reach of a proctoscope, and this portion of bowel is usually within the pelvis. In this location the bowel is in a more or less fixed position, is separated from highly radiosensitive or critical structures, and under some circumstances could perhaps be

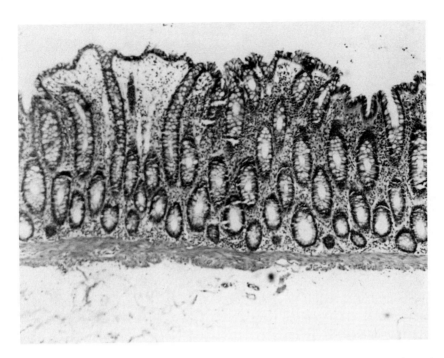

Fig. 12-16. Section of large bowel from patient given preoperative irradiation for rectal carcinoma (3800 rad in 24 elapsed days, 19 fractions, ^{60}Co). The section was obtained 1 day after completion of preoperative irradiation. The epithelium is intact, and the only noticeable abnormalities are focal edema of lamina propria and diffuse submucosal edema.

given high doses. Nearly all these are adenocarcinomas and are occasionally radio-curable. Papillon reported a 78% 5-year survival rate for a *highly selected* group of limited, well-differentiated rectal cancers treated by irradiation with a contact apparatus. Properly fractionated doses of radiation are tolerated by adjacent uninvolved large bowel (Fig. 12-16).

There are few preoperative criteria by which to judge prognostic features in carcinoma of the colon. The size of the lesion does not correlate with any other features, although in the usual instance a biopsy can be obtained and the degree of differentiation is of definite prognostic significance. Appropriate clinical and laboratory procedures should be performed to exclude the possibility of metastases in a patient with biopsy-proven colon cancer. For purposes of discussion we prefer the pathologic stage system as originally proposed by Duke and modified by Astler and Coller:

Stage A	Limited to mucosa or submucosa
Stage B1	Extension into but not through muscularis
Stage B2	Extension to or through serosa; negative nodes
Stage C1	Limited to serosa; positive nodes
Stage C2	Extension through serosa; positive nodes
Stage D	Distant metastases

Table 12-4. Anatomic sites of failure following curative resection
for cancer of the rectum*

Anatomic site of failure	Percent failure only in one site	Percent failure in more than one site
Local or regional	25–48.1 (33.8)	48–92.3 (64.9)
Distant metastases	4– 7.7 (5.4)	26–50.0 (35.1)
Peritoneal seeding	0	3– 5.8 (4.1)

*Modified from Gunderson, L. L.: Clin. Gastroenterol. **5:**743-776, 1976.

The results of surgery for carcinoma of the rectum and pelvic colon, Stages A and B1, are excellent. Once tumor has penetrated through the serosa or lymph node metastases appear, the chance of local recurrence, distant metastases, or a combination of the two increases with each advancing stage. Of 100 newly diagnosed patients with carcinoma of the colon, only 70% will be eligible for a curative resection at the time of surgery, and of these roughly one half will survive more than 5 years. It is thus apparent that although surgery is the primary modality of treatment, it fails in its intent more than 60% of the time. Cass and associates reviewed the outcome of 280 patients who underwent surgery for adenocarcinoma of the colon and rectum and had complete tumor resection. Thirty-seven percent of the patients developed recurrence during the period of observation. Of the 105 patients with recurrence, sixty-three had local recurrence only, fifteen had local recurrence and distant metastases, and twenty-seven had distant metastases only (Table 12-4). In this series, recurrence of cecal lesions was as common as those of the rectum. Walz and associates and Gunderson and Sosin reported similar results. In all such series the depth of penetration of the tumor through the bowel and the presence or absence of lymph node metastases are strong determinants in the likelihood of subsequent *local* failure. When the tumor extends through the bowel wall (B2 and C2 lesions), local failure may occur in 40% to 60% of the patients. Local recurrence is the cause of death in at least 50% of those who die from the disease (Withers and Romsdahl). The implications for postoperative irradiation in these stages are obvious. For the more limited lesions or those with no invasion through the wall and minimal lymph node disease, the likelihood of local failure diminishes and there is no clear indication for postoperative irradiation. In large collected series the incidence of extension through the bowel wall (B2 and C2) is approximately 70%.

Lymph drainage through the middle and inferior hemorrhoidal vessels may spread cancer to the pelvis. However, spread through superior hemorrhoidal vessels is not uncommon with node involvement at the level of the origin of the inferior mesenteric artery. These facts have led to a search for adjuvant measures to improve the results of surgery, particularly in those cases with local spread. In view of the relative ease of irradiating the whole pelvis and the relative frequency of carcinoma in this region, preoperative irradiation has been administered in the hope of rendering more cases resectable and improving survival (Chapter 2). Stearns has reported the

Memorial Hospital experience with this approach. In this retrospective analysis there was an apparent increase in survival attributed to irradiation for those patients with Duke's C lesions. Maximum tumor doses were considerably less than 2000 rad (orthovoltage). The resectability rates of 69% and 86% with or without preoperative irradiation, respectively, indicate the influence of clinical selection. This fact was recognized by Stearns and led him to undertake a prospective study, the results of which failed to support the value of preoperative irradiation.

Stevens and associates reported an experience with ninety-seven patients given high-dose preoperative irradiation (at least 5000 rad). Fifty-seven of those patients had carcinoma that was judged clinically resectable, and in forty the adenocarcinoma was deemed inoperable. Of the forty patients judged operable and who had a curative resection after preoperative irradiation, the 5-year survival was 53%. No patients who received preoperative irradiation and curative resection had pelvic recurrence. As has been the case in other studies of preoperative irradiation of adenocarcinoma of the colon, a high proportion (50%) of the resected specimens were classified as Stage A and less than 20% as Stage C lesions. Stevens and associates (1978) have also reported an experience with *anterior resection* and primary anastomosis for patients given preoperative irradiation of at least 5000 rad for carcinoma of the rectum. All of the thirteen patients in that group had tumors at least 12 cm above the anal verge. None of these patients developed local recurrence, and only one died of metastases (follow-up 10 months to 16 years).

Hayes and associates reported preliminary findings in thirty-one patients randomized to surgery alone or preoperative irradiation. A dose of 4500 rad was given preoperatively to the rectal lesions and the regional lymphatics, including those of the level of the inferior mesenteric artery. Of the sixteen patients randomized to surgery only, eleven patients had involvement of resected lymph nodes, whereas only three of the thirteen patients receiving preoperative irradiation had positive resected lymph nodes. These studies indicate that adenocarcinoma of the rectum and rectosigmoid is a relatively radiosensitive lesion and that lymph node metastases may be sterilized with the doses employed (Fig. 12-17). In addition preoperative irradiation would appear to reduce the incidence of local recurrence and improve resectability rates (Table 12-5). It should be borne in mind that cure infrequently follows resection of locally advanced initially nonresectable cancers given preoperative irradiation. The potential of preoperative irradiation in the initially unresectable lesion has been emphasized by Pilepich and associates. Nevertheless, there is increasing evidence that local preoperative or postoperative irradiation will increase the incidence of long-term tumor-free survival in a significant proportion of patients.

As mentioned previously, the pathologic findings at the time of curative resection for carcinoma of the colorectum make it possible to select those patients most likely to fail locally (B2 and C2). In an analysis of thirty-one such patients selected for postoperative irradiation between 1971 and 1976 at the Latter Day Saints Hospital, Gunderson reported local failure in only one patient. In patients with residual disease following resection, clinical evidence of recurrence developed in five of twenty

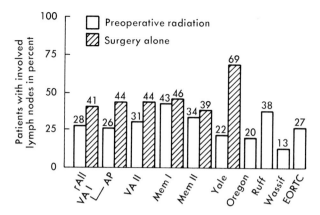

Fig. 12-17. Percentage of patients with cancer of the colon showing involved lymph nodes following resection. Various trials show a consistently smaller percentage in those patients having preoperative radiotherapy compared to those having surgery alone for treatment of colorectal cancer. (Modified from Higgins, G. A., and Rosewit, B.: The role of radiotherapy in the surgical treatment of large bowel cancer. In Ariel, I. M., editor: Progress in clinical cancer, vol. 7, New York, 1978, Grune & Stratton, Inc.

Table 12-5. Local recurrence in clinically resectable rectosigmoid adenocarcinoma with curative resection*

Author	Institution	Surgery only (%)	Radiation and surgery (%)
Gilbertsen	University of Minnesota	37	
Cass	University of Florida	28	
Morson	St. Marks (London)	10	
Ree	University of Chicago	24	
Stearns	Memorial Hospital, New York (2000 R)	—†	—†
Roswit	VA hospitals (2000-2500 rad)	40	29
Boulis-Wassif	Rotterdam (3450 rad)		10
Stevens	University of Oregon (5000 rad anterior resection)	9	0
Gunderson	Latter Day Saints Hospital (4500-5500 rad postoperative irradiation)		6 (geographic misses)
Withers	M. D. Anderson Hospital	21	4

*From Stevens, K. R., Fletcher, W. S., and Allen, C. V.: A review of the value of radiation therapy for adenocarcinoma of the rectum and sigmoid, Proceedings of the International Conference of Gastrointestinal Cancer held in Tel Aviv, Basel, Switzerland, 1979, S. Karger, A. G.
†Decreased recurrence in those patients with regional metastases receiving radiation therapy prior to surgery.

patients. Mendiondo and associates also reported an increased incidence of local control for patients with Stages B and C lesions of the rectum irradiated postoperatively compared to control obtained in similar patients treated by surgery only. Based on these and other observations we recommend postoperative irradiation for all patients with Stages B2 and C2 lesions. In view of the high incidence of local recurrence in carcinomas arising in the cecum, we also favor postoperative irradiation for these tumors. If the anticipated disease is microscopic only, a dose of 5000 rad is sufficient. For patients with gross residual disease in the pelvis a higher dose is recommended. Postoperative irradiation is more likely to gain acceptance with our surgical colleagues than is preoperative irradiation. In addition the actual stage of the disease, as determined from the surgical specimen, can guide us in determining the need for postoperative irradiation. This obviously permits elimination of patients with A, B1, and limited C1 lesions.

IRRADIATION OF NONRESECTABLE PRIMARY RECTAL CARCINOMA AND OF POSTOPERATIVE PELVIC RECURRENCE. Fifteen to twenty-five percent of patients with carcinoma of the colon will be found to be nonresectable at the time of surgery. In addition, the incidence of local recurrence at the suture line after resection varies from 10% to 15% (Cole and associates), and regional lymph node involvement or distant metastases will be present half the time. Overall 5-year survival of resectable cases ranges between 30% and 40%. It is thus apparent that a large number of patients with carcinoma of the colon will be seen with either nonresectable lesions, local recurrence, or symptomatic metastases. Surprisingly, there has been little interest in attempting palliative irradiation in these patients.

Recurrence in the pelvis or perineum after surgery (usually abdominoperineal resection) for carcinoma of the rectum or pelvic colon may present as a palpable mass with pelvic pain, pain radiating into the thighs, or bleeding and discharge. Wang and Schulz reported that 60% of these recurrences appear within 2 years after surgery. Irradiation produced significant palliation of pain in sixty-three of seventy-six patients, shrinkage of tumor in twelve of twenty, and arrest of bleeding or discharge in nineteen of twenty patients. Wang and Schulz emphasize the possibility of long-term control in patients with disease confined to the pelvis. Six of fifty patients in this category survived 5 years, and two had initially been judged inoperable. Rao and associates reported that five of thirty-seven patients treated radically for recurrent or inoperable lesions were free of disease 24 to 84 months following treatment. Thus the possibility of long-term tumor-free survival should be kept in mind in planning irradiation for what is ordinarily considered a hopeless group of patients.

Although pain and bleeding may be arrested in some patients with doses of 2000 rad, we believe that a dose of 4500 to 5500 rad in 5 to 6 weeks is justified when the known disease is confined to the pelvis. Smedal and associates have emphasized the importance of including the perineum in the treatment field when there is posterior pelvic pain or pain radiating down the legs.

In those patients with potentially curable carcinoma of the pelvic colon who are not suitable candidates for surgery, we recommend vigorous irradiation of the primary cancer and regional pelvic lymph nodes. Techniques similar to those for other primary pelvic cancers are employed. The contribution of irradiation of the lymph nodes along the mesenteric vessels is uncertain, and we have not included this region in the treatment volume. Preirradiation colostomy is not routinely justified in the absence of obstruction. Doses of 5000 to 5500 rad in 5 to 6 weeks to the regional lymph nodes and 6500 rad in 7 to 8 weeks to a limited primary lesion are well tol-

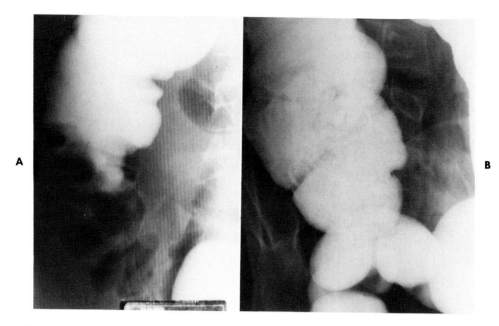

Fig. 12-18. A, Constricting lesion of the ascending colon in patient with known Hodgkin's disease. **B,** Barium enema in the same patient after 4000 rad ⁶⁰Co to lesion shown in **A.**

erated. Doses of 4500 to 5000 rad can eradicate some lymph node metastases and reduce the incidence of local recurrence in the bowel.

Malignant lymphoma of the colon

The colon may be involved as the primary site of malignant lymphoma, but, as in other areas of the gastrointestinal tract, it is most often associated with more advanced disease. The principles discussed for gastric and small bowel lymphomas apply to the large bowel. When a patient with known lymphoma presents with a detectable lesion involving the colon, irradiation is preferable to surgery except in patients with significant symptoms of obstruction (Fig. 12-18).

REFERENCES

Akakura, I., Nakamura, Y., Kakegawa, T., Nakayama, R., Watanabe, A., and Yamashita, H.: Surgery of carcinoma of the esophagus with preoperative irradiation, Chest **57**:47-57, 1970.

Allen, A. W., Donaldson, G., Sniffen, R. C., and Goodale, F.: Primary malignant lymphoma of gastrointestinal tract, Ann. Surg. **140**:428-438, 1954.

Allen, C. V.: High dose preoperative radiation therapy in carcinoma of the rectosigmoid colon. In Vaeth, J. M., editor: The interrelationship of surgery and radiation therapy in the treatment of cancer, Baltimore, 1970, University Park Press.

Allen, C. V., and Fletcher, W. S.: Observations on preoperative irradiation of rectosigmoid carcinoma, Am. J. Roentgenol. **108**:136-140, 1970.

Astler, V. B., and Coller, F. A.: The prognostic significance of direct extension of carcinoma of the colon and rectum, Ann. Surg. **139**:846-851, 1954.

Baker, D. G., and Mitchell, R. I.: Studies of intestines during acute radiation syndrome, Gastroenterology **44**:291-300, 1963.

Berger, I. R., Gay, B. B., and Whorton, C. M.: Malignant lymphoma of the stomach, Radiology **62**:527-535, 1954.

Berkson, J., Walters, W., Gray, H. K., and Priestly, J. T.: Mortality and survival in cancer of the stomach: a statistical summary of the experience of the Mayo Clinic, Proc. Staff Meet., Mayo Clin. **27**:137-151, 1952.

Bloedorn, F. G., and Kasdorf, H.: Radiotherapy in squamous cell carcinoma of the esophagus. In Clark, R. L., Cumley, R. W., McCay, J. E., and Copeland, M. M., editors: Oncology 1970, Proceedings of the Tenth International Cancer Congress, vol. 4, Chicago, 1971, Yearbook Medical Publishers, Inc.

Bowers, R. F., and Brick, I. B.: Surgery in radiation injury of the stomach, Surgery **22**:20-40, 1947.

Brick, I. B.: Effects of million volt irradiation on the gastrointestinal tract, Arch. Intern. Med. **96**: 26-31, 1955.

Burnett, H. W., and Herbert, E. A.: The role of irradiation in the treatment of primary malignant lymphoma of the stomach, Radiology **67**:723-728, 1956.

Bush, R. S., and Ash, C. L.: Primary lymphoma of the gastrointestinal tract, Radiology **92**:1349-1354, 1969.

Cass, A. W., Million, R. R., and Pfaff, W. W.: Patterns of recurrence following surgery alone for adenocarcinoma of the colon and rectum, Cancer **37**:2861-2865, 1976.

Cole, W. H., Roberts, S. S., and Strehl, F. W.: Modern concepts in cancer of the colon and rectum, Cancer **19**:1347-1358, 1966.

Concannon, J. P., Summers, R. E., Cole, G., Werl, C., Kopp, U., and Sigdestad, C. P.: Effects of x-radiation and actinomycin D on intestinal epithelium of dogs, Radiology **97**:157-164, 1970.

Cox, J. D.: Prognostic factors in malignant lymphoreticular tumors of the small bowel and ileocecal region, Int. J. Radiat. Oncol. Biol. Phys. **5**:185-190, 1979.

Crile, G., Hazard, J. B., and Allen, K. L.: Primary lymphosarcoma of the stomach, Ann. Surg. **135**: 39-43, 1952.

Dawson, A. B.: Histological changes in the gastric mucosa of the dog following irradiation, Am. J. Roentgenol. **13**:320-326, 1925.

del Regato, J. A., and Spjut, H. J.: Ackerman and del Regato's cancer—diagnosis, treatment, and prognosis, ed. 5, St. Louis, 1977, The C. V. Mosby Co.

Dickson, R. J.: Radiation therapy in carcinoma of the esophagus: a review, Am. J. Med. Sci. **241**: 662-677, 1961.

Doggett, R. L., Guernsey, J. N., and Bagshaw, M. A.: Combined radiation and surgical treat-

ment of carcinoma of the thoracic esophagus. In Vaeth, J. M.: The interrelationship of surgery and radiation therapy in the treatment of cancer, Baltimore, 1970, University Park Press.

Fenton, P. F., and Dickson, H. M.: Changes in some gastrointestinal functions following x-irradiation, Am. J. Physiol. **177**:528-530, 1954.

Fleming, J. A. C., and Barrett, N. R.: Carcinoma of the oesophagus and stomach. In Carling, E. R., Windeyer, B. W., and Smithers, D. W.: Practice in radiotherapy, London, 1955, Butterworth & Co., Ltd.

Fox, B. W., Littman, A., Grossman, M. I., and Ivy, A. C.: Effect of intragastric irradiation on gastric acidity in the dog, Gastroenterology **23**: 517-534, 1953.

Fraser, R. W., Wara, W. M., Thomas, A. N., Mauch, P. M., Fishman, N. H., Galante, M., Phillips, T. L., and Buschke, F.: Combined treatment methods for carcinoma of the esophagus, Radiology **128**:461-465, 1978.

Friedman, A. I.: Primary lymphosarcoma of the stomach, Am. J. Med. **26**:783-800, 1959.

Gaitan-Gaitan, A., Rider, W. D., and Bush, R. S.: Carcinoid tumor—cure by irradiation, Int. J. Radiat. Oncol. Biol. Phys. **1**:9-13, 1975.

Goldgraber, M. B., Rubin, C. E., Palmer, W. L., Dobson, R. L., and Massey, B. W.: The early gastric response to irradiation, a serial biopsy study, Gastroenterology **27**:1-20, 1954.

Goodner, J. T.: Surgical and radiation treatment of cancer of the thoracic esophagus, Am. J. Roentgenol. **105**:523-528, 1969.

Green, N., Beron, E., Melbye, R. W., and George, F. W., III.: Carcinoma of pancreas—palliative radiotherapy, Am. J. Roentgenol. **117**: 620-622, 1973.

Groves, L. K., and Rodriquez-Antunez, A.: Treatment of carcinoma of the esophagus and gastric cardia with concentrated preoperative irradiation therapy followed by early operation. A progress report, Ann. Thorac. Surg. **15**:333-345, 1973.

Guernsey, J. M., and Knudsen, D. F.: Abdominal exploration in the evaluation of patients with carcinoma of the thoracic esophagus, J. Thorac. Cardiovasc. Surg. **59**:62-66, 1970.

Gunderson, L. L.: Combined irradiation and surgery for rectal and sigmoid carcinoma, Curr. Probl. Cancer **5**:40-53, 1976.

Gunderson, L. L., and Sosin, H.: Areas of failure found at reoperation (second or symptomatic look) following "curative surgery" for adenocarcinoma of the rectum, clinicopathologic correlation and implications for adjuvant therapy, Cancer **34**:1278-1292, 1974.

Haslam, J. B., Cavanaugh, P. J., and Stroup, S. L.: Radiation therapy in the treatment of irresectable adenocarcinoma of the pancreas, Cancer **32:** 1341-1345, 1973.

Hamilton, F. E.: Gastric ulcer following radiation, Arch. Surg. **55:**394-399, 1947.

Hayes, M. A., Khoerman, M. M., and Vidone, R.: Preoperative radiation therapy in carcinoma of the rectum, Am. J. Proctol. **23:**289-295, 1972.

Jenkinson, E. L., Epperson, K. D., and Pfisterer, W. H.: Primary lymphosarcoma of the stomach, Am. J. Roentgenol. **72:**34-44, 1954.

Jennings, F. L.: Acute radiation effects in the esophagus, Arch. Pathol. **69:**407-413, 1960.

Krishnamurthi, S.: Cobalt 60 beam therapy in cancer of the thoracic esophagus, Indian J. Cancer **2:** 115-117, 1965.

Littman, A., Fox, B. W., Schoolman, H. M., and Ivy, A. C.: Lethal effect of intragastric irradiation in the dog, Am. J. Physiol. **174:**347-351, 1953.

Loeb, M. T.: Carcinoma of the esophagus, Lancet **85:**425-427, 1965.

Marcial, V. A., Tome, J. M., Ubinas, J., Bosch, A., and Correa, J. N.: The role of radiation therapy in esophageal cancer, Radiology **87:**231-238, 1966.

Marcial-Rojas, R. A., and Castro, J. R.: Irradiation injury to elastic arteries in the course of treatment for neoplastic disease, Ann. Otol. **71:**945-958, 1962.

Marks, R. D., Scruggs, H. J., and Wallace, K. M.: Preoperative radiation therapy for carcinoma of the esophagus, Cancer **38:**84-89, 1976.

Mendiondo, O. A., Wang, C. C., Welch, J. P., and Donaldson, G. A.: Postoperative radiotherapy in carcinomas of the rectum and distal colon, Radiology **119:**673-676, 1976.

Millburn, L., Hendrickson, F. R., and Faber, P.: Curative treatment of epidermoid carcinoma of the esophagus, Am. J. Roentgenol. **103:**291-299, 1968.

Montagna, W., and Wilson, J. W.: Cytologic study of intestinal epithelium of mouse after total body x-irradiation, J. Natl. Cancer Inst. **15:**1703-1736, 1955.

Nakayama, K., Orihata, H., and Yamaguchi, K.: Surgical treatment combined with preoperative concentrated irradiation for esophageal cancer, Cancer **20:**778-788, 1967.

Nakayama, K., and Kinoshita, Y.: Surgical treatment combined with preoperative concentrated irradiation, J.A.M.A. **227:**174-181, 1974.

Palmer, W. L., and Templeton, F.: The effects of radiation therapy on gastric secretion, J.A.M.A. **112:**1429-1434, 1939.

Papillon, J.: Resectable rectal cancers, treatment by curative endocavitary irradiation, J.A.M.A. **231:**1385-1387, 1975.

Parker, E. F., and Gregorie, H. B.: Carcinoma of the esophagus, long-term results, J.A.M.A. **235:** 1018-1020, 1976.

Pearson, J. G.: The radiotherapy of carcinoma of the oesophagus and postcricoid region in southeast Scotland, Clin. Radiol. **17:**242-257, 1966.

Pearson, J. G.: The value of radiotherapy in the management of esophageal cancer, Am. J. Roentgenol. **105:**500-513, 1969.

Pearson, J. G.: The value of radiotherapy in the management of squamous oesophageal cancer, Br. J. Surg. **58:**794-798, 1971.

Pearson, J. G.: The present status and future potential of radiotherapy in the management of esophageal cancer, Cancer **39:**882-890, 1977.

Phillips, T. L., and Margolis, L.: Radiation pathology and the clinical response of lung and esophagus. In Vaeth, J. M., editor: Radiation effect and tolerance normal tissue, Baltimore, 1972, University Park Press.

Pierquin, B., Wambersie, A., and Tubiana, M.: Cancer of the thoracic oesophagus: two series of patients treated by 22 Mev betatron, Br. J. Radiol. **39:**189-192, 1966.

Pilepich, M. V., Munzenrider, J. E., Tak, W. K., and Miller, H. H.: Preoperative irradiation of primarily unresectable colorectal carcinoma, Cancer **42:**1077-1081, 1978.

Postlethwait, R. W., Sealy, W. C., Emlet, J. R., and Zavertnik, J. J.: Squamous cell carcinoma of the esophagus, Surg. Gynecol. Obstet. **105:**465-472, 1957.

Rao, A. R., Kagan, A. R., Chan, P. Y., Gilbert, H. A., and Nussbaum, H.: Effectiveness of local radiotherapy in colorectal carcinoma, Cancer **42:** 1082-1086, 1978.

Redd, B. L.: Lymphosarcoma of the stomach, Am. J. Roentgenol. **82:**634-650, 1959.

Roswitt, B., Malsky, S. J., and Reid, C. B.: Radiation tolerance of the gastrointestinal tract. In Vaeth, J. M., editor: Front. Radiation Ther. Oncology **6:**160-181, 1971.

Ruff, C. C., Dockerty, M. B., Fricke, R. E., and Waugh, J. M.: Preoperative radiation therapy for adenocarcinoma of the rectum and rectosigmoid, Surg. Gynecol. Obstet. **112:**715-723, 1961.

Scanlon, E. F., Morton, D. R., Walker, J. M., and Watson, W. L.: The case against segmental resection for esophageal carcinoma, Surg. Gynecol. Obstet. **101:**290-296, 1955.

Schein, P. S., Lavin, P. T., Moertel, C. G., et al.: Pandomized Phase II clinical trial of adriamycin, methotrexate and actinomycin-D in advanced measurable pancreatic carcinoma, Cancer **42:** 19-22, 1978.

Shedd, D. P., Crowley, L. G., and Lindskog, G. F.: A ten year study of carcinoma of the esophagus, Surg. Gynecol. Obstet. **101:**55-58, 1955.

Smedal, M. I., Wright, K. A., and Siber, F. J.: The palliative treatment of recurrent carcinoma of rectum and rectosigmoid with 2 MV. radiation, Am. J. Roentgenol. **100:**904-908, 1967.

Smoron, G. L.: Radiation therapy of carcinoma of gallbladder and biliary tract, Cancer **40:**1422-1424, 1977.

Snoddy, W. T.: Primary lymphosarcoma of the stomach, Gastroenterology **20:**537-553, 1952.

Stearns, M. W., Jr.: Low dose preoperative roentgen therapy for cancer of the rectum. In Rush, B. F., Jr., and Greenlaw, R. H., editors: Cancer therapy by integrated radiation and operation, Springfield, Ill., 1968, Charles C Thomas, Publisher.

Stevens, K. R., Jr., Allen, C. V., and Fletcher, W. S.: Preoperative radiotherapy for adenocarcinoma of the rectosigmoid, Cancer **37:**2866-2874, 1976.

Stevens, K. R., Jr., Fletcher, W. S., and Allen, C. V.: Anterior resection and primary anastomosis following high dose preoperative irradiation for adenocarcinoma of the recto-sigmoid, Cancer **41:**2065-2071, 1978.

Stevens, K. R., Fry, R., and Stone, C.: A new technique for irradiating thoracic inlet tumors, Int. J. Radiat. Oncol. Biol. Phys. **4:**731-734, 1978.

Swift, M. N., Taketa, S. T., and Bond, V. P.: Delayed gastric emptying in rats after whole and partial body x-irradiation, Am. J. Physiol. **182:** 479-486, 1955.

Tanner, N. C., and Smithers, D. W.: Tumours of the oesophagus, Edinburgh, 1961, E. & S. Livingstone, Ltd.

Tepper, M., Vidone, R. A., Hayes, M. A., Lindenmuth, W. W., and Kligerman, M. W.: Preoperative irradiation in rectal cancer; initial comparison of clinical tolerance, surgical and pathologic findings, Am. J. Roentgenol. **102:**587-595, 1968.

Tepper, J., Nardi, G., and Suit, H.: Carcinoma of the pancreas, review of MGH experience from 1963 to 1973, analysis of surgical failure and implications for radiation therapy, Cancer **37:**1519-1524, 1976.

Vander Vennert, K. R.: Epidermoid carcinoma of the esophagus—a review of 150 cases, Am. Surg. **31:**487-492, 1965.

Walz, B. J., Lindstrom, E. R., Butcher, H. R., Jr., and Baglan, R. J.: Natural history of patients after abdominal-perineal resection; implications for radiation therapy, Cancer **39:**2437-2442, 1977.

Wang, C. C., and Schulz, M. D.: The role of radiation therapy in the management of carcinoma of the sigmoid, rectosigmoid, and rectum, Radiology **79:**1-5, 1962.

Watson, T. A.: Radiation treatment of cancer of the esophagus, Surg. Gynecol. Obstet. **117:**346-354, 1963.

Watson, T. A., and Brown, E. M.: X-ray therapy in carcinoma of the esophagus, J. Thorac. Surg. **22:** 216-218, 1951.

White, D. C.: An atlas of radiation histopathology, Springfield, Va., 1975, National Technical Information Service, Publisher.

Withers, H. R., and Romsdahl, M. M.: Postoperative radiotherapy for adenocarcinoma of the rectum and rectosigmoid, Int. J. Radiat. Oncol. Biol. Phys. **2:**1069-1074, 1977.

Wolferth, C. C., Brady, L. W., and Enterline, H. T.: Primary lymphosarcoma of the stomach, Surg. Gynecol. Obstet. **109:**755-761, 1959.

13

The kidney

RESPONSE OF THE NORMAL KIDNEY TO IRRADIATION

Radiations produce renal lesions both directly by their effect on the kidneys and indirectly from the products of tissues destroyed elsewhere in the body. Irradiation of a large volume of tissue exclusive of the kidneys may produce an elevated blood uric acid level, and the kidneys may show temporary hyperemia, edema, and tubular damage. Under such circumstances, renal function tests reveal a transient decrease in tubular function (Huang and associates). The return to normal is generally rapid without any sequelae. However, if renal function is already impaired, this additional damage may be serious. Indeed, massive tissue breakdown under these circumstances may be fatal. Patients with lymphoma will occasionally present an elevated blood urea nitrogen level secondary to leukemic infiltration of the kidneys. They may also present an increased blood uric acid level and uric acid crystals in the urine even before treatment is given (Fisher and associates). The management of this problem is simplified by the use of allopurinol.

ACUTE CHANGES. The *common* renal function studies fail to show any consistent changes either early or late after *fractionated* renal doses of 1000 to 2000 rad. Yet special studies including measurement of glomerular filtration rate, renal plasma flow, and tubular excretory capacity show changes (Avioli and associates). These and other studies were performed on ten patients before, during, and after abdominal irradiation for cancer. Prior to irradiation all patients had normal renal function. Total renal doses of 2000 to 2400 rad were given in 3 to 4 weeks. A decrease in renal plasma flow was found after only 400 rad. This test proved to be the most sensitive and consistent index of radiation-induced renal damage. Glomerular filtration rate was slightly decreased by renal doses of 400 rad, rose to above normal with doses up to 1625 rad, and decreased to subnormal values with still higher doses. This decrease persisted for at least 12 months. Tubular function (Tm_{PAH}) decreased irregularly until rather high doses had been given. In spite of changes in these functions, no changes were detected in the common renal function studies. Mendelsohn and Caceres performed a unilateral nephrectomy in dogs and then studied the acute effects of irradiating the remaining hypertrophied kidney. Doses to the kidney were 2010, 2750, and 3780 rad in 13 days. The severity of the response increased with the larger doses. Glomerular function measured by inulin clearance and renal blood flow showed a

366

transient increase followed by a rapid decrease to below normal. Gradual and incomplete improvement occurred subsequently. These workers proposed that the increased renal blood flow may be a consequence of a reactive hyperemia, but the contribution of radiation-induced vascular damage to this change is unknown. Tubular function, measured as Tm_{PAH}, decreased steadily for 8 to 9 weeks. By the thirty-second week this function approached the normal level. Blood urea nitrogen increased as tubular function decreased and then returned to normal, as might be expected.

Gup and associates performed differential function studies on explanted dog kidneys 5 to 7 months after unilateral irradiation. The doses given were 2000 rad fractionated in 20 days, 1000 rad fractionated in 10 days, and single doses of 1000 and 500 rad. The control kidneys received less than 2 rad from scattered radiations. There was a significant decrease in glomerular filtration rate and renal plasma flow of the irradiated kidney compared to the control kidney at all doses given. When the dogs were sacrificed, no significant difference in weight was noted between the irradiated and nonirradiated kidneys. Histologically, no radiation-induced changes were observed.

By microscopic examination, the pathogenesis of this acute phase of renal damage has been difficult to define. By electron microscopy, the first detectable changes are those of the glomerular endothelial cells. They swell, and the basement membrane blends with large quantities of material on its endothelial aspect (Rosen and associates). At this point the tubules and interstitial tissues appear unchanged. Mostofi and associates found the glomeruli relatively undamaged at this time, and Maier and Casarett found changes appearing first in the arterioles. They point out that the direct continuity of the internal elastic membrane of the afferent arteriole with the glomerular basement membrane permits us to explain the changes in both by an injury common to both endothelia.

Higher doses used experimentally and clinically produce severe damage to all renal structures. With such doses microscopic findings during this acute phase are those of an atrophic organ with fibrotic zones, destroyed or atrophic tubules, and glomeruli (Mendelsohn and Caceres). Work by Flanagan indicates that with single doses of 2800 rad to the rabbit's kidney, tubular damage from both a histologic and a functional viewpoint reaches its peak in 4 weeks. Slow, incomplete recovery follows (Figs. 13-1 and 13-2).

The administration of doses in excess of 2300 rad in 5 weeks to both kidneys will produce the clinical picture of acute radiation nephritis in about half the patients (Luxton). The earliest clinical findings consist of proteinuria, hypertension, anemia, and cardiomegaly. Hypertension is indicative of severe changes and is the most serious finding. Although the kidneys may recover and the hypertension may disappear, this is not usually the case. Of the twenty patients with acute radiation nephritis reviewed by Luxton, ten died. Within a month or two the so-called chronic or late changes begin to appear, and all survivors will have some degree of chronic nephritis. Six of the ten died of malignant hypertension in 12 months from onset. Three died of

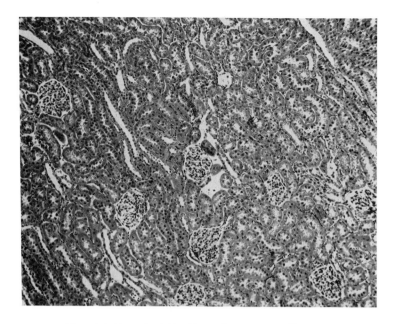

Fig. 13-1. Normal rabbit kidney. Compare with Fig. 13-2.

renal failure 7 to 11 years from onset. Microscopic findings consist of widespread glomerular, tubular, and arteriolar injury. The care of these patients is supportive and should be directed toward helping the patient through the acute phase with hypotensive drugs, transfusions, rest, dietary guidance, and, if necessary, long-term renal dialysis.

CHRONIC CHANGES. Inseparable from the previously described acute changes are a series of serious changes developing over a period of several months, and as pointed out previously, these changes may result in death years later. A history of acute radiation nephritis is not a prerequisite for chronic radiation nephritis. The most obvious changes are impaired renal function with albuminuria and inability to concentrate. Hypertension and anemia are usually present.

In their excellent analysis, Kunkler and associates defined the limit of renal radiation tolerance in man. Patients with seminoma of the testis had sites of probable abdominal metastases irradiated through large ports. The kidneys were included in the treated volume. When a dose of 2500 to 3250 rad in 3 to 6 weeks was delivered to the whole of both kidneys in fifty-five patients, 40% were known to have developed renal damage and seven patients died from radiation-induced renal damage. Further clinical developments in this group of patients were reported by Luxton and by Kunkler and associates. Thus, of twenty-four patients with chronic radiation nephritis, nine were normotensive for 8 years. More often, the patients develop the clinical picture of chronic glomerular nephritis (hypertension, proteinuria, anemia, casts in the urine, and elevated blood urea nitrogen). As might be expected, the kidneys became small and fibrotic.

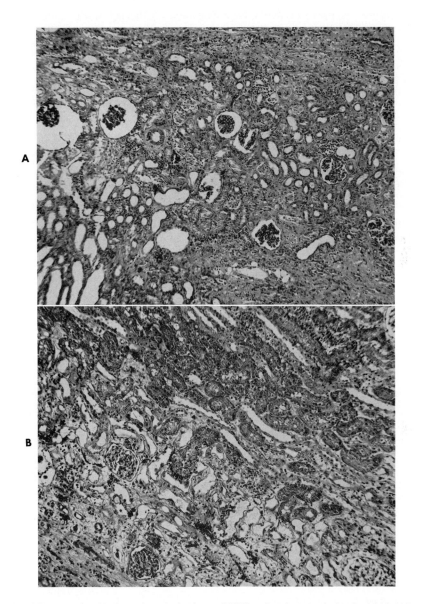

Fig. 13-2. Microscopic changes after single dose of 2800 rad to the exteriorized rabbit's kidney (220 kv; hvl, 1.2 mm Cu; TSD, 52 cm). **A,** One month after irradiation. Every glomerulus shows extensive damage. There is widespread tubular necrosis and atrophy. Round cells have inflltrated interstitial tissues. Vascular damage is not evident except in glomeruli. **B,** Representative changes 4 months later. Incomplete recovery of all elements has occurred. Some glomeruli have recovered strikingly. Tubular damage is still severe, although noticeable recovery has occurred. The initial infiltration has decreased. Associated studies revealed some recovery of function. (Courtesy Dr. C. L. Flanagan.)

It is important here to realize that irradiation of only one kidney can produce malignant hypertension and that the hypertension may disappear after nephrectomy. Therefore any patient developing hypertension after upper abdominal irradiation should be investigated for the possibility of radiation-induced renal damage. If the damage is unilateral, nephrectomy should be considered.

Asscher's fascinating studies throw light on the puzzle of radiation-induced hypertension and indeed on the late effects of radiations in all areas of the body. Hypertension secondary to renal irradiation appears earlier the higher the renal dose and the less the fractionation. Furthermore, its severity is not so much dependent on the absolute amount of renal tissue irradiated as it is on the proportion of total renal mass irradiated. Hypertension from any cause produces profound hypertensive vascular damage in *irradiated* blood vessels, whereas unirradiated vessels subjected to the same hypertension may remain normal in appearance for months. In other words, the radiations "sensitize" the blood vessels to hypertensive changes. In the kidney, this "sensitization" of vessels to hypertensive damage has serious implications, especially considering that hypertension is an expected sequela of high renal doses. However, the "sensitization" of vessels to hypertensive damage is not confined to the kidney. It develops in all irradiated tissues. Asscher and Anson pointed out that a patient who previously had vital tissues irradiated—brain, spinal cord, bowel, or lung—can, because of the developing hypertension, develop vascular necrosis leading to heretofore unexplained sequelae. These laboratory findings should be kept in mind in weighing the radiation "tolerances" in hypertensive patients or the causes of necrosis in patients who have recently become hypertensive.

As demonstrated by Asscher, the pathogenesis of radiation-induced hypertension from renal irradiation may be summarized as follows. In rats, renal arteries manifest their "sensitization" within 60 days after a single dose of 1200 rad to both kidneys. About 90 days after renal irradiation, hypergranulation of the juxtaglomerular cells can be seen. This is recognized as one of the first morphologic changes related to subsequent hypertension, and it is apparently a consequence of decreased renal artery flow, even though at this point the vessels appear normal. About 5 months after irradiation, hypertension is well developed, and necrosis of the "sensitized" arteries develops.

An explanation of the anemia of these patients is lacking, although Asscher suggested that the radiation damage might decrease renal erythropoietin and increase hemolysis. The anemia, however, is like that seen in chronic renal insufficiency of any etiology.

Microscopic examination of the kidneys during this chronic phase reveals marked tubular destruction with interstitial fibrosis and glomerular hyalinization (Fig. 13-3). Characteristic postirradiation vascular changes are seen—subendothelial fibrous connective tissue proliferation in the medium and smaller arteries—but the most impressive changes are those of tubular destruction. Since the glomerular efferent vessels subdivide to form the microvasculature of the tubules, damage to the glomerular circulation will also affect the blood supply of the tubules (White). This

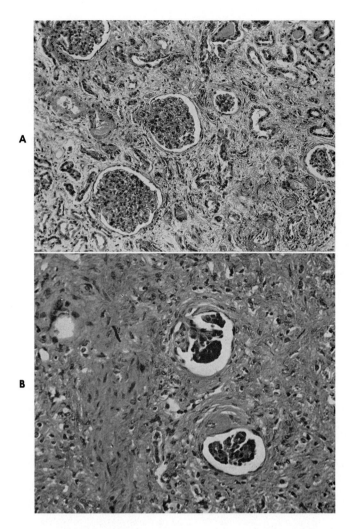

Fig. 13-3. Radiation nephritis. **A,** Thirteen months after delivery of a calculated 3000 rad minimum to left kidney. Glomerular changes are moderately severe, and tubular damage is very severe. Interstitial edema, round cell infiltration, and fibrosis are striking. **B** reveals findings in a patient irradiated repeatedly for upper abdominal Hodgkin's disease who died from radiation nephritis. Dose-time relationship is not known. Glomeruli are almost completely destroyed. No tubules are left. (W. U. neg. 57-4651A; courtesy Dr. L. V. Ackerman.)

direct effect of vascular damage accounts for the atrophy of kidneys seen following doses of radiation sufficient to affect the afferent arterioles.

On those rare occasions when both kidneys must be included in the irradiated volume, the maximum dose delivered to the kidneys should not exceed 2300 rad in 5 weeks, or its biologic equivalent, unless the risk of late renal damage is justified.

Either a part or all of the left kidney has often been included in the high-dose volume used for encompassing the spleen in the irradiation of patients with Hodg-

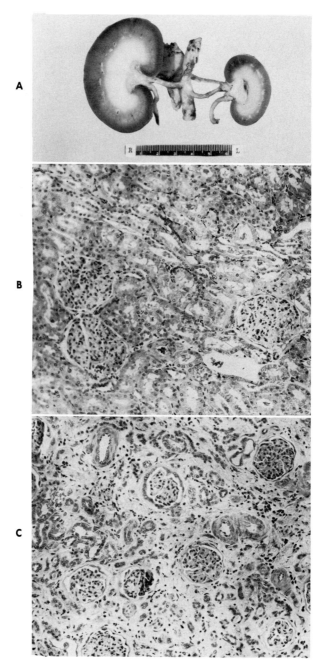

Fig. 13-4. A, Autopsy specimen 3 months after single dose of 1500 rad (^{60}Co) to both kidneys of a dog. Right renal artery was infused with epinephrine at the time of irradiation. Atrophic left kidney was essentially nonfunctioning when differential urine collections were made prior to sacrifice. The infused right kidney excreted normal amounts of urine and showed no gross radiation effects. **B** and **C,** Photomicrographs of sections from kidneys shown in **A. B,** Essentially normal-appearing right kidney (infused with epinephrine at time of irradiation). **C,** Unprotected left kidney. There are severe tubular damage, interstitial fibrosis, and arteriolar and glomerular changes. (From Johnson, R. E., Doppman, J. L., Harbert, J. C., Steckel, R. J., and MacLowry, J. D.: Radiology **91:**103-108, 1968.)

kin's disease. The dose given is often as high as 4000 rad in 4 to 5 weeks. One would imagine that this dose would be associated with frequent left kidney malfunction. Studies performed in our own institution and by Birkhead and associates have failed to demonstrate any significant renal dysfunction in these patients. This is not likely to be the case in children (Donaldson and associates).

As might be expected when chemotherapy is given with renal irradiation, nephritis will appear earlier and with a lower dose (Churchill and associates).

The precautions necessary to prevent radiation-induced renal failure are obvious. Renal irradiation should be avoided when possible. This implies accurate definition of tumor extent and recognition of the presence of congenital variation in number and position of the kidneys. An intravenous pyelogram, at least, should be available to meet these needs. When renal irradiation is judged unavoidable, as much renal tissue as possible should be shielded and the dose limited to 2000 rad in 2 weeks. In rare instances this can be accomplished by redefining the tumor volume after the initial dose (for example, in the case of massive involvement of the para-aortic lymph nodes by lymphoma or seminoma). It may be possible to deliver a high dose to the kidney and prevent radiation nephritis by selective infusion of the renal artery with vasoconstrictors to produce local ischemia and hypoxia (Johnson and associates) (Fig. 13-4). The possibility of this technique has been demonstrated experimentally in dogs and has been applied to patients with upper abdominal neoplasms. The possibility of shifting a kidney to the iliac fossa with reimplantation of the vessels should be considered if doses greater than the kidney tolerance are necessary. When neither of these alternatives is possible and chronic renal insufficiency is an accepted sequela of treatment, then considerations of long-term renal dialysis or kidney transplantation are not unreasonable if cure by irradiation is obtainable.

CARCINOMA OF THE KIDNEY

Primary carcinomas of the kidney are divided into three major categories—adenocarcinomas of the renal parenchyma, Wilms' tumors, and carcinomas of the renal pelvis. These must be separated from carcinomas metastatic to the kidney and rare primary sarcomas.

Adenocarcinomas of the renal parenchyma in adults

Adenocarcinomas of the renal parenchyma arise from the epithelium of renal tubules. Electron microscopic study (Oberling and associates) revealed the presence of brush border structures in renal cell carcinoma, laying to rest the theory of adrenal origin and rendering the term *hypernephroma* obsolete. As pointed out previously, moderately high doses of radiations can be given to the normal tubular epithelium before physiologic or morphologic injury is obvious. For the most part adenocarcinomas arising from these cells present a similar or even greater tolerance to irradiation. Doses of 2000 to 3000 rad to the tumor in 3 weeks produce few significant gross or microscopic changes (Flocks and Kadesky). The unresected primary lesion and proved postoperative persistence have rarely been reported as being eradicated by irradiation alone.

A major factor in determining prognosis is tumor grade. High-grade and anaplastic malignancies frequently invade the renal vein and perirenal tissues and metastasize to regional lymph nodes. In Riches' series of 110 patients, thirty with low-grade neoplasms had no evidence of spread to lymph nodes, renal vein, or perirenal extension. The 5- and 10-year survival rates were 86% and 60%, respectively. In those patients with high-grade neoplasms, the 5- and 10-year survival rates were 29% and 18%, respectively. The addition of postoperative irradiation in cases locally confined could not be expected to improve results significantly. When the renal vein was grossly invaded, postoperative irradiation did not improve results. Lymph node metastases were present in 8.2% and perirenal extension in 21%, and in these cases tumor grade was more important than the addition of postoperative irradiation in determining the outcome.

Adenocarcinomas of the renal parenchyma are usually regarded as radioincurable. Surgery, when possible, is the primary treatment of choice. However, Riches and associates point out that 28% of the patients have nonresectable lesions.

Adenocarcinomas of the kidney usually grow silently until they become locally advanced or until they produce symptomatic metastases. Vein invasion leading to hematogenous metastasis is common. Invasion of perirenal fat or neighboring organs leads to frequent local recurrence. The recurrence rate remains high even after 5 years. Among patients clinically well at the end of 5 years, between a third and a half will die of recurrence (Mintz and Gaul). The striking similarities between the natural history of this tumor and carcinoma of the breast are obvious.

The only possible contribution of the frequently recommended routine postoperative irradiation is one of temporarily suppressing recurrent tumor growth. We do not believe that the collected figures reviewed by Riches and associates or reviews like those of Flocks and Kadesky prove the value of routine postoperative irradiation. In his retrospective analysis of patients given postoperative irradiation after nephrectomy, Rafla demonstrated improvement in survival only in those patients with capsular invasion and no other bad prognostic features. Finney reported the results of a prospective trial of postoperative irradiation following nephrectomy in which all gross disease was removed. He could not attribute benefit to postoperative irradiation, and there was no difference in the incidence of local recurrences or distant metastasis between the irradiated and nonirradiated groups. Van der Werf-Messing found no improvement in survival in a prospective trial of preoperative radiation using 3000 rad in 3 weeks. There did, however, appear to be an increase in rate of resectability in patients given irradiation. At present we advise postoperative irradiation only in those patients with known persistence of the disease.

TECHNIQUE OF IRRADIATION. In the irradiation of the locally nonresectable cancer, large opposing ports are usually sufficient. The recommended dose will rarely be greater than 4500 rad in 5 to 6 weeks. The same technique is used for irradiation of postoperative persistence of the disease. In view of the discussion given earlier, it is questionable if higher doses are indicated when cure is not possible and palliation is the sole aim. Portions of many organs may be included in the irradiated volume—that is, the spleen, stomach, large bowel, small bowel, lung, and liver.

Radiation injury to these organs must be weighed in the treatment of renal carcinomas.

Metastases may respond to doses similar to those given for metastatic breast lesions. Such treatment may be particularly helpful by arresting the growth of osseous metastases in weight-bearing bones. In general, however, the response will be less frequent than for carcinoma of the breast.

PROGNOSIS AND RESULTS. There are few reports in the literature proving without question that irradiation alone can cure a patient with adenocarcinoma of the renal parenchyma. Some inoperable or partially resected primary lesions will show a good temporary radiation-induced regression. The frequency with which this can be accomplished is not known. The shrinking of painful space-occupying renal masses and the arrest of destruction of osseous defects are the aims and, at times, the results of palliative irradiation.

Adenocarcinomas of the renal parenchyma in children

Adenocarcinoma of the renal parenchyma is uncommon in children and is rarely seen in the first 5 years of life. Although the tumor may present as an abdominal mass, pain and hematuria are more common than in Wilms' tumor. Surgical removal is the treatment of choice; the rationale for irradiation is probably the same as discussed for adenocarcinoma of the renal parenchyma in adults. In a review of eighty-four childhood cases, approximately 50% were cured (Castellanos and associates).

Wilms' tumor

Wilms' tumor occurs almost exclusively in children, is highly malignant, and metastasizes early, particularly to the lungs. Since these tumors possess both malignant epithelial and malignant connective tissue elements, they are thought to represent embryonic renal tissues; hence the terms *"embryoma"* and *"nephroblastoma."*

Mesoblastic nephroma of infancy is a benign tumor of the newborn that must be separated from the general category of Wilms' tumors (Bolande and associates). It is mostly stromal in nature, the rare epithelial nests probably representing trapped elements. It might be difficult to differentiate at times from a sarcomatous Wilms' tumor.

D'Angio and associates reported six cases of mesoblastic nephroma among 606 children registered in the National Wilms' Tumor Study (NWTS). A similar incidence has been noted by Lemerle and associates in their report of a clinical trial conducted by the International Society of Pediatric Oncology (SIOP).

In the usual Wilms' tumor the epithelial elements recapitulate various stages of nephronic differentiation with tubules and abortive glomeruli. Other epithelial types, uncommon to the normal kidney, may be present. The stromal component is equally mixed with fibrosarcomatous, leiomyosarcomatous, and frequently skeletal muscle differentiation as well. Adipose, cartilaginous, and osseous differentiation may also be present. Under different circumstances these tissue types are usually regarded as relatively radioresistant, yet after irradiation of Wilms' tumor, striking early regres-

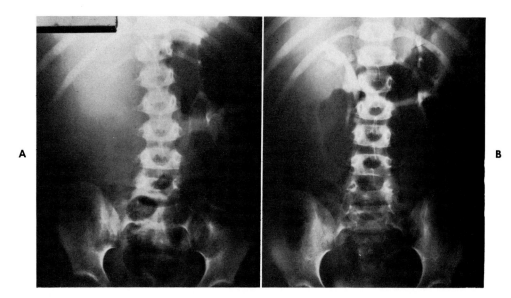

Fig. 13-5. A, IVP showing large mass in right abdomen with distortion and displacement of the collecting system of right kidney in a 5-year-old child. A dose of approximately 2800 rad was given through three 10 × 16 ports (140 kv; 8 ma, 0.25 mm Cu plus 1.0 mm Al added filter). **B,** Repeat IVP 1 month after **A,** showing significant shrinkage. Diagnosis of Wilms' tumor confirmed by nephrectomy. (Courtesy Dr. Harvey White.)

sion is the rule (Fig. 13-5). Doses to the tumor of no more than 1000 rad may reduce the tumor to less than half its original dimensions. The epithelial elements respond less to irradiation than do the sarcomatous elements (Bothe). A tumor with a predominance of epithelial cells will be less affected than one composed predominantly of connective tissue cells. Lemerle and associates reported a significant correlation between a favorable prognosis and the number of epithelial differentiated elements seen in the tumor. Regardless of the relative cellular composition of these tumors, studies done after preoperative irradiation generally reveal persistent disease. Permanent control usually depends on complete surgical resection. Survival is definitely superior in children under 2 years of age. This effect of age is even apparent in the early study by Gross and Neuhauser that showed a survival of 70% to 80% in children under the age of 12 months. The relationship of age and prognosis has been documented in both the NWTS and the SIOP clinical trials. Garcia and associates found that survival was better with small tumors than with large ones. They also found survival was better in the absence of local infiltration of perirenal tissue, the absence of vessel invasion, and the absence of local and distant metastases. The staging system used in the NWTS is as follows:

Group I Tumor limited to kidney and completely resected. The surface of the renal capsule is intact. The tumor was not ruptured before or during removal. There is no residual tumor apparent beyond the margins of resection.

Group II Tumor extends beyond the kidney but is completely resected. There is local extension of the tumor, that is, penetration beyond the pseudocapsule into the perirenal soft tissues, or para-aortic lymph node involvement. The renal vessels outside the kidney substance are infiltrated or contain tumor thrombus. There is no residual tumor apparent beyond the margins of resection.

Group III   Residual nonhematogenous tumor confined to abdomen. Any one or more of the following occur: (a) The tumor has been biopsied or ruptured before or during surgery. (b) There are implants on peritoneal surfaces. (c) There are involved lymph nodes beyond the abdominal periaortic chains. (d) The tumor not completely resectable because of local infiltration into vital structures.

Group IV   Hematogenous metastases. Deposits beyond Group III to, for example, lung, liver, bone, and brain.

Group V   Bilateral renal involvement either initially or subsequently.

Platt and Linden and others have demonstrated the significance of a 2-year survival free of Wilms' tumor. Wolff and associates reported the long-term results of a single versus multiple courses of actinomycin D in the treatment of Wilms' tumor. The use of multiple courses of actinomycin D significantly improved relapse-free survival, but with the addition of salvage therapies in those children with recurrence or metastases there was no significant effect on ultimate survival rate. This modification of the natural history of Wilms' tumor must be considered in evaluating the results of current therapy. In children not given maintenance chemotherapy, the risk of developing pulmonary metastases varies between 30% and 50%, and the mean interval from recognition of metastasis and treatment of the primary tumor is approximately 6 months. This fact is important in planning the follow-up management of children with Wilms' tumor.

PREOPERATIVE IRRADIATION. The diagnosis of Wilms' tumor is not usually made until the infant's mother feels the large abdominal mass or notices the distended abdomen. The tumor is usually large. Removal of such a large tumor was formerly accompanied by a high surgical mortality. Many surgeons, particularly those using the extraperitoneal posterior approach, found the procedure simplified if, before resection, the mass could be diminished by irradiation. With nephrectomy by way of the transperitoneal route, the mere size of the lesion has not been a serious obstacle. Gross did not use preoperative irradiation and had no operative deaths in 20 years.

We believe that the arguments for or against preoperative irradiation do not depend on tumor size per se. Rather the large size is usually an index of duration of growth and correlated with degree of advancement. The arguments relative to preoperative irradiation in general were discussed in Chapter 2. That discussion applies to Wilms' tumor also. However, with Wilms' tumor the diagnosis cannot be assured without biopsy. The SIOP controlled clinical trial of preoperative versus postoperative radiation therapy evaluated 195 randomized patients. Two thousand rad administered preoperatively significantly reduced the number of "surgical spill" cases (three versus twenty cases) and obviated the need for whole abdominal irradiation given postoperatively in a significant number of patients. Unfortunately at surgery no cancer was present, and a diagnosis other than Wilms' tumor was established in 4% of the total group. Apparently, a large number of young children with Group I tumors were needlessly irradiated. There was no significant difference in survival between the two groups. Thus, if irradiation is to be avoided whenever possible, preoperative irradiation has no place in the management of Wilms' tumor.

POSTOPERATIVE IRRADIATION. Despite its remote curative possibilities, routine postoperative irradiation has been practiced by leading treatment centers and is widely advocated. Gross, at Boston Children's Hospital, emphasized his faith in such irradiation by recommending its initiation prior to the patient's recovery from anesthesia. He reported a 2-year survival of 47%. Prior to adjuvant chemotherapy, this was the highest published survival rate of a large number of patients and had a significant influence on treatment planning at other institutions. Rarely are persistent or previously untreated tumors controlled by irradiation alone. In our experience only about 10% of children with pulmonary metastases are controlled by irradiation alone, whereas 50% survive when irradiation is administered in combination with actinomycin D.

In the NWTS report by D'Angio and associates children under the age of 2 years, with Group I tumors were not benefited by routine administration of postoperative irradiation. In the Group I cases of children over 2 years of age there is a slight tendency, but no statistically significant difference, toward improved local control and survival with the administration of postoperative irradiation. It should be borne in mind that the initial reports of this study permit only a review of relapse-free survival, and as noted above, this may not be a meaningful measure of ultimate outcome in the current treatment of Wilms' tumor. There is no question of the importance of postoperative irradiation in Group II and Group III cases. In a review of the NWTS experience with Group III cases, Tefft and associates reported control of abdominal disease in all but eight of fifty-eight evaluable children. Although there is clear evidence that the use of actinomycin D reduces the incidence of distant metastases, it is impossible to determine what role postoperative irradiation plays in reducing such distant spread.

The sequelae from tissue doses of 2000 rad or more in these young patients are quite predictable and must be accepted when irradiation is recommended. If the child is less than 9 years old and the dose to the vertebrae is 2000 rad (orthovoltage) or more in 4 to 6 weeks, permanent radiographic abnormalities inevitably develop (Neuhauser and associates). In the same period such changes will be less frequent with doses from 1000 to 2000 rad, whereas none will appear when doses are below 1000 rad. The younger the child, the more severe the defect. It was formerly thought that inclusion of the entire transverse width of the vertebral column would eliminate the risk of scoliosis. Unfortunately, this has not been the case. In fact, some of the worst deformities have followed irradiation of the entire vertebral width (Rubin and associates; Vaeth and associates). Atrophy of the irradiated flank muscle is not uncommon and may contribute to the degree of scoliosis (Fig. 13-6). However, at times we see such atrophy of muscles with barely detectable scoliosis. Bowel injury is usually

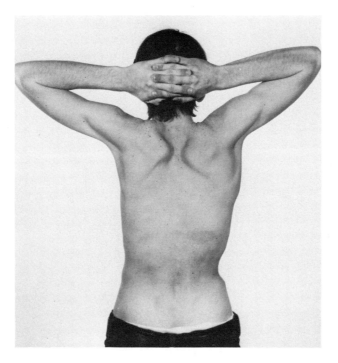

Fig. 13-6. Marked muscle atrophy of right flank of a 15-year-old boy irradiated at age 4 for Wilms' tumor of the right kidney. There is no detectable scoliosis.

in the form of a transient diarrhea without any serious permanent sequelae. We have, however, observed several young adults irradiated in childhood who have significant reduction in size of the irradiated colon and in one case manifestations of a localized chronic ulcerative colitis (Fig. 13-7). Concannon and associates have shown an apparent threshold of daily dose to produce severe intestinal damage when irradiation is combined with actinomycin D (Chapter 12).

Li and Stone evaluated late sequelae in 142 young adults who received treatment of malignancies in childhood. Of the total, 70% had been given orthovoltage radiation and 87% had received chemotherapy. Ten developed second malignancies (7%), and eight of these ten malignancies arose in previously irradiated tissues. Two patients died as a result of the second malignancies. While half of these young adults had major defects attributable to their treatment in childhood, most of those surveyed expressed satisfaction with the quality of their life.

It is our belief that definite curative benefits from routine postoperative irradiation must be clear-cut and outweigh such sequelae before irradiation can be accepted as a significant adjunct to surgery. The fact that irradiation alone has cured some patients with Wilms' tumor certainly justifies postoperative irradiation when disease is known to have been left behind or when metastases are detected.

TECHNIQUE OF IRRADIATION. In infants and small children, simple anterior and posterior parallel opposing ports, together with a lateral port, are sufficient. The

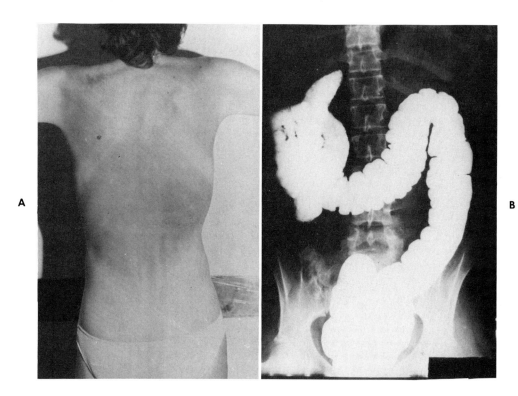

Fig. 13-7. A, Skin changes and muscle atrophy in the right flank of 20-year-old woman given post-operative irradiation at age 10 months after resection of a malignant tumor of the adrenal gland. **B,** Colon x-ray film of same patient showing atrophy and mucosal irregularities of previously irradiated right hemicolon (cecum and appendix were identified on spot films). The remaining unirradiated colon is entirely normal.

ports should encompass the known disease plus a generous margin of apparently normal tissues (Fig. 13-8). Care should be taken to avoid irradiation of the opposite kidney. When whole abdominal irradiation is necessary, the dose to the contralateral kidney should be kept below 1500 rad, including the contribution of scatter. The optimum dose to be delivered to the center of the tumor is not established with any certainty. We recommend a dose of 3000 rad in 3½ weeks when gross tumor has been left behind at surgery or lymph node metastases are found. There is scant evidence to recommend postoperative irradiation for Group I cases, regardless of the child's age. Garcia and associates confirmed the suspicion that children under 2 years of age are diagnosed at an earlier stage than children over 2 years of age. Thus clinical stage and not chronologic age should form the rationale for the recommendation of postoperative irradiation. When pulmonary metastases are present, both lungs are irradiated, using anterior and posterior ports to a total dose of 1200 rad combined with actinomycin D. We formerly thought this dose difference a paradox. However, if one considers that the combination of total lung irradiation with actinomycin D results in control in only 50% of the cases, compared with control of abdominal

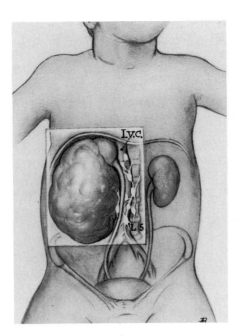

Fig. 13-8. Diagram of volume usually included in irradiation of Wilms' tumor. Compare with Fig. 13-6.

Table 13-1. Doses recommended for the National Wilms' Tumor Study

Age	Total tumor dose
Birth to 18 months	1800 to 2400 rad
19 to 30 months	2400 to 3000 rad
31 to 40 months	3000 to 3500 rad
41 months or more	3500 to 4000 rad

disease in 86% of the cases in Group III lesions when higher doses are delivered, this is not paradoxic but rather indicative of a dose response when the normal tissue volume permits a higher dose to be employed. The dose recommendations of the NWTS are shown in Table 13-1.

COMBINATION CHEMOTHERAPY AND IRRADIATION. Surgery alone is highly successful in controlling Wilms' tumor locally confined to the kidney. Unfortunately, the fact that more than half the children with this disease will present with or develop distant metastases makes any chance of improving survival dependent on the prevention or successful treatment of distant metastases. There is no definite evidence that preoperative irradiation can prevent metastases from Wilms' tumor, and there are all too few survivors whose metastatic lesions were controlled by surgery or irradiation alone. Evidence is available that actinomycin D and vincristine modify the frequency of metastases.

Farber has reviewed the work leading to clinical trials with actinomycin D as a

Table 13-2. Two-year survival studies in patients treated for Wilms' tumor metastases to the lungs*

Reference	Radiotherapy only	Radiotherapy and actinomycin D
Burgert	8% (2/25)	36% (9/25)
Farber		
Group A		58% (18/31)
Group B		26% (11/43)
Johnson	(0/8)	43% (3/7)
Maier	14% (1/7)	50% (4/8)
Pearson	14% (1/7)	
Reiquam	43% (3/7)	(0/5)
Sukarochama	20% (2/10)	14% (1/7)
Vietti		57% (8/14)
Wagget		78% (7/9)
Westra	4% (1/25)	
Monson		47% (9/19)
TOTAL	11% (10/89)	42% (70/168)

*From Monson, K. J., Brand, W. N., and Boggs, J. D.: Radiology **104:**157-160, 1972.

useful agent in the prevention and treatment of metastases. Of fifty-three children without evidence of metastases on admission to Boston Children's Hospital who received postoperative irradiation and actinomycin D, forty-seven (89%) survived 2 years. There is no evidence that actinomycin D and vincristine produce relapse-free survival superior to that of either drug alone. In the final report of the Children's Cancer Study Group A evaluation of single versus multiple courses of actinomycin D, relapse-free survival is definitely superior in those children given multiple courses (Wolff and associates). There was, however, no difference in the ultimate survival of children in either arm when additional therapy was given those who developed metastases or local recurrence. It is important to note that only one child receiving multiple courses of chemotherapy developed metastases, whereas twelve who received only the initial course developed metastases to the lung. Although subsequent therapies will salvage some of these children, we believe that the value of maintenance chemotherapy has been proven.

The overall survival for children with pulmonary metastases now approaches 50% with combination therapy. Similar results have not been attained with irradiation alone or actinomycin D alone. Published survival data for treated pulmonary metastases are shown in Table 13-2. Monson and associates have shown the importance of bilateral whole lung irradiation even when a solitary metastasis is suspected.

BILATERAL WILMS' TUMOR. Bilateral involvement of the kidneys by Wilms' tumor occurs in about 5% of cases (Ragab and associates; D'Angio and associates). Ehrlich and Goodwin have emphasized the surgeon's responsibility in exploring the contralateral kidney during the surgical treatment of an abdominal mass believed to be a Wilms' tumor. Such an exploration is possible only with a transverse transperitoneal incision. It is usually possible in most simultaneously occurring bilateral Wilms' tumors and some metachronous lesions to remove the primary mass and perform a partial nephrectomy on the contralateral, less involved kidney. We have not recommended routine irradiation to the bed of the partially nephrectomized kidney in those cases when partial nephrectomy is not adequate to encompass the disease. A dose of radiation under 2000 rad with concomitant actinomycin D may lead to cure in some children. Concannon and associates have noted that combinations of irradiation and actinomycin D do not lower the tolerance of the kidneys below that expected from irradiation alone. Richards and associates have reported their experience with one child whose contralateral disease was treated with 4000 rad to the involved part of the kidney in conjunction with actinomycin D and vincristine. Their patient survived over 5 years without evidence of recurrence or renal failure. Despite this apparent success, we believe that the primary management of a partially involved contralateral kidney should be surgical.

CARCINOMA OF THE RENAL PELVIS

Tumors of the renal pelvis may be either transitional cell carcinomas or epidermoid carcinomas. In either case they resemble the same cell types seen in the urinary bladder and are best treated by surgery. Although one may speculate on the radiosensitivity of these tumors, they are rarely controlled by irradiation (Rafla; Johansson and associates). The rarity of these lesions also forbids any meaningful statement relative to the palliative value of irradiation.

SUMMARY

Although there is considerable variation in the radiosensitivity of the three types of carcinomas found in the kidney, surgery is unquestionably the treatment of choice. The control of any of these lesions by irradiation alone is rare. For this reason the curative value of routine postoperative irradiation is often questioned. Wilms' tumor is the most radiosensitive of all renal carcinomas, and postoperative irradiation is recommended when there is a high risk of local residual cancer, when local tumor is known to have been left behind, and in the treatment of metastases. There is now evidence that actinomycin D and vincristine may prevent or, in combination with irradiation, control metastases from Wilms' tumor.

REFERENCES

Asscher, A. W., and Anson, S. C.: Arterial hypertension and irradiation damage to the nervous system, Lancet **2:**1343-1346, 1962.

Asscher, A. W.: The delayed effects of renal irradiation, Clin. Radiol. **15:**320-325, 1964.

Avioli, L. V., Lazor, M. Z., Cotlove, E., Grace, K. C., and Andrews, J. R.: Early effects of radiation on renal function in man, Am. J. Med. **34:** 329-337, 1963.

Birkhead, B. M., Dobbs, C. E., Beard, M. F.,

Tyson, J. W., and Fuller, E. A.: Assessment of renal function following irradiation of the intact spleen for Hodgkins disease, Radiology **130:** 473-476, 1979.

Bolande, R. P., Brough, A. J., and Izant, R. J., Jr.: Congenital mesoblastic nephroma of infancy, Pediatrics **40:**272-278, 1967.

Bothe, A. E.: Tissue changes in mixed tumors of the kidney after roentgen therapy, J. Urol. **33:** 434-442, 1935.

Castellanos, R. D., Aron, B. S., and Evans, A. T.: Renal adenocarcinoma in children, J. Urol. **111:** 534-539, 1974.

Churchill, D. N., Hong, K., and Gault, M. H.: Radiation nephritis following combined abdominal radiation and chemotherapy, Cancer **41:** 2162-2164, 1978.

Concannon, J. P., Summers, R. E., Cole, C., and Weil, C.: Effects on renal function: x-radiation combined with systemic actinomycin D, Am. J. Roentgenol. **108:**141-148, 1970.

Concannon, J. P., Summers, R. E., Cole, G., Werl, C., Kopp, U., and Sigdestad, C. P.: Effects of x-radiation and actinomycin D on intestinal epithelium of dogs, Radiology **97:**157-164, 1970.

D'Angio, G. J., Evans, A. E., Breslow, B., Beckwith, B., Bishop, H., Feigl, P., Goodwin, W., Leape, L., Sinks, L. F., Sutow, W., Tefft, M., and Wolff, J.: The treatment of Wilms' tumor, Cancer **38:**633-646, 1976.

Donaldson, S. S., Moskowitz, P. S., Canty, E. L., and Efron, B.: Radiation induced inhibition of compensatory renal growth in weanling mouse kidney, Radiology **128:**491-495, 1978.

Ehrlich, R. M., and Goodwin, W. E.: The surgical treatment of nephroblastoma (Wilms' tumor), Cancer **32:**1145-1149, 1973.

Farber, S.: Chemotherapy in the treatment of leukemia and Wilms' tumor, J.A.M.A. **198:**826-836, 1966.

Finney, R.: An evaluation of postoperative radiotherapy in hypernephroma treatment—a clinical trial, Cancer **32:**1332-1340.

Fisher, M. S., Torre, A. V., and Wohl, G. T.: Fatal uremia due to uric acid crystals in a case of lymphosarcoma, Radiology **70:**84-88, 1958.

Flanagan, C. L.: Personal communication, 1958.

Flocks, R. H., and Kadesky, M. D.: Malignant neoplasms of the kidney: an analysis of 353 patients followed five years or more, J. Urol. **79:** 196-201, 1958.

Garcia, M., Douglass, C., and Schlosser, J. V.: Classification and prognosis of Wilms' tumor, Radiology **80:**574-580, 1963.

Gross, R. E.: Surgery in infancy and childhood, Philadelphia, 1953, W. B. Saunders Co.

Gup, A. K., Schlegel, J. U., Caldwell, T., and Schlosser, J.: Effect of irradiation on renal function, J. Urol. **97:**36-39, 1967.

Huang, K., Almand, J. R., and Hargan, L. A.: The effect of total body x-irradiation on hepatic and renal function in albino rats, Radiat. Res. **1:**426-436, 1954.

Johansson, S., Angervall, L., Bengtsson, U., and Wahlquist, L.: A clinicopathologic and prognostic study of epithelial tumor of the renal pelvis, Cancer **37:**1376-1383, 1976.

Johnson, R. E., Doppman, J. L., Harbert, J. C., Steckel, R. J., and MacLowry, J. D.: Prevention of radiation nephritis with renal artery infusion of vasoconstrictors, Radiology **91:**103-108, 1968.

Kunkler, P. B., Farr, R. F., and Luxton, R. W.: The limit of renal tolerance to x-ray, Br. J. Radiol. **25:**190-200, 1952.

Kunkler, P. B.: The significance of radiosensitivity of the kidney. In Buschke, F., editor: Progress in radiation therapy, New York, 1962, Grune & Stratton, Inc.

Lemerle, J., Tournade, M. F., Gerard-Marchant, R., Flamant, R., Sarrazin, D., Flamant, F., Lemerle, M., Jundt, S., Zucker, J. M., and Schweisguth, O.: Wilms' tumor: natural history and prognostic factors, Cancer **37:**2557-2566, 1976.

Lemerle, J., Vonte, P. A., Tournade, M. F., Delemarse, J. F. M., Jereb, B., Ahstrom, L., Flamant, R., and Gerard-Marchant, R.: Preoperative versus postoperative radiotherapy, single versus multiple courses of actinomycin D, in the treatment of Wilms' tumor, Cancer **38:**647-654, 1976.

Li, F. P., and Stone, R.: Survivors of childhood cancer, Ann. Intern. Med. **84:**551-553, 1976.

Luxton, R. W.: The clinical and pathological effects of renal irradiation. In Buschke, F., editor: Progress in radiation therapy, New York, 1962, Grune & Stratton, Inc.

Maier, J. G., and Casarett, G. W.: Patho-physiologic aspects of radiation nephritis in dogs, The University of Rochester Atomic Energy Project, UR-626, 1963.

Mendelsohn, M. L., and Caceres, E.: X-ray and renal function, Am. J. Physiol. **173:**351-354, 1953.

Mintz, E. R., and Gaul, E. A.: Kidney tumors; some causes of poor end results, N.Y. State J. Med. **39:**1405-1411, 1939.

Monson, K. J., Brand, W. N., and Boggs, J. D.: Results of small-field irradiation of apparent solitary metastasis from Wilms' tumor, Radiology **104:**157-160, 1972.

Mostofi, F. K., Pani, K. C., and Ericsson, J.: Effects of irradiation on canine kidney, Am. J. Pathol. **44:**707-725, 1964.

Neuhauser, E. B. D., Wittenborg, M. H., Berman, C. Z., and Cohn, J.: Irradiation effects of roentgen therapy on the growing spine, Radiology **59:**637-651, 1952.

Oberling, C., Riviere, M., and Haguenau, F.: Ultrastructure of the clear cells in renal carcinomas and its importance for the demonstration of their renal origin, Nature (Lond.) **186:**402, 1960.

Platt, B. B., and Linden, G.: Wilms' tumor—a comparison of 2 criteria for survival, Cancer **17:**1573-1578, 1964.

Rafla, S.: Renal cell carcinoma: natural history and results of treatment, Cancer **25:**26-40, 1970.

Rafla, S.: Tumors of the upper urothelium, Am. J. Roentgenol. **123:**540-551, 1975.

Ragab, A. H., Vietti, T. J., Crist, W., Perez, C., and McAllister, W.: Bilateral Wilms' tumor, a review, Cancer **30:**983-988, 1972.

Richards, M. J. S., Miller, R. C., and Joo, P.: Radical partial renal irradiation, Cancer **38:**2093-2095, 1976.

Riches, E. W., Griffiths, I. H., and Thackray, A. C.: New growths of the kidney and ureter, Br. J. Urol. **23:**297-356, 1951.

Riches, E. W.: Factors in the prognosis of carcinoma of the kidney, J. Urol. **79:**190-195, 1958.

Riches, E.: The place of radiotherapy in the management of parenchymal carcinoma of the kidney, J. Urol. **95:**313-317, 1966.

Rosen, S., Swerdlow, M. A., Muehrcke, R. C., et al: Radiation nephritis: light and electron microscope observations, Am. J. Clin. Pathol. **41:**487-502, 1964.

Rubin, P., Duthie, R. B., and Young, L. W.: The significance of scoliosis in postirradiated Wilms' tumor and neuroblastoma, Radiology **79:**539-559, 1962.

Tefft, M., D'Angio, G. J., and Grant, W.: Postoperative radiation therapy for residual Wilms' tumor, Cancer **37:**2768-2772, 1976.

Vaeth, J. M., Levitt, S. H., Jones, M. D., and Holtfreter, C.: Effects of radiation therapy in survivors of Wilms' tumor, Radiology **79:**560-567, 1962.

van der Werf-Messing, B.: Carcinoma of the kidney, Cancer **32:**1056-1061, 1973.

White, D. C.: An atlas of radiation histopathology, United States Energy and Research Administration, 1975.

Wolff, J. A., D'Angio, G., Hartmann, J., Krivit, W., and Newton, W. A., Jr.: Long-term evaluation of single versus multiple courses of actinomycin D therapy of Wilms' tumor, N. Engl. J. Med. **290:**84-86, 1974.

14

The urinary bladder

RESPONSE OF THE NORMAL URINARY BLADDER TO IRRADIATION

The normal urinary bladder is unavoidably irradiated during conventional treatment for carcinoma of the cervix and of the prostate. Since a large proportion of patients receiving such treatment survive many years, much information has been accumulated relative to both early and late irradiation reactions and tolerances in the bladder. Much of this information applies to irradiation of the normal bladder that is accomplished principally by intravaginal and intracervical radium therapy. With the Manchester or Paris technique, the dose of radiations delivered to the posterior bladder wall is six to eight times greater than that delivered to the anterior wall. For this reason, areas of significant reaction are invariably well localized in the lower posterior portion of the bladder wall, which is that portion nearest the radium. Individual variations in bladder tolerance, together with striking dissimilarity in individual radium positioning, make any pretext at precision difficult in ascribing a given dose of radium to a given bladder reaction. Such information is of limited value in defining bladder tolerances, such as encountered in treating carcinoma of the bladder. Other data from Hueper and associates, from Wallace, and from patients treated for carcinoma of the prostate assist us in defining the limit of normal bladder tolerance to external irradiation. Finally, we have the spectrum of radiation-induced effects found in preoperatively irradiated bladders and in postmortem studies.

In developing a guide to the tolerance of patients being treated for carcinoma of the bladder we must appreciate the fact that postirradiation sequelae are much more frequent if high bladder doses of radiations are preceded by ulceration, infection, old fibrotic changes, and previous segmental resection or extensive cauterization. Table 14-1 may serve as a guide for determining tissue tolerance to radiation doses given for carcinoma of the bladder.

EARLY REACTIONS. A mild early mucosal reaction may be produced by levels of 3000 rad delivered to the bladder in 3 to 4 weeks. This will generally pass unnoticed. In addition to a slight reduction in bladder capacity due to increased bladder irritability, there may be a blanching of the irradiated mucosa. We believe this may be secondary to edema not unlike that observed on the buccal mucosa after the first

Table 14-1. Correlation of bladder dose and incidence of radiation-induced bladder sequelae in patients with cancer of the bladder*

	Percent patients with sequelae in particular dose range								
	3600	3660-4170	4228-4800	4860-5400	5460-6000	6066-6620	6680-7200	7260	Total
Number of patients	27	52	18	63	93	81	122	38	533
Bladder (27)†			6	5	8	6	5	5	5
Rectum (13)				5	1	1	2	16	2
Kidney (10)	4	3		3	2	2		3	2
Small bowel (8)		4			1	4		5	1.5
Subcutaneous tissue (1)								3	
Bladder and rectum (7)					1		3	5	1
Bladder and kidney (6)					3	2	1		1
Rectum and small bowel (1)								3	
Bladder and rectum and small bowel (1)							1		
Rectum, small bowel and bone (1)							1		
Bladder, subcutaneous tissue and bone (1)								1	
TOTAL‡ (76)	4	6	6	13	16	16	12	42	14

*Modified from Miller, L. S.: Cancer **39**:973-980, 1977.
†Total number of patients with particular sequela(e) = number in parentheses.
‡Cardiovascular excluded.

few days of oral cavity irradiation. Occasional submucosal petechiae are seen. At this stage individual blood vessels are still cystoscopically recognizable. A somewhat higher dose level may still further reduce bladder capacity. Later, the mucosa has been reported to present an intense, red, velvet-like appearance. We have not found such changes in spite of serial cystoscopic examination. Severe, acute reactions usually but not invariably appear with cancerocidal levels of irradiation. With local radium, this may occur 2 weeks after 7000 to 9000 rad in 6 to 8 days. After external pelvic irradiation with crossfiring beams or rotational techniques, this may mean 7000 rad in 7 to 8 weeks. The more acute symptoms may develop near the end of irradiation and last for 3 weeks. Intense urinary frequency and incontinence occasionally appear. Cystoscopically, the bladder mucosa appears as it would in an acute cystitis. Desquamation is rarely seen. Microscopically, the findings are those of acute inflammation of the bladder mucosa and submucosa. Engorged capillaries, round cell infiltration, and edema characterize this phase.

From the experience gained in treating carcinoma of the cervix and of the prostate by external irradiation alone, it has been shown that the normal whole bladder can tolerate high doses—that is, 6500 to 7500 rad midpelvis given over 7 to 8 weeks. The patient develops the transient symptoms described previously. However, late bladder complications with such doses are few. Radiation-induced bladder injuries are more common when these high doses are given to patients with pre-

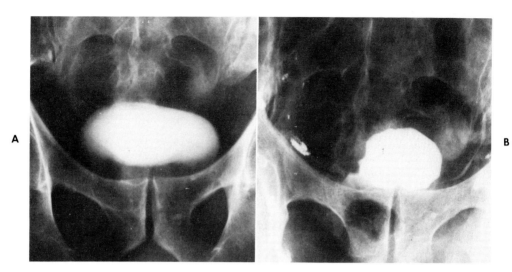

Fig. 14-1. A, Radiographically normal bladder in patient with Hodgkin's disease. **B,** Surface irregularities and reduced volume in same patient after 1600 rad (moving-strip technique) to the bladder with concomitant cyclophosphamide. Patient had symptoms of severe cystitis and histologic changes of acute cystitis with mucosal ulceration.

existing bladder damage such as carcinoma or if a surgical procedure or extensive fulguration preceded the irradiation.

The bladder shows a remarkable ability to reepithelize severely involved areas if irradiation is discontinued and the patient is placed on bed rest and given sedatives, urinary antiseptics, and antibiotics. Chemotherapeutic agents, notably cyclophosphamide, will increase the severity of the acute bladder reaction when used during bladder irradiation and severely limit the tolerance of the bladder to irradiation (Fig. 14-1).

LATE REACTIONS. When doses of 6000 to 7000 rad in 7 to 8 weeks are delivered to the posterior bladder wall or to the whole bladder, the late reaction is no different from that seen in similar tissue elsewhere (Fig. 14-2). Since the changes are slow in making their appearance (1 to 4 years), symptoms are confined primarily to the cured patients. Dean and Slaughter found that the higher the dose, the earlier and more frequently symptoms of late radiation cystitis appear. Watson and associates admitted the logic of this conclusion, but their data failed to substantiate it. They found that the occurrence as well as the severity of late radiation changes in the bladder were not necessarily in direct proportion to the dosage delivered unless amounts in excess of 10,000 mg-hr (an average of 7000 rad to the bladder mucosa in the region of the trigone) were given.

Microscopically, interstitial fibrosis occurs in the heavily irradiated area. Accompanying this is an obliterative endarteritis and telangiectasia (Wallace). On cystoscopic examination the blood vessels may present a tuftlike appearance, or they may be dilated and tortuous (Watson and associates). Occasionally, such a thin-walled

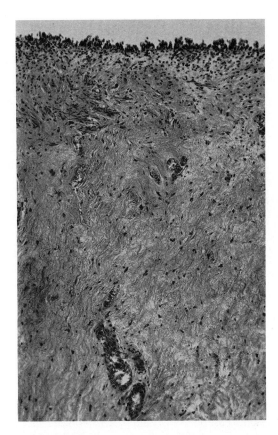

Fig. 14-2. Low-power enlargement of bladder mucosa 3 years after delivery of a calculated dose of 2900 rad by radium in 48 hours and 5800 rad in 5 weeks by external irradiation. The epithelium is atrophic. The submucosa shows marked edema and fibrosis. Symptoms were those of small bladder capacity.

vessel will rupture and may result in painless hematuria. At times this may be severe. If the vitality of these tissues is excessively impaired, or if trauma is applied to such an area of decreased vitality, ulceration or fistula may follow. After many months the bladder epithelium covering heavily irradiated segments appears thin, pale, and atrophic but may be locally hyperplastic. The epithelium readily ulcerates, and at times this may occur without obvious preceding trauma or infection. The diameters of such ulcers vary from a few millimeters to several centimeters. Mucosa revealing bullous edema and telangiectases borders the densely adherent necrotic center (Watson and associates). Often the urologist finds it difficult to distinguish these late radiation sequelae from tumor recurrence. Biopsy is useful in these cases. Radiation-induced atypia of submucosal mesenchymal cells is often present, and the pathologist might experience difficulty in differentiating them from isolated tumor cells. When the necrosis becomes extensive, secondary infection with urea-splitting organisms follows. These organisms are responsible for calcareous deposits and even calculi that aggravate the patient's symptoms. The prolonged secondary infection may lead to an ascending pyelonephritis and its accompanying renal damage. Most ulcers will heal slowly under conservative management. Ureteral transplantation, preferably with the construction of an ileal bladder, should be considered for the severely injured bladder in a patient who is in relatively good physical condition otherwise.

On p. 458 we mentioned the frequent concern for radiation-induced ureteral damage from the treatment given for carcinoma of the cervix. Obviously the ureters are exposed to high doses during irradiation for carcinoma of the bladder. If such treatment is responsible for ureteral narrowing or obstruction, it must be very rare indeed (Edsmyr and Nilson). It follows that until proven otherwise, postirradiation development of ureteral obstruction should ordinarily be considered a consequence of recurrent cancer.

CARCINOMA OF THE BLADDER

Just as in other sites, the technique of treatment and prognosis of carcinoma of the bladder varies with the clinical extension of the disease. One sees in the bladder a striking diversity in position, size, and shape of carcinomas, as well as all degrees of differentiation from the highly invasive early metastasizing lesions to the highly curable papillomas. The limited treatment proved sufficient for Grade I lesions is hopelessly inadequate for infiltrative lesions, whereas radical therapy required for extensive infiltrative lesions carries much too great a morbidity and mortality to be applied to the former. Between these two extremes is a variety of procedures equally incapable of application to all bladder cancers. In radiotherapy, highly flexible techniques are readily adaptable to the clinical characteristics of bladder tumors. A thorough understanding of these clinical characteristics is a major prerequisite to proper technique.

Factors affecting treatment decisions and end results

The basic techniques of irradiating cancer of the bladder are well standardized. However, some variation in technique and certainly some variation in risks should be considered according to cell type, clinical stage, microscopic grade, the presence or absence of lymphatic permeation, and the risks of metastases to regional nodes. Data referable to all these factors may not be available to the radiation oncologist after biopsy alone, but when available, they relate to radioresponsiveness, extent of disease, and prognosis. This relationship assists in defining dose-time-volume factors and whether anticipated benefits justify probable sequelae.

CELL TYPES AND GRADES. Tumors of the bladder are classified according to cell type into urothelial (transitional), squamous, and glandular. According to their growth characteristics they are subdivided into papillary and nonpapillary.

Papillary tumors account for almost 90% of all bladder tumors and are further subdivided into four histologic grades depending on cellularity, organization, nuclear pleomorphism, and number of mitotic figures. Since it is not unusual for several histologic grades to coexist, care must be taken to biopsy multiple areas of a tumor and to report the highest grade found.

Nonpapillary carcinomas range from in situ urothelial carcinoma to invasive urothelial, squamous, and adenocarcinoma. Rarer types are adenosquamous and spindle cell carcinomas. Rhabdomyosarcomas are found almost exclusively in children. Extensive, multifocal, in situ changes not infrequently accompany invasive bladder cancer and create a dilemma in the local treatment of this condition. In situ carcinoma of the bladder is the only intraepithelial cancer of which we are aware that may be symptomatic. The weakened neoplastic mucosa denudes easily, and the patient develops a chemical cystitis as a presenting symptom (Utz and Zincke; Moloney and associates).

The gross appearance of the cancer on cystoscopy—that is, papillary, sessile, or infiltrating with ulceration—correlates with the degree of anaplasia. The papillary cancers are more often well differentiated, whereas the flat infiltrating cancers are more often anaplastic.

LYMPHATIC PERMEATION AND LYMPH NODE METASTASES. Lymphatic or venous permeation in any site worsens the prognosis. For example, Jewett and associates found lymphatic permeation in seven of nineteen patients who died with Stage A and Stage B1 cancers and in none of twenty-nine survivors. Of 114 patients in Stage B2 and Stage C who died of cancer, lymphatic permeation was seen in forty. Of a total of fifty-four patients with lymphatic permeation, forty-seven died of cancer. Furthermore, when lymphatic permeation is found in the bladder wall, lymph node metastases will be present in about 90% of the patients. When no lymphatic permeation is found in the surgical specimen, metastases will be found in about 50% of the patients. Lymphatic permeation occurs only in close proximity to the cancer and is not thought to be the cause of what is recognized as multiple foci of origin (Simon and associates).

The lymph drainage from the bladder empties into the hypogastric and external iliac chains of nodes. The incidence of lymph node metastases in the various clinical stages is not well defined. In Stage A and small Stage B1, lymph node metastases are unusual, and for these stages the treatment plan need not encompass the regional lymph nodes. In autopsy studies on patients with Stage B2 and Stage C cancers, regional lymph nodes contain metastases 60% of the time (Jewett and associates). In these stages, external iliac and hypogastric lymph node chains should be encompassed in the irradiated volume. Just how frequently the lymph node metastases can be eradicated by irradiation is unknown, but judging from data available from patients with carcinoma of the cervix we believe a significant proportion of metastases is controlled. Lymphadenectomy for metastatic disease is occasionally curative (Dretler and associates), and there is every reason to believe that irradiation of involved nodes can also be curative.

CLINICAL STAGES. Two major clinical stage classifications are available for carcinomas of the bladder. They are comparable in many respects. The descriptions published by the American Joint Committee are given in the following listing. The somewhat comparable surgically determined stages recommended by Jewett are shown. The staging used by Jewett was designed primarily for the surgeon at the time of operation. Involvement of the lymph nodes of the pelvis or aortic areas and a precise measurement of depth of invasion into the bladder wall cannot be determined without operation. Except for the biopsy and cystoscopy, the American Joint Committee staging procedure can be completed by nonoperative means. Following is the American Joint Committee TNM Classification for carcinoma of the urinary bladder (1978). Jewett's lettered staging and the comparable numerical staging are referred to throughout this chapter.

SURGICAL STAGES (JEWETT)		TNM CLASSIFICATION*
	T— Primary tumor	
		The suffix "m" should be added to the appropriate T category to indicate multiple lesions. Papilloma is classified as "GO."
	TX	Minimum requirements cannot be met
	T0	No evidence of primary tumor
	TIS	Sessile carcinoma in situ
	Ta	Papillary noninvasive carcinoma
A	**T1**	On bimanual examination a freely mobile mass may be felt—this should not be felt after complete transurethral resection of the lesion, and/or there is papillary carcinoma without microscopic invasion beyond the lamina propria
B1	**T2**	On bimanual examination there is induration of the bladder wall, which is mobile. There is no residual induration after complete transurethral resection of the lesion, and/or there is microscopic invasion of superficial muscle of bladder
B2 and C	**T3**	On bimanual examination there is induration or a nodular mobile mass is palpable in the bladder wall which persists after transurethral resection
	T3a	Microscopic invasion of deep muscle
	T3b	Invasion through the full thickness of bladder wall
D1 and D2	**T4**	Tumor fixed or invading neighboring structures and/or there is microscopic evidence of invasion of the prostate and in the other circumstances listed below at least muscle invasion
	T4a	Tumor invading substance of prostate, uterus, or vagina
	T4b	Tumor fixed to the pelvic wall and/or infiltrating the abdominal wall
	N— Nodal involvement	
		The regional lymph nodes are the pelvic nodes just below the bifurcation of the common iliac arteries. The juxtaregional lymph nodes are the inguinal nodes, the common iliac, and para-aortic nodes†
	NX	Minimum requirements cannot be met
	N0	No involvement of regional lymph nodes
	N1	Involvement of a single homolateral regional lymph node

*From the American Joint Committee for Cancer Staging and End Results Reporting: Manual for staging of cancer, Chicago, 1978, Whiting Press.

†Subsequent data regarding the histologic assessment of the regional lymph nodes may be added to the N category thus: "N−" for nodes with no microscopic evidence of metastasis, or "N+" for those with microscopic evidence of metastasis, for example, N0+, etc.

N2   Involvement of contralateral, bilateral, or multiple regional lymph nodes

N3   There is a fixed mass on the pelvic wall with a free space between this and the tumor

N4   Involvement of juxtaregional lymph nodes

M—Distant metastasis

MX   Not assessed

M0   No (known) distant metastasis

M1   Distant metastasis present

HISTOPATHOLOGY

Predominant cancer is a transitional cell cancer.

STAGE GROUPING

No stage grouping is recommended at this time.

GRADE

Well-differentiated, moderately well-differentiated, poorly to very poorly differentiated, or numbers 1, 2, 3-4

The differentiation between T2 and T3 is not always readily made on clinical examination. As stated, superficial muscle infiltration in one area does not exclude deep infiltration in another area. The magnitude of the error in clinical assessment of extent is summarized in Table 14-2. In a more detailed description Prout reported that the extent of disease was frequently more advanced than was assessed clinically. Thus twenty-six of fifty-five clinical Stage B1 lesions were a higher stage on cystectomy: 12 were B2, 5 were C, and 9 were D. Twenty-nine of sixty-three clinical Stage B2 were higher on cystectomy: 19 were C and 10 were D. Seven of twenty-seven clinical Stage C lesions were higher on cystectomy: six were D1 and one was D2. This limitation of clinical staging must be taken into consideration during treatment planning. We now believe that pelvic nodes and bladder should be encompassed in the treatment volumes in most patients with clinical Stages B1 and higher.

Table 14-2. Accuracy of clinical staging in patients with carcinoma of the urinary bladder*

Author	Clinical stage	Number of patients	Number of patients in each pathologic stage					
			<B1	B1	>B1	<B2	B2	>B2
Varkarakis	B1	21	3	4	14			
	B2	15					5	10
Whitmore†	B1	22	5	5	10			
	B2	43				10	14	19
Prout	B1	47	12	14	21			
	B2	53				8	18	27

*Modified from Prout, G. R.: Cancer Res. **37**:2764-2770, 1977.
†Two thousand rad in five treatments immediately preceding cystectomy.

Two techniques of irradiation are available for consideration:

1. Interstitial irradiation with radium needles or artificially produced radioactive sources such as tantalum wire, gold grains, or iridium sources
2. External pelvic irradiation crossfiring the bladder and generally including regional lymph nodes

Interstitial irradiation

Interstitial techniques for cancer of the urinary bladder, like interstitial techniques elsewhere, provide a means for administering a well-localized high dose to the implanted volume. The dose at the edge of the implant decreases quickly so that adjacent tissues receive a low dose. The successful exploitation of this distribution of dose in the treatment of carcinomas of the bladder depends on one's ability to select patients in which the cancer of the bladder is well localized and implantable. In the bladder it is impractical to implant a cancer larger than 5 cm in diameter (van der Werf-Messing). Multiple planes and volume implants are not practical in the bladder. Single-plane implants effectively irradiate a slab only 1 cm thick. A 1 cm margin in depth cannot be attained if there is any clinically detectable infiltration. Therefore this method cannot be used alone with a curative intent on any but superficial lesions of small areas. The fungating portion of the tumor may be removed by diathermy prior to implantation in order to bring thicker lesions within the limitations of a single-plane implant. The uncertainty of depth of infiltration demands other techniques when muscle is more than superficially infiltrated. The wall of the bladder dome is thin and not suitable for implantation. Finally, multiple cancers usually make implantation impractical. These criteria for selecting patients for interstitial implants assure a group of patients with a relatively good prognosis.

When the criteria are followed and the sources are inserted according to the Paterson-Parker system, local control is excellent with good bladder function and a low complication rate (van der Werf-Messing).

Interstitial techniques in combination with surgery and external pelvic irradiation have been used for selected patients to preserve bladder function. Miller selects patients with T2 carcinomas who might ordinarily be suitable for segmental resection. Two thousand rad is delivered to the whole bladder in 10 fractions of external beam therapy prior to segmental resection. Immediately after the bladder incision is closed, 0.66 mg/cm strength radium needles are implanted in the bladder parallel to the wound. An additional dose of 5000 rad is thus delivered to fingers of tumor that might have been left behind. The effectiveness of this bladder-sparing attempt has not been reported, but it is a rational approach toward extending the local effectiveness of segmental resection.

For T3 carcinomas less than 5 cm in diameter, preimplant external pelvic irradiation (3 daily fractions of 350 rad each) has been reported to decrease the rate of local recurrence (van der Werf-Messing). However, this combination has not been widely employed, since it does not irradiate draining lymph nodes adequately and must be restricted to single small primary lesions. A more rational approach for T3 lesions combines preradium whole-pelvis irradiation of 4000 rad in 4 weeks with about one half the usual dose from an implant.

The Grade 1, Stage I carcinomas of the bladder are generally treated by cauterization. The more invasive lesions are considered for partial or total cystectomy, whole bladder irradiation using external techniques, or combinations of these.

External pelvic irradiation

Once the muscle wall of the bladder is invaded, the incidence of metastases to regional lymph nodes increases and cure rates diminish rapidly. When the risk of such spread is high, the choice of treatment lies between radical cystectomy, irradiation alone, and preoperative irradiation followed by cystectomy. In a randomized study, Prout and associates found that if muscle invasion is present, preoperative irradiation followed by cystectomy improves survival over that obtained by *cystectomy alone*. In a separate randomized study Miller found that if deep muscle is invaded, preoperative irradiation followed by cystectomy is superior to *irradiation alone* (Table 14-3). Although these two studies may not settle unequivocally the superiority of preoperative irradiation followed by cystectomy, they have persuaded us to recommend it for the majority of patients with Stage II and III lesions. This does not mean that irradiation alone or cystectomy alone has no place in the care of these patients.

External pelvic irradiation given with ^{60}Co or megavoltage beams provides the means for homogeneously irradiating the bladder and its draining lymph nodes. Dose-limiting critical organs in this volume include the sigmoid colon, rectum, loops of small bowel, and the bladder itself. The major postirradiation complications that develop in these patients are shown in Tables 14-1 and 14-4. Some of the complica-

Table 14-3. Comparison of preoperative irradiation plus cystectomy with radiation therapy alone—randomized clinical trial*

Treatment	Number of patients	5-year survival (%)
Radiation therapy alone	32	16
Preoperative irradiation plus cystectomy	35	46

*Modified from Miller, L. S.: Cancer **39**:973-980, 1977.

Table 14-4. Incidence of complications after radiation therapy alone in 533 patients with carcinoma of the bladder*

Organ	Complication (%)
Bladder	8
Rectum	4.3
Kidney	3
Small bowel	2.1

*From Miller, L. S.: Cancer **39**:973-980, 1977.

tions, especially those related to the urinary bladder, are undoubtedly augmented by ulceration, infection, and fibrosis produced by the cancer and by unsuccessful surgical intervention. Renal complications were secondary to urinary tract infections or ureteral obstructions. The high incidence of rectal complications after 7000 rad in 35 fractions in 7 weeks reported by Miller establishes an upper limit for that fractionation pattern and volume and provides a major guide for technical factors.

EXTERNAL PELVIC IRRADIATION ALONE. Papillomas of the bladder are not usually eradicated by external pelvic irradiation. Their inclusion in a volume irradiated because of coincidental infiltrating cancer confirms their relative radioresistance.

Stage A or Stage I cancers involving areas less than 3 cm in diameter hardly justify the demands of external pelvic irradiation. Fulguration or limited excision seems adequate. Larger areas, even if superficial, or multiple small foci justify serious consideration of external pelvic irradiation; however, the request for irradiation for this is rare.

Small Stage B1 or Stage II cancers, when confirmed as such by sectioning the biopsy specimen, do well with partial or total cystectomy or with irradiation. However, uncertainty of the depth of muscle infiltration cautions the radiation oncologist to irradiate the entire bladder and, for larger lesions, the regional lymph nodes as well. Should these more superficial cancers be treated by fulguration, close observation is extremely important. At the first sign of persistence, vigorous irradiation is given to prevent deeper muscle or perivesicle infiltration. If a persistence is diagnosed while still in a limited stage, the prognosis is reasonably favorable (Buschke and Jack; Crigler and associates). The greatest curative contribution of external pelvic irradiation alone will be in patients with these limited Stages I and II lesions.

Large Stage II lesions and B2 or Stage III lesions that are *not* suitable for combined radiotherapy and cystectomy should also be considered for irradiation alone. For these the entire bladder and the hypogastric and iliac lymph node chains (12 to 16 cm wide and 12 to 14 cm vertically) should be encompassed. Volumes, such as those used in the treatment of carcinoma of the cervix, are not generally necessary in males and contribute seriously to the sequelae when used indiscriminately (Cordonnier and Seaman).

PREOPERATIVE IRRADIATION. It has been a uniform observation that preoperative irradiation of 4000 to 4500 rad in 4 to 5 weeks often diminishes the depth of cancer invasion into the muscle of the bladder wall. Thus Prout reported that one third of the patients given the dose mentioned above had no histologic evidence of residual cancer in their bladders. Another one third had reduction of the depth of muscle invasion that "reduced" their clinical stage. Patients with no residual cancer in their resected bladder had a higher 5-year survival rate than those found to have cancer in their cystectomy specimens (Table 14-5). Patients responding with a "reduction" in clinical stage had a higher 5-year survival rate than those failing to show such a response (van der Werf-Messing, 1975) (Fig. 14-3).

With the aim of diminishing the time and expense of preoperative irradiation,

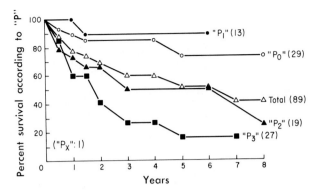

Fig. 14-3. Actuarial survival of patients treated with preoperative irradiation (4000 rad in 4 weeks) and cystectomy. All lesions were classified as T3 before irradiation. The depth of infiltration was diminished following irradiation in keeping with the "P" categories indicated. Survival is plotted according to depth of infiltration found on cystectomy specimen. (From van der Werf-Messing, B.: Cancer **36:**718-722, 1975.)

Table 14-5. Data on 5-year survival of patients treated with preoperative irradiation and cystectomy

Author	No cancer in cystectomy specimen (%)	Cancer in cystectomy specimen (%)
Prout	44	34
Miller	54	25

total doses of 2000 rad in 5 daily fractions have been advocated. Cystectomy is performed within a few days. No valid comparison of this technique has been made with the conventional technique described before. However, it should be pointed out that the shortened schedule offers patients few, if any, of the advantages of more conventional fractionation, that is, tumor reoxygenation, normal cell repopulation, intracellular repair, and radiation-induced synchrony. One can also be assured that for a given radiation-induced cancerocidal effect, normal tissue damage will almost certainly be greater with the shortened schedule. Finally, if for any reason cystectomy is not done or if at the time of cystectomy cancer is left behind, the administration of additional radiation therapy to treat to tolerance is made very difficult. Such shortened preoperative schedules used in other anatomic sites have sooner or later been abandoned. Four thousand to 4500 rad in 4 to 5 weeks is, in our opinion, only marginally adequate for microscopic foci of carcinoma of the bladder. Few therapists have considered the possibility of identifying patients at high risk for metastases in pelvic nodes who might benefit from postcystectomy "boosting" doses to the nodal areas. Such information is being utilized in the irradiation of other pelvic tumors such as carcinoma of the endometrium and prostate. Despite the observation that many of these patients will already have developed occult systemic spread of their cancer, we

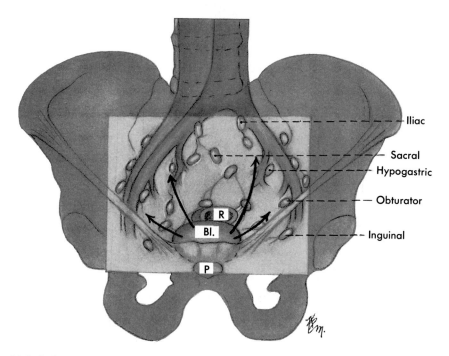

Fig. 14-4. Outline of volume to be considered in the irradiation of carcinoma of the bladder. A volume of this proportion is necessary if regional nodes are to be irradiated. However, only the bladder with a small margin of pericystic tissues is now being carried to high doses.

believe adequate attention has not been given to the possible benefits of post-cystectomy boosting doses. This concept is being studied.

TECHNIQUE. In planning external pelvic irradiation as the sole treatment, the bladder alone is encompassed if no muscle infiltration has occurred. The bladder plus the hypogastric and iliac nodes are encompassed if muscle has been invaded (Fig. 14-4). Bimanual examination defines the location of the bladder neck and the status of any gross extravesicle infiltration. It also assists in defining extensions above the pelvis. Cystographs supplement the information obtained by cystoscopy in defining the size and position of the cancer with regard to external landmarks. Enlargement of the volume to encompass regional nodes extends the volume primarily superiorly and laterally. This adds significantly to the volume of bowel irradiated. At least in the male, it is inadvisable to try to spare the anterior wall of the rectum. Margins are too narrow. If extravesicle extension is present, the anterior one half of the rectum will also be included in the high-dose volume. For the more advanced cancers of the bladder, more bowel must be treated superiorly and laterally as well as posteriorly.

Should the bladder be treated empty, full, or overdistended? If the bladder is full or overdistended, normal bowel is displaced. This is especially important if regional

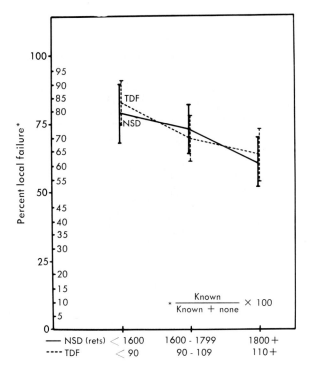

Fig. 14-5. Effect of radiation dose to cancer of bladder on percent of local failure. Incidence of local failure decreases as time-dose-fractional factor and NSD increase. (From Miller, L. S.: Cancer **39:** 973-980, 1977.)

nodes are to be encompassed. For those patients whose bladder only is the target of irradiation, the bladder should be emptied.

There is little choice as far as technique is concerned. Megavoltage or ^{60}Co beams must be used. The simplicity and the rectum-sparing possibilities of a three-beam arrangement (one anterior and two oblique posterior beams) and of the four-port "box" technique make them by far the most often used. Other arrangements include rotational techniques either with arcs or segmental blocks, which provide rectal sparing. Combinations of these techniques may be used to supply whole pelvic irradiation plus the boosting dose to the bladder.

Dose-time-volume factors. Postirradiation recurrence in the bladder is a common cause of failure. This is true even after 7000 rad in 7 to 8 weeks. Also, local control is dose related (Fig. 14-5). Therefore the optimum dose is, in large part, dictated by the maximum doses tolerated by the bladder and adjacent bowel. These were defined in Table 14-1. When it is necessary to encompass regional nodes as well as the bladder, a volume 12 to 16 cm wide, 12 to 14 cm vertical dimension, and 9 to 10 cm in anteroposterior dimension is usually adequate. Occult metastases in regional nodes are given 5000 to 5500 rad in 5 to 6 weeks. When tolerance permits, the bladder is given an additional boosting dose of 2000 rad in 2 weeks.

The technique for giving preoperative irradiation is similar to that described above except that efforts should be made to spare somewhat the site of the anticipated abdominal incision. A "box" technique or rotational technique is satisfactory in this respect.

Of those patients with Stage I and II cancers selected for radiotherapy alone, Whitmore and associates reported 50% were surviving at 5 years. Caldwell and associates also obtained 50%. However, the range of results is wide, indicating the importance of patient selection and wide variation in clinical extent in this apparently limited cancer.

When bladder muscle has been infiltrated with cancer, regional nodes will contain cancer about 50% of the time. When perivesicle connective tissue is invaded with cancer, regional nodes will contain cancer 100% of the time. The question of whether the irradiated volume should be extended to encompass retroperitoneal nodes in these advanced stages has not yet been answered.

Results of radiation therapy alone

A wide and meaningful experience of treating cancer of the bladder with megavoltage and ^{60}Co beams has now been acquired and reported. Control of the primary lesion varies with clinical stage and microscopic grade. Sixty percent of the patients in the heterogeneous series reported by del Regato were either living and well at 5 years or had no detected cancer in the bladder at autopsy. In an evaluation of precystectomy irradiation, Crigler and associates sectioned the bladder carefully after doses of 6000 rad in 6 weeks. At various intervals after this dose, no cancer could be found in six of nineteen cystectomy specimens. Most of the patients had muscle invasion demonstrated in the preirradiation biopsy. A conservative estimate is that in Stage B1 and Stage B2 the doses recommended previously will eradicate all cancer in the bladder and in at least half the patients. Or, stated another way, Miller found postirradiation local persistence within the treated volume in about 45% of his patients. The cancer-free 5-year survival rate will be lower than this because of occult spread beyond the bladder. Just how often extravesicle extension or pelvic lymph node metastases can be controlled is unknown. In our series with apparently localized but nonresectable biopsy-proved *extravesicle* extension, none of thirty-two patients lived 5 years and most were dead at 2 years. However, a few patients with palpable extravesicle masses have been cured (Morrison and Deeley). In Table 14-6 the data reported by Miller are shown. He found that about 7% of patients with extension to the pelvic wall or other types of extravesicle extension could be cured. It is Buschke's opinion that, despite their greater tendency to metastasize, the advanced but less differentiated cancers were more likely to be sterilized locally than the advanced but well-differentiated cancers; this is not supported by van der Werf-Messing. Table 14-7 lists a spectrum of 5-year survival rates.

Postoperative irradiation

To our knowledge systematic postcystectomy irradiation using modern concepts has not been adequately tested for patients with large Stage II lesions or for all

Table 14-6. Stage D1: effect of extracystic extension on survival after radiotherapy*

Type of extension	Number of patients	5-year survival (%)
Invasion of pelvic wall	40	5
Invasion of prostate	22	0
Both	29	14
Other	25	8
TOTAL	116	7

*Modified from Miller, L. S.: Clinical evaluation and therapy for urinary bladder: radiotherapy. In Oncology 1970, Proceedings of the Tenth International Cancer Congress, Chicago, 1971, Year Book Medical Publishers, Inc.

Table 14-7. Result of radiation therapy alone in the treatment of carcinoma of the bladder (%)

Author	Follow-up	Stage I	Stage II	Stage III
Laing	5 years	52	16	0
		OA,B1		**B2,C**
Crigler	5 years	32		28
Caldwell	5 years	50		20
		A,B1		**B2,C**
Buschke	5 years	44		14
Morrison	4 years	37		21
			Irradiation alone	
Miller	5 years	27		23

patients with Stage III lesions. It is clear that when postcystectomy irradiation is reserved for patients with proven recurrences or for patients with known residual extracystic cancer, the results are very poor. It is also clear that postoperative irradiation will cure very few patients who have recurrence after segmental resection. It is entirely possible that systematic postcystectomy whole pelvis irradiation to a dose level of 5000 rad in 25 fractions over 5 to 6 weeks could improve disease-free survival rates. Postoperative dose levels much higher than this have produced unacceptable complication rates (Miller).

SUMMARY

Carcinoma of the urinary bladder presents us with a variety of gross morphologic types, microscopic patterns, and stages of advancement, all affecting prognosis. Lesions of small diameter that have not invaded muscle will usually be treated surgically. In several independent clinical studies (Prout; Miller; van der Werf-Messing) preoperative irradiation followed by cystectomy for patients with B1 and B2 lesions produced disease-free survival rates equal to or greater than the rates obtained by other methods of treatment. Patients with such cancers who are otherwise unsuitable for cystectomy should be considered for radiation therapy alone.

The technique employed in treating these patients should be adequate to encompass the regional pelvic lymph nodes. Megavoltage techniques permit this with a minimum of patient discomfort.

REFERENCES

Buschke, F., and Jack, G.: Twenty-five years' experience with supervoltage therapy in the treatment of transitional cell carcinoma of the bladder, Am. J. Roentgenol. **99**:387-392, 1967.

Caldwell, W. L., Bagshaw, M. A., and Kaplan, H. S.: Efficacy of linear accelerator x-ray therapy in cancer of the bladder, J. Urol. **97**:294-303, 1967.

Caldwell, W. L.: Cancer of the urinary bladder, St. Louis, 1970. W. H. Green, Inc.

Cordonnier, J. J., and Seaman, W. B.: Betatron therapy in advanced carcinoma of the urinary bladder, J. Urol. **76**:256-262, 1956.

Crigler, C. M., Miller, L. S., Guinn, G. A., and Schillaci, H. G.: Radiotherapy for carcinoma of the bladder, J. Urol. **96**:55-60, 1966.

Dean, A. L., and Slaughter, D. P.: Bladder injury subsequent to irradiation of the uterus, J. Urol. **46**:917-924, 1941.

del Regato, J. A., and Chahbazian, C. M.: Radiotherapy of transitional cell carcinoma of the urinary bladder with Cobalt 60, Radiology **87**: 1054-1056, 1966.

DeWeerd, J. H., and Colby, M. Y.: Bladder carcinoma, combined radiotherapy and surgical treatment, J.A.M.A. **199**:109-111, 1967.

Dretler, S. P., Ragsdale, B. D., and Leadbetter, W. F.: The value of pelvic lymphadenectomy in the surgical treatment of bladder cancer, J. Urol. **109**:414-416, 1973.

Edsmyr, F., and Nilson, A. E.: Vesico-ureteric reflex in connection with supervoltage therapy for bladder carcinoma, Acta Radiol. (Ther.) **3**:449-451, 1965.

Herger, C. C., and Sauer, H. R.: A consideration of the response of bladder tumors to external radiation, J. Urol. **50**:310-321, 1943.

Hueper, W. C., Fisher, V. C., de Carvajal-Forero, J., Thompson, M. R.: The pathology of experimental roentgen-cystitis in dogs, J. Urol. **47**: 156-167, 1942.

International Union Against Cancer: Malignant tumours of the urinary bladder, 1963-1967.

Jewett, H. J.: Carcinoma of bladder: influence of depth of infiltration on 5-year results following complete extirpation of primary growth, J. Urol. **67**:672-676, 1952.

Jewett, H. J., King, L. R., and Shelley, W. M.: A study of 365 cases of infiltrating bladder cancer: relation of certain pathological characteristics to prognosis after extirpation, J. Urol. **92**:668-678, 1964.

Laing, A. H., and Dickinson, K. M.: Carcinoma of the bladder treated by supervoltage irradiation, Clin. Radiol. **16**:154-164, 1965.

Miller, L. S.: Clinical evaluation and therapy for urinary bladder: radiotherapy, Oncology 1970, Proceedings of the Tenth International Cancer Congress, Chicago, 1971, Year Book Medical Publishers, Inc.

Miller, L. S.: Bladder cancer: superiority of preoperative irradiation and cystectomy in clinical Stages B2 and C, Cancer **39**:973-980, 1977.

Moloney, P. J., Elliot, G. B., McLouglin, M., and Sinclair, A. D.: In situ transitional carcinomas and non-specifically inflamed contracting bladder, J. Urol. **111**:162-164, 1974.

Morrison, R., and Deeley, T. J.: The treatment of carcinoma of the bladder by supervoltage x-rays, Br. J. Radiol. **38**:449-458, 1965.

Prout, G. R.: The surgical management of bladder carcinoma, Urol. Clin. North Am. **3**:149-175, 1976.

Prout, G. R.: The role of surgery in the potentially curative treatment of bladder carcinoma, Cancer Res. **37**:2764-2770, 1977.

Sagerman, R. H., Veenema, R. J., Guttmann, R., Dean, A. L., and Uson, A. C.: Preoperative irradiation for carcinoma of the bladder, Am. J. Roentgenol. **102**:577-580, 1968.

Simon, W., Cordonnier, J. J., and Snodgrass, W. T.: The pathogenesis of bladder carcinoma, J. Urol. **88**:797-802, 1962.

Utz, D. C., and Zincke, H.: The masquerade of bladder cancer in situ as interstitial cystitis, J. Urol. **111**:160-161, 1974.

van der Werf-Messing, B.: Telecobalt treatment of carcinoma of the bladder, Clin. Radiol. **16**: 165-172, 1965.

van der Werf-Messing, B.: Carcinoma of the bladder T3NxMo treated by preoperative irradiation followed by cystectomy, Cancer **36**:718-722, 1975.

van der Werf-Messing, B.: Cancer of the urinary

bladder treated by interstitial radium implant, Int. J. Radiat. Oncol. Biol. Phys. **4:**373-378, 1978.

Wallace, D. M.: The ill-effects of radiotherapy, Br. J. Urol. **26:**364-368, 1954.

Wallace, D. M.: Clinical assessment of bladder tumour. In Wallace, D. M., editor: Tumours of the bladder, London, 1959, E. & S. Livingstone, Ltd.

Walton, R. J.: Therapeutic uses of radioactive isotopes in the Royal Cancer Hospital, Br. J. Radiol. **23:**559-566, 1950.

Watson, E. M., Herger, C. C., and Sauer, H. R.: Irradiation reactions in the bladder: their occurrence and clinical coures following the use of x-ray and radium in the treatment of female pelvic disease, J. Urol. **57:**1038-1050, 1947.

Whitmore, W. F., Grabstald, H., Mackenzie, A. R., Iswariah, J., and Phillips, R.: Preoperative irradiation with cystectomy in the management of bladder cancer, Am. J. Roentgenol. **102:** 570-576, 1968.

15

The prostate gland

The prostate gland lies directly posterior to the pubis, is easily palpated on digital rectal examination, and is intimately related to the bladder neck and the rectum. The margins of the normal gland are readily identified as is at least the more inferior portion of the seminal vesicles.

The lymphatic drainage of the prostate gland is divided into three major pathways. Intraglandular lymphatics in the inferior portion of the gland unite to form major trunks that pass posterosuperiorly, lateral to the rectum, to empty into the presacral nodes. Some of these vessels bypass the presacral nodes to empty directly into low para-aortic nodes. Lymph channels emerging from the superior portion of the gland drain laterally to obturator and hypogastric nodes and also superolaterally to external iliac nodes (Fig. 15-1). McLaughlin and associates found that the obturator-hypogastric group of nodes are by far the most commonly involved nodes, but external iliac and common iliac nodes also contain metastases in a substantial proportion. Obturator, hypogastric, or presacral nodes are not ordinarily visualized at the time of the foot lymphangiogram. For this reason the "negative" lymphangiogram has limited significance in patients with carcinoma of the prostate gland.

The normal prostate gland tolerates high doses of radiations with destruction of glands, production of dense fibrous tissue, and damage to blood vessels (Bulkley and associates). High doses are commonly given to this volume during irradiation of carcinoma of the bladder. There is no record of symptom-producing radiation damage of the prostate gland. The interstitial injection of colloidal ^{198}Au into the prostate produces necrosis of the gland, but symptoms develop only after bladder, prostatic urethra, or bowel injury. There are no data indicating whether the level of serum acid phosphatase is elevated during or after a high dose of radiations delivered to the normal prostate gland. There are questions as to the effect of irradiation of the prostate gland on libido and sexual function (Table 15-5).

Glandular hyperplasia coexists in about half of the patients with carcinoma of the prostate gland. In such cases irradiation may decrease infection and often results in shrinking of the gland.

CARCINOMA OF THE PROSTATE GLAND

Cancer of the prostate gland is almost exclusively adenocarcinoma, although rarely transitional cell carcinoma may arise in the larger prostatic ducts (Rubenstein

404

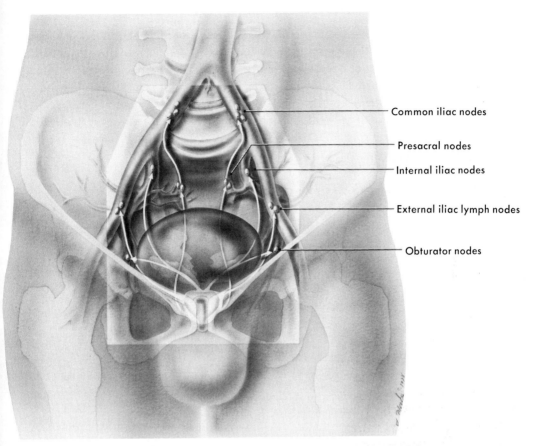

Common iliac nodes

Presacral nodes

Internal iliac nodes

External iliac lymph nodes

Obturator nodes

Fig. 15-1. Lymphatic drainage of prostate. Compare to Table 15-3.

and Rubnitz). The majority of carcinomas of the prostate gland originate in the peripheral part of the gland and are often in the subcapsular zone. In this location the tumor nodule is readily palpated, but not readily biopsied through the cystoscope. Biopsy through the perineum or anterior rectal wall is more common. In its peripheral, subcapsular location early capsular infiltration and direct extension beyond the prostate gland occur in about one half of those patients judged clinically to have limited disease. Adenocarcinoma will be an unsuspected coincidental finding in 5% to 10% of patients subjected to transurethral resection for benign prostatic hypertrophy. By the time the clinical diagnosis is suspected, carcinoma of the prostate gland will have spread in every instance to perineural spaces within the gland. Extension to the perivesicle fascia, the bladder, and pelvic lymph nodes usually occurs in that order. Denonvilliers' fascia is a major barrier to its extension posteriorly. Blood vessel invasion is not uncommon. It is presumed that hematogenous spread by way of the veins accounts for early osseous metastases, but this is by no means certain.

Clinical staging of carcinoma of the prostate gland

There is perhaps no anatomic site for which there is more diversity and confusion in clinical staging than there is for carcinoma of the prostate gland. This compounds the difficulty in sorting out the treatment of choice from the many recommended methods of management. Hopefully, the American Joint Committee's recommendations (1978) will crystalize the opinions so that staging will become uniform. Until this occurs, workers must be well acquainted with TNM categories as well as criteria for other clinical staging systems. Both are used in the following discussion.

TNM CLASSIFICATION*

T— Primary tumor

TX	Minimum staging requirements cannot be met
T0	No tumor palpable; includes incidental findings of cancer in a biopsy or operative specimen; assign all such cases a G, N, or M category
T1	Tumor intracapsular surrounded by normal gland
T2	Tumor confined to gland, deforming contour, and invading capsule, but lateral sulci and seminal vesicles are not involved
T3	Tumor extends beyond capsule with or without involvement of lateral sulci and/or seminal vesicles
T4	Tumor fixed or involving neighboring structures. Add suffix (m) after "T" to indicate multiple tumors (e.g., T2m)

N— Nodal involvement†

NX	Minimum requirements cannot be met
N0	No involvement of regional lymph nodes
N1	Involvement of a single regional lymph node
N2	Involvement of multiple regional lymph nodes
N3	Free space between tumor and fixed pelvic wall mass
N4	Involvement of juxta-regional nodes

M—Distant metastasis

MX	Not assessed
M0	No (known) distant metastasis
M1	Distant metastasis present

HISTOPATHOLOGY

Almost always adenocarcinoma, grades variable

STAGE GROUPING

No stage grouping is recommended at this time.

GRADE

Well-differentiated, moderately well-differentiated, poorly to very poorly differentiated, or numbers 1, 2, 3-4

Similar diverse views exist when considering histologic grading of prostatic carcinoma. This is in part because of the frequent occurrence of different patterns of

---

* From the American Joint Committee for Cancer Staging and End Results Reporting: Manual for staging of cancer, Chicago, 1978, Whiting Press.

† If N category is determined by lymphangiography or isotope scans, insert "1" or "i" between "N" and appropriate number (e.g., N12 or Ni2). If nodes are histologically positive after surgery, add "+"; if negative, add "−".

tumor growth in the same case. Sampling problems are particularly a hazard of small needle biopsies, which may be minimized by obtaining multiple biopsies. The two most reliable parameters are presence or absence of gland formation and degree of nuclear anaplasia. We usually combine these two parameters to determine the grade of prostatic carcinoma. Other variables such as size of acini, quantity and quality of stroma, type of cell borders, etc. may have a bearing on prognosis, but this is still unproven. The impact of histologic grade on cure rates has been dramatically illustrated by Harisiadis and associates. The 5-year survival rate was 64.4% for patients with Stage C well-differentiated cancers but only 28.7% for patients with Stage C undifferentiated tumors.

In an analysis of microscopic findings in 208 prostates removed during radical prostatectomy for early carcinoma of the prostate, Byar and Mostofi found the extent of *primary* lesion as described on rectal examination was in reasonable agreement with the microscopic description of the extent of the primary cancer in 74.5% of the patients. In addition they found the cancer was located peripherally or peripherally and centrally in 97% of the patients. They judged the peripheral origin an important factor in early capsular involvement. The cancer extended across the midline of the gland in 80% of the patients and appeared to be multifocal in origin in 85%. Thirty of 175 patients (17%) who showed no clinical evidence of invasion of seminal vesicles or capsule showed such extension on microscopic examination. Nine of thirty-two patients who were suspected of having such extension did not show it on microscopic examination. Finally, extension of the cancer to the seminal vesicles reduced the postradical prostatectomy 7-year survival rate from 66% to 32%. Penetration of the capsule reduced the 7-year postsurgical survival rate from 69.4% to 33%. Whether such extensions also modify survival after radical radiotherapy is unknown.

The frequency of unexpected extracapsular extension in clinical Stage B (T1 and T2) varies rather widely. Representative percentages are given in Table 15-1. In Jewett's experience no patient was cured by prostatectomy if the operative specimen revealed extension of the cancer beyond the capsule (Jewett and associates). A very significant proportion of such patients are curable by radiation therapy. The need to identify patients with a high risk of occult extracapsular extension is obvious.

Metastases of carcinoma of the prostate to regional lymph nodes may be early in

Table 15-1. Incidence of occult extraprostatic extension of adenocarcinoma of the prostate gland in clinical Stage B (T1 and T2)

Author	Percent occult extension
Berlin (1958)	19
Byar (1972)	18
Jewett (1972)	
(UICC) B1	16
(UICC) B2	50
Williams (1975)	37

Table 15-2. Incidence of unsuspected metastases to pelvic lymph nodes in carcinoma of the prostate gland*

UICC stage	Number of patients	Number of patients with positive nodes	Percent with positive nodes
B1	19	4	21
B2	17	5	30
C	24	12	50
TOTAL	60	21	35

*Modified from McLaughlin, A. P., Saltzstein, S. L., McCullough, D. L., and Gittes, R. F.: J. Urol. **115**:89-94, 1976.

Table 15-3. Distribution of metastases to pelvic lymph nodes in carcinoma of the prostate*

Location	Clinical Stages B1, B2	Clinical Stage C	Total
Obturator-hypogastric (alone)	3	3	6
Obturator–hypogastric–external iliac	2	2	4
Obturator–hypogastric–external iliac–common iliac	1	4	5
Obturator–hypogastric–common iliac	0	3	3
External iliac (alone)	2	0	2
Common iliac (alone)	1	0	1
TOTAL	9	12	21

*Modified from McLaughlin, A. P., Saltzstein, S. L., McCullough, D. L., and Gittes, R. F.: J. Urol. **115**:89-94, 1976.

the evolution of the disease. The incidence according to clinical stage and anatomic distribution is given in Tables 15-2 and 15-3. In addition the incidence of nodal involvement increases as the histologic grade increases. Thus, of thirty-nine differentiated prostatic cancers, eight (20%) yielded positive pelvic nodes on lymph node dissection. Of twenty-three undifferentiated cancers, twelve (56%) had positive pelvic nodes (Saltzstein and McLaughlin). These figures are in general agreement with those of Flocks and associates, Arduino and Glucksman, and Pistenma and associates. Here, as in the case of extracapsular extension, we find a strong argument for external pelvic irradiation, especially for all high-grade lesions and for patients with clinical Stages B and C. It is also clear that draining lymph nodes will not be encompassed in the high-dose volume when portals are planned to irradiate only the gland with a narrow margin. Thus two of the major justifications for radiation therapy for carcinoma of the prostate, that is, extracapsular extension and metastases to regional lymph nodes, require that generous volumes be encompassed in the zone of high dose.

LYMPHANGIOGRAM. The foot lymphangiogram often helps in developing the plan of treatment even though it fails to agree with the microscopic findings in about 30% of the patients. Thus Pistenma and associates reported that for clinical Stages A and B the false positive rate was 12.5% and the false negative rate was 16.3%. For Stage C the false positive rate was 4%, and the false negative rate was 23.1%. We generally use the positive lymphangiogram as if it were a definite indication of metastases to lymph nodes. We are less inclined to accept the negative lymphangiogram as a definite indication of the absence of regional metastases. Many urologists use the positive lymphangiogram in Stages A and B (T1 and T2) as a contraindication to prostatectomy, whereas the negative lymphangiogram is one of their prerequisites for prostatectomy.

From the foregoing data it is clear that, currently, clinical evaluation of extent of the primary cancer and the metastases is not precise. These limitations of clinical staging must be appreciated and irradiation planned accordingly.

Technique of irradiation

Numerous early attempts to treat carcinoma of the prostate by irradiation were so discouraging that it became a general belief that the disease was indeed radioincurable. These early attempts, made with intracavitary, interstitial, or medium-voltage techniques, were handicapped by inhomogeneous distribution of radiations or inadequate depth dose. ^{60}Co and megavoltage beams provided the first means for consistent homogeneous high-dose irradiation of carcinoma of the prostate gland.

There is ample proof from several institutions that carcinomas of the prostate gland may be eradicated by external irradiation in a large proportion of patients. The rate of success depends on the clinical stage, technique of irradiation, and the end point one selects. The status of the postirradiation needle biopsy has been a popular end point. The outcome of this type of biopsy will vary with clinical stage, radiation technique, and the duration of the interval between irradiation and biopsy. If one biopsies predominantly the most suspicious lesions or shortly after irradiation, a high proportion of biopsies will be positive. Cox and Tijerina found that for Stage C lesions 60% of forty-three patients had positive biopsies 3 to 9 months postirradiation. This was reduced to 24% of twenty-five patients at 12 to 30 months postirradiation (Fig. 15-2). Malignant nodules may remain palpable in the prostate gland for 9 to 12 months. Even at 12 months not all residual palpable nodules will yield positive needle biopsies. Seventeen of forty-one patients (41%) yielded a positive needle biopsy when the gland had returned to normal on palpation, whereas twenty-eight of thirty-six patients (78%) yielded a positive needle biopsy when the nodule in the gland remained palpable (Mollenkamp and associates). Overall, 12 months or more after 7000 rad have been delivered to clinical Stage C carcinoma of the prostate gland, 50% will show no residual local cancer. Dose-response data are otherwise rather poorly developed.

There is no detectable correlation between the presence of a postirradiation positive biopsy with treatment factors, either hormonal or radiotherapeutic. For the individual patient the presence of the postirradiation positive biopsy seems to have little significance and is no longer recommended as a guide to management (Cox and Stoffel).

The selection of patients for irradiation has been generous. This is a result of limited knowledge of the radiocurability of the various clinical stages, the palliation

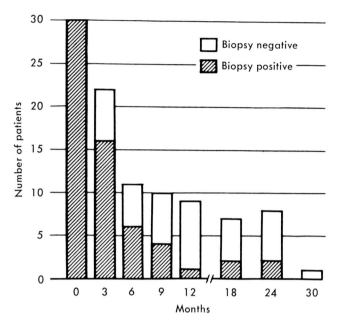

Fig. 15-2. Correlation of biopsy results with postirradiation interval. Dose to prostate was 7000 rad in 6 to 7 weeks. (From Cox, J. D., and Tijerina, A.: Radiology **112**:215-216, 1974.)

Table 15-4. Frequency of prostatic carcinoma as the principal cause of death related to clinical stage*

Clinical stage	Number of patients	Prostatic carcinoma as principal cause of death (%)
I	32	14.3
II	37	25.8
III	117	48.6
IV	158	84.0

*Modified from Schoonees, R., Palma, L. D., Gaeta, J. F., Moose, R. H., and Murphy, G. P.: N.Y. J. Med. **72**(part 1): 1021-1027, 1972.

provided when cure is not obtained, and an acceptable incidence of high-dose effects. Except as mentioned subsequently, we irradiate any patient with T1, T2, or T3 lesions whose cancer is confined to the pelvis and whose general condition justifies this major effort. Some consideration must be given to the fact that few patients with clinical T0 histologic Grades I and II cancers die from their cancer. Schoonees and associates reviewed 352 patients with histologically verified adenocarcinomas of the prostate. The frequency with which cancer causes death in these patients is tabulated in Table 15-4. Of the patients with clinical T0, cancer was the principal cause of death in 14%. All this 14% had histologic Grade III or IV adenocarcinomas. These data cast serious doubt on the necessity of treating all patients with well-differentiated T0 cancers. In some patients the cancer may originate deep in the gland and be impalpable for a sufficiently long period to permit *diffuse* intraglandular spread (Barnes and associates). The prognosis in this instance becomes more that of clinical T2 rather than T0. However, there is as yet no routine procedure short of prostatectomy to determine such diffuse occult spread. Other than the well-differentiated cancers mentioned before, microscopic grading has not been used to influence radiation therapy technique (Mostofi).

The prostate gland, sandwiched between the pubis and rectum and encircling the bladder neck, can be irradiated by the technique described for cancer of the bladder. We do not know how frequently regional lymph node metastases can be eradicated or what effect such eradication might have on survival. However, the incidence of regional metastasis to lymph nodes in the various stages is shown in Tables 15-2 and 15-3. Furthermore, at the time of prostatectomy, half of all Stage II (T1 and T2) lesions will have already extended beyond the gland. This fact, coupled with the fact that such a small proportion of cancers will be diagnosed during the early stages, means that larger volumes will be required for most patients. The lymph node drainage of the prostate gland is illustrated in Fig. 15-1. The primary cancer and regional metastasis can be encompassed by anteroposterior and posteroanterior beams 15 × 15 cm. Lateral beams for the "box" technique can be 15 × 9 cm if the presacral nodes are not to be encompassed. The precise location of the prostate and its relation to the opacified bladder and rectum, along with the relative position of the draining lymph nodes, are best defined by simulation. If a rotational technique is to be used for the boosting dose, the simulation is usually repeated. An alternative technique makes use of a single anterior and two oblique posterior beams. A perineal beam is particularly useful for irradiating the large prostatic masses that bulge inferiorly toward the anus. Tissue tolerances in the irradiated volume are similar to those found in treating carcinoma of the urinary bladder and, to a lesser extent, in treating carcinoma of the cervix.

DOSE-TIME RELATIONSHIPS. We generally try to deliver a minimum of 5000 rad (at the rate of 160 to 180 rad per fractions per day) to the node-bearing region (hypogastric, obturator, and external and common iliac nodes). An additional 2000 rad boost in 2 to 3 weeks through reduced ports encompassing the primary cancer may be added after a 2-week split. The importance of maintaining a low daily dose cannot be overemphasized if total doses are to be in the range of 7000 rad. There is no question but that the para-aortic nodes are involved in a proportion of patients. However, treating this area adds considerably to the risks of the procedure and a planned clinical trial has not yet indicated it to be of value. Shrinkage of the cancer may be slow. Nine to 12 months may be required for it to reach its minimal size, although notable shrinkage generally occurs during irradiation. If the cancer is large in comparison to the size of the normal gland, shrinkage may seem more dramatic than if the cancer is small. The dose mentioned will probably eradicate the primary lesion in at least half the patients. Diarrhea and dysuria are common, and they are managed symptomatically.

COMBINATIONS OF RADIATION THERAPY AND ANTIANDROGENS. Antiandrogen therapy shrinks the primary and metastatic masses in over 70% of the patients treated. If it is true that the larger the tumor mass the higher the dose of radiations necessary for its eradication, then antiandrogen-induced shrinkage could conceivably diminish the dose of radiations required for eradication of the intrapelvic disease. This line of reasoning has led to the combined use of these therapies for carcinoma of the prostate gland. It also led surgeons to combine antiandrogen therapy with prostatectomy. Although Scott and Boyd recommend this combination, the randomized clinical trials conducted by the Veterans Administration have failed to substantiate any benefit from combining antiandrogen therapy with prostatectomy (Byar). The value of adding antiandrogen therapy to radiation therapy has not been determined. Lipsett and associates and Cosgrove and Kaempf concluded from their nonrandomized clinical experience that the combination is superior to radiation therapy alone. By contrast, in a small randomized clinical trial van der Werf-Messing and associates and Neglia and associates found the combination resulted in no improvement over radiation therapy alone. Obviously, further clinical trials are indicated. Until this question is settled, we do not routinely recommend antiandrogen therapy be given with "curative" irradiation. However, we have not refused to administer "curative" irradiation because of previous castration or concurrent hormonal therapy.

INTERSTITIAL IRRADIATION. Interest in interstitial irradiation has been prompted by four considerations.

1. Interstitial irradiation enables the delivery of a high dose to a well-defined prostatic volume without delivering a concomitant high dose to the rectum or major segment of the bladder.
2. When the disease is limited, good local control is possible.
3. The procedure requires little of the patient's time and can be performed at the time of a node sampling procedure.
4. In contrast to prostatectomy, the procedure is less demanding on the patient and does not usually produce a loss of potency.

EXTERNAL PELVIC IRRADIATION. External pelvic irradiation has the following advantages as compared to interstitial irradiation (Harisiadis and associates).

1. In addition to the primary lesion, the periprostatic tissues and regional nodes can be homogeneously irradiated with external beams.
2. Laparotomy is not necessary; thus the complications associated with surgery are reduced.
3. Local control of the primary lesion is excellent with external pelvic irradiation. Most patients who fail do so not because of local recurrence alone, but because of distant metastases or distant metastases and local disease.
4. Even when an implant is performed, external irradiation must often be given anyway to encompass periprostatic tissues and regional nodes.

Thus, there are but a few patients for whom implant alone is a suitable treatment, that is, patients with a primary lesion limited to the prostate with minimal risk of

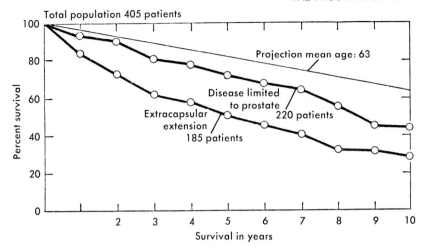

Fig. 15-3. Percent survival in patients irradiated for carcinoma of the prostate (total population = 405 patients). (From Bagshaw, M. A., Ray, G. R., Salzman, J. R., and Meares, E. M.: Cancer Chemother. Rep. **59:**165-173, 1975.)

spread to periprostatic tissues or regional nodes. In most institutions such lesions are now being treated by surgery.

RESULTS. A major obstacle to establishing the treatment of choice for the various clinical stages of cancer of the prostate gland is its uncertain natural history. Most patients with limited disease and many patients with moderately advanced disease survive for long asymptomatic periods even when untreated. Thus, even if cancer has extended beyond the capsule but has not metastasized distantly, the 5-year survival exceeds 50% with hormonal treatment alone (van der Werf-Messing). The effect of irradiation on length of survival has been difficult to ascertain. This is especially the case since studies have not usually been conducted by prospectively randomizing patients. The survival rates for the Stanford experience are shown in Fig. 15-3 and those of Lipsett and associates in Fig. 15-4. These are representative of results of current radiation therapy techniques. A wide variety of factors affect prognosis including clinical stage, histologic grade, pretreatment obstructive changes on the excretory pyelogram, delay in initiation of irradiation, and various factors related to dose (Harisiadis and associates).

Of those vigorously irradiated patients who eventually die from widespread metastases, half will have no symptoms referable to their primary lesion; of those who have had vigorous irradiation, half will show no residual local cancer at autopsy. The results of needle biopsies were mentioned previously.

COMPLICATIONS. Acute radiation-induced diarrhea and dysuria are to be expected in about half the patients during the last half to last third of the treatment period. As pointed out, these symptoms should be treated just as in patients with carcinoma of the cervix.

Late sequelae have been surprisingly few considering the high doses used. The delivery of 7000 rad in 7 to 8 weeks to the region of the prostate gland using mega-

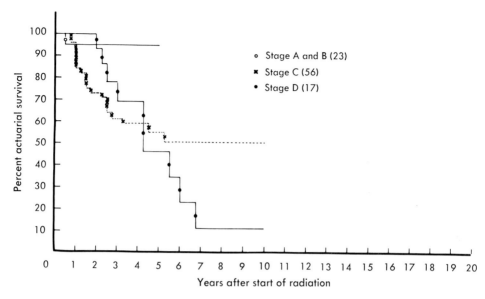

Fig. 15-4. Percent of postirradiation actuarial survival according to clinical stage of cancer of prostate. (From Lipsett, J. A., Cosgrove, M. D., Green, N., et al.: Int. J. Radiat. Oncol. Biol. Phys. **1**:1049-1058, 1976.)

voltage beams requires the use of several techniques if serious subcutaneous fibrosis is to be avoided. This is especially true in fat patients or patients with large dimensions. Furthermore, if the cancer has extended inferiorly and is within a centimeter or so of the anus, it may be impossible to deliver an adequate dose to the cancer without delivering a similar dose to the anus and perineal skin. The fear of high-dose sequelae in the abdominal or perineal skin has prompted us to place a limit of 5000 rad in 5 or 6 weeks or its equivalent as the maximum given dose delivered through each portal. Since we ordinarily shrink the irradiated volume after a depth dose of 5000 rad in 5 or 6 weeks, we take that point to start a rotational technique for delivering the boosting dose of 2000 rad.

Late rectal and bladder sequelae are similar to those described after treatment for carcinoma of the cervix. One cannot avoid a certain number of serious rectal ulcerations and strictures if the above-mentioned doses are used. An occasional colostomy or urinary diversion may be necessary. Small bowel is usually irradiated during the initial part of the treatment, but with care it can be excluded from the boosting dose. We do not know how to identify patients in which these serious sequelae are likely to develop and therefore must accept the risks. However, these sequelae will be reduced by daily doses no greater than 180 rad. Reported incidences are given in Table 15-5.

PALLIATIVE IRRADIATION OF METASTASES. Hormonal management of the patient with widespread metastases is well established. The patient will eventually escape from the benefits of hormones. Local irradiation of symptom-producing

Table 15-5. Incidence of late gastrointestinal and genitourinary complications following radiation therapy for carcinoma of the prostate gland

Author	Number of patients	Complications (%)		
		Rectal	Bladder or urethra	Impotence
Pistenma (1976)	430	12	3.7	41
van der Werf-Messing (1976)	60	6.7	6.7	
Mollenkamp (1975)	88	3.4	3.4	23
Perez (1976)	59	5.2	8.5	10

metastases can be of great benefit. One should appreciate the fact that some of these patients will live for years. The dose of radiations should be planned with this in mind. If the patient's course has been slow and his general condition remains relatively good, we recommend relatively high palliative doses of 4500 rad in 3 weeks if dose-limiting critical organs, that is, spinal cord, are not in the treated volume. When we have not used doses of this level and survival has been long, retreatment two or three times has been necessary. Relief of pain will be obtained in half or more of the patients. If a short life is anticipated, about two thirds of this dose should be adequate. Estrogen therapy produces the sometimes painful and often embarrassing enlargement of the male breast. This enlargement can be prevented by administering 1500 rad in three doses of 500 rad each to a circle 3 cm in diameter centered on the nipple (Alfthan and Kettunen; Gagnon and associates). We have been impressed with the efficacy of this irradiation.

SUMMARY. The availability of megavoltage and telecobalt beams has brought carcinoma of the prostate into the group of diseases curable by external pelvic irradiation. Few cancers of the prostate are diagnosed sufficiently early to be cured by surgery. We believe primary high-dose external pelvic irradiation is the treatment of choice for all cancers of the prostate gland apparently confined to the pelvis except for the Stage I, Grade 1 and 2 lesions.

REFERENCES

Alfthan, O., and Kettunen, K.: The effect of roentgen ray treatment of gynecomastia in patients with prostatic carcinoma treated with estrogen hormones: a preliminary communication, J. Urol. 94:604-606, 1965.

Arduino, L. J., and Glucksman, M. A.: Lymph node metastasis in early carcinoma of the prostate, J. Urol. 88:91-93, 1962.

Bagshaw, M. A., Ray, G. R., Salzman, J. R., and Meares, E. M.: Extended-field radiation therapy for carcinoma of the prostate: a progress report, Cancer Chemother. Rep. 59:165-173, 1975.

Barnes, R., Hirst, A., and Rosenquist, R.: Early carcinoma of the prostate: comparison of Stages A and B, J. Urol. 115:404-405, 1976.

Budhrajar, S. W., and Anderson, J. C.: An assessment of the value of radiotherapy in the management of carcinoma of the prostate, Br. J. Urol. 36:535-540, 1964.

Bulkley, G. J., Cooper, J. A., and O'Conor, V. J.: Intraprostatic injections of radioactive colloids. II. Distribution within the prostate and tissue changes following injection in the dog. Trans. Am. Assoc. Genitourin. Surg. 45:57-65, 1953.

Byar, D. P., and Mostofi, F. K.: Carcinoma of the prostate: prognostic evaluation of certain pathologic features in 208 radical prostatectomies, Cancer 30:5-13, 1972.

Byar, D. P.: The Veterans Administration Cooperative Urological Research Group's studies of cancer of the prostate, Cancer 32:1126-1130, 1973.

Cosgrove, M. D., and Kaempf, M. J.: Prostatic cancer revisited, J. Urol. 115:79-81, 1976.

Cox, J. D., and Tijerina, A.: Preliminary results of biopsies following irradiation for locally advanced adenocarcinoma of the prostate, Radiology 112:215-216, 1974.

Cox, J. D., and Stoffel, T. J.: The significance of needle biopsy after irradiation for Stage C adenocarcinoma of the prostate, Cancer 40:156-160, 1977.

del Regato, J. A.: Radiotherapy in the conservative treatment of operable and locally inoperable carcinoma of the prostate, Radiology 88:761-766, 1967.

del Regato, J. A.: Cancer of the prostate, J.A.M.A. 235:1727-1730, 1976.

Flocks, R. H., Culp, D., and Porto, R.: Lymphatic spread from prostatic cancer, J. Urol. 81:194-196, 1959.

Gagnon, J. D., Moss, W. T., and Stevens, K. R.: Pre-estrogen breast irradiation for patients with carcinoma of the prostate: a critical review, J. Urol. 121:182-184, 1979.

Harisiadis, L., Veenema, R. J., Senyszn, J. J., Puchner, P. J., and Tretter, P.: Carcinoma of the prostate, Cancer 41:2131-2142, 1978.

Jewett, H. J., Bridge, R. W., Gray, G. F., and Shelley, W. M.: The palpable nodule of prostatic cancer, J.A.M.A. 203:403-406, 1968.

Jewett, H. J., Eggleston, J. C., and Yawn, D. H.: Radical prostatectomy in the management of carcinoma of the prostate: probable causes of some therapeutic failures, J. Urol. 107:1034-1040, 1972.

Lipsett, J. A., Cosgrove, M. D., Green, N., et al.: Factors influencing prognosis in the radiotherapeutic management of carcinoma of the prostate, Int. J. Radiat. Oncol. Biol. Phys. 1:1049-1058, 1976.

McLaughlin, A. P., Saltzstein, S. L., McCullough, D. L., and Gittes, R. F.: Prostatic carcinoma: incidence and location of unsuspected lymphatic metastases, J. Urol. 115:89-94, 1976.

Mollenkamp, J. S., Cooper, J. F., and Kagan, A. R.: Clinical experience with supervoltage radiotherapy in carcinoma of the prostate, J. Urol. 113:374, 1975.

Mostofi, F. K.: Problems of grading carcinoma of prostate, Semin. Oncol. 3:161-169, 1976.

Neglia, W. J., Hussey, D. H., and Johnson, D. E.: Megavoltage radiation therapy for carcinoma of the prostate, Int. J. Radiat. Oncol. Biol. Phys. 2:873, 1977.

Nesbit, R. M., and Baum, W. C.: Serum phosphatase determinations in diagnosis of prostatic cancer: a review of 1,150 cases, J.A.M.A. 145:1321-1324, 1951.

Perez, C. A., Ackerman, L. V., Silber, I., and Royce, R. K.: Radiation therapy in the treatment of localized carcinoma of the prostate, Cancer 34:1059-1068, 1974.

Pistenma, D. A., Ray, G. R., and Bagshaw, M. A.: The role of megavoltage radiation therapy in the treatment of prostatic carcinoma, Semin. Oncol. 3:115-122, 1976.

Rubenstein, A. B., and Rubnitz, M. E.: Transitional cell carcinoma of the prostate, Cancer 24:543-546, 1969.

Saltzstein, S. L., and McLaughlin, A. P.: Clinicopathologic features of unsuspected regional lymph node metastases in prostatic adenocarcinoma, Cancer 40:1212-1221, 1977.

Schoonees, R., Palma, L. D., Gaeta, J. F., Moose, R. H., and Murphy, G. P.: Prostatic carcinoma treated at categorical center, N.Y. J. Med. 72(part 1):1021-1027, 1972.

Scott, W. W., and Boyd, H. L.: Combined hormone control therapy and radical prostatectomy in the treatment of selected cases of advanced carcinoma of the prostate: a retrospective study based upon 25 years of experience, J. Urol. 101:86-92, 1969.

van der Werf-Messing, B., Sourek-Zikova, V., and Blonk, D. I.: Localized advanced carcinoma of the prostate: radiation therapy versus hormonal therapy, Int. J. Radiat. Oncol. Biol. Phys. 1:1043-1048, 1976.

Veterans Administration Cooperative Urological Research Group: Treatment and survival of patients with cancer of the prostate, Surg. Gynecol. Obstet. 124:1011-1017, 1967.

16

The testicle

RESPONSE OF THE NORMAL TESTICLE TO IRRADIATION

The wide variety of tissues constituting the testicle, together with its importance and accessibility, have made it a favorite site of study among radiobiologists. This was as true in 1903 as it is today. The germinal epithelium itself presents a wide variation of radiosensitivities from that of the mitotically active spermatogonia to that of the mature spermatozoa. The interstitial cells and the Sertoli cells, although intimately associated with the germinal cells, present still different radiosensitivites. Histologic, hormonal, genetic, and fertility studies have all contributed to the understanding of the radiation response of these cell types. A major concern here is to define to what extent irradiation of the testicle alters the quantity and quality of offspring. This is not a simple determination. There are objective changes in the irradiated testicle indicative of the great sensitivity of this organ. There are quantitative changes in semen reflecting the suppression of germinal activity with corresponding microscopic changes in the seminiferous tubules. Finally, there are alterations in fertility, a decrease in number of offspring, and genetic mutations. Functional changes in offspring have also been considered. Only a small part of this voluminous material can be reviewed here. The reader is referred to the excellent review by Mandl for a more detailed account and to Zuckerman for a summary.

After a single dose of 600 to 1000 rad to the testicle of a rat, the organ becomes soft, smaller, and lighter (Kohn and Kallman, 1955). These gross changes continue for 3 to 4 weeks. Then, if the dose has not been too great, regeneration begins. Several months may be required for return to preirradiation weights. Serial microscopy during the postirradiation period reveals the reasons for these gross changes (Fig. 16-1). Dead spermatogonia begin to appear a few hours after irradiation. The majority of primitive spermatogonia (Type A) are thought to have an LD_{50} of about 600 rad, whereas some of their daughter cells (Type B spermatogonia), which subsequently form spermatocytes, are thought to have an LD_{50} of 21 to about 100 rad (Lushbaugh and Ricks). By the eighth or ninth day, no spermatogonia can be found. It should be recalled that spermatogonia are the source of spermatocytes, which in turn become spermatids and then spermatozoa. In man, testicular depletion of sperm through maturation (and failure of spermatogonia to supply replacement cells) takes 46 days, and an additional 21 days are required for the sperm count to drop to zero

417

(Rowley and associates). Any decrease or subsequent increase in the number of cells of the germinal epithelium is largely determined by the radiosensitivity of the spermatogonia. However, with doses greater than 400 rad some of the spermatids are killed and the interval to azoospermia is decreased. The chromosomal number is reduced from the diploid number of 46 to haploid during meiosis occurring in the

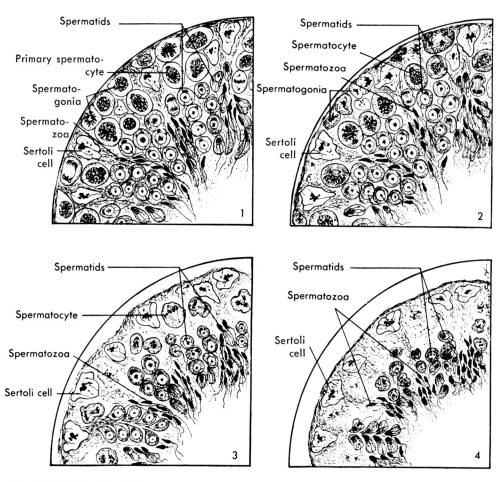

Fig. 16-1. Effects of irradiation on the testis. **1,** Diagram of a *normal seminal tubule* containing all the different cells and stages of spermatogenesis. **2,** *Two hours after irradiation:* many spermatogonia are missing; others are undergoing abnormal mitosis. **3,** *Four days after irradiation:* no spermatogonia are left; Sertoli cells have closed ranks at the base; all other cells have continued their development so that there are fewer primary spermatocytes, some of them showing abnormal mitosis; more mature cells are unchanged. **4,** *Eight days after irradiation:* all primary spermatocytes have disappeared; the cellular column has diminished in height. Some secondary spermatocytes show abnormal mitosis. **5,** *Twenty-one days after irradiation:* no spermatocytes are left. The cellular column is reduced to a layer of Sertoli cells. There remain a few spermatids, some of which show abnormally shaped heads. **6,** *Thirty-four days after irradiation:* no spermatids are left. The tube has shrunk further. Only Sertoli cells and new spermatogonia are seen. (From del Regato, J. A., and Spjut, H. J.: Ackerman and del Regato's cancer: diagnosis, treatment, and prognosis, ed. 5, St. Louis, 1977, The C. V. Mosby Co.)

progression from the primary spermatocyte to the secondary spermatocyte. In contrast to the multiple critical targets of cells with a diploid number (Chapter 1), cells with a haploid number respond to radiations as if they had only one critical target; there is no shoulder on the cell survival curve, and recovery from sublethal injury is not evident. This does not mean that serious genetic changes are not occurring in irradiated living cells. Spermatids are somewhat more resistant to the induction of morphologic abnormalities and cell death than spermatogonia. However, they are sensitive to the production of chromosomal aberrations and mutations.

After the dose mentioned previously, no spermatogonia are visible by the ninth day, but complete aspermia does not develop for several weeks. The more radioresistant elements continue their process of maturation until they are eliminated as mature sperm. Spermatozoa are more radiosensitive to mutation production after insemination than in the testes or seminal vesicles. Radiation aspermia may be complete, incomplete, or of short or long duration, depending on the total dose and technique of administration. If the dose has not been too high, Type A spermatogonia reappear at first sparsely, and some soon produce Type B spermatogonia, which in turn produce spermatocytes even before the tubules are completely repopulated by spermatogonia. Recovery is usually incomplete. The source of these spermatogonia, which initiate tubular repopulation, is not established. It has been suggested that they may originate from as yet unidentified undifferentiated cells, Sertoli cells, or modified spermatogonia in Sertoli syncytium (Momigliano and Essenberg). Oakberg believes that certain spermatogonia (Type A) are of heterogeneous sensitivity, depending on their mitotic activity and stage of development. An occasional Type A spermatogonium is radioresistant, and this initiates the repopulation of the tubules. Repopulation after severe depletion takes approximately three times longer than unirradiated spermatogenesis. Neither the severity of the radiation injury nor the rate of recovery is modified significantly by hormonal administration before, during,

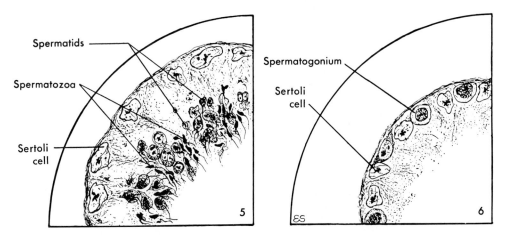

Fig. 16-1, cont'd. For legend see opposite page.

or after the exposure (Binhammer). Years may be required before repopulation and the sperm count reach their maximums.

During the period of aspermia after the previously mentioned dose, neither the interstitial hormone-producing cells nor the syncytial cells of Sertoli appear significantly altered morphologically. In young animals when the interstitial cells are still undergoing proliferation and maturation, their growth is suppressed by irradiation, and the adult animal will be hormonally deficient. In the adult animal, Binhammer found that a single dose of 1000 rad reduced androgen production but did not eliminate it. By contrast, Rowley and associates found that as the sperm count decreased, the total urinary gonadotropins increased presumably as a compensatory response. In the presence of a complete and permanent aspermia, there is no gross regression of secondary sex characteristics. This emphasizes the difference between radiation-induced and surgical castration in the male and confirms the function of each cell type in the process of reproduction.

The effects of irradiation vary with the total dose and the type of fractionation, oxygen tension of cells in question, temperature of the testicle, and type of radiations. Similar effects are produced on the testicle whether the irradiation is localized or total body (Fogg and Cowing). Total body irradiation given with the testicles shielded produces no effect on spermatogenesis (Kohn). A single dose of 50 to 100 rad to the rodent's testicle decreases the rate of spermatogonia production slightly. A dose of 250 to 500 rad destroys many spermatogonia. Still higher single doses produce the effects described. A wide range of wavelengths is of similar biologic effectiveness (Bane and associates). Species differences are striking and may result from differences in the length of the cell cycle and the length of spermatogenesis, the duration of the entire reproductive period, and the basic differences in the sensitivity of spermatogonia. The sensitivity of the germ cell fluctuates widely with its developmental stage at the time of the irradiation. In general, mitotically active spermatogonia are very sensitive. As mentioned previously, the final premeiotic generation, when the primary spermatocyte is formed, is more sensitive than preceding generations. Spermatids are relatively resistant to induction of morphologic abnormalities and cell death but are sensitive to chromosomal aberrations and mutations.

The possibilities of fractionated irradiation as a clinical technique were first realized during Regaud's classic study of the effects of irradiation on spermatogenesis. He inserted radon needles into rams' testicles. In one case, 4.5 millicuries were destroyed over a period of 28 days, and in other cases similar or even higher doses were given in 30 to 42 hours. The more protracted irradiation produced more nearly complete and more lasting depressions of spermatogenesis. This was later confirmed using fractionated roentgen irradiation (Ferroux and associates; Casarett and Eddy). The latter produced complete and permanent aspermia in dogs with 3 R per day (x rays) to a total dose of 475 R, whereas a single dose of 2000 R did not cause this effect. Such fractionation decreased the damage to scrotal skin but increased the destruction of germinal epithelium. The differences between the biologic effectiveness of single doses and fractionated radiations were discussed in Chapter 1. The *cumulative* damage of small fractionated doses of total body irradiation is greater in the germinal epithelium of the testicle than in any other male tissue (Bloom and Bloom).

Even before the sperm count decreases, the morphologically normal, irradiated sperm manifest their injury by producing smaller than normal litters (Gowen and Stadler). Sexes of offspring are affected equally. A discussion of radiation-induced genetic changes is beyond the scope of this review. However, several important conclusions should be recognized by anyone using radiations.

1. Ionizing radiations produce genetic mutations.
2. These mutations are cumulative to a high degree.
3. The frequency of radiation-induced genetic mutations depends on the dose. Presumably, the relationship is a straight line without a threshold. The incidence of chromosomal abnormalities and genetic mutations subsequent to testicular irradiation is reduced with time due to selective elimination.
4. A low dose rate may produce fewer mutations than a high dose rate even though total doses are equal (Russell, 1961). The apparent discrepancies between this and items 2 and 3 are yet to be clarified.
5. Radiation-induced mutations are almost entirely harmful. If they are not the cause of death of the developing or developed first-generation offspring, they will be passed on to future generations. This will increase the mutation load of race in such a way as to contribute to the death of one individual just as surely as if it had caused the death of a first- or second-generation offspring.

Although the previously mentioned findings have been described for *Drosophila* and mice, there are almost no significant genetic data for man. Eight men accidentally exposed to radiations of nuclear origin were studied for several years. Doses estimated at 236 to 365 rad produced transient sterility. Serial sperm counts and testicular biopsies revealed initial decreases in counts. Within 41 months semen had apparently returned to normal. In some men reproduction was accomplished (MacLeod and associates). Fifty to 70 rad delivered to the remaining testicle during radiotherapy for carcinoma of the testicle does not prevent reproduction (Smithers and Wallace; Krantz and associates). Apparently the genetic changes occur in man, but there are likely to be quantitative differences that make it impossible to know their relative importance. When using megavoltage beams for Stage I seminoma of the testicle, about 150 rad scatter from the usual "dog-leg" shaped ports to the remaining testicle. After such doses to the remaining testicle, patients are capable of fathering children. van der Werf-Messing reported thirty-one such patients who had fathered normal children. During radiation therapy for carcinoma of the prostate gland, the dose scattered to the testicles may be several times this, but because such patients infrequently desire to father children, the dose is less significant than for patients mentioned before. During the irradiation of pelvic nodes through an inverted Y portal used in treating Hodgkin's disease, the testicles may be given doses of 140 to 300 rad. Such fractionated total doses may cause prolonged aspermia (Speiser and associates; Hahn and associates). How hazardous is the present permissible dose with various proportions of the population exposed? How much patient exposure is justified during the solution of a given diagnostic problem? Except to say that exposure should be kept to the minimum compatible with good medical care, no rules are available.

Other types of external irradiation (electron and neutron beams), like internally administered radioisotopes, produce damage similar to that described previously, but the distribution of the cellular destruction depends entirely on the distribution of the radiant energy.

The epididymis, the ductus deferens, and the seminal vesicles show no striking changes after moderate irradiation (Coliez and Bourdon). These findings are of no therapeutic significance.

LYMPH DRAINAGE OF THE TESTICLES. From the hilum of the testicle four to eight collecting lymphatics drain by way of the spermatic cord through the inguinal ring along the general course of the right and left testicular veins. These lymphatics empty in nodes related to the aorta and inferior vena cava. On the right most of the draining nodes are lateral, anterior, and medial to the inferior vena cava and anterior to the aorta. Occasionally, drainage will empty into the more superior right common iliac nodes. On the left most of the draining nodes are lateral and anterior to the aorta. On both sides there are extensive collateral and intercommunicating lymphatics. Contralateral drainage commonly occurs above the level of the renal veins. Disruption of draining lymphatics, as might occur during herniorrhaphy or vasectomy, may reroute lymph drainage through the subcutaneous lymphatics of the inferior-anterior abdominal wall into contralateral iliac nodes. The epididymis drains into ipsilateral iliac nodes, and the lymph drainage of the scrotal skin and subcutaneous tissue is into inguinal and iliac nodes.

CARCINOMA OF THE TESTICLE

Only the lymphomas and those testicular tumors arising from germinal epithelium are of radiotherapeutic significance. For the most part, the rare tumors arising from interstitial cells and those arising from testicular connective tissues are not sufficiently radiosensitive to be radiocurable and will not be discussed further. The clinical aspects of the disease vary with the histologic type. A simple histologic classification of testicular carcinomas has been devised by Friedman and Moore.

A. Germinal tumors
   1. Seminoma
   2. Embryonal tumors
      a. Embryonal carcinoma
      b. Teratocarcinoma
      c. Adult teratoma
      d. Choriocarcinoma
   3. Combinations of 1 and 2
B. Nongerminal tumors

The following tentative classification of germinal tumor by the World Health Organization Panel on testicular tumors appeared recently (Mostofi). Although it is similar to the preceding classification, it includes some variants not considered in the Friedman and Moore classification.

Tumors showing single histologic pattern
    Seminoma
        Classic
        Anaplastic
        Spermatocytic
    Embryonal carcinoma
        Adult
        Polyembryoma
        Infantile
    Choriocarcinoma
    Teratoma
        Mature
        Immature
Tumors showing mixed histologic types
    Embryonal carcinoma and teratoma (teratocarcinoma)
    Others

Several of these histologic types may occur in the same testicle, resulting in fifteen possible combinations. However, on the basis of clinical behavior, only five groups are worthy of recognition. These five groups, ranging from best to poorest prognosis, are listed:

1. Seminoma, pure
2. Embryonal carcinoma, pure or with seminoma
3. Teratoma, pure or with seminoma
4. Teratoma, with either embryonal carcinoma or choriocarcinoma or both, and with or without seminoma
5. Choriocarcinoma, pure or with seminoma or embryonal carcinoma or both*

Dixon and Moore emphasize that pure seminoma is the least malignant, its presence in combination with other types does not improve prognosis. In contrast the presence of teratoma with embryonal carcinoma or choriocarcinoma warrants a better prognosis than either of the latter two alone.

The term *embryonal* has been used to mean different types of tumors in different histologic classifications. To avoid confusion the British classification has avoided the term altogether. However, the majority of classifications accept the Dixon and Moore use of the term.

Natural steps in the spread of this disease are recognized in clinical staging, and the following seems rational. This staging system is similar to that proposed by Castro, but it includes some of the features of the system proposed by Maier and associates (1969). With minor exceptions the two are similar.

---

*From Dixon, F. J., and Moore, R. A.: Tumors of the male sex organs, Section VIII, Fascicles 31b and 32, Washington, D.C., 1952, Armed Forces Institute of Pathology, p. 52.

Stage I   The cancer is confined to the testicle. This determination is made by clinical and radiographic studies and by orchiectomy. Should subsequent retroperitoneal node dissection reveal microscopic foci of cancer in nodes, the clinical stage does not change, but subgroups should be formed (Maier and Van Buskirk).

Stage II   There is clinical or radiographic evidence of metastases to para-aortic, iliac, or inguinal lymph nodes or microscopic evidence in the orchiectomy specimen of invasion beyond the testicle.

Stage III There is clinical or radiographic evidence of metastases to mediastinal, supraclavicular, or pelvic lymph nodes.

Stage IV   Metastases are more widespread than in Stage III.

The TNM classification of the American Joint Committee (1978) is not given here because it is certain to create confusion in regard to spread to inguinal nodes with or without previous inguinal or scrotal surgery and with or without nodal fixation. In addition, it is a major departure from the more widely used clinical staging mentioned before and needs to be tested in many clinical and therapeutic situations.

In addition to the usual history and physical examination, staging requires that a special search be made for retroperitoneal, pelvic, mediastinal, and supraclavicular metastases. Many recently published series are composed of patients staged and treated in the 1950s and early 1960s as well as patients staged and treated since the availability of the lymphangiogram, chest tomograms, and the like. Some series include in Stage II those patients with no clinical or radiographic evidence of metastases but who are found to have metastases in retroperitoneal nodes at the time of surgery. This creates a difficult problem in comparing the results of surgery, chemotherapy, and radiation therapy.

The degree of agreement between the clinical and pathologic staging is, of course, critical in deciding modality and extent of treatment. In this regard the lymphangiogram is paramount in establishing pretreatment extent of retroperitoneal spread. Of eighteen patients with nonseminomatous tumors and positive lymphangiograms, 16 (88.9%) were verified as having metastases to retroperitoneal nodes (Hussey and associates). The experience of others is similar (Table 16-1).

Table 16-1. Correlation between lymphangiographic and histologic status of retroperitoneal lymph nodes in patients with nonseminomatous carcinoma of the testicle

Lymphangiographic status	Author	Histologic status of retroperitoneal nodes (%)	
		Positive	Negative
Lymphangiogram positive	Hussey	88.9	11.1
	Wallace	81	19
	Maier	93	7
Lymphangiogram normal	Hussey	17	83
	Wallace	15	85
	Maier	25	75

Wallace and Jing reported that out of eighty-three lymphangiograms performed on patients with seminoma (all stages), twenty were positive. Similarly, of 131 lymphangiograms performed on patients with nonseminomatous carcinomas, fifty-three were positive.

The incidence of false negative lymphangiograms in patients with nonseminomatous tumors is also well established. Retroperitoneal lymphadenectomy revealed that of sixty-five such patients whose lymphangiograms were normal, ten had cancer in nodes (Wallace and Jing). Also, of 106 patients with normal lymphangiograms, 17% were found to have occult metastases in retroperitoneal nodes (Hussey and associates) (Table 16-1).

Of those patients with Stage II nonseminomatous tumors who have verified metastases to retroperitoneal nodes, 42% will develop more distant metastases during follow-up care. Of similar patients (Stage II tumors) whose retroperitoneal nodes are in fact negative on removal, only 11% will develop more distant metastases (Hussey and associates).

Lymphadenectomy is seldom indicated in patients with seminomas, but there is no reason to believe that positive lymphangiograms in patients with seminomas are any less or more precise than they are in patients with nonseminomatous cancers. Of those patients with Stage I seminomas (including those who had negative lymphangiograms), very few develop mediastinal or extranodal metastases even when no irradiation is given above the diaphragm (Table 16-2). Of those patients with Stage II seminomas who were given no irradiation above the diaphragm, two of eleven developed supradiaphragmatic metastases (Doornbos and associates).

Summary of clinical characteristics of significance in formulating a treatment policy

Most patients will have had an inguinal orchiectomy before being seen by the radiation oncologist. The referring physician may not have obtained baseline alpha fetoprotein, chorionic gonadotropin, or carcinoembryonic antigen levels. The establishment of preorchiectomy levels of these markers may assist in subsequent management and posttreatment follow-up.

Table 16-2. Cause of eighteen failures in 132 patients irradiated for seminoma Stages I to III*

Cause of failure	Number of failures
Marginal recurrence	3
Metastases above diaphragm	3
Metastases of mixed histologic types	4
Dead of intercurrent disease	3
Recurrence in irradiated field	1
Extranodal metastases	1
Second testicular cancer	1
Complications to therapy	1
Lost to follow-up	1

*Modified from Doornbos, J. F., Hussey, D. H., and Johnson, D. E.: Radiology **116:**401-404, 1975.

Preradiation therapy levels should be obtained. Additional work-up should include the usual complete history and physical examination, the usual laboratory data and chest films, chest tomograms, excretory urogram, and bilateral pedal lymphangiogram.

Seminoma

STAGE I. If there is no evidence of extension beyond the testicle, there is no greater than a 10% chance that there are occult metastases in retroperitoneal nodes and little chance that there is spread to the mediastinal or supraclavicular nodes.

STAGE II. If abdominal disease is present but not bulky (less than 10 cm in diameter), there is about a 20% chance that occult spread has occurred above the

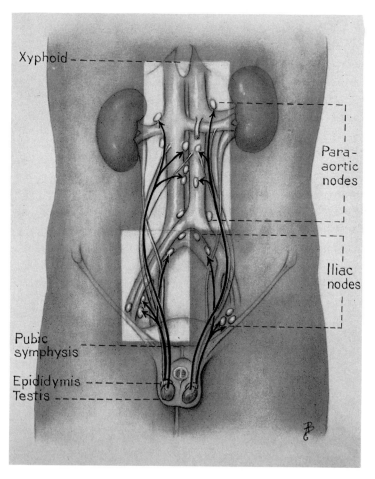

Fig. 16-2. Lymph node drainage of testicles and the usual position of associated structures serving as guides in planning irradiation for malignant tumors of the testicle. Above the aortic bifurcation the anteroposterior and posteroanterior fields should extend bilaterally to the medial portions of both kidneys. Below the bifurcation of the aorta only the ipsilateral nodes usually need irradiating.

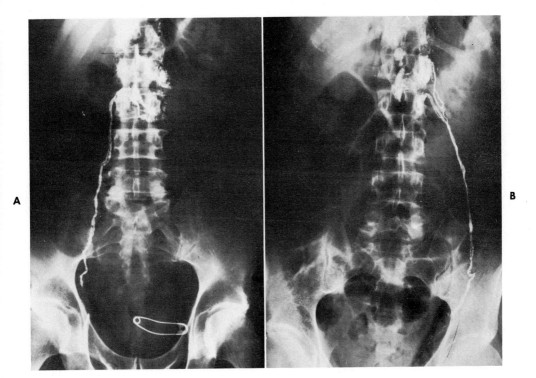

Fig. 16-3. Direct filling of para-aortic lymph nodes draining the testicle, demonstrated by testicular lymphangiograms of the right, **A,** and left, **B,** sides. The iliac nodes are bypassed. (Courtesy Dr. F. M. Busch.)

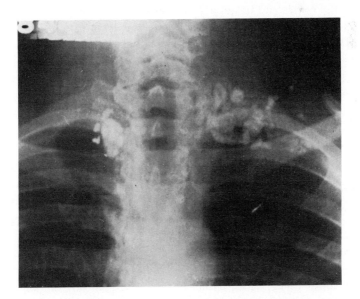

Fig. 16-4. Bilateral filling of supraclavicular lymph nodes from a foot lymphangiogram. There was no filling of mediastinal nodes. Ease with which supraclavicular lymph nodes fill suggests the need for their inclusion in the zones of irradiation in treatment of seminoma of the testicle.

diaphragm and a remote chance that more distant occult metastases are present. If the abdominal metastases are greater than 10 cm in diameter, there is a greater but as yet poorly defined risk of more extensive nodal and extranodal metastases above and below the diaphragm.

STAGE III. Few patients present with obvious metastases in mediastinal structures without having clinically obvious advanced disease. Most patients with Stage III seminoma will already have developed occult widespread metastases, and their management should be planned with this presumption in mind.

STAGE IV. The few patients who present with widespread metastases from seminoma will require planned combinations of systemic chemotherapy and local irradiation from the start.

Cancers other than seminomas

Data on each of the other four groups are scanty due to the small number of patients available for analysis. It is recognized that patients with Stage I teratomas, pure or with seminoma (Group 3), rarely develop extranodal metastases (Hussey and associates). Patients in Groups 2 and 4 have been pooled and are presented in Table 16-3. It is clear that if retroperitoneal nodes are involved, the chance of extranodal metastases is high and systemic as well as local treatment should be considered.

Techniques of irradiation

In establishing a treatment policy, one must weigh the radiocurability of the tumor type, the routes and frequency of spread, and the sequelae associated with a "curative" irradiation. Seminoma, whether in the testicle or metastatic to lymph nodes or other soft tissue, is highly radiosensitive, and if all the seminoma can be encompassed in the usual portals, it can be cured in almost every instance. As little as 1000 rad in 2 weeks may eradicate this tumor in retroperitoneal nodes. Embryonal carcinoma responds less well, but its lymph node metastases usually shrink with irradiation and they are radiocurable if small (Maier; Fayos and Kim; Hussey and associates). Large masses of teratocarcinomas and of embryonal carcinomas usually respond poorly to irradiation unless they contain large elements of seminoma. Teratocarcinomas have been rarely cured by radiotherapy alone. However, radiotherapy can hardly be expected to sterilize the large, bulky, inoperable masses for which it is often given. At the same time it has been difficult to evaluate the role of radiotherapy in the limited or occult disease generally treated by retroperitoneal lymph node dissection, either alone or in combination with irradiation and chemotherapy.

Patients with seminoma should have irradiation of the para-aortic and ipsilateral iliac nodes even if there are no clinically or radiographically demonstrable metastases. When para-aortic nodes are known to be involved by seminoma, the abdominal irradiation should be followed by irradiation of the mediastinum and both supraclavicular regions. We lack data necessary to justify routine irradiation of the medi-

Table 16-3. Incidence of widespread metastases in patients with Groups 2 and 4 nonseminomatous cancers of the testicle*

Clinical stage	Incidence of extranodal metastases according to status of retroperitoneal nodes	
	Negative nodes	Positive nodes
I	10/93 (10.8%)	5/18 (27.8%)
II	2/17 (11.7%)	14/27 (57.8%)

*Modified from Hussey, D. H., Luk, K. H., and Johnson, D. E.: Radiology **123:**175-180, 1977.

Table 16-4. Metastases from seminoma of the testicle*

Site involved	Number of patients	Percent of sixty patients†
Para-aortic lymph node	52	86.7
Mediastinal lymph node	5	8.3
Left supraclavicular lymph node	11	18.3
Lung	15	25.0
Liver	5	8.3
Bone	4	6.7
Brain	2	3.3
Inguinal lymph node	1	1.7

*Modified from Martin, L. S., Woodruff, M. W., Webster, J. H., and Pickren, J. W.: Arch. Surg. **90:**306-312, 1965.
†Of 179 patients, sixty had metastases on admission. The distribution of metastases is shown. Some patients had more than one organ involved.

astinum and supraclavicular areas when the lymphangiogram is normal. Of seventy-one patients with clinical Stage I seminoma, forty-nine were given irradiation of the retroperitoneal nodes plus irradiation of the mediastinum and left supraclavicular nodes. Twenty-two were given irradiation of the retroperitoneal nodes only. There was no persistent cancer in either group, and the 5-year tumor-free survival rate was the same in both groups (Ytredal and Bradfield; Doornbos and associates). There is nothing in the literature to support routine irradiation of the mediastinum and supraclavicular nodes in clinical Stage I seminoma. This decision to withhold mediastinal irradiation should be based on a normal lymphangiogram and chest film, among other considerations.

To assist in defining the volumes of interest, the pretreatment work-up should include careful abdominal and supraclavicular palpation, chest films, and an excretory urogram to rule out ureteral displacement and to define kidney position. The information gained from the lymphangiogram is so valuable in these patients that we insist it be performed in every patient who does not already have obvious abdominal metastases. The venogram may also assist in positioning ports.

DOSAGE CONSIDERATIONS FOR SEMINOMA OF THE TESTICLE. The dose required to eradicate seminoma is consistently low; therefore the field arrangement can be simple. Precautions should be taken to avoid irradiation of significant renal tissue (Chapter 13). This can be accomplished by securing an excretory urogram, which defines the size and position of the kidneys and ureters and by taking appropriate beam verification films. Parallel opposing anterior and posterior ports using landmarks shown in Fig. 16-2 are sufficient. The rapid treatment of this volume is accompanied by frequent anorexia and occasionally nausea and vomiting, so the daily dose must be kept relatively low. Four to 5 weeks are nearly always required to deliver midabdominal tissue doses of 3000 rad, which is the upper limit indicated for seminoma. In the rare event that more extensive or large abdominal metastases are present, the moving-strip technique with kidney shielding is well tolerated and effective (Chapter 19). The same moving-strip technique in combination with chemotherapy is also useful when the disease is metastatic to the lungs (Simon and associates). Boosting doses of 1000 to 1500 rad may be given through reduced ports for residual large tumor masses (Doornbos and associates).

Since many of these patients will want to have children, adequate shielding of the remaining testicle must be accomplished if possible. In the usual patient in which orchiectomy has been performed by a high ligation, the entire scrotum is encased in a "clam shell" lead shield 2 cm thick during each treatment. If the testicle was removed through a scrotal incision, then that hemiscrotum must be treated. Since the remaining testicle would be difficult to shield under these circumstances, it has been proposed that a hemiscrotectomy be performed on these patients.

In patients with Stage II seminomas the irradiation of retroperitoneal nodes should be followed by irradiation of the mediastinal and supraclavicular areas to doses of at least 2500 rad in 3 weeks. Overlap of beam edges should be avoided by calculation of gap areas. Medial aspects of both pulmonary hilar areas should be included.

NONSEMINOMATOUS CARCINOMAS OF THE TESTICLE. The management of patients with nonseminomatous carcinomas of the testicle is not as clear-cut as that outlined for seminomas. Because they respond less well to irradiation, surgery is used more often to remove retroperitoneal metastases in nodes. Because these cancers spread extranodally more frequently than seminomas, chemotherapy has assumed a major role in their management. The role of radiation therapy is therefore often debated, but the data presented by Maier and associates, Hussey and associates, and Fayos and Kim, form a solid clinical data base on which we may evaluate the contribution of external irradiation.

The dose required for the eradication of these carcinomas is greater than that required for seminoma. The scanty data available suggest that small foci are controlled in the great majority by doses of 4500 to 5000 rad given by the sandwich technique described in the following paragraph (Table 16-5). Larger masses of 4 to 6 cm are not dependably controlled by such doses, and masses 10 cm in diameter are seldom, if ever, controlled by such doses. For large masses we are limited by the tolerance of the bowel. The poor response of these tumors requires that large tumors be excised and that the maximum tolerated dose be given when known disease is left behind.

The so-called sandwich technique combines initial preoperative irradiation of ipsilateral iliac and retroperitoneal nodes (2500 to 3000 rad given in 3 to 4 weeks) with bilateral retroperitoneal dissection and finally postoperative irradiation of this nodal

Table 16-5. Dose-response data for nonseminomatous carcinoma
of the testicle in para-aortic lymph nodes*

	Subsequent recurrence in para-aortic nodes			
		Irradiation dose (rad)		
Initial status of nodes	No irradiation	2000-3000	3000-4500	4500-5500
No known cancer in nodes	3/92	0/14	0/10	0/7
Cancer initially present but all known cancer resected	5/9	1/2	0/5	1/28
Gross cancer remaining	3/4	4/4	4/4	3/7

*Modified from Hussey, D. H., Luk, K. H., and Johnson, D. E.: Radiology **123**:175-180, 1977.

Table 16-6. Three-year disease-free survival rate for patients
with nonseminomatous cancers of the testicle*

	3-year survival		
Therapy	Stage I	Stage II	Total
Orchiectomy plus radiation therapy only†	25/29 (86%)	9/11 (82%)	30/40 (85%)
Orchiectomy with "sandwich" technique‡	29/30 (97%)	17/21 (81%)	46/51 (90%)
TOTAL	54/59 (92%)	26/32 (81%)	80/91 (88%)

*Modified from Maier, J. G., and Mittemeyer, B.: Cancer **39**:981-986, 1977.
†Minimum of 4000 rad in 4 weeks given sequentially to iliac-retroperitoneal nodes and to mediastinal-supraclavicular nodes.
‡Minimum of 3000 rad in 3 weeks to iliac-retroperitoneal nodes followed by retroperitoneal lymphadenectomy and an additional 1500 rad in 8 days. The mediastinal-supraclavicular nodes are then given 4000 rad.

region (1500 to 2000 rad in 2 to 3 weeks). There may be a temptation to withhold the second irradiation of the sandwich technique if on examination of the radically resected retroperitoneal nodes, no evidence of disease is found (the preoperative irradiation alone reduces the incidence of histologically positive nodes in Stage I from 17% to 3% and in Stage II from 88.9% to 52% [Hussey and associates]). However, the usual node dissection does not remove all nodes, and the usual resected specimen is not studied by serial sections. Therefore full dose postoperative irradiation is added for all patients treated. This combined course has produced the excellent cure rates for patients with Stage I and good cure rates for patients with Stage II nonseminomatous carcinomas (Maier and Mittemeyer) (Table 16-6). It is probable that these results can be improved still further by placing the patients with several retroperitoneal nodes (more than three or four) on chemotherapy following the postoperative irradiation. Chemotherapy should be the initial treatment for patients with retroperitoneal nodes greater than 10 cm and for all patients with Stages III and IV lesions. With this latter group irradiation or surgery is used locally for persistent masses of tumor.

Chemotherapy

As was indicated earlier, a substantial proportion of patients with nonseminomatous carcinomas metastatic to retroperitoneal and supradiaphragmatic nodes will already have developed occult distant metastases, that is, at least 42% of this group will develop widespread metastases. Multidrug chemotherapy—especially combinations of vinblastine (Velban), actinomycin D, and bleomycin (VAB), with *cis*-dichlorodianmine platinum (CDDP)—produce partial shrinkage in 20% to 35% and at least transient clinical disappearance of all metastases in 30% to 70% (Cheng and associates). Relapses in the various series occur in 30% to 100%. The scarcity of nonseminomatous cancers makes accumulation of data slow, especially when the clinical stages and histologic groups are considered separately. However, it is now quite clear that metastases, if small and few, can be controlled by chemotherapy in 30% to 40% of patients for as long as 2 years and perhaps permanently. It is thus critical that patients at high risk for occult distant metastases, that is, those with more than two or three metastases to retroperitoneal or supradiaphragmatic nodes and those with elevated hormonal markers, receive chemotherapy as a routine planned part of their combined care. The optimum sequence of radiation therapy, node dissection, and chemotherapy remains unsettled. However, until any single or any two of these modalities control 100% of the metastases in the retroperitoneal nodes, the use of all three modalities seems indicated in the high-risk categories mentioned before. We recommend the "sandwich technique" reported by Maier followed by chemotherapy. In contrast to earlier reports, more recent experience verifies the patients' tolerance to this sequence. It also verifies that prior irradiation does not seriously diminish response to chemotherapy as had been suggested in the earlier clinical trials.

Carcinoma of the testicle in children

Infantile embryonal carcinoma differs significantly in histologic pattern from embryonal carcinoma of the adult. The tendency for the tumor cells to grow and form structures reminiscent of the yolk sac has resulted in the widely used synonym *yolk sac tumor*. Similar histologic features may be seen in teratocarcinomas of the adult and less often in pure embryonal carcinoma of the adult type.

Almost all tumors of the testicle that occur before puberty are embryonal adenocarcinomas and have a better prognosis than adult types. It is not possible to determine the precise role of irradiation or lymphadenectomy in the management of these rare tumors. This is particularly true of infants when cure can be expected for 80% to 90% with orchiectomy alone or supplemented by irradiation or lymphadenectomy. Staubitz and associates reported a cure of all four of their patients treated by orchiectomy and bilateral retroperitoneal lymph node dissection. Two of the four patients had positive nodes. Ise and associates gave retroperitoneal node irradiation after orchiectomy to thirty-nine children with localized disease and thirty-four (89%) survived. An average dose of 3000 rad was given. In the series reported by Tefft and associates, six children were subjected to lymphadenectomy, none had nodal metastases, and all survived. Jeffs described the Toronto Hospital for Sick Children experience where eleven of thirteen children were cured. Only two had lymphadenectomy (nodes negative), and two had retroperitoneal irradiation.

These reports suggest that orchiectomy alone, with careful follow-up and chest x-ray films every 3 months, is sufficient for children less than 2 years of age. Retroperitoneal nodes and distant metastases are more likely in older boys, and irradiation of the retroperitoneal areas should be considered in such cases. The role of lymphangiography or computed axial tomography in management decisions is yet to be defined.

Rhabdomyosarcoma, lymphoma, and leukemia all may present as painless testicular masses. Treatment of these tumors is discussed in other chapters.

Extratesticular seminoma

There is the rare circumstance of a retroperitoneal mass that on biopsy appears microscopically like seminoma of the testicle, but on physical examination the testicles are perfectly normal. There is a temptation to remove the ipsilateral testicle, and an occult primary cancer may be present. However, it is now accepted that such cancers may arise primarily from the urogenital remnants in the retroperitoneal area. We believe the clinically normal testicle should not be removed (Abell and associates).

Radiation therapy techniques for extratesticular seminomas must be tailored according to anatomic site of origin and the anticipated lymph drainage. Optimum doses are the same as for testicular seminomas.

Prognosis and results

Survival rates vary sharply with the pathologic diagnosis. Several reports indicate that the 5-year survival rate for seminoma should appraoch 90% (Table 16-7). Lymphoid stroma is found in varying amounts between the masses of seminoma cells. This is thought to be related to host reaction to the cancer. Abundant lymphoid stroma justifies an even better prognosis. Thus, of eighty patients whose seminoma showed no lymphoid stroma, 53% were living at 5 years. Of seventy patients whose seminoma showed lymphoid stroma, 80% were living at 5 years (Martin and associates).

Spermatocytic seminoma is a clinically and histologically distinctive variant of

Table 16-7. Control rates for seminoma treated by orchiectomy followed by irradiation

Author	Number of patients	Clinical stages	5-year survival (%)
Ekman and associates	47	I-III	87
Host and Stokke	56	I-III	84
Kurohara and associates	30	I	100 (3 years)
MacKay and Seders	116	I	89
Maier and associates (1968)	106	I-II	87
Castro	113	I-III	75 (3 years)
Doornbos and associates	141	I-IV	81 (3 years)
Kademian and associates	30	I-IV	93

seminoma. In contrast to classic seminoma, there is maturation of the tumor cells, and cells resembling secondary spermatids and even spermatocytes may be found. Glycogen, lymphocytic infiltration, and fibrous stroma are less conspicuous in spermatocytic seminoma, making differential diagnosis with malignant lymphoma difficult at times. Clinically, it is seen mostly in the elderly and is seldom associated with other cellular components such as terotoma or embryonal carcinoma. It has not been described in extratesticular sites (Talerman). It constitutes about 7% of all seminomas. Data relative to metastasizing capabilities and its radioresponsiveness and radiocurability are not available. With such data as are available, we believe it should be treated no differently from the classic seminoma of the same clinical stage. Cure rates are at least as high as those for classic seminoma.

It appears likely that examples of widely metastasizing spermatocytic seminoma are in reality misdiagnosed malignant lymphoma (Mostofi and Price; Rosai and associates).

Anaplastic seminoma comprises 10% to 12% of all seminomas. It responds similarly to classic seminoma and should be treated as classic seminoma. Data are scanty but apparently patients with anaplastic seminoma are diagnosed with a slightly higher clinical stage than the patients with classic seminoma. This probably accounts for the fact that the overall cure rate for anaplastic seminoma averaged 77%, whereas that for classic seminoma averaged 93% (Maier and associates, 1968).

It should be emphasized that, even when seminoma recurs in a previously irradiated zone or when, after treatment, it metastasizes to extra-abdominal tissues, an aggressive treatment policy should be followed. Cures are possible in situations that would be utterly hopeless with most other cell types. There is a danger that nonradiologic physicians who do not appreciate these facts lose the opportunity to cure. About 50% of the patients with recurrent seminoma will be living and well at 5 years if an aggressive retreatment policy is followed (Friedman and Purkayashtha).

The causes of failure to cure patients with seminoma of the testicle are highly

Table 16-8. Tumor-free survival rates at 3 years (all stages)*

Cell type	Number of patients treated	Percent of total number in subgroup	Number and percent living NED at 3 years
Seminoma, pure	113	39	85 (75%)
Embryonal carcinoma, pure or with seminoma	78	26	28 (36%)
Teratoma, pure or with seminoma	24	8	16 (66%)
Teratoma with embryonal carcinoma, or choriocarcinoma, or seminoma	56	18	28 (50%)
Choriocarcinoma, pure or with seminoma or embryonal carcinoma or both	13	5	1

*Modified from Castro, J. R.: In Johnson, D. E., editor: Testicular tumors, Flushing, N.Y., 1972, Medical Examination Publishing Co., Inc.

Table 16-9. Ten-year survival probability (Berkson and Gage method)*

Cell types	Stage I				Stage II		Stages III and IV or Stage III (Maier)		Totals	
	Nodes clinically or microscopically negative		Nodes clinically negative but microscopically positive							
	Number of patients	Survival	Number of patients	Survival	Number of patients	Survival	Number of patients	Survival	Number of patients	Survival
Seminoma (pure)	262	98%	22	76%	34	75%	18	7%	336	90%
Embryonal carcinoma alone or with seminoma	51	77%	81	36%	20	15%	52	6%	204	36.5%
Teratocarcinoma pure or with seminoma	106	76.5%	81	51%	29	63%	45	4.5%	261	49.5%
Teratocarcinoma with embryonal or choriocarcinoma or both with or without seminoma	5	4 of 5	3	1 of 3	0		14	0	22	22%
Choriocarcinoma pure or with seminoma or embryonal carcinoma or both	3	3 of 3	2	0	0		11	0	16	18%

*Modified from Maier, J. G., and Van Buskirk, K. V.: J.A.M.A. **213**:44-45, 1970.

Table 16-10. Three-year disease-free survival rates for patients with various histologic types of nonseminomatous carcinomas of the testicle*

Histologic type	Number of patients treated	3-year NED rate (all stages)
Embryonal carcinoma, pure or with seminoma (Group II)	120	37/120 (39%)
Teratoma, pure or with seminoma (Group III)	45	28/45 (62%)
Teratoma with embryonal carcinoma and/or embryonal carcinoma (Group IV)	91	50/91 (55%)
Choriocarcinoma, pure or with seminoma and/or embryonal carcinoma (Group V)	23	6/23 (26%)
TOTAL	279	131/279 (47%)

* Modified from Hussey, D. H., Luk, K. H., and Johnson, D. E.: Radiology **123:**175-180, 1977.

varied (Table 16-2). It is clear from this type of analysis that careful attention to technique will reduce the failure rate.

Even before the advent of chemotherapy, of twenty patients with embryonal carcinoma metastatic to resected retroperitoneal nodes, eleven were alive at 5 years (Patton and Mallis). More recent results are shown in Table 16-10. Most of these data were accumulated prior to current chemotherapy, and these results should be compared with 5-year disease-free survival rates based on current treatment as these rates become available.

The therapy of malignant lesions in the undescended testicle, stage for stage, is no different from that previously described. Excisions of the primary lesion should be followed by irradiation of the para-aortic nodes as indicated previously. Most such lesions will be seminomas, but some will be teratocarcinomas. Control rates are the same as those for cancers developing in the scrotum.

Primary malignant lymphomas of the testicle are rare and should probably be treated as lymphomas elsewhere by irradiation of the primary lesion using generous fields. However, orchiectomy is usually done for diagnostic purposes. Subsequent involvement of the remaining testicle is common—that is, nine of twenty-five cases reported by Fergusson. A small proportion of these patients will live 5 years if the disease is clinically and radiographically limited to the testicle (Eckert and Smith). The value of prophylactic abdominal irradiation in malignant lymphomas remains unknown (Varney). However, we believe it is appropriate to treat the iliac and retroperitoneal nodes to a dose of 4000 rad in 4 weeks even in the absence of a positive lymphangiogram.

Summary

Carcinomas of the testicle present a wide variety of radiosensitivities with closely correlated radiocurabilities. Irradiation contributes to the care of these patients through its ability to eradicate the lymph node metastases in many seminomas, some embryonal carcinomas, and an occasional teratocarcinoma. When the radiosensitivity is poor or wide dissemination of the metastases is present, irradiation in combination with retroperitoneal node dissection and chemotherapy are available for producing a substantial proportion of long-term cancer-free survivors.

REFERENCES

Abell, N. R., Fayos, J. V., and Lampe, I.: Retroperitoneal germinomas (seminomas) without evidence of testicular involvement, Cancer 18:273-290, 1965.

Bane, H. N., Tyree, E. B., Thompson, P. A., Nickson, J. J., and Shapiro, G.: Decrease in mouse testes weight after exposure to 180-kv, 250-kv, and 22.5 Mev x-rays, Radiat. Res. 3:213, 1955.

Binhammer, R. T.: Effect of increased endogenous gonadotropin on the testes of irradaited immature and mature rats, Radiat. Res. 30:676-686, 1967.

Bloom, W., and Bloom, M. A.: Histological changes after irradiation. In Hollaender, A., editor: Radiation biology, New York, 1954, McGraw-Hill Book Co.

Boden, G., and Gibb, R.: Radiotherapy and testicular neoplasms, Lancet 2:1195-1197, 1951.

Casarett, G. W., and Hursh, J. B.: Effects of daily low doses of x-rays on spermatogenesis in dogs, vol. II, Proceedings of the International Conference on the Peaceful Uses of Atomic Energy, New York, 1956, United Nations.

Casarett, G. W., and Eddy, H. A.: Effect of x-irradiation on spermatogenesis in dogs, Report U. R. 668, Atomic Energy Commission, 1965.

Castro, J. R.: Lymphadenectomy and radiation therapy in malignant tumors of the testicle other than pure seminoma, Cancer 1:87-91, 1969.

Castro, J. R., and Gonzalez, M.: Results in treatment of pure seminoma of the testis, Am. J. Roentgenol. 111:355-359, 1971.

Cheng, E., Cvitkovic, E., Wittes, R. E., and Golley, R. B.: Germ cell tumors. II. Cancer 42:2162-2168, 1978.

Coliez, R., and Bourdon, R.: Action biologique des rayons-x des rayonnements emis par les corps radioactifs. In Delherm, L.: Electro-radiotherapie, Paris, 1951, Masson et Cie.

Dixon, F. J., and Moore, R. A.: Tumors of the male sex organs, Section VIII, Fascicles 31b and 32, 1952, Armed Forces Institute of Pathology.

Doornbos, J. F., Hussey, D. H., and Johnson, D. E.: Radiotherapy for pure seminoma of the testis, Radiology 116:401-404, 1975.

Eckert, H., and Smith, J. P.: Malignant lymphoma of the testis, Br. Med. J. 2:891-894, 1963.

Ekman, H., Giertz, G., Johnson, G., and Notter, G.: Tumors of the testicle: XIII, Congres de la Societe Internationale d'Urologie 1:26-28, 1964.

Fayos, J. V., and Kim, Y. H.: Treatment of testicular tumors, Radiology 128:471-475, 1978.

Fergusson, J. D.: Tumours of the testes, Br. J. Urol. 34:407-421, 1962.

Ferroux, R., Regaud, C., and Samssonow, N.: Effects des rayons de roentgen administres sans fractionnement de la dose sur les testicules du rat au point de vue de la sterilisation de l'epithelium seminal, Compt. rend Soc. de biol. 128:170-173, 1938.

Fogg, L. C., and Cowing, R. F.: The changes in cell morphology and histochemistry of the testis following irradiation and their relation to other induced testicular changes, Cancer Res. 11:23-28, 1951.

Friedman, N. B., and Moore, R. A.: Tumors of the testis: a report on 922 cases, Millit. Surgeon 99:573-593, 1946.

Friedman, M., and Purkayashtha, M. C.: The management of late metastasis, recurrence, or a second primary tumor, Am. J. Roentgenol. 83:25-42, 1960.

Gowen, J. W., and Stadler, J.: Acute irradiation effects on reproductivity of different strains of mice. In Carlson, W. D., and Gassner, F. X., editors: Effects of ionizing radiation on the reproductive system, New York, 1964, The Macmillan Co.

Hahn, E. W., Feingold, S. M., and Nisce, L.: Aspermia and recovery of spermatogenesis in cancer patients following incidental gonadal irradiation during treatment, Radiology 119:223-225, 1976.

Hussey, D. H., Luk, K. H., and Johnson, D. E.: The role of radiation therapy in the treatment of germinal cell tumors of the testis other than pure seminoma, Radiology 123:175-180, 1977.

Ise, T., Ohtsuki, H., Matsumoto, K., and Sano, R.: Management of malignant testicular tumors in children, Cancer 37:1539-1545, 1976.

Jeffs, R. D.: Management of embryonal adenocarcinomas of the testis in childhood: an analysis of 164 cases. In Godden, J. O., editor: Cancer in childhood, New York, 1973, Plenum Publishing Corp.

Kademian, M. T., Bosch, A., and Caldwell, W. L.: Seminoma: results of treatment with megavoltage irradiation, Int. J. Radiat. Oncol. Biol. Phys. 1:1075-1079, 1976.

Kohn, H. I., and Kallman, R. F.: Testes weight loss as a quantitative measure of x-ray injury in the mouse, hamster, and rat, Br. J. Radiol. 27:586-591, 1954.

Kohn, H. I.: On the direct and indirect effects of x-rays on the testis of the rat, Radiat. Res. 3:153-156, 1955.

Kohn, H. I., and Kallman, R. F.: The effect of fractionated x-ray dosage upon the mouse testis, J. Natl. Cancer Inst. 15:891-899, 1955.

Krantz, S., Ward, J. A., Mendeloff, J., and Haltiwanger, E.: Germinal cell tumors of the testis, Am. J. Roentgenol. 93:138-144, 1965.

Kurohara, S. S., George, F. W., Dykhuisen, R. F., and Leary, K. L.: Testicular tumors: analysis of 196 cases treated at the U.S. Naval Hospital in San Diego, Cancer 20:1089-1098, 1967.

Lewis, L. C.: Testis tumors: report on 250 cases, J. Urol. 59:763-772, 1948.

Lushbaugh, C. C., and Ricks, R. C.: Some cytokinetic and histopathologic considerations of irradiated male and female gonadal tissues. In Vaeth, J. M., editor: Radiation effect and tolerance, normal tissue, Baltimore, 1972, University Park Press.

MacKay, E. N., and Seders, A. H.: A statistical review of malignant testicular tumours based on the experience of the Ontario Cancer Foundation Clinics, 1938-1961, Can. Med. Assoc. J. 94:889-899, 1966.

MacLeod, J., Hotchkiss, R. S., and Sitterson, B. W.: Recovery of male fertility after sterilization by nuclear radiation, J.A.M.A. 187:637-641, 1964.

Maier, J. G., Sulak, M. H., and Mittemeyer, B. T.: Seminoma of the testis: analysis of treatment success and failure, Am. J. Roentgenol. 102:596-602, 1968.

Maier, J. B., Van Buskirk, K. E., Sulak, M. H., Perry, R. H., and Schamber, D. T.: An evaluation of lymphadenectomy in the treatment of malignant testicular germ cell neoplasms, J. Urol. 101:356-359, 1969.

Maier, J. G., and Van Buskirk, K. E.: Treatment of testicular germ cell malignancies, J.A.M.A. 213:97-98, 1970.

Maier, J. G., and Mittemeyer, B.: Carcinoma of the testis, Cancer 39:981-986, 1977.

Mandl, A. M.: The radiosensitivity of germ cells, Biol. Rev. 39:288-371, 1964.

Martin, L. S., Woodruff, M. W., Webster, J. H., and Pickren, J. W.: Testicular seminoma, Arch. Surg. 90:306-312, 1965.

Merren, D. D., Vest, S. A., and Lapton, C. H.: Treatment of malignant tumors of the testis, J. Urol. 65:128-135, 1951.

Momigliano, E., and Essenberg, J. M.: Regenerative processes induced by gonadotropic hormones in irradiated testes of the albino rat, Radiology 42:273-282, 1944.

Mostofi, F. W., and Price, E. B.: Tumors of the male genital system. In Armed Forces Institute of Pathology: Atlas of tumor pathology, 1973, Second series, No. 8.

Oakberg, E. F.: Sensitivity and time of degeneration of spermatogenic cells irradiated in various stages of maturation in the mouth, Radiat. Res. 2:369-391, 1955.

Parker, R. G., and Holyoke, J. B.: Tumors of the testis, Am. J. Roentgenol. 83:43-65, 1960.

Patton, J. F., and Mallis, N.: Tumors of testicle, J. Urol. 81:457-461, 1959.

Regaud, C.: Influence de la duree d'irradiation sur les effets determines dans le testicule par le radium, Compt. rend Soc. de biol. 86:787-790, 1922.

Rosai, J., Silber, I., and Khodadouse, K.: Spermatocytic seminoma I: clinicopathologic study of six cases and review of the literature, Cancer 1:92-102, 1969.

Rowley, M. J., Leach, D. R., Warner, G. A., and Heller, C. G.: Effect of graded doses of ionizing radiation on the human testis, Radiat. Res. 59:665-678, 1974.

Russell, W. L.: Genetic effects of radiation in mammals. In Hollaender, A., editor: Radiation biology, New York, 1954, McGraw-Hill Book Co.

Russell, W. L.: Effect of radiation dose rate on mutation in mice, J. Cell Comp. Physiol. (suppl. 1) 58:183-187, 1961.

Schwartz, J. W., and Mallis, N.: Teratoma testis: report of 100 consecutive cases, J. Urol. 72:404-410, 1954.

Simon, N., Winsberg, F., Rotman, M., and Silverstone, S. M.: Radiotherapy with moving strip technique for testicular tumors, metastatic to the lungs, J.A.M.A. 197:759-761, 1966.

Smithers, D. W., and Wallace, E. N.: Radiotherapy in the treatment of patients with seminomas and teratomas of the testicle, Br. J. Urol. 34:422-435, 1962.

Speiser, B., Rubin, P., and Casarett, G.: Aspermia following lower truncal irradiation in Hodgkin's disease, Cancer 32:692-698, 1973.

Staubitz, W. J., Magoss, I. V., Oberkircher, O. J., Lent, M. H., Mitchell, F. D., and Murphy, W. T.: Management of testicular tumors, J.A.M.A. 166:751-758, 1958.

Staubitz, W. J., Jewett, T. C., Magoss, I. V., Schenk, W. G., and Phalakornhule, S.: Management of testicular tumors in children, J. Urol. 94:683-686, 1965.

Staubitz, W. J.: The place of nodal dissection, J.A.M.A. 213:99-100, 1970.

Talerman, A.: Spermatocytic seminoma, J. Urol. 112:212, 1974.

Tefft, M., Vawter, G. F., and Mitus, A.: Radiotherapeutic management of testicular neoplasms in children, Radiology 88:457-465, 1967.

van der Werf-Messing, B.: Radiotherapeutic treatment of testicular tumors, Int. J. Radiat. Oncol. Biol. Phys. 1:235-248, 1976.

Varney, D. C.: Lymphosarcoma of the testis, J. Urol. 73:1081-1088, 1955.

Wallace, S., and Jing, B.-S.: Lymphangiography: diagnosis of nodal metastases from testicular malignancies, J.A.M.A. 213:94-96, 1970.

Whittle, J. M.: Tumors of the testicle, Br. J. Radiol. 30:7-13, 1957.

Ytredal, D. O., and Bradfield, J. S.: Seminoma of the testicle: prophylactic mediastinal irradiation versus periaortic and pelvic irradiation alone, Cancer 3:628-633, 1972.

Zuckerman, S.: The sensitivity of the gonads to radiation, Clin. Radiol. 26:1-15, 1965.

17

The cervix

CARCINOMA OF THE CERVIX

Three major biologic factors are critical in planning irradiation for carcinoma of the cervix: the site of origin and routes of spread, the radiation tolerance of neighboring organs, and the radiosensitivity of the primary lesion and its extensions. These factors vary from patient to patient, and they can be determined in a given patient with only limited precision. A realization of this uncertainty is likewise important in planning the irradiation of the individual patient. These biologic factors must be appreciated before the physical problems involved in external and internal irradiation are discussed.

Site of origin and routes of spread

The great majority of carcinomas of the cervix are of squamous cell origin. Most of these are the poorly differentiated nonkeratinizing large cell type. Well-differentiated, highly keratinizing tumors are less frequent. Tumors made up of small cells growing in sheets are generally regarded as a small-celled variant of squamous cell carcinoma, but some of these may be of neuroendocrine origin as are oat cell carcinomas of the lung (Tateishi and associates).

Primary adenocarcinoma of the cervix comprises less than 5% of all cervical cancers. The majority are made of mucin-producing columnar cells resembling endocervical lining, similar to those most common in the salivary gland. Tumors with scant mucin production are difficult to differentiate from endometrial cancers. A form of adenosquamous carcinoma is occasionally encountered in the cervix. A rare variant of adenocarcinoma of the cervix is the so-called adenoid cystic carcinoma (Gordon and associates).

Squamous cell carcinoma of the cervix usually originates at the junction of the columnar and squamous epithelia in the endocervical canal or at the external os, but it may not be visible until spread occurs through the external os and over the posterior lip. The extension of the primary tumor is rarely symmetric and often involves the parametrium before presenting at the cervical os (Gusberg and associates). The growth may infiltrate early and appear on initial examination as a hard plaque or sleeve, or the mucosa may ulcerate and a necrotic defect may form in the cervix and the vaginal vault. The tumor may proliferate in an exophytic fashion from the surface of the cervix. The resulting papillary columns of tumor may grow several times larger

440

than the cervix itself and may even present at the vaginal orifice. Necrosis, with infection and bleeding, is invariable with the exophytic type. In other patients the cancer may be more infiltrative, producing a stony hard cervix with relatively less ulceration. Extensive growth in the endocervix may enlarge the cervix several times its normal diameter, creating the so-called barrel-shaped cervix. As will be noted later, the administration of radiations must be tailored to fit these clinical patterns of growth.

Although the possible directions of spread are limited, no reliable sequence is followed in the progression of this lesion. The cancer usually extends into the lateral fornices, somewhat less frequently into the anterior fornix, and only occasionally into the posterior fornix. Later, infiltration of the anterior and lateral vaginal walls is to be expected. Simultaneous extension upward in the cervical canal and into the lower uterine segment may occur. Such extension is difficult to ascertain clinically, and its presence or absence is not a criterion for staging. However, an analysis of 302 patients with cancer of the cervix revealed that those having extension of the cancer into the endometrium had a worsening of the prognosis (Table 17-1). One must be aware of the possibility of myometrial destruction produced by this ascending infiltration of tumor. Even the most cautious radium insertion attempted in the presence of myometrial infiltration may end in perforation of the uterus and perhaps in peritonitis.

The pathways remaining for direct extension are anteriorly into the bladder, posteriorly into the rectum, or laterally into the parametrium. Extension into the bladder or rectum occurs late and is infrequent. Parametrial extension occurs early and frequently and is of major importance both from a prognostic and from a therapeutic viewpoint. A discussion of the anatomy of the paracervical tissue is therefore important.

PARACERVICAL TISSUES. The uterus is suspended in a midpelvic position by anterior, posterior, and posterolateral ligaments. The ligaments and their associated connective tissues are normally elastic, allowing relatively free movement of the uterus. Chronic inflammatory processes as well as infiltration by cancer often limit uterine mobility. The vesicouterine tissues pass from the lateral aspects of the vagina and uterus to the lateral aspects of the bladder and then to the pubis. The uterosacral ligaments pass posteriorly, lateral to the rectum, to the sacrum. The cardinal

Table 17-1. Prognostic significance of endometrial extension from primary carcinoma of the cervix*

Stage	Patients tumor free at 3 years	
	D and C initially positive	D and C initially negative
I	33/45 (73%)	89/110 (81%)
II	28/47 (59.5%)	48/65 (73.8%)

*From Perez, C. A., Zivnuska, F., Askin, F., Kumar, B., Camel, H. M., and Powers, W. E.: Cancer **35:**1493-1504, 1975.

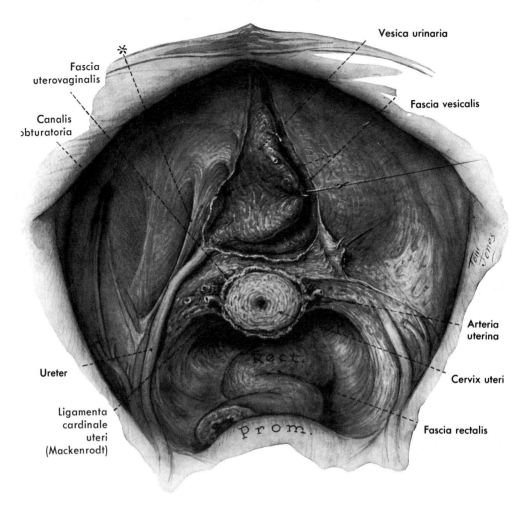

Fig. 17-1. View from above of pelvic ligaments that form pathways of spread of carcinoma of the cervix. Note the proximity of the ureter embedded in the parametrium. (From Anson, B. J.: An atlas of human anatomy, Philadelphia, 1950, W. B. Saunders Co.)

ligaments sweep inferomedially, as well as anteriorly, from the pelvic wall to the lateral aspects of the cervix. These ligaments represent the pathways of major uterine and vaginal arteries, veins, and lymphatics. Similarly, these ligaments form the usual pathways of tumor infiltration and metastases from the paracervical tissues to lymph nodes and the circulatory system (Figs. 17-1 and 17-2). In addition to the structures in the parametrium mentioned previously, the ureters pass anteroinferiorly and medially through the parametrium to the bladder. As they course through the parametrium, the ureters are but 1.5 cm lateral to the cervix, and in this position they are highly vulnerable to compression by infiltrating tumor. Rarely, however, does actual ureteral infiltration occur. Although tumor infiltration of the uterosacral ligaments may occur, this is apparently less frequent and usually considered a later manifestation of the disease.

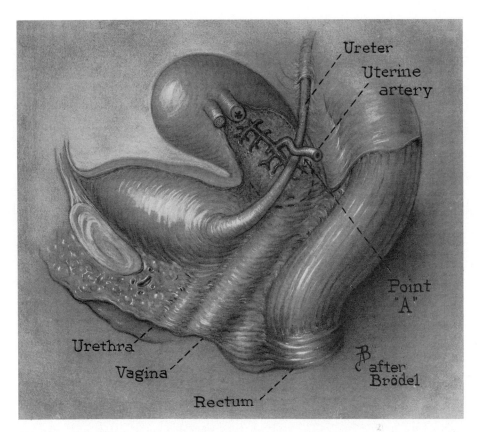

Fig. 17-2. Lateral view of pelvic viscera. Note point "A" and the relations of the peritoneum to cervix and fornices. Also note proximity of cervix to bladder and rectum.

Direct extension into the bladder and rectum occurs only after the adjacent fornices and vaginal walls have been infiltrated. Since the anterior fornix is shallow and the vesicovaginal septum is thin, bladder infiltration occurs more frequently than rectal infiltration. In either case, infiltration is indicative of a particularly aggressive tumor and a poor prognosis. The initial phase of bladder invasion produces obstruction of perivesical lymphatics. Like the peau d'orange effect seen with extensive involvement of cutaneous lymphatics in cancer of the breast, the bladder mucosa becomes edematous, manifested as bullous edema. Bullous edema, however, may have additional etiologies, so it alone cannot be taken as unquestioned evidence of bladder wall invasion. Positive biopsy is essential before one can make a certain diagnosis of bladder invasion. Invasion of the anterior rectal wall is easier to diagnose. Simple digital examination, with one finger in the vagina and one finger in the rectum, is generally sufficient to define thickening of the septum and fixation of rectal mucosa.

LYMPHATIC SPREAD. The lymph drainage of the cervix is formed as the subendothelial lymphatic plexus unites with stromal lymphatics and the resulting vessels

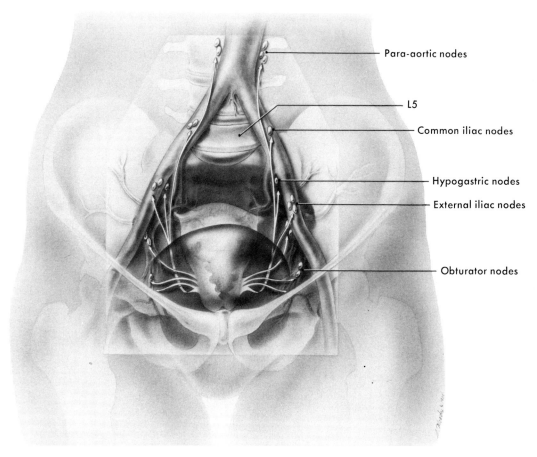

Para-aortic nodes

L5

Common iliac nodes

Hypogastric nodes

External iliac nodes

Obturator nodes

Fig. 17-3. Lymph node drainage of cervix and the usual relationship of the nodes to bony pelvis. Note extension of the field superiorly used in selected patients to encompass nodes as high as the aortic bifurcation.

join subserosal channels to form three major collecting trunks at the lateral aspects of the cervix (Fig. 17-3).

The more superior channels follow the path of the uterine artery laterally through the broad ligament to nodes near the junction of the hypogastric and external iliac arteries. The middle lymphatics drain into the obturator nodes. The channels originating from the most inferior aspect of the cervix drain toward the posterior pelvic wall to the hypogastric, common iliac, and para-aortic nodes. Lymph channels from the posterior aspect of the cervix drain through the uterosacral ligament to hypogastric, common iliac, superior rectal, and para-aortic nodes (Plentl and Friedman). As cancer infiltrates beyond the cervix into the uterine corpus or inferiorly into the vagina or vulva, the lymphatic spread expands to include the patterns of drainage recognized for those particular anatomic sites.

There are a few lymph nodes occasionally found in the tissues immediately

Table 17-2. Incidence of biopsy-proven metastases in para-aortic lymph nodes according to initial clinical stage*

Stage	Buchsbaum	Averette	Nelson	Total
I	0/23	3/40	—	3/63 (4.7%)
IIa	—	2/9	—	2/9
IIb	—	2/9	5/31	7/40 (17%)
III	7/20	2/20	13/28	22/68 (32%)
IV	1/2	1/2	—	2/4

*Modified from Chism, S. E., Park, R. C., and Keys, H. M.: Cancer **35:**1505-1509, 1975.

Table 17-3. Distribution of 2090 positive pelvic lymph nodes from 744 patients with carcinoma of the cervix (all stages included)*

Node group	Number	Percent of total
Obturator	398	19
Hypogastric	363	17.4
External iliac	479	22.9
Common iliac	266	12.7
Parametrial	231	11.1
Paracervical	213	10.2
Paravaginal	9	0.4
Sacral	28	1.3

*Modified from Plentl, A. A., and Friedman, E. A.: Lymphatic system of the female genitalia, Philadelphia, 1971, W. B. Saunders Co.

surrounding the cervix, but these are variable and, except for ureteral lymph nodes, have not been given much consideration in the treatment of cancer of the cervix.

The anatomic location and distribution of commonly involved pelvic lymph nodes are illustrated in Fig. 17-3. The overall incidence of involvement of the various pelvic nodal groups is given in Table 17-3. These figures should not be taken too seriously, since the number of positive nodes found in an operative specimen depends on the type of surgery and the persistence of the pathologist in dissecting the surgical specimen. However, the obturator, hypogastric, and external iliac nodes are more frequently involved, whereas the common iliac and parametrial nodes are less frequently involved. As the disease progresses, these nodal groups are not involved in a predictable stepwise fashion such as to permit systematic inclusion or exclusion of pelvic nodal groups according to clinical stage. The incidence of metastases to pelvic lymph nodes according to clinical stage is summarized in Table 17-4. The wide variation between the reporting institutions is striking. By averaging a large number of reports, positive pelvic lymph nodes were found in 16.5% of patients with Stage I carcinoma, in 31.9% of those with Stage II carcinoma, and in 46.7% of those with Stage III carcinoma (Morton and associates).

Data relative to the incidence of metastases to para-aortic lymph nodes stage by stage are scanty and, as yet, entirely inadequate. However, one set of data is given in Table 17-2. The incidence shown for Stage III is almost certain to be higher than shown. Probably a third to half the patients with Stage III lesions have metastases to para-aortic nodes.

LYMPHANGIOGRAPHY IN CARCINOMA OF THE CERVIX. The presence or absence of metastases in pelvic and para-aortic lymph nodes cannot be determined by the usual clinical examination. Without this information, radiotherapy planning must be based on the probability of the presence or absence of disease (Table 17-4). Lymphangiography provides the radiation oncologist with a means for defining lymph node involvement in some patients and, at least when the study is positive, a possibility of tailoring the beam sizes and positions to cover those presumed metastases. Thus, of forty-one positive lymphograms obtained in patients with carcinoma of the cervix, forty were verified as being positive on biopsy at laparotomy (Piver and associates). By contrast, of sixty-one negative lymphograms, twelve were shown on laparotomy to have metastases in lymph nodes. Of a total of fifty-three patients proved to have metastases to lymph nodes, 77.7% were diagnosed by the lymphogram. However, it is unusual that a lymphangiogram will yield the "whole truth and nothing but the truth" as far as nodal involvement is concerned. A positive lymphangiogram may yield positive nodes on laparotomy, but it is rare that the full extent of nodal involvement is thus defined. Those patients with positive lymphangiograms whose positive nodes are left unirradiated will almost invariably die of cancer (Tawil and Belanger). Radiation therapy is foremost among the few options left for such patients.

Table 17-4. Proportion of pelvic lymph nodes involved in various stages

Author	Stage I	Stage II	Stage III	Number of patients
Lange (1960)	28.8	43.8		174
Mitani and associates (1962)	30.2	33.6		159
Morton and associates (1964)	23.7			38
Parsons and associates (1960)	13.4	22.0		87
Riva and associates (1961)	19.0	35.0	64.3	74
Welch and associates (1961)	11.7	24.2	37.1	486
Yagi (1962)	12.0	23.7	50.0	116

Table 17-5. Correlation of lymphangiographic and biopsy findings in the various node groups*

Lymph node group	Rad. positive Hist. positive	Rad. negative Hist. negative	Rad. negative Hist. positive
Para-aortic	14	69	6
Common iliac	10	41	0
External iliac	20	45	7
Internal iliac	1	37	0
Obturator	0	36	3
Inguinal	2	0	0
TOTAL	47	228	16

*From Piver, M. S., Wallace, S., and Castro, J. R.: Am. J. Roentgenol. **111**:278-283, 1971.

Whether the lymphangiogram is positive or negative for metastases, the still further refinement of staging by adding routine laparotomy to the diagnostic work-up has not contributed information leading to increased patient survival rates (Keys and Park). The distribution of confirmed positive nodes in a group of patients representing all clinical stages as determined by lymphangiography is shown in Table 17-5.

CLINICAL STAGING. The curability and treatment of carcinoma of the cervix is strongly influenced by the type of extension. The clinical classification given is that of the American Joint Committee for Cancer Staging and End Result Reporting (1978).

STAGING CLASSIFICATION*

Stage 0   Carcinoma in situ, intraepithelial carcinoma
Stage I   The carcinoma is strictly confined to the cervix (extension to the corpus should be disregarded)
      Stage Ia   Microinvasive carcinoma (early stromal invasion)
      Stage Ib   All other cases of stage I; occult cancer should be marked "occ"
Stage II   The carcinoma extends beyond the cervix but has not extended to the pelvic wall. The carcinoma involves the vagina, but not as far as the lower third.
      Stage IIa   No obvious parametrial involvement
      Stage IIb   Obvious parametrial involvement
Stage III   The carcinoma has extended to the pelvic wall. On rectal examination, there is no cancer free space between the tumor and the pelvic wall. The tumor involves the lower third of the vagina. All cases with a hydronephrosis or nonfunctioning kidney are included, unless they are known to be due to other cause
      Stage IIIa   No extension to the pelvic wall
      Stage IIIb   Extension to the pelvic wall and/or hydronephrosis or nonfunctioning kidney
Stage IV   The carcinoma has extended beyond the true pelvis or has clinically involved the mucosa of the bladder or rectum. A bullous edema as such does not permit a case to be allotted to stage IV
      Stage IVa   Spread of the growth to adjacent organs
      Stage IVb   Spread to distant organs

Clinical staging must be concluded before treatment is initiated, and it must not be modified regardless of subsequent findings. For the sake of standardizing clinical staging, certain commonly available studies are used, including palpation, inspection, endocervical curettage, intravenous urography, and x-ray examinations of the lungs and bones. Highly useful but less commonly performed lymphograms, venograms, and laparotomies cannot be used for clinical staging purposes.

The pelvic examination, preferably under an anesthetic, is by far the most important single examination. The supplementary studies mentioned before are important but will infrequently yield abnormal findings that justify modification of the impressions acquired from the pelvic examination. This point was strikingly illustrated by Griffin and associates and is obvious in their tables (Tables 17-6 and 17-7). The low yield of these supplementary procedures must not be taken to mean

---

*International Federation of Gynecology and Obstetrics nomenclature. From the American Joint Committee for Cancer Staging and End Results Reporting: Manual for staging of cancer, Chicago, 1978, Whiting Press.

Table 17-6. Tumor-related abnormalities found during routine work-up*

Clinical stage	Number of patients	Positive findings by procedure				
		Cystoscopy	Proctoscopy	Barium enema	Intravenous pyelogram	Chest x-ray film
I	111	0	0	0	0	0
IIa	123	0	0	0	0	0
IIb	44	0	0	0	2	1
IIIa	8	0	0	0	2	0
IIIb	37	2	5	3	24	1
IV	4	2	4	4	3	0
TOTAL	227	4	9	7	31	2

*Modified from Griffin, T. W., Parker, R. G., and Taylor, W. J.: Am. J. Roentgenol. Radium Ther. Nucl. Med. **127:**825-827, 1976.

Table 17-7. Supplementary diagnostic procedures resulting in change of clinical stage*

Initial clinical stage	Positive diagnostic procedure justifying upstaging
IIb	Chest x-ray film
IIIb	Cystoscopy
IIIb	Proctoscopy
IIIb	Proctoscopy, barium enema
IIIb	Proctoscopy, barium enema
IIIb	Proctoscopy, cystoscopy
IIIb	Proctoscopy, cystoscopy, barium enema, chest x-ray film

*Modified from Griffin, T. W., Parker, R. G., and Taylor, W. J.: Am. J. Roentgenol. Radium Ther. Nucl. Med. **127:**825-827, 1976.

that they need not be performed. Even when they are negative, they provide a valuable baseline study to assist in future patient evaluation.

At present there is no obvious consensus as to the value of the lymphangiogram as a *routine* staging procedure for patients with Stages IIb and III. This is because the rate of false "negatives" is substantial, and even when positive, the full extent of nodal involvement is rarely defined. For these reasons the decision to irradiate or not to irradiate retroperitoneal nodes is often based on the probability of nodal involvement as illustrated in Table 17-4.

Like all clinical staging procedures, the staging of carcinoma of the cervix has its limitations. In Stage I no extension beyond the cervix can be palpated; yet 16.5% of patients with Stage I disease have pelvic lymph node metastases. This will vary within Stage I. Few patients with lesions less than 1 cm in diameter will have developed lymph node metastases, a fact taken into consideration when intracavitary radium is used as the sole treatment. Kottmeier (1955) pointed out that 60% of surgically treated patients with Stage I disease may show parametrial extension on microscopic examination of the surgical specimen. Gusberg and associates reported a much

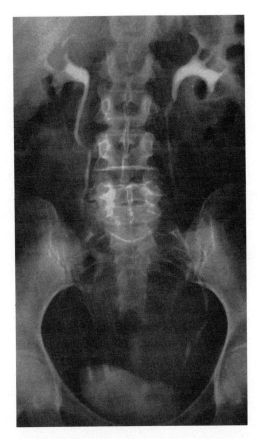

Fig. 17-4. Pretreatment excretory urogram of patient with Stage II carcinoma of the cervix.

lower but still significant proportion (14.6%). Similarly, surgical specimens from patients with Stage II disease may show regional lymph node involvement that cannot be detected clinically (31.9%). In contrast, parametrial induration that is generally assumed to be due to cancer may not be caused by cancer. Of fifty-one patients with induration of the parametrium, only twelve were shown at surgery to contain cancer (Dearing). Although a much higher percentage of involvement is usually reported, it is well to remember that not every parametrial induration is due to cancer.

These limitations of clinical staging must be weighed in planning irradiation. As mentioned previously, the ureters are in a vulnerable location while coursing through the parametrium. It would appear on inspection of the relationship of the cervix to the ureter that little lateral spread of carcinoma is necessary to displace or compress the ureter. It is a surprising fact that ureteral obstruction does not occur more often in patients with early disease and that it does not occur in all patients with advanced disease. It has been recognized that such abnormalities warrant a poor prognosis even though the disease may not appear advanced otherwise. When control of the primary cancer is not obtained, the majority of patients will die of uremia secondary to carcinoma obstructing the ureters.

The prognosis implied by ureteral abnormalities depends not only on the extent of spread otherwise—that is, the clinical stage—but also on the treatment given. In patients with Stage III and Stage IV disease, the prognosis is much worse if ureteral obstruction is present. The degree of ureteral obstruction, whether mild or severe, is not so important as the presence or absence of obstruction (Iliya and associates).

Treatment to the parametrium must be vigorous; otherwise control of spread to these tissues cannot be expected. Not infrequently, patients with initially abnormal pyelograms will show normal ureters by the end of irradiation (Figs. 17-4 and 17-5). Kottmeier (1964) performed 1502 preirradiation pyelograms on 3484 patients

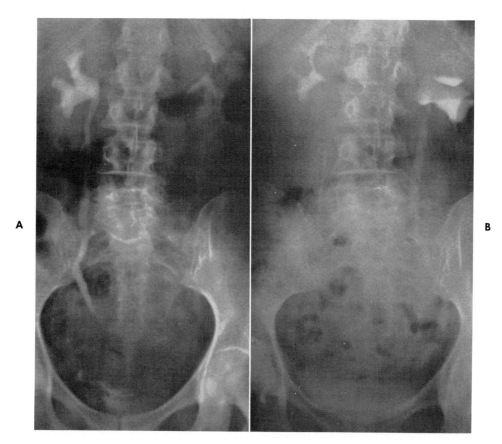

Fig. 17-5. A, Same patient as in Fig. 17-4. Obstruction of right ureter 10 months after 4600 mg-hr of radium (distribution unknown) and a calculated 2000 rad in 4 weeks to the midpelvis delivered by external pelvic split-field technique. At the time this obstruction was diagnosed, an additional 2000 rad was delivered to site of obstruction by external means. **B,** Same patient 2 years after initial irradiation. Right ureteral obstruction was relieved by irradiation. Left ureter has since become obstructed.

evaluated. Of the 1502 patients, 268 pyelograms were diagnosed as showing hydro-nephrosis or nonfunction. A 5-year survival of 32.8% was obtained in patients with abnormal pyelograms, whereas 55.6% survival was obtained in those with normal pyelograms. Of fifty-seven patients with preirradiation hydronephrosis who survived at least 5 years after treatment and were then reevaluated, forty-one were found to have been restored to normal and sixteen remained asymptomatic but hydronephrot-ic (Kottmeier, 1964). Out of 1749 patients, Slater and Fletcher diagnosed ureteral obstruction in 194 prior to irradiation. The ureters returned to normal in seventeen after radiotherapy. Radical pelvic surgery has not produced survival rates superior to those obtained by irradiation in this selected group of patients. If obstruction has progressed to the point of producing a high BUN, the patients invariably die. We have not found that ureteral transplants can frequently reverse the process.

SURGICAL STAGING BY LAPAROTOMY. Laparotomy has been used in *experimental studies* to determine the distribution and incidence of metastases to lymph nodes in various clinical stages and to determine the validity of positive and negative lymphangiograms. Irradiation has cured some patients with biopsy-proven metastases in common iliac and para-aortic nodes. There is merit in determining the pretreatment status of these nodes if the information obtained will modify treatment technique and survival. At present the lymphangiogram—at least in Stages IIb, III, and IVa—is of help in determining lymph node status. There seems to be little to gain by routine staging laparotomy if one encompasses not only the lymphangio-graphically abnormal nodal groups, but also the apparently normal nodal groups at substantial risk for involvement in the irradiated volume (Kademian and Bosch; Su-darsnam and associates; Keys and Park). The techniques for this irradiation are given on p. 470.

Radiation tolerance of pelvic organs

The radiation response of pelvic structures, like the response of most other tissues, depends not only on dose-time relationships, but to a lesser degree also on age and race of the patient, volume and distribution of the dose within that volume, previous treatment, whether it be surgery or irradiation, stage of disease, and quality of the beam. The practical problem of anticipating a given reaction in a given patient or of assessing tolerance prior to a curative attempt is not always simple or reliable. A certain percentage of radiation-induced complications is unavoidable. Experience has established guidelines from which the radiation oncologist must extrapolate for the individual patient.

The tolerance of pelvic structures may be at one radiation dose level if external pelvic irradiation and radium are administered according to the Paris technique but at an entirely different level if external pelvic irradiation and transvaginal irradiation are used in the treatment of carcinoma of the cervical stump. The dose distribution and the fractionation are different in these two techniques. Also, Kottmeier (1951) pointed out that there were important differences in tolerances between two differ-ent radium techniques. This was because of differences in radium distribution and dose rate. As will be shown later, technique should be modified in keeping with the clinical stage. However, the dose from intracavitary radium must be integrated with that from external pelvic irradiation if one is to keep sequelae within acceptable limits and obtain maximum control rates. Simple addition of the doses received at a point in the parametrium from intracavitary sources and from external pelvic irradiation may give equal sums but may produce different reactions. The tolerances of pelvic viscera and cancer cure rates for these various combinations have been established by extensive clinical use and must serve as our guides.

The more advanced the cancer of the cervix, the greater the dose necessary for it's eradication. Regardless of technique, it is evident that as the clinical stage becomes more advanced, the proportion of favorable responses decreases. The advanced stages require not only larger ports but also higher doses. With advanced disease, higher risks of injury are therefore anticipated and justified. This, coupled with the fact that the advanced cancer has often already compromised the integrity of the bladder and bowel, means that the most serious sequelae develop in patients with Stage III and Stage IV lesions. Most data available apply only to the tolerances of pelvic structures to the combined use of external pelvic irradiation and intracavitary sources (Chapter 14).

CERVIX AND CORPUS. Tissues composing the cervix and corpus of the uterus can tolerate high doses of radiations. In fact they withstand higher doses than any other comparable volume of tissues in the body. Doses of 20,000 to 30,000 rad in about 2 weeks are routinely tolerated. This high tolerance permits a high dose that leads to control of the cervical lesion in practically all early cases (Jampolis and associates; Kottmeier, 1953). Indeed, the success of radium in the treatment of cervical lesions is due almost entirely to this unusual radiation tolerance of the uterus. The epithelia of the uterus and vagina have a remarkable ability to recover from radiation injury, and the dense, smooth muscle and stroma of the uterus seem little affected by the doses just mentioned (Fig. 17-6). It should be remembered that the cervix is not called on to function appreciably after irradiation. For this reason fibrotic changes that would be symptom-producing in the rectum or in the bladder pass unnoticed in the cervix.

Slow-healing postirradiation ulcers of the cervix or of the vaginal vault occasionally develop 6 to 12 months after treatment. These rarely develop unless the original cervical cancer was advanced with an extensive local ulceration. Months may be required for reepithelization. These ulcers are relatively asymptomatic and are difficult to distinguish from persistent cancer. There is real danger that such ulcers may progress to form a fistula. Kottmeier (1964) reported that twenty-six postirradiation ulcers developed in 3484 patients when the Stockholm technique was used. Chau and associates found vault necrosis in thirty-two of 741 patients treated with radium and megavoltage beams. A modification of the Paris technique was used. Although it seems logical to expect that malpositioned radium could be related to the incidence of such ulcers, this has not been the case. Conservative management consisting of simple cleanliness, good nutrition, and specific antibiotics for any proved sensitive causative organism will usually suffice.

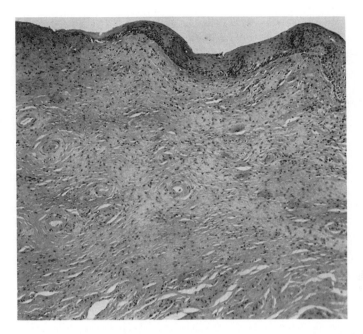

Fig. 17-6. Low-power enlargement of a section through a cervix that had received 20,000 to 30,000 rad by the Manchester radium technique. There is surprisingly little edema or fibrosis. The epithelium is thin and is absent in one area. (W. U. neg. 57-4779A; courtesy Dr. L. V. Ackerman.)

RECTOSIGMOID AND RECTUM. Since radiation injury of the large bowel is encountered most often after radiotherapy of carcinoma of the cervix, the detailed description of large bowel response is included in this section. Some of the types of injury presented are obviously also produced by radiotherapy of cancer of the bladder and prostate.

The sigmoid, rectosigmoid, and rectum are more susceptible to radiation injury than other pelvic organs. The frequency of large bowel injury is dependent on its relationship to and the distribution of the radium, as well as on the total dose from radium and external pelvic irradiation (Kagan and associates, 1976; Lee and associates, 1976). With external pelvic irradiation, again the large bowel will show the most frequent significant reaction of any of the pelvic organs. This susceptibility of the large bowel to radiation injury has been a major factor in determining which of the many techniques is preferable. Two types of large bowel reaction are recognized—the acute early reaction and the more chronic late reaction (Figs. 17-7 to 17-9).

The early reaction consists of diarrhea, tenesmus, and occasional minor hemorrhage. It appears near the end of external pelvic irradiation or within a few days of radium removal. The irradiation acts as a local irritant on the bowel mucosa and thus stimulates increased motility. If irradiation has been particularly vigorous, the diarrhea may be bloody. On proctoscopic examination the mucosa appears edematous and inflamed with a number of small bleeding points, but at this stage there is nothing to distinguish the reaction from that produced by other irritating agents.

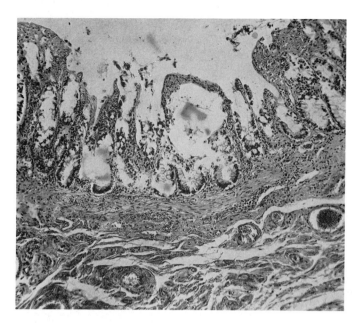

Fig. 17-7. Section through large bowel of patient who, 3 years before, received a calculated 6000 rad to the rectum during two radium insertions 2 weeks apart. There is moderate edema with some fibrosis and atypical cells. There was no ulceration. The patient had no bowel symptoms.

Such a reaction is to be expected in modern therapy of carcinoma of the cervix. Indeed, if there is no such reaction with conventional techniques, one might question the adequacy of the treatment. The diarrhea may be checked with paregoric or diphenoxylate (Lomotil), bed rest, and a low-residue diet. Rarely will other measures be necessary. A few days after irradiation, the bowel habits return to normal, and there are usually no serious sequelae.

The late bowel reaction is an infrequent complication that may appear 6 months to 2 years after irradiation. Microscopic examination of the rectum in all adequately irradiated patients will show a thickening of the bowel wall from edema and a less pliable bowel from fibrosis. Symptoms are not usually sufficiently severe as to be alarming. With the more serious reaction, the symptoms are those of severe bowel irritation—that is, diarrhea, tenesmus, bleeding, and perhaps a burning sensation in the rectum.

The relationship of this reaction to the early reaction is not clear, although both are more frequent with higher doses, decreased fractionation, and larger irradiated volumes. It should be pointed out that vigorous early reactions are not necessarily followed by late reactions. Occasionally patients with mild acute reactions may develop late reactions. Late rectal reactions may be divided into the localized lesions of the anterior wall of the rectum (at the level of the high dose from vaginal radium) and the more diffuse changes involving that segment of rectum or sigmoid colon encompassed by the external pelvic irradiation.

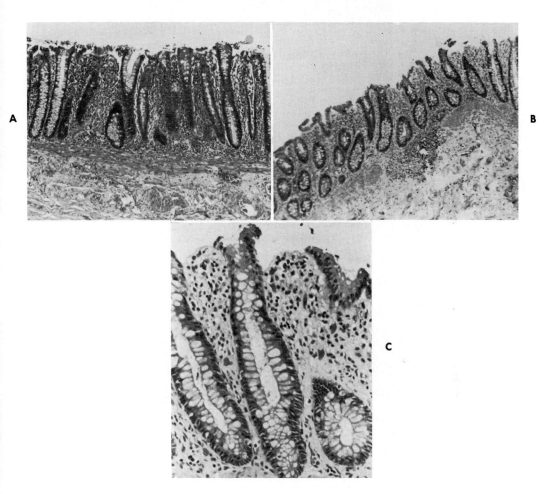

Fig. 17-8. Acute radiation reaction of large bowel. **A,** The histologic appearance of a normal colon. The hemopoietic cells, mainly plasma cells and lymphocytes, appear as tiny black dots between the glandular tissue. (H & E; magnification ×78.) **B,** Section from colon given 2000 rad in 12 days, 10 days prior to colectomy. This section is from the colonic mucosa uninvolved by cancer. The most marked change is the depletion of the hemopoietic cells normally present in the colonic mucosa and submucosa. Near the center of the picture beneath the mucosa is a remnant of lymphoid nodule. The mucosa is thinned. (H & E; magnification ×78.) **C,** A higher power photograph of section shown in **B.** The irradiated colonic mucosa shows clearly the paucity of lymphocytes and plasma cells in connective tissue stroma. (H & E; magnification ×137). (Courtesy Dr. K. Schneider.)

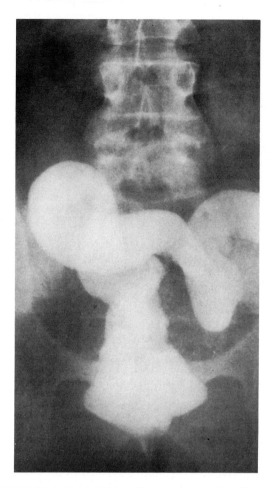

Fig. 17-9. On barium enema the rectum is rigid and has a ragged outline. Five years earlier the patient was irradiated for carcinoma of the cervix, Stage III. By external pelvic ⁶⁰Co irradiation (18 × 14 cm anterior and posterior portals), a midpelvic dose of 4500 rad was given in 5 weeks. Intracavitary uterine and vaginal radium was used once for 5000 mg-hr. The tandem was 10 cm long. The patient developed occasional mild blood-streaked diarrhea but was otherwise asymptomatic.

Excessive rectal doses from radium may follow inadequate packing separating the vaginal radium from the rectovaginal septum, a uterine retroflexion that has not been taken into account, an unusually long uterine tandem filling an enlarged uterine canal, excessive doses by vaginal radium, a narrowed vagina, misplacement of a vaginal source into the posterior fornix, or the slipping of the uterine tandem into the vagina. The necessity of careful radium placement and immobilization followed by roentgenographic confirmation of the placement is obvious. It is equally clear that a certain small proportion of severe radiation-induced large bowel complications will develop even after taking all recognized precautions.

Local late rectal ulceration will generally heal with conservative management.

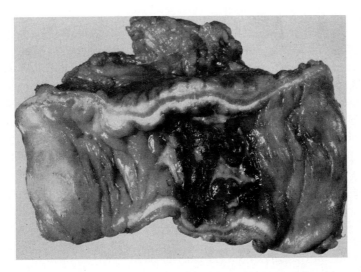

Fig. 17-10. Gross specimen of obstructed bowel. The dose to the segment is not known exactly but probably exceeded 6000 rad in 6 weeks. The proximal dilated bowel extended to the right. Note thickened edematous walls. No cancer was present in the ulcer. (W. U. neg. 57-447; courtesy Dr. L. V. Ackerman.)

Mineral oil to soften the stool and paregoric to decrease bowel motility, along with a low-residue diet and bed rest, will promote healing in the majority of patients. The complications of perforation either into the vagina or into abdominal organs, severe hemorrhage, and obstruction are unusual and are considered surgical problems.

The less frequent large bowel reaction from high-dose external pelvic irradiation appears as a woody induration completely encompassing a segment of rectum or rectosigmoid and presents symptoms similar to that described before (Fig. 17-9). Almost from the beginning there is a narrowing of the bowel lumen that may become so severe that colostomy is necessary. The etiology of this type of reaction has never been definitely established, although bowel epithelium, submucosa, small and large blood vessels, and surrounding connective tissues all show radiation-induced changes (Fig. 17-10).

The bowel superior to the rectum may also develop signs of radiation damage. This is particularly likely when a loop of the sigmoid colon falls into the cul-de-sac or remains relatively fixed in the volume of high dose. Symptoms consist of those of partial low bowel obstruction, bright blood and mucus in the stool, and alternate diarrhea and constipation. Barium enema reveals a narrowed segment with rigid walls (Fig. 17-9). This may progress to complete obstruction requiring surgical relief.

In the preceding discussion it is immediately clear that a precise statement of radiation tolerance of the large bowel is difficult. A variety of individual factors modifies individual tolerance. However, as a baseline from which one may extrapolate, we accept the following. When external pelvic megavoltage or ^{60}Co beams are used as the sole treatment for advanced cancers of the cervix, 7000 rad midpelvis in

7 to 8 weeks is near the limit of tolerance (skin portal 16 × 15 cm). When radium is used and a dose of 6500 rad divided in two increments is delivered to point A (8000 to 9000 mg-hr), an additional parametrial dose of 4000 to 5000 rad given by external irradiation using a split field is near the maximum. Finally, an initial whole pelvis dose of 4000 rad given by external pelvic irradiation without a midline shield should be supplemented by no more than 5000 mg-hr of radium. With the more advanced clinical stages, high doses are necessary and greater risks of bowel damage are justified. Most of the bowel wall thickening, bowel obstruction, and fistulae will develop in patients who have large central cancers or Stage III or IV lesions. In these patients, not only are maximum tolerated doses necessary to achieve maximum cure rates, but parametrial infiltration by cancer and secondary infection also contribute to decreased radiation tolerance of the connective tissues.

SMALL BOWEL. Since irradiation for carcinoma of the cervix consists of irradiating the pelvic contents, only limited portions of small bowel are included. The normal motility of the small bowel usually prevents the administration of excessive doses to any one segment. However, previous pelvic surgery, pelvic inflammatory disease, or the extension of cancer to the peritoneal surface increases the frequency of adhesions, and as a result the incidence of small bowel radiation injuries increases sharply. Friedman was unable to confirm the importance of adhesions experimentally, but clinically there can be no question of the correlation between small bowel radiation damage and previous pelvic surgery. In our experience, at least a fourth of the patients giving a history of previous surgery develop postirradiation signs and symptoms of late small bowel damage. The clinical picture is usually that of progressive intestinal obstruction. The loop of bowel fixed in the irradiated area will present a narrowed lumen with or without associated mucosal ulceration (Fig. 17-10). Surgical relief of this obstruction is generally required.

Carefully fractionated irradiation of the smallest possible volume will assure a minimum of such accidents, but the risk must otherwise be accepted. The effects of irradiating large segments of the small bowel are rarely a concern in treating limited carcinoma of the cervix. However, with the identification of metastases in common iliac and para-aortic nodes and the fact that these metastases can be controlled by irradiation, longer segments of small bowel are now being irradiated. Doses of about 5000 rad in 5 or more weeks delivered to para-aortic nodes are associated with serious subsequent small bowel damage in 10% to 20% of the patients (Lepanto and associates, 1975). Doses this high or higher delivered to the retroperitoneal area should probably be delivered over a longer period of time and through a combination of portals with the patient in several different positions in order to lessen the risk of small bowel damage. (See Chapter 12.)

URETER. In its course through the parametrium, the ureter lies a scant 1.5 cm from the lateral vaginal fornix. High doses exceeding the usual cancerocidal level are routinely delivered to this portion of the ureter. The tolerance of the ureter is emphasized by the rarity of late ureteral complications. Corscaden found but two patients presenting possible ureteral radiation injuries out of 900 irradiated patients.

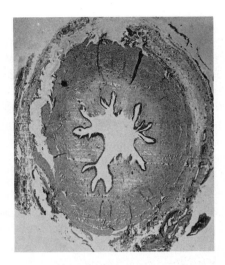

Fig. 17-11. Ureter damage by interstitial parametrial [198]Au. Dosage to the ureter is impossible to calculate. Grossly the wall was strikingly thickened and hard. The patient had no persistent cancer. (Courtesy Dr. Harvey Butcher.)

In the absence of recurrent cancer, hydronephrosis developed during the follow-up period in twenty of 3484 patients irradiated (Kottmeier, 1964). Radiations were presumed to be the responsible etiologic agent. However, six of the twenty patients received parametrial [198]Au. The usual Stockholm technique (without [198]Au) produced significant ureteral damage in fourteen of 1888 symptom-free, 5-year survival patients. Out of 1416 patients with normal pretreatment pyelograms and 139 patients without pyelograms, 134 ureters became obstructed after irradiation (Slater and Fletcher). In 108 of these instances, active pelvic cancer was present along the lymphatics near the ureter. Only five of the remaining twenty-six had ureteral obstruction resulting from radiation-induced periureteral fibrosis. Irradiation followed by hysterectomy seems to increase the risk of ureteral damage (Rotman and associates). The dose delivered to the ureter and to the parametrium is, of course, highly important in the etiology of ureteral stricture. Yet stricture seems to occur at the lower dose levels as well as at the higher levels (Chau and associates). The conclusion is therefore justified that whole pelvis irradiation alone is not conducive to excessive fibrosis and stricture (Fig. 17-11). With conventional Stockholm and Paris techniques and their modifications, late ureteral obstruction is indicative of recurrence in the parametrium until proved otherwise (Figs. 17-4 and 17-5).

The mechanism of radiation-induced ureteral stricture is not understood. It is speculated that necrosis of the cancer with subsequent parametrial fibrosis, coupled with parametritis, is responsible. If recurrent cancer cannot be found in such a patient, the stricture should receive the same attention as in any other noncancerous patient.

FEMORAL HEAD AND NECK. Because skin-tumor distances are great, all available ports were utilized when medium-voltage beams were employed. The direct lateral port unavoidably irradiates the femoral head and neck. If, with medium-voltage radiations, skin doses of 3000 rad were given in 6 weeks, there was real risk that fractures of the femoral neck would occur a year or so later. These were usually preceded by moderately severe hip pain and then an obvious subcapital fracture. This medium-voltage technique is mentioned only to be condemned in modern radiation therapy. Microscopic changes in irradiated bone are discussed in Chapter 21. The actual mechanism by which the bone is weakened remains somewhat obscure, but osteoporosis secondary to vascular resorption and osteoclastic activity are thought to be chiefly responsible. Although the marrow is usually fibrotic, other vascular elements are little affected (Stephenson and Cohen). The radiation-induced fracture must be differentiated from a fracture secondary to metastasis, since in one patient irradiation might help and in the other it would be contraindicated. Healing of the fracture depends on the severity of radiation damage of the bone-forming cell. The blood supply to the femoral head is not generally seriously affected, and avascular necrosis of the femoral head is uncommon.

With megavoltage beams, the proportion of the dose absorbed in bone is much less than with medium-voltage beams. The lateral portal can be safely used with the cobalt or betatron x-ray beam. Except for such a lateral megavoltage beam, however, the femoral neck should not be included in the volume of significant dose. No more than a small portion of the femoral head need be included in the anterior and posterior beams. Only four instances of change in the femoral head developed in 741 patients reported by Chau and associates. In only one of these four patients was the damage severe, and in this instance radium and 250 kv radiations were used. We have seen no radiation-induced damage of the femoral head or neck since ^{60}Co and megavoltage have become available.

Radiosensitivity of carcinoma of the cervix and its extensions

RADIOSENSITIVITY OF THE PRIMARY CANCER. The dose of radiations required to control the primary cervical lesion is widely variable. Midpelvic doses of 4000 to 5000 rad are capable of destroying the primary lesion in a significant percentage of patients. Yet in other patients, doses of 20,000 to 30,000 rad to the cervix have failed. Several attempts have been made to establish optimum dose-time levels (Tod; Nolan and associates; Garcia; Fletcher, 1971). It is now evident that the cure rate does increase as the dose increases up to the tolerance levels described previously. Beyond this level, little, if any, increase in control of the primary lesion can be expected, but a serious increase in the incidence of complications will occur. In the face of this wide variation in the radiosensitivity of the primary lesion, the optimum dose to the primary lesion is established by the tolerance of the rectum, rectosigmoid, bladder, and small bowel. When radium is the sole treatment for limited cancers, the dose at point A as delivered by the Manchester technique should be about 7600 rad (Cole). All techniques exploit the great radiation tolerance of the cervix by giving high doses to this area.

Fletcher (1971) has emphasized the pitfalls of using the summation of doses at a given point as a guide for either optimum or maximum doses. Instead, he has detailed the radium distribution, the milligram-hours, and the external pelvic doses found to be optimum for the various clinical stages. This concept emphasizes the variations of dose with clinical stage and thus the variation of risks of late sequelae with clinical stage. These maximum tolerated doses were listed previously.

As in other anatomic sites, large, bulky, cancerous masses of the cervix exhibit a relatively greater radioresistance and manifest this resistance with an increased local recurrence rate. Durrance and associates describe this tendency for large cancers to develop recurrences. In addition to more cancer cells and more severe hypoxia, a contributing factor is the great distance between the central uterine tandem and the more deeply invading cancer cells as exemplified in the barrel-shaped cervix. A combination of radiotherapy and surgery is particularly effective in this infrequent situation. Durrance and associates recommend a whole pelvis dose of 4000 rad in 4 weeks plus a limited radium dose of 4000 to 5000 mg-hr and, finally, a "conservative total hysterectomy." The rationale here is to accept 5000 rad as an adequate dose for small foci in the periphery of the pelvis and remove the central bulk by a limited resection. Rotman and associates have not found hysterectomy under these circumstances to be necessary for local control unless the diameter of the cervix exceeds 7 cm.

RADIOSENSITIVITY OF METASTASES TO REGIONAL LYMPH NODES. The effectiveness of irradiation in controlling metastases to pelvic lymph nodes is no longer controversial. The dose of radiations must be in keeping with knowledge of dose requirements for eradication of squamous cell carcinoma in nodes elsewhere. From our irradiation of tumors of the head and neck we know that a high proportion of small foci are controlled by doses of 4500 to 5000 rad in 5 to 6 weeks. A similar proportion of clinically palpable nodes up to 2 cm in diameter are controlled by doses of about 6000 rad in 6 to 7 weeks. Nodes 2 to 4 cm are often controlled by doses up to 7500 rad in 8 weeks. The accumulated evidence, although scanty, indicates that metastases to pelvic and para-aortic nodes respond quite similarly to those described previously. Since pelvic and para-aortic nodes cannot be clinically evaluated relative to size, the dose must be the highest tolerated by normal structures if the chances for control are to be maximum. This usually implies 1500 to 2000 rad in 5 to 6 days to the pelvic nodal areas from radium and 3500 to 5000 rad in 6 weeks or more delivered by external pelvic irradiation. For the more advanced stages, radium dosage is decreased, and the dose given by external irradiation to the pelvic nodes may be greatly increased (p. 472). Doses of 4500 to 5000 rad external irradiation can be tolerated in volumes greater than those enclosing the primary pelvic node areas if the risks are accepted. The radiation tolerance of the small bowel limits the maximum dose that can be delivered to the para-aortic nodes. Although Fletcher and associates set this limit at 4500 rad, others have given higher doses with acceptable sequelae (Silberstein and associates). When lower doses and inadequate ports have been used, the frequency of "apparent radioresistance" has increased. For this reason a careful analysis of time-dose-volume relationships is essential in evaluating reports of the radioincurability of patients with metastases to pelvic and para-aortic lymph nodes.

To determine the capability of radiations to sterilize cancer metastatic to pelvic lymph nodes, several clinical experiments have been performed. These studies fall into two large categories.

1. Irradiation of those patients who, on preirradiation laparotomy, were proved by biopsy to have metastases to pelvic lymph nodes. Radiotherapy was the sole treatment of these patients. Yet Kottmeier (1953) proved that, even when cancer was known to have been left behind, some patients were living and well more than 5 years after irradiation.

2. Comparison of the incidence of pelvic lymph node metastases with and without previous pelvic irradiation. Many studies of this type have been reported. Brown and associates irradiated the pelvic lymph nodes vigorously in twenty-four patients. On removal of the pelvic lymph nodes there was no evidence of metastases in eighteen patients, whereas three had widespread pelvic disease and one had one positive obturator node. The expected rate of metastases for a comparable stage would be at least twice this rate.

Rutledge and Fletcher performed lymphadenectomy after 4000 to 6000 rad whole pelvis irradiation plus the contribution from radium. The incidence of metastases to pelvic lymph nodes is shown in Table 17-8. Although there is considerable variation in the incidence of positive nodes found in unirradiated patients, an average from the literature is shown in Table 17-4. The difference is dramatic and permits no conclusion other than that sterilization of metastases to lymph nodes is frequently accomplished.

Morton and associates reported the results of a prospective study intended to define the capability of radiations to sterilize cancer in pelvic lymph nodes. Alternate patients with Stage I carcinoma were given irradiation before lymphadenectomy, and the others were given a similar dose after lymphadenectomy. The irradiation consisted of the administration of 8999 rad to point A and 4500 rad to point B. Combined external pelvic and radium irradiation was used. The nature of fractionation was not given. Lymphadenectomy was performed 8 weeks after irradiation. The results are shown in Table 17-9.

There are several criticisms to the type of studies just described. Doses of radiations reaching the nodes are difficult to evaluate. The type of lymph node dissection performed after irradiation may not remove the same total number of nodes as is removed when surgery is used alone. In addition, radiations shrink all lymph nodes, including those with cancer. The pathologist will therefore have more difficulty dissecting nodes from the operative specimen when radiation therapy has been given.

The effectiveness of radiations on metastases to pelvic lymph nodes has been measured in still another way. A group of patients treated by radiation therapy alone was compared with a group treated by combined radiation therapy and subsequent lymphadenectomy (Table 17-10). No significant difference in survival rates could be detected (Rutledge and associates, 1965). This fact, coupled with the frequent complications of the combined procedure, demonstrates clearly that routine post-irradiation lymphadenectomy is not indicated. Para-aortic lymph nodes have been

Table 17-8. Value of irradiation in the treatment of carcinoma of the cervix metastatic to pelvic lymph nodes (100 patients with Stage III cancer)*

Treatment	Percentage of instances in which positive nodes present in operative specimen
Irradiation and then surgery	In irradiated volume only, 5% Beyond irradiated volume only, 8% Both in and beyond irradiated volume, 9% Total, 22%
Surgery only	66% to 43%

*Modified from Rutledge, F. N., and Fletcher, G. H.: Am. J. Obstet. Gynecol. **76**:321-324, 1958. One hundred patients with Stage III cancer were given vigorous irradiation by the method described by Fletcher.

Table 17-9. Value of irradiation in the treatment of carcinoma of the cervix metastatic to pelvic lymph nodes*

Procedures	Number of patients	Positive nodes (%)
Lymphadenectomy before irradiation	38	22.7
Lymphadenectomy after irradiation	32	12.5

*Modified from Morton, D. G., Lagasse, L. D., Moore, J. G., Jacobs, M., and Amromin, G. D.: Am. J. Obstet. Gynecol. **88**:935, 1964. This prospective randomized study was planned to define the value of irradiation in Stage I cancer of the cervix (see text).

Table 17-10. Comparison of irradiation alone with irradiation followed by lymphadenectomy for carcinoma of the cervix (a prospective randomized study)*

Clinical stage	Irradiation alone		Irradiation plus lymphadenectomy	
	Number	Surviving 5 years (%)†	Number	Surviving 5 years (%)†
I	30	86	39	93
IIa	39	77	39	89
IIb	25	54	28	62
IIIa	23	54	28	33
IIIb	25	54	35	63

*From Rutledge, F. N., Fletcher, G. H., and MacDonald, E. J.: Am. J. Roentgenol. **93**:610, 1965.
†Life table method.

biopsied, found to contain cancer, and then irradiated. Fletcher (1971) reported two such patients living after 5 years without evidence of cancer. Silberstein and associates found no evidence of residual cancer in three of six patients 3 to 11 years after they were given 6000 rad in 6 weeks for biopsy-proved metastasis to the para-aortic nodes. Of twenty-eight patients with involved common iliac or para-aortic nodes or both who had irradiation with curative intent, sixteen (57%) were alive and well at 2 to 13 years. Of fifteen patients who had known nodal disease left at the time of

Table 17-11. Irradiation of patients with involved para-aortic nodes

Author	Dose	Number of patients	Years of follow-up	Percent survivors
Vongtama	2000-4000	21	2	19 (4/21)
	6000	20	2	30 (6/20)
Lepanto	5000	26	2	42 (11/26)
Silberstein	6000	6	3-11	50 (3/6)

preirradiation laparotomy or hysterectomy, eight (53%) were living and well at 2 to 13 years (Keys and Park, 1976). Additional survival data are scanty (Table 17-11).

We believe that such evidence, coupled with statistics given in Tables 17-8 and 17-9, justifies a vigorous course of treatment planned to irradiate the nodal areas that are likely to harbor metastases. In limited stages such irradiation has at least as much to offer as radical hysterectomy with lymph node dissection. In Stages II, III, and IV surgery cannot compete with irradiation.

Adenocarcinoma of the cervix

Adenocarcinoma of the cervix usually arises in the endocervix and presents the same clinical manifestations as squamous cell carcinoma of the cervix. However, Weiner and Wizenberg (1975) pointed out that surgery alone or surgery followed by irradiation is advocated routinely by some who believe that

1. Adenocarcinomas are less radiosensitive than squamous cell carcinomas.
2. This cancer grows within the endocervix to produce a central mass of tumor similar to the "barrel-shaped cervix."
3. These cancers often represent extensions from adenocarcinomas of the corpus.

Although there may be clinical situations in which each of these is true, there is ample evidence to verify that stage for stage adenocarcinoma of the cervix is as curable by radiation therapy as is squamous cell carcinoma. Of course one must identify the patient with the large central cervical mass or barrel-shaped cervix. This is treated by preoperative irradiation and surgery just as is squamous cell carcinoma presenting with the same clinical findings. If the bulk of the adenocarcinoma is curetted from the cavity of the corpus, and a nonmucinous histologic cell type is present, the patient should probably be treated as if she had adenocarcinoma of the endometrium with cervical invasion. By contrast mucin-producing cancers originate more often from the cervix. The radiocurability of adenocarcinoma of the cervix is confirmed by the reports of Sala and associates, Wildermuth and Melhorn, and Weiner and Wizenberg (Table 17-12).

We recommend that with the exceptions mentioned before, adenocarcinoma of the cervix should be treated the same as squamous cell carcinoma of the cervix. Comparable results can be expected.

Radiation techniques for carcinoma of the cervix

The discussion to follow is a summary of several techniques that have evolved over many years. Thousands of patients have been treated by these techniques and

Table 17-12. Radiocurability of adenocarcinoma of the cervix*

Stage	Number of patients	Percent surviving 5 years
I	26	84.6
II	26	76.9
III	10	33
IV (palliative)	4	0
I, II, III	66	64.8

*Modified from Weiner, S., and Wizenberg, M. J.: Cancer **35:**1514-1516, 1975.

their value is well established. However, as more knowledge is acquired, treatment with these techniques will no doubt continue to improve. Regardless of the technique adopted, one cannot emphasize too strongly the necessity for individualization of therapy. Rarely will two patients present exactly the same cancer problem. The most important single factor in clinical radium therapy is the skill of the physician in handling individual patients. The techniques and doses to be quoted are average figures. To attempt to reproduce this average in every patient is inexcusable. When possible, indications for varying technique and dose are given, but these are the details acquired only through training and experience with patient problems.

The radiation oncologist must shift emphasis from intracavitary radium to external pelvic irradiation in patients with advanced carcinoma, appreciate the limitations of radium and the advantages of transvaginal irradiation in carcinoma of the cervical stump, plan a combination of surgery and irradiation in certain pregnant patients developing carcinoma of the cervix and in patients with bulky midline lesions in clinical Stages I and II, and finally adapt his treatment to the treatment already administered by the referring physician. He must have a working knowledge of all the techniques mentioned before. He must be capable of adapting treatment to the clinical findings rather than using a single radium technique and inflexible doses, field sizes, and periods of fractionation. This individualization of treatment is true in all radiotherapeutic procedures but seems to have become most frequently abused in the treatment of carcinoma of the cervix.

INTRACAVITARY RADIUM OR CESIUM. The most commonly used technique employs intracavitary radium usually supplemented by external pelvic irradiation. Since the reaction in midline structures limits the dose that may be given by radium, there is a definite advantage in separating the vaginal radium into two sources, one for each lateral fornix. The magnitude of the physical advantage of using separated vaginal sources is seen in the table published by Ter-Pogossian and associates. All modern techniques take advantage of this concept to reduce the midline dose while slightly increasing the dose laterally. It must be remembered that the linear source used as a uterine tandem produces a dose distribution that decreases rapidly with depth. Cancers that infiltrate deeply into the substance of the middle and upper parts of the cervix may well extend beyond the zone effectively irradiated by the tandem. Fletcher has emphasized this point and has recommended a "conservative hysterectomy" for selected patients falling into this category. An example of this rapid

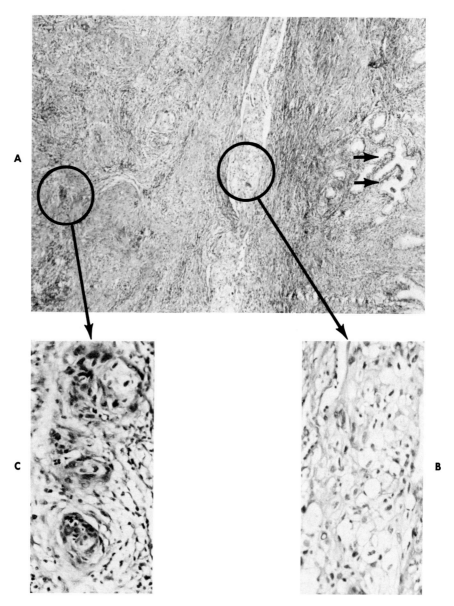

Fig. 17-12. Section of superior segment of a "barrel-shaped" cervix harboring postirradiation persistent invasive squamous cell carcinoma. Initial clinical Stage IIb with extension into the left parametrium. Treatment of 5600 rad whole true pelvis in 43 total days, ^{60}Co, 16 × 14 cm. AP and PA portals supplemented after the initial 4000 rad in 30 days by 4560 mg-hr of radium (standard loaded tandem and vaginal sources). Limited hysterectomy was performed 6 weeks after treatment was completed. Cervical canal is on the right near arrows in **A.** The focus of cancer nearest the canal, **B,** shows cells with extensive ballooning degeneration of the cytoplasm. The focus of cancer, **C,** is deep in the wall and at a greater distance from the canal. It shows much less radiation effect.

decrease in dosage from the tandem and the findings on conservative hysterectomy are shown in Fig. 17-12. When radioactive sources are used, preloaded systems are no longer acceptable. Afterloading systems not only reduce the exposure of personnel, but, more importantly, also permit precise tailoring of lengths and strengths of sources to the patient's anatomy.

In the development of modern intracavitary techniques for the treatment of carcinoma of the cervix, two schools of therapy led the way. The Stockholm technique was characterized by two intensive, short radium treatments delivering a relatively high dose to the cervix, corpus, and vaginal vault. The radium was placed in small lead boxes that varied in size and content. The boxes were packed against the cancerous mass and away from the bladder and rectum. The uterine tandem containing 50 to 75 mg of radium delivered about half the dose.

The second technique was developed in Paris. It was characterized by much less intense radium sources inserted for a longer treatment time. The vaginal sources were placed in corks, which were packed into the lateral fornices. One additional midline cork was sometimes used. Equal amounts of radium were used in the corpus and in the vagina. Both techniques have been modified to fit modern megavoltage capabilities. The tolerances have been established by years of experience.

Expression of dose. The precise expression of dose from intracavitary sources used in the treatment of carcinoma of the cervix has been and to a large extent continues to be difficult and often impractical. Early workers established normal tissue tolerances and local cancer control rates in terms of the product of the amount of radium inserted and the duration of the insertion. This expression is, of course, related to dose absorbed at various points but lacks precision for individual patients because the normal anatomy and the size, shape, and extent of the cancer require variations in the amount and distribution of radium. At the same time the position of critical organs varies widely. The mere multiplication of milligram-hours by a fixed factor in an attempt to express dose at a certain point does nothing to improve our understanding of the dose absorbed by movable, distensible normal tissues or cancers. However, computer-aided dosimetry is now readily available for routine calculation of dose at any point. Furthermore, the relation of the bladder and rectum to the radium can be determined by films taken with the radium applicators in place. Correlations of precise dose distributions with critical organ tolerances and local cancer control rates may now be possible. However, the clinical justification for these additional dosimetry procedures has not been sufficiently convincing to provoke their widespread adoption. Until such time as their clinical value is clear, radium doses will continue to be expressed in milligram-hours by most radiation oncologists. However, we urge the use of computer-aided dosimetry and the routine calculation of maximum dose to critical organs (bowel and bladder). In the meantime in our discussions of tissue tolerances we must use milligram-hours because all reported experience is based on milligram-hours as the "unit" of dose.

Rather than expressing dose in terms of milligram-hours or millicuries destroyed, the Manchester system, before the availability of computer-aided dosimetry, enabled one to express the dose in terms of rad at several representative points in relation to the position of the radium. Although the locations of these points are now often defined in terms of anatomic sites, the actual specification is by necessity related to the position of the radium. The necessary variation in the position and distribution of the radium significantly changes the anatomic structures in which points A and B are located. Instead of corks, rubber or plastic ovoids are used in the Manchester system. The surface of the ovoid represents an area of equal dose for a source of radium (1.5 cm active length) placed along the axis of the ovoid. All tissues in contact with the ovoid will receive an equal dose of known magnitude. Its rotation produces insignificant variations in dose. Three sizes of ovoids are available—2, 2.5, and 3 cm in diameter. By the original Manchester technique, the ovoids are held apart by cupped "spacers" or "washers," depending on the degree of separation desired. A conventional intrauterine linear source is also inserted. Mechanical devices have become available that make insertion easier, more flexible, and with less exposure to personnel (Fletcher and associates, 1952). In some patients it is possible to maintain a known fixed relationship between the uterine tandem and the vaginal sources. However, it is dangerous to force all uteri to conform to the rigid type of device, and in none of the more widely used techniques (Stockholm, Paris, Manchester, or M. D. Anderson) has it been found that such a change is advisable.

To have meaning, the dose from radium to selected points within the pelvis must be related to the effectiveness of treatment or the reaction of normal tissues. Tod and Meredith believed that point A fulfilled these requirements better than any other. It is located clinically by measuring 2 cm superiorly and 2 cm laterally from the inferior end of the intrauterine radium source (presumed to be at the cervical os). Point B is 3 cm lateral to point A. The dose at point A is assumed to be representative of the dose to the paracervical triangle and to correlate with the incidence of sequelae as well as the 5-year control rate (Paterson). There are serious limitations in using the dose at two such points as a measure of the dose to this large volume. The objection to point A is its nearness to the radium sources. Rather minor variations in radium placement may produce appreciable fluctuations in the dose at point A. Point B, together with the tissue superior to it, is thought to be of significance in considering the dose to the node-bearing tissues. The node-bearing volume is large and the dose at a single point near the inferomedial edge of this volume can hardly be representative. This is especially true for the nodes above the obturator nodes. Computer-aided dosimetry made these limitations of points A and B obvious. Just how these detailed data made available by computer-aided dosimetry might best be used is still to be defined. The limitation is no longer definition of dose, but specification of dose in sensitive normal organs when the precise location of those normal organs is poorly defined and the dose in them varies widely because of the sharp gradient in dose with small differences in distance from the radium. However, computer-aided dosimetry permits specific calculation of dose at points along the pelvic wall regardless of applicator position and loading. It also assists in identifying areas of low dose or excessively high dose. It is of special value in considering the adequacy of dose to external and common iliac nodes in comparison to the dose to obturator nodes. Dose rates from intracavitary sources are major determinants of normal tissue tolerances (Kagan and associates). These rates vary markedly from one point to another within the pelvis. Computer assistance also makes the routine calculation of dose rates practical.

With full recognition of the aforementioned limitations implied in using the concepts of points A and B, Tables 17-13 and 17-14 summarize the Manchester system. These tables are useful only in those practices in which computer-aided dosimetry is not available.

The *dose rate* will naturally depend on the amount of radium. The *distribution of dose* depends on the radium distribution. To permit flexible dose rates within the Manchester system of radium distribution, the proportion of radium in each applicator is expressed in *units*. If one wishes a higher dose rate, the unit of radium must be increased. For the typical Manchester treatment, the unit of radium is 2.5 mg, producing a dose rate of 57 R per hour at point A. Tables 17-13 and 17-14 give the ideal radium distribution for the Manchester technique.

Table 17-13. Loadings in terms of units for the Manchester system*

Intrauterine applicators (left to right, fundus to cervix)		
Long tandem	3 radium tubes	6–4–4 units
Medium tandem	2 radium tubes	6–4 units

Vaginal ovoids (in pairs across the vagina)	
Large ovoids	9 units each
Medium ovoids	8 units each
Small ovoids	7 units each

Nonstandard treatments

  a. Short intrauterine tandem—1 radium tube, 8 units
  b. Vaginal ovoids used in "tandem" are loaded as above

*From Tod, M., and Meredith, W. J.: Br. J. Radiol. **26**:252-257, 1953.

Table 17-14. A practical loading system for the revised Manchester system*

Intrauterine tubes			
Loading—mg	Long	Medium	Short (nonstandard)
From fundus to cervix	15–10–10	15–10	20

Vaginal ovoids			
Loading—mg	Large or one 5+, two 10	Medium or one 20	Small or one 10+, two 5
Alternatively	One insertion one 20	One insertion one 15	One insertion one 15
	One insertion one 25	One insertion one 25	One insertion one 20

Time for 8000 R at point A	140 hours
Time for 6500 R at point A	114 hours

*From Tod, M., and Meredith, W. J.: Br. J. Radiol. **26**:252-257, 1953.
Notes:
1. Range of dose rate at point A for standard insertions, 57 R per hour ± 1.5%
2. Dose at point A in 140 hours with short intrauterine applicator and standard ovoids, 7000 R.
3. Dose at point A in 140 hours if ovoids are "in tandem," 7500 R.
4. Dose at point A in 140 hours if short intrauterine applicator is used with ovoids "in tandem," 6500 R.

As mentioned previously, younger patients tolerate higher doses than do elderly patients. With the Manchester technique the optimum dose in patients under 65 years of age who are not to receive external pelvic irradiation is 7600 rad to point A delivered in two sessions of 3 days each with a 4- to 7-day interval between. For patients over 65 years of age, this should be reduced to 6300 rad given in a similar fashion. About three fifths of the dose at point A comes from the intrauterine radium and two fifths from the vaginal source. External pelvic irradiation is added to the dose laterally. The knowledge that cancer in the parametrium and cancer metastatic to pelvic nodes can be sterilized, as cited previously, prompts us to recommend external pelvic irradiation in all but the earliest Stage I cancers.

Although anatomic variations in the uterus dictate to a large extent the position of the tandem, manipulation at the time of insertion can alter the relationship of the vaginal radium to the tandem. Perhaps the most common error is to separate the vaginal sources too forcefully. This tends to shift them inferiorly away from the cervix. Tension on the cervix with a tenaculum should never be maintained during placement of the vaginal sources. Release of the tension permits the uterus to retract superiorly, pulling away from the vaginal radium. If vaginal packing is forced too strongly superiorly, the uterus may increase its tilt, and the resulting relationship between the vagina and uterine radium increases the risk of inadequate dose in the posterior lip and excessive dose in the anterior lip. The opposite defect may follow if the corpus is posterior. Also, when the radium is packed too firmly upward, it tends to slide into the posterior fornix and away from the middle position. These easily corrected common technical defects can be related to local recurrence and high-dose sequelae in a high proportion of cases (Sherman and associates). Others have confirmed the fact that the local recurrence rate increases sharply and bowel and bladder injuries increase if vaginal sources cannot be placed in their usual lateral positions or if a short tandem must be used (Bourne and Mead; Kagan and associates). In our experience the most common causes of a poor radium placement are a narrowed vaginal vault and too much upward pressure before adequate packing is placed posteriorly. For Stage I and limited Stage II cancers, a poor intracavitary implant might well signal the need for one of several alternatives, that is, (1) the insertion of a cylinder of needles into the substance of the cervix and lower uterine segment, (2) a boosting dose to central structures using a rotational or box technique, (3) hysterectomy after irradiation as is performed for the patient with a barrel-shaped cervix, or (4) radical hysterectomy.

The fact that a high proportion of patients in whom the intracavitary implant is suboptimal develop local recurrence makes it critical that these alternatives be available and are considered.

External pelvic irradiation

The aims and justification for external pelvic irradiation have been presented previously and may be summarized as follows.

1. Intracavitary sources cannot, with safety, deliver cancerocidal doses beyond 3 to 3.5 cm from the external cervical os.

2. The volume usually requiring high doses includes not only the uterus, upper vagina, and medial portions of the parametrium, but also the lateral portions of the broad ligament, the uterosacral ligaments, and the frequently involved pelvic lymph nodes. Lymphangiographic evidence of metastases to common iliac and para-aortic nodes occurs surprisingly often in the more advanced stages. The advisability of encompassing these nodes in the treated volume must now be considered.

3. Intracavitary sources as described for any of the previously mentioned techniques deliver a high dose to the normal sized cervix (20,000 to 30,000 rad). This dose is sufficient to be lethal to any radioresponsive carcinoma. This dose diminishes rapidly so that an adequate dose is not delivered to the periphery of a lesion that is bulky and of a size and shape to place its periphery beyond about 3.5 cm. Irradiation of the tissues beyond the uterus, vagina, and medial parametrium must be accomplished without overirradiation of midline structures, the bowel, the skin, or femoral necks.

The importance of external pelvic irradiation in patients with extension of cancer to the parametrium or regional nodes cannot be too strongly emphasized. As del Regato has stated: "Our greatest present possibility of improving results, particularly in the treatment of the advanced cases of carcinoma of the cervix, lies in the understanding of the role and in the adequate utilization of external pelvic irradiation."[*] External pelvic irradiation is the only proved method capable of delivering an effective dose homogeneously throughout the large volume defined previously.

Films taken with either the simulator or the therapy unit will assist in defining port size and position. The relative position of the cervix within this volume can be defined by special devices (Fletcher and associates, 1956) or by placing an air-filled test tube the length of the vagina when the localization film is taken.

The sequence of combining external pelvic irradiation and intracavitary sources is not as simple as it may first appear. It has been advocated for years that external pelvic irradiation should precede the radium implant. This will shrink a large central mass or cauliflower-like growth, diminish the infection, and assist in returning a displaced uterus to its normal position. Each of these changes will permit a better radium implant. However, to shed further light on the proper sequence, Paterson and Russell (1962) performed a prospective randomized clinical study. They compared the 5-year survival rates of patients given external pelvic irradiation first with those given radium first. Standard Manchester techniques were used. The majority of patients had Stage III lesions. The results are shown in Table 17-15. Although the difference here (P = 0.2) is not of the generally accepted significant level, it certainly suggests that external pelvic irradiation should be given first.

With these facts in mind, we believe that a policy similar to that recommended by Fletcher (1971) is excellent. No external irradiation is given in the more limited Stage I lesions or if the lesions are 1 cm or less in diameter. Treatment consists of two radi-

---

[*] From del Regato, J. A.: The role of roentgen therapy in the treatment of cancer of the cervix uteri, Am. J. Roentgenol. **68**:63-66, 1952.

Table 17-15. Comparison of 5-year survival rates of the sequence of radium plus external pelvic irradiation with that of external pelvic irradiation plus radium*

Sequence	Number of patients	5-year survival rate (%)
Radium, then x ray	116	35.3
X ray, then radium	105	45.7

*Modified from Paterson, R., and Russell, M.: Clin. Radiol. **13**:313-315, 1962.

um implants 7 to 10 days apart. Each implant consists of 4500 to 5000 mg-hr, with a source distribution similar to that recommended by Paterson.

If the lesion is somewhat more advanced but has minimal necrosis and has not yet produced appreciable deformity of the cervix or fornices, radium may be implanted initially (4000 mg-hr). External irradiation given by the split-field technique starts immediately thereafter. This is interrupted in 10 days for the second radium implant (4000 mg-hr). External irradiation is then continued for a midparametrial dose of at least 4500 rad in an overall period of 6 weeks.

External irradiation is the initial therapy regardless of stage when deformity of the cervix or fornices has occurred. This includes most patients with Stage II and Stage III lesions. No midline shield should be used initially. The more advanced the primary lesion, the greater the preradium dose of external pelvic irradiation. Thus, in a patient with limited cervical and fornical deformity the preradium dose of external pelvic irradiation will usually be about 2000 rad in 2½ weeks. This is followed by a radium implant of 4000 mg-hr and additional external pelvic irradiation with a midline shield. The additional dose from external beams is usually 2500 rad to the midparametrium. A second radium implant equal to the first completes the treatment. When the vault deformity is severe or the central mass is large, a midpelvis dose of 3500 rad is given in 4 to 5 weeks. If, at that time, regression has been good, a single radium implant of 4000 to 5000 mg-hr is made. After this, external irradiation is resumed but with the split-field technique, and an additional midparametrial dose of 2000 rad is given. With the advanced stages, 4000 rad in 4 weeks may not produce good shrinkage. When this is the case, whole pelvis irradiation is continued without interruption to a minimum of 6000 rad in 6 to 8 weeks. A radium implant of 4000 mg-hr is then attempted, or transvaginal irradiation with the del Regato–type cones is performed (4000 rad at the level of the cervix in 10 days using 200 kv radiations, hvl 1 mm Cu at the shortest possible cervix-target distance). If neither of these are practical, boosting doses are delivered to the central structures using a rotational or box technique.

External pelvic irradiation is the sole treatment in advanced lesions that produce bilateral frozen pelvis or extensively necrotic lesions with rectal or bladder infiltration. Since no midline shield is used, we favor a single anterior port and two oblique posterior ports or preferably the four-port box technique. This minimizes the risk of a reaction in the cleft between the buttocks. A dose of 7000 rad in 7 to 8 weeks has

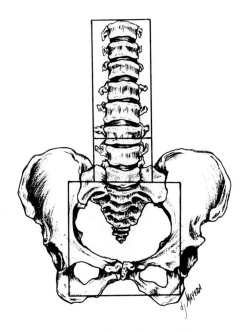

Fig. 17-13. Bony landmarks used as guides for various portal arrangements in treating carcinoma of cervix. For limited stages, upper margin passes through L5. For Stages IIb and III an extension is used, the upper border of which is near upper margin of L4. When para-aortic nodes are to be encompassed, a portal is placed above L4 to D1.

been given (4 to 5 mv with source-skin distance 80 to 100 cm through a 16 × 15 cm portal anteriorly and posteriorly and two 15 × 9 cm opposed lateral portals). A good dose distribution can be obtained by such a four-port box technique with sparing of posterior rectal wall and the anterior bladder wall.

FIELD SIZE AND POSITION. Field size is, of course, tailored to the likely extent of the cancer. Fortunately, the walls of the true pelvis usually restrict lateral, anterior, and posterior spread. The inferior margin of the beam should encompass all vaginal extension and the obturator fossae. The level of the superior margin varies with the assessment of upward spread. For most patients with limited cancers, simple anterior and posterior beams 16 cm wide and 16 cm in vertical dimension encompass all necessary tissues. For these patients (Stages Ib and IIa), the superior margin of the treated volume is usually placed above the promontory at the level of L5 (Fig. 17-16). A 3 to 4 cm wide midline lead shield at least for the inferior half to two thirds of the field is suspended above those patients who have had or are about to have a full dose from radium. This lead is positioned to shield the rectum from external pelvic beams. It should therefore be centered to shield the rectum and not necessarily shifted in keeping with the position of the radium implant. A midparametrial dose of 4500 to 7000 rad over 5 to 8 weeks can be given with acceptable skin reaction. The late subcutaneous fibrosis seen especially in fat patients with large dimensions should be reduced by treating each field each day using four fields when possible and a higher energy photon beam.

These ports should be modified for more advanced cancers that require treating common iliac nodes or a long segment of vagina. A variety of beam types and wedges has been tailored to produce what was presumed to be improved dose distributions. However, no single arrangement has proved superior.

The incidence of metastases to para-aortic lymph nodes in the various clinical stages is defined in Table 17-2. When a lymphangiogram has been performed, involved para-aortic nodes should be encompassed. We also recommend irradiation of apparently normal para-aortic nodes if the common iliac nodes show involvement on the lymphangiogram. Until more data are obtained, we have recommended the following guidelines. When common iliac nodes only are positive on the lymphogram, nodes up to the lower edge of T11 are encompassed. Also when lower or midaortic nodes are positive, nodes up to T11 are encompassed. If a lymphangiogram is not available, any decision to irradiate more than pelvic lymph nodes must be based on the probabilities expressed in Table 17-2. Extensions of the treated volume to encompass para-aortic lymph nodes rarely need to be wider than 8 cm. Ideally, when para-aortic nodes are to be irradiated, one half to two thirds of the dose can be given through large anterior and posterior spade-shaped ports. These avoid the risk of overlap or of an underirradiated gap. The remainder of the dose to the para-aortic nodes can be given through lateral or rotating beams. Regardless of the dose planned for the primary lesion and pelvic nodes, the dose to the para-aortic nodes should seldom exceed 5000 rad in 5 weeks. Higher doses with considerably greater fractionation and sharply reduced ports can be used to boost total doses to larger metastases. More specific guidelines are yet to be defined. The remainder of the dose to the pelvic volume can be given by a box technique.

The use of external irradiation alone in the treatment of advanced carcinoma of the cervix has been discussed by several authors (Baclesse; Fletcher and associates, 1956). As has been seen, however, the cervix and corpus definitely tolerate higher doses than do other pelvic structures. A dose distribution as achieved with external irradiation and intracavitary radium or external irradiation with either transvaginal irradiation or a boosting dose from a reduced external beam technique takes advantage of these differences in tolerance in those groups of patients cited previously. The use of external pelvic irradiation alone is therefore reserved for those advanced cancers in which the centrally located portion of the disease is but a fraction of the total problem or for those patients to whom, for one reason or another, neither radium nor transvaginal irradiation can be given. In such circumstances there are two alternatives if cure is the aim of treatment. For locally advanced cancers, a whole pelvis dose of 6000 to 7000 rad is given. Reduced fields may be used after 5000 rad. The irradiation of choice for the more limited cancers consists of a whole pelvis dose of 5000 to 5500 rad in 5 to 6 weeks followed by a small-port rotational technique bringing the dose to the uterus, the vault, and paracervical tissues to 7000 rad in about 8 weeks.

The possibilities of a volume implant using interstitial needles in the parametrium are severely limited, particularly when viewed with a knowledge of Paterson and Parker rules and the size and shape of the volume of potential spread. Efforts to systematically implant the volume using elaborate means for radium or ^{60}Co needle placement or, more recently, afterloading techniques using ^{192}Ir have been periodically revived and abandoned because of increased complications with no increase in cure rates.

Chemotherapy

Perhaps the most encouraging recent finding in the care of patients with Stages III and IV cancer of the cervix limited to the pelvis is the fact that hydroxyurea administered during external pelvic irradiation seems to increase the incidence of complete tumor regression, increase length of tumor-free survival, and indeed increase the probability of survival (Hreshchyshyn and associates). The toxicity of the drug seems acceptable. We anticipate rapid adoption of this combination treatment for patients with locally advanced disease.

Transvaginal irradiation

Transvaginal irradiation alone has few, if any, indications in the treatment of carcinoma of the cervix. Only the most limited lesions can be completely encompassed by transvaginal cones. As was discussed previously, the clinical impression of tumor extent is frequently inaccurate. This uncertainty, coupled with the fact that most lesions cannot be encompassed by the transvaginal cone, demands that external irradiation complement the internal irradiation. With transvaginal irradiation, the centrally located segment of tissue can be irradiated with little risk of overirradiating the rectum and bladder. Vigorous external irradiation is necessary to control the disease beyond the limits of the transvaginal cone. The external irradiation should be given first for reasons previously listed. Transvaginal irradiation is then given using a cone transparent to x rays and of maximum tolerated diameter (del Regato, 1952; Caulk). A short target-cervix distance (about 25 cm) will assure a maximum divergence of rays through the walls of the cone and a good dose to the vaginal walls. This divergence of the rays through the walls of the cone is highly desirable if there is extension of the cancer onto the vaginal walls. However, as the peripheral portion of this small beam passes through the cone wall and through the tissues, its percentage depth dose decreases rather rapidly. One should therefore not assume that any tumor outside that included within the opening of the cone is receiving the stated dose. Usually at the level of the cervix a 4 cm circle of adequate irradiation can be achieved with a cone 4 cm in diameter. Radiations produced at 110 to 280 kv are satisfactory. Fractionation over 2 weeks with daily doses of 350 to 400 rad (mucosa) to a total of 3500 to 4000 rad plus the contributions from external irradiation will raise the midline dose to a maximum tolerated level in most patients.

Surgery for carcinoma of the cervix

It is evident from the previous discussion that *simple* hysterectomy alone has little place in the treatment of invasive carcinoma of the cervix. On microscopic examination of the surgical specimen, about 60% of all patients with Stage I carcinoma have been reported as showing occult paracervical extension (Kottmeier, 1953). This figure may be too high, but the argument against simple hysterectomy is obvious. A simple total hysterectomy alone in patients with carcinoma of the cervix will be followed by frequent recurrence—a fact regretfully learned by many surgeons inexperienced with this disease. Such paracervical disease demands that more than the uterus and vaginal cuff be removed. On the other hand, the proximity of paracervical extension to the ureter, and in the more advanced carcinomas the proximity to the bladder and rectum, may demand the removal of these organs if a curative cancer operation is to be performed. Thus the ureteral-sparing radical hysterectomy at best can be successfully applied only to selected patients with limited disease.

Although the path of potential spread must be entered when the ureter is spared, the ureter poses no problem for modern radiotherapeutic procedures. The often mentioned advantages of hysterectomy over irradiation for selected patients with limited lesions follow.

1. Ovarian function is preserved in young women. (Following radiation therapy, hormones can be prescribed to accomplish most of the benefits of ovarian preservation.)

2. The vagina will not be stenosed by the colpostats. (The vagina will, however, be shortened significantly if an adequate cuff is resected.)

3. Radioresistant cancers will be removed. (The incidence of postirradiation local recurrence in the limited stages is less than 3% when modern techniques are used. This figure is probably very close to the incidence of postoperative recurrence in comparable limited stages.)

4. Radiation-induced bowel and bladder injury will not be a problem. (The operative mortality and morbidity, that is, ureteral, bladder, and bowel dysfunction, are, on balance, twice that produced by radiation therapy [Di Saia and associates].)

In summary, no convincing randomized clinical trial using modern concepts is available to assist us in identifying which *individual* patient with limited disease might profit more from one modality than the other. However, it is now the consensus that if the surgeon selects favorable lesions in favorable patients (thin and in good general condition), he can obtain control rates equal to those obtained by irradiation of a much wider spectrum of patients. However, the morbidity from surgery tips the balance in favor of radiation therapy for all except the very limited lesion, that is, no more than the occult lesion showing microscopic evidence of invasion or the well-delineated lesion less than 1 cm in diameter.

Carcinoma of the cervical stump

If subtotal hysterectomy has been performed for a benign condition at least 2 years prior to the onset of symptoms leading to the diagnosis of carcinoma of the cervix, we assume that the surgery was not performed in the presence of the carcinoma. These patients are diagnosed as having carcinoma of the true cervical stump. On the other hand, if less than 2 years has elapsed, we are justified in assuming that the subtotal hysterectomy was performed in the presence of carcinoma of the cervix. These we call *coincident cases*. As has been seen for other sites, inadequate surgery usually makes the prognosis worse. This finding is borne out in all published studies of coincident cases; therefore it is important to establish the interval between surgery and onset of symptoms. Some workers (Sala and Leon) have recommended that a 3-year symptom-free interval be used instead of 2 years. This may eliminate a few cases that might otherwise be questionable. The same clinical stages are used in classifying carcinoma of the cervical stump as are used for other carcinomas of the cervix. The same pretreatment studies should be carried out.

TREATMENT. The fact that the corpus is not present eliminates the possibility of inserting a tandem of the usual length. This means that more emphasis must be placed on vaginal radium, transvaginal irradiation, and external irradiation. When radium is to be used, the tandem can rarely be over 2 cm. This offers little more than can be delivered by a midline ovoid placed at the external os. The dose administered by vaginal radium cannot be increased significantly over that usually given vaginally in the uncomplicated case. For these reasons the dose delivered to the parametrium by radium will be less. Furthermore, the dose to the depth of the canal of the stump will often be inadequate if only vaginal radium can be used.

Usually the stump can be included in a beam directed transvaginally. The risk of missing fundal extension does not exist in these cases. The rectum and bladder can, if indicated, be readily shielded, and external irradiation can be added to bring the dose laterally to the desired level. For these reasons we believe transvaginal irradiation is particularly useful in these cases. The technique and doses recommended are similar to those described previously. As previously described, the transvaginal irradiation should be given after vigorous whole pelvis irradiation. With the megavoltage beams, we use the four-port box technique. The whole pelvis is included in each port. A dose of 4000 to 6000 rad midpelvis in 6 weeks is followed by 3000 to 4000 rad given transvaginally. For comparable clinical stages, the sizes of the ports for external pelvic irradiation are the same for cancer of the stump and the intact uterus. The absence of the corpus does not justify using a smaller port. For a patient with a Stage I lesion 2 to 3 cm in diameter, a whole pelvis dose of 4000 to 4500 rad in 4 weeks should be followed by a cervical dose by transvaginal irradiation of 4000 rad in 10 days. For a patient with a Stage III lesion extending inferiorly along the vaginal wall and laterally into the parametrium, a whole pelvis dose of 6000 rad in 6 to 7 weeks should be followed by a transvaginal dose of 3000 to 4000 rad in 10 days. Although there may be some concern that the vaginal mucosa deep to the plastic cone is underdosed, this has not been experienced clinically. In fact the mucosal reaction is invariably intense, and failure, when it occurs, is rarely in the vault or vagina.

PROGNOSIS AND RESULTS. The 5-year survival rate of patients treated for carcinoma of the true cervical stump is approximately the same as for the usual carcinoma of the cervix (Table 17-16). Sala and Leon reported a 90% 5-year survival for Stage I, 35% for Stage II, 49% for Stage III, and 14% for Stage IV. In contrast, if

Table 17-16. Comparison of survival rates obtained by treating cancer of the cervix of the intact uterus and that of the cervical stump*

Clinical stage	1705 patients treated for cancer of intact uterus: 5-year survival (%)	189 patients treated for cancer of cervical stump: 5-year survival (%)
I	91.5	97.0
IIa	83.5	93.0
IIb	66.5	67.0
IIIa	45.0	61.0
IIIb	36.0	32.0
IV	14.0	0

*Modified from Fletcher, G. H.: Am. J. Roentgenol. **111**:225-242, 1971.

the subtotal hysterectomy was performed less than 2 years before the onset of symptoms of recurrence, the control rate is greatly decreased. Fricke and Decker reported only four of thirteen such patients living at 5 years. In our own group, if the operation was performed at the time cancer was present and if irradiation was delayed until recurrence was clinically obvious, only two out of forty-two patients were living after 5 years. More recently Deutsch and Parsons reported six of thirty-eight patients were living and well 2.5 years after irradiation of clinically palpable postoperative local recurrences.

To eliminate carcinoma of the true stump entirely, it is now the policy to perform a total hysterectomy instead of a supracervical hysterectomy for selected benign diseases of the fundus. This policy is fully justified in the light of the low morbidity and mortality after total hysterectomy. The steps necessary to eliminate coincident cases are obvious. The error is usually a result of the surgeon being unable to conceive that two diseases might exist in the presence of vaginal bleeding.

A similar although less serious situation is created in the patient who has a simple hysterectomy for a benign process, only to have a coincident carcinoma of the cervix discovered in the resected specimen. To withhold irradiation until a palpable recurrence develops is inviting disaster. Once palpable recurrence develops, cure is almost impossible. On the other hand, vigorous irradiation soon after hysterectomy produces sufficiently good results to recommend such irradiation as a routine precautionary procedure. Full cancerocidal doses are given. External pelvic irradiation coupled with transvaginal irradiation is used. Durrance (1968) showed that such a policy yields a high proportion of cured patients. Eleven of eleven patients treated were living and well at 3 years, and nine of nine patients at 5 years when there was microscopic evidence of transection of cancer. It should be remembered that after total hysterectomy the small or large bowel may be in direct contact with the vaginal vault. The depth dose from transvaginal irradiation to the bowel may be considerable. With this knowledge, we limit the dose to the vault from transvaginal irradiation to 3000 rad in 10 days. The dose from external pelvic irradiation is the same as previously outlined.

Carcinoma of the cervix during pregnancy

Carcinoma of the cervix is found in one of 2500 deliveries. Pregnancy is found in 1% to 2% of all patients diagnosed as having carcinoma of the cervix. Although it is often difficult to conceive of the two different conditions being present at one time, it appears that there is no significant delay in making the diagnosis of cancer. Indeed, pregnancy itself prompts the physician to take a smear and make an adequate pelvic examination. As a result, the proportion of cases now appearing in the earlier stages is greater than that in series of nonpregnant women. Thus Thompson and associates reported that thirty-five of forty-two patients presented with Stage I lesions. Twenty one of these thirty-five had Stage Ia and fourteen had Stage Ib. Five of the forty-two had Stage II, and only two had Stage III lesions. As we shall see, this striking shift toward the limited clinical stages influences the common modality of management. Furthermore, as the time from conception lengthens, the proportion of advanced clinical stages increases. This trend continues up to 6 months postpartum (Creasman and associates). The average age of pregnant patients with carcinoma of the cervix is 10 to 15 years younger than nonpregnant ones.

When carcinoma of the cervix and pregnancy occur together, there is not only the problem of curing the mother, but also that of saving the child. The problems vary with both the stage of pregnancy and the clinical stage of the carcinoma. Carcinoma of the cervix has classically been regarded as producing a harmful effect on the course of pregnancy, on cervical dilation during labor, and on healing during the postpartum period. Some workers believe that pregnancy accelerates the growth of carcinoma of the cervix. However, this belief is poorly substantiated (Waldrop and Palmer). Results now verify that, stage for stage, prognosis is about the same. Once the diagnosis of microscopically invasive carcinoma is made and a decision is made to proceed with definitive treatment, the work-up of the patient should be as for a nonpregnant patient. However, treatment has been deferred for a few selected patients with clinically occult invasive carcinoma in which the depth of invasion as measured on the conization specimen does not exceed 3 mm. Although it is difficult to see how this sequence can be followed without serious risks, it has been used by Thompson and associates in seven patients with no deaths.

If a clinically obvious invasive carcinoma of the cervix is diagnosed during the first trimester of pregnancy, the chances of the mother delivering a viable baby are remote. Such patients are usually treated as if they were not pregnant. Thus, if the disease is limited Stage I, either irradiation or surgery may be considered. If irradiation is to be used, it is generally wise to start treatment with external irradiation. With the daily doses mentioned previously, abortion will occur in 4 to 6 weeks. If it should not occur, the pregnancy must be interrupted surgically. In early pregnancy this can be done vaginally. The treatment of the carcinoma should proceed just as if there had been no pregnancy, starting with external pelvic irradiation to a dose of 4000 rad in 4 weeks. Reevaluation at that point is necessary to decide if involution is sufficient to proceed with radium implantation.

Table 17-17. Carcinoma of the cervix coincident with pregnancy of at least 7 months' duration (comparison of patient survival after vaginal delivery and after cesarean section)*

	Vaginal		Abdominal	
Stage	Number of patients treated	5-year survival (%)	Number of patients treated	5-year survival (%)
I	47	70.2	8	75.0
II	48	43.8	7	0
III	40	20.0	12	25.0
IV	11	15.3	7	0
TOTAL	148	43.3	34	26.5

*Modified from Waldrop, G. M., and Palmer, J. P.: Am. J. Obstet. Gynecol. **86:**202-212, 1963.

Table 17-18. Carcinoma of the cervix coincident with pregnancy (comparison of survival rates obtained by irradiation)*

	Pregnant		Nonpregnant	
Stage	Number of patients treated	5-year survival (%)	Number of patients treated	5-year survival (%)
I	54	70.4	572	66.9
II	56	39.3	1303	46.5
III	52	21.2	1411	28.1
IV	20	10.0	1167	4.9
TOTAL	182	40.1	4452	32.4

*Modified from Waldrop, G. M., and Palmer, J. P.: Am. J. Obstet. Gynecol. **86:**202-212, 1963. Included are patients who received some treatment elsewhere.

Table 17-19. Two-year absolute tumor-free survival rate according to time of diagnosis*

	Two-year tumor-free survival rate according to clinical stage	
Time of diagnosis	I	II
Trimester of pregnancy		
1	9/9	4/5
2	8/8	8/9
3	5/5	1/2
TOTAL	22/22 (100%)	13/16 (81%)
Postpartum		
0-3	14/16	9/15
4-6	7/9	5/6
TOTAL	21/25 (84%)	14/21 (67%)

*From Creasman, W. T., Rutledge, F. J., and Fletcher, G. H.: Obstet. Gynecol. **36:**495-501, 1970.

If the carcinoma is diagnosed in the second trimester of pregnancy, hysterotomy should be carried out, and this should be followed by treatment as outlined before.

If the lesion is diagnosed in the last trimester of pregnancy and it is early or moderately advanced, treatment should be delayed until a viable baby can be delivered by cesarean operation. Then treatment can proceed as before. If the carcinoma is advanced, there is still a temptation to defer therapy until a viable baby can be obtained by cesarean operation. This is not always possible. Bleeding may be severe. The use of vaginal radium has been advocated for growth restraint, but about 20% of the viable babies delivered after such therapy will show damage to the head. We have not used this technique and we do not recommend it. At this stage of pregnancy, if a well and viable baby is insisted on, treatment must be deferred.

Waldrop and Palmer supported the practice of vaginal delivery in these patients (Table 17-17). Although most clinics will probably continue to deliver by cesarean section, the excellent results cited in Table 17-17 justify a consideration of vaginal delivery. Postpartum whole pelvis irradiation can be started 10 days to 2 weeks after delivery. Ports should include the corpus and can be decreased as the uterus shrinks. Doses are the same as those recommended for nonpregnant patients.

If the carcinoma is diagnosed at term, cesarean operation should be performed immediately, and irradiation should be carried out as indicated previously. Surgery has the same indications and contraindications as for nonpregnant patients, except that the abdomen must be opened for the cesarean section and the temptation to proceed with hysterectomy is greater. Surgery has a predominant role in the treatment of many of these patients with limited disease.

The control rates obtained by hysterectomy for the Stage Ia and Ib lesions are good. These patients are, of course, young and usually in good general physical condition, and they tolerate the surgery. Results reported by Sall and associates and Thompson and associates argue for the consideration of hysterectomy for very limited lesions. However, the presence of extracervical spread and metastases to regional lymph nodes was reported by Thompson and associates. We, therefore, use the same indications for radiation therapy in the clinically obvious cancers in recently pregnant patients as we use in the nonpregnant patients.

PROGNOSIS AND RESULTS. The rich vascular bed present in the pregnant uterus is reported to contribute to the rapid growth of carcinoma of the cervix. We doubt that this is true. In contrast to the usual poorer prognosis sometimes reported in these patients, the data in Table 17-18, taken from Palmer's data, and Table 17-19 from Creasman suggest that this is not true. Similar good results have been reported by Lucci. Fetal mortality depends on the stage of pregnancy, but the mortality rate will be considerable in all babies even if the given policies are adopted.

Summary

The cervix, corpus, and paracervical tissues tolerate high doses of radiations. The primary lesion of carcinoma of the cervix is moderately radiosensitive. This combination enables the radiation oncologist to control a high proportion of carcinomas of the cervix. There is indisputable evidence that metastases in pelvic and retroperitoneal nodes can be controlled by irradiation in a significant proportion of patients. The exact percentage is not established, and the effect of such control on long-term survival is even less well understood. This does not imply, however, that lymphadenectomy with or without radical hysterectomy is superior.

The type of irradiation must be tailored to the clinical extent and the associated circumstances (pregnancy, cervical stump, narrow or large vagina, and so forth), and no single method is best in all circumstances.

When intracavitary techniques are to be used, we prefer the flexibility of an afterloading technique, using a Manchester-type distribution. However, it is possible to produce good results with other intracavitary techniques when they are applied with an appreciation of all factors involved.

External irradiation is the most important single technique in the control of lesions in the advanced stages. It is the most practical and effective way of bringing the dose in the lateral part of the pelvis to the desired level.

Results of irradiation are good and have continued to improve as limits and aims have been defined.

REFERENCES

Averette, H. E., Dudan, R. C., and Ford, J. H., Jr.: Exploratory celiotomy for surgical staging of cervical cancer, Am. J. Obstet. Gynecol. 113: 1090-1096, 1972.

Baclesse, F.: Roentgen therapy in the treatment of advanced cervico-uterine cancer, including extensive postoperative recurrences, Am. J. Roentgenol. 63:252-254, 1950.

Baud, J.: Results of radiotherapy in 124 epithelioma cases of stump of the cervix, treated from 1919 to 1944 at the Curie Foundation, J. Fac. Radiologists 3:203-207, 1952.

Bickel, W. H., Childs, D. S., and Poretta, C. M.: Postirradiation fractures of the femoral neck, J.A.M.A. 175:204-212, 1961.

Bosch, A., and Marcial, V. A.: Evaluation of the time interval between external irradiation and intracavitary curietherapy in carcinoma of the uterine cervix: influence on curability, Radiology 88:563-567, 1967.

Bourne, R. G., and Mead, K. W.: A proposed method of selecting patients with carcinoma of the cervix for radiotherapy or surgery, Radiology 90:139-141, 1968.

Brown, W. E., Meschan, I., Kerekes, E., and Sadler, J. M.: Effect of radiation on metastatic pelvic lymph node involvement in carcinoma of the cervix, Am. J. Obstet. Gynecol. 62:871-889, 1951.

Brunschwig, A.: The surgical treatment of cancer of the cervix State I and II, Am. J. Roentgenol. 102: 147-151, 1968.

Caulk, R. M.: Review of seventeen years' experience with transvaginal roentgen therapy in cervical cancer, Am. J. Roentgenol. 76:965-970, 1956.

Chau, P. M., Fletcher, G. H., Rutledge, F. N., and Dodd, G. D.: Complications in high dose whole pelvis irradiation in femoral pelvic cancer, Am. J. Roentgenol. 87:22-40, 1962.

Cole, M. P.: Radiotherapy for cervical cancer—radium. In Easson, E. C.: Cancer of the uterine cervix, Philadelphia, 1973, W. B. Saunders Co.

Cole, M. P. Radiotherapy for cervical cancer—x-rays. In Easson, E. C.: Cancer of the uterine cervix, Philadelphia, 1973, W. B. Saunders Co.

Corscaden, J. A.: Gynecologic cancer, Baltimore, 1956, The Williams & Wilkins Co.

Creasman, W. T., Rutledge, F. N., and Fletcher, G. H.: Carcinoma of the cervix associated with pregnancy, Obstet. Gynecol. 36:495-501, 1970.

Cuccia, C. A., and Bloedorn, F. G.: Treatment of primary adenocarcinoma of the cervix, Am. J. Roentgenol. 99:371-375, 1967.

Dearing, R.: Study of renal tract in carcinoma of cervix, Am. J. Obstet. Gynecol. 60:165-174, 1953.

del Regato, J. A.: The treatment of carcinoma of the cervix, Radiology 46:579-582, 1946.

del Regato, J. A.: The role of roentgen therapy in the treatment of cancer of the cervix uteri, Am. J. Roentgenol. 68:63-66, 1952.

del Regato, J. A.: Comparative results of surgery and radiotherapy in carcinoma of the cervix, Lancet 77:454-457, 1957.

del Regato, J. A.: Cancer of the female genital organs (cancer of the cervix). In del Regato, J. A., and Spjut, H. T.: Ackerman and del Regato's cancer: diagnosis, treatment, and prognosis, ed. 5, St. Louis, 1977, The C. V. Mosby Co.

Deutsch, M., and Parsons, J. A.: Radiotherapy for carcinoma of the cervix recurrent after surgery, Cancer 34:2051-2055, 1974.

Di Saia, P. J., Morrow, C. P., and Townsend, D. E.: Synopsis of gynecologic oncology, New York, 1975, John Wiley & Sons, Inc.

Durrance, F. Y.: Radiotherapy following simple hysterectomy in patients with Stage I and II carcinoma of the cervix, Am. J. Roentgenol. 102: 165-169, 1968.

Durrance, F. Y., Fletcher, G. H., and Rutledge, F. N.: Analysis of central recurrent disease in Stages I and II squamous cell carcinomas of the cervix on intact uterus, Am. J. Roentgenol. 106: 831-838, 1969.

Easson, E. C.: A comprehensive approach to cervical cancer, Clin. Radiol. 18:337-348, 1967.

Emge, L. A.: The influence of pregnancy on tumor growth, Am. J. Obstet. Gynecol. 28:682-697, 1934.

Finger, J. G., and Post, M.: Spontaneous femoral neck fracture following pelvic irradiation, Arch. Surg. 81:545-552, 1960.

Fletcher, G. H., Shalek, R. J., Wall, J. A., and Bloedorn, F. G.: A physical approach to the design of applicator in radium therapy of carcinoma of the cervix, Am. J. Roentgenol. 68:935-947, 1952.

Fletcher, G. H., Wall, J. A., Bloedorn, F. G., Shalek, R. J., and Wootton, P.: Direct measurements and isodose calculations in radium therapy of carcinoma of the cervix, Radiology 61:885-901, 1953.

Fletcher, G. H., and Calderon, R.: Positioning of pelvic portals for external irradiation in carcinoma of the uterine cervix, Radiology 67:359-370, 1956.

Fletcher, G. H., Brown, T. C., and Rutledge, F. N.: Clinical significance of rectal and bladder dose measurements in radium therapy of cancer of the uterine cervix, Am. J. Roentgenol. 79:421-450, 1958.

Fletcher, G. H., Rutledge, F. N., and Chau, P. M.: Policies of treatment in cancer of the cervix uteri, Am. J. Roentgenol. 87:6-21, 1962.

Fletcher, G. H.: Cancer of the uterine cervix, Am. J. Roentgenol. 111:225-242, 1971.

Fricke, R. E., and Decker, D. G.: Late results of radiation therapy for cancer of the cervical stump, Am. J. Roentgenol. 79:32-35, 1958.

Friedman, N. B.: Pathogenesis of intestinal ulcers following irradiation, Arch. Pathol. 59:2-4, 1955.

Garcia, M.: Further observation on tissue dosage in cancer of the cervix uteri, Am. J. Roentgenol. 73:35-58, 1955.

Gordon, H. W., McMahon, N. J., Agliozzo, C. M., Rao, P. R., and Rogers, J.: Adenoid cystic (cylindromatous) carcinoma of the uterine cervix, Am. J. Clin. Pathol. 58:51-57, 1972.

Graham, R. M.: Is cytology a reliable prognosticator of radiosensitivity? J.A.M.A. 193:825, 1965.

Gusberg, S. B., Fish, S. A., and Wang, Y.: The growth pattern of cervical cancer, Obstet. Gynecol. 2:557-561, 1953.

Gusberg, S. B.: Choice of treatment for cervix cancer, J.A.M.A. 193:826, 1965.

Harris, W., and Silverstone, S. M.: Radiation therapy for cancer of the cervix with an analysis of the fundamental dosimetry, J. Mt. Sinai Hosp., N.Y. 14:369-382, 1947.

Hayden, G. E.: Carcinoma of the cervix associated with pregnancy, Am. J. Obstet. Gynecol. 71: 780-789, 1956.

Heyman, J.: Staging in carcinoma of the uterine cervix: a reply of Dr. del Regato, Am. J. Roentgenol. 70:840-841, 1953.

Heyman, J.: Annual report of results of radiotherapy, vol. 9, Stockholm, 1954, P. A. Norstedt, & Söner.

Hirst, J. C.: Cancer of the cervix during pregnancy, Am. J. Obstet. Gynecol. 61:860-871, 1951.

Hreshchyshyn, M. M., Aron, B. S., Boronow, R. C., Franklin, E. W., and Shingleton, H. M.: Hydroxyurea or placebo combined with radiation to treat Stages III B and IV cervical cancer confined to the pelvis, Int. J. Radiat. Oncol. Biol. Phys. 5:317-322, 1979.

Iliya, F. A., O'Leary, J. A., and Frick, H. C.: Prognostic significance of ureteral obstruction in carcinoma of the cervix, Cancer 19:689-690, 1966.

Jampolis, S., Andras, J., and Fletcher, G. H.: Analysis of sites and causes of failure of irradiation in invasive squamous cell carcinoma of the intact uterine cervix, Radiology 115:681-685, 1975.

Javert, C. T.: The lymph nodes and lymph channels of the pelvis. In Meigs, J. V., editor: Surgical treatment of cancer of the cervix, New York, 1954, Grune & Stratton, Inc.

Kademian, M. T., and Bosch, A.: Is staging laparotomy in cervical cancer justifiable? Int. J. Radiat. Oncol. Biol. Phys. 2:1235-1238, 1977.

Kagan, A. R., Di Saia, P. J., Woolin, M., Nussbaum, H., and Tawa, K.: The narrow vagina, the antecedent for irradiation injury, Gynecol. Oncol. 4:291-298, 1976.

Keys, H., and Park, R. C.: Treatment and survival of patients with cancer of the cervix and nodal metastasis, Int. J. Radiat. Oncol. Biol. Phys. **1:** 1091-1097, 1976.

Kline, J. C., Buchler, D. A., Boone, M. L., Peckham, B. M., and Carr, W. F.: The relationship of reactions to complications in radiation therapy of cancer of the cervix, Radiology **105:**413-416, 1972.

Kottmeier, H. L.: Studies of the dosage distribution in the pelvis in radium treatment of carcinoma of the uterine cervix according to the Stockholm method, J. Fac. Radiologists **2:**312-319, 1951.

Kottmeier, H. L.: Carcinoma of the female genitalia, Baltimore, 1953, The Williams & Wilkins Co.

Kottmeier, H. L.: The places of radiation therapy and of surgery in the treatment of uterine cancer, Am. J. Obstet. Gynecol. **62:**737-751, 1955.

Kottmeier, H. L.: Complications following radiation therapy in carcinoma of the cervix, Am. J. Obstet. Gynecol. **88:**854-866, 1964.

Lee, K. H., Kagan, A. H., Nussbaum, H., Wollin, M., Winkley, J. H., and Norman, A.: Analysis of dose, dose-rate and treatment time in the production of injuries by radium treatment for cancer of the uterine cervix, Br. J. Radiol. **49:**430-440, 1976.

Lepanto, P., Littman, P., Mikuta, J., Davis, L., and Celebre, J.: Treatment of para-aortic nodes in carcinoma of the cervix, Cancer **35:**1510-1513, 1975.

Leucutia, T.: The question of ureteral obstruction by irradiation, Am. J. Roentgenol. **53:**291-295, 1945.

Llusia, J. B., Ortiz, F. N., Gimenez-Tebar, V., and Crespo, J. Z.: Effect of radiotherapy of tumor-bearing lymph nodes in carcinoma of the cervix uteri, Am. J. Obstet. Gynecol. **84:**508-514, 1962.

Lucci, J. A.: Carcinoma of the cervix and pregnancy: an analysis of 111 cases. In M. D. Anderson Hospital Report: carcinoma of the uterine cervix, endometrium, and ovary, Chicago, 1962, Year Book Medical Publishers, Inc.

McDuff, H. C., Jr., Carney, W. I., and Waterman, G. W.: Carcinoma of cervix and pregnancy, Obstet. Gynecol. **8:**196-202, 1956.

Martin, C. L., and Rogers, F. T.: The effect of irradiation on the ureter, Am. J. Roentgenol. **16:** 215-218, 1926.

Meigs, J. V.: Cancer of the cervix, an appraisal, Am. J. Obstet. Gynecol. **72:**467-478, 1956.

Morton, D. G., Lagasse, L. D., Moore, J. G., Jacobs, M., and Amromin, G. D.: Pelvic lymphadenectomy following radiation in cervical carcinoma, Am. J. Obstet. Gynecol. **88:**932-938, 1964.

Nolan, J. F., Costolow, W. E., and DuSault, L.:

Radium treatment of carcinoma of the cervix uteri, Radiology **54:**821-831, 1950.

Palmer, J. P.: Quoted in Eastman, N. J.: Williams obstetrics, New York, 1956, Appleton-Century-Crofts.

Paterson, R.: Radiotherapy in cancer of the cervix, Acta Radiol., suppl. 116, pp. 395-404, 1954.

Paterson, R., and Russell, M. H.: Clinical trials in malignant disease. VI. Cancer of the cervix uteri: is x-ray therapy more effective given before or after radium? Clin. Radiol. **13:**313-315, 1962.

Paterson, R., and Russell, M. H.: Clinical trials in malignant disease. VII. Cancer of the cervix uteri, evaluation of adjuvant x-ray therapy in Stages I and II, Clin. Radiol. **14:**17-19, 1963.

Perez, C. A., Zivnuska, F., askin, F., Kumar, B., Camel, H. M., and Powers, W. E.: Prognostic significance of endometrial extension from primary carcinoma of the uterine cervix, Cancer **34:** 1493-1504, 1975.

Piver, M. S., Wallace, S., and Castro, J. R.: The accuracy of lymphangiography in carcinoma of the uterine cervix, Am. J. Roentgenol. **111:**278-283, 1971.

Plentl, A. A., and Friedman, E. A.: Lymphatic system of the female genitalia, Philadelphia, 1971, W. B. Saunders Co.

Rhamy, R. K., and Stander, R. W.: Postradiation in ureteral stricture, Surg. Gynecol. Obstet. **113:** 615-622, 1961.

Rotman, M., John, M. J., Moon, S. H., Choi, K. N., et al.: Limitations of adjunctive surgery in carcinoma of the cervix, Int. J. Radiat. Oncol. Biol. Phys. **5:**327-329, 1979.

Rutledge, F. N., and Fletcher, G. H.: Transperitoneal pelvic lymphadenectomy following supervoltage irradiation for squamous cell carcinoma of cervix, Am. J. Obstet. Gynecol. **76:**321-324, 1958.

Rutledge, F. N., Fletcher, G. H., and MacDonald, E. J.: Pelvic lymphadenectomy as an adjunct to radiation therapy in treatment for cancer of the cervix, Am. J. Roentgenol. **93:**607-614, 1965.

Rutledge, F. N., Gutierrez, A. G., and Fletcher, G. H.: Management of Stage I and II adenocarcinomas of the uterine cervix on intact uterus, Am. J. Roentgenol. **102:**161-164, 1968.

Sala, J. N., Gleason, J. A., and Spratt, J. S.: Adenocarcinoma of the cervix uteri: report of 104 cases, Mo. Med. **59:**1168-1173, 1962.

Sala, J. N., and Leon, A. D.: Treatment of carcinoma of the cervical stump, Radiology **81:**300-306, 1963.

Sall, S., Rini, S., and Pineda, A.: Surgical management of invasive carcinoma of the cervix in pregnancy, Obstet. Gynecol. **118:**1-5, 1974.

Sherman, A. I., Bonebrake, M., and Allen, W. M.:

Application of radioactive colloidal gold in the treatment of pelvic cancer, Am. J. Roentgenol. **66**:624-638, 1951.

Sherman, A. I., and Camel, H. M.: A review of diagnosis, treatment and complications for carcinoma of the cervix uteri, Am. J. Obstet. Gynecol. **89**:439-453, 1964.

Silberstein, A. B., Aron, B. S., and Alexander, L. L.: Para-aortic lymph node irradiation in cervical carcinoma, Radiology **95**:181-184, 1970.

Silverstone, S. M., and Melamed, J. L.: Effective irradiation with radium for cancer of the cervix, Radiology **69**:360-371, 1957.

Slater, J. M., and Fletcher, G. H.: Ureteral strictures after radiation therapy for carcinoma of the uterine cervix, Am. J. Roentgenol. **111**:269-272, 1971.

Stephenson, W. H., and Cohen, B.: Post-irradiation fractures of the neck of the femur, J. Bone Joint Surg. **38B**:830-845, 1956.

Stockbine, M. F., Hancock, J. E., and Fletcher, G. H.: Complications in 831 patients with squamous cell carcinoma of the intact cervix treated with 3,000 rads or more whole pelvis irradiation, Am. J. Roentgenol. **108**:293-304, 1970.

Sudarsnam, A., Charyulu, K., Belinson, J., Averette, H., et al.: Influence of exploratory celiotomy on the management of carcinoma of the cervix, Cancer **41**:1049-1053, 1978.

Tateishi, R., Wada, A., Hayakawa, K., Hengo, J., Ishii, S., and Terakawa, N.: Argyrophil cell carcinomas (apudomas) of the uterine cervix, Virchows Arch. a (Pathol. Anat.) **366**:257-274, 1975.

Tawil, E., and Belanger, R.: Prognostic value of the lymphangiogram in carcinoma of the uterine cervix, Radiology **109**:597-599, 1973.

Taylor, H. C.: Controversial points in the treatment of carcinoma of the cervix, Cancer **5**:435-441, 1952.

Ter-Pogossian, M., Sherman, A. I., and Arneson, A. N.: An expanding fixed tandem-ovoids colpostat for the treatment of carcinoma of the cervix, Am. J. Obstet. Gynecol. **64**:937-941, 1952.

Ter-Pogossian, M., and Sherman, A. I.: Radiation dosimetry in the treatment of carcinoma of the cervix uteri by intraperitoneal radioactive gold and radium, Am. J. Roentgenol. **74**:116-122, 1955.

Thomas, W. L., Carter, B., and Parker, R. T.: Radical panhysterectomy (Wertheim) and radical pelvic lymphadenectomy; a preliminary report of 75 operations, South. Med. J. **41**:895-902, 1948.

Thompson, J. D., Caputo, T. A., Franklin, E. W., and Dale, E.: The surgical management of invasive cancer of the cervix in pregnancy, Am. J. Obstet. Gynecol. **121**:853-863, 1975.

Tod, M. C.: Optimum dosage in treatment of carcinoma of uterine cervix by radiation, Br. J. Radiol. **14**:23-29, 1941.

Tod, M. C., and Meredith, W. J.: Treatment of cancer of the cervix uteri—a revised "Manchester method," Br. J. Radiol. **26**:252-257, 1953.

Todd, T. F.: Rectal ulceration following irradiation treatment of carcinoma of the cervix uteri, Surg. Gynecol. Obstet. **67**:617-631, 1938.

Twombly, G. H., and Taylor, H. C.: The treatment of cancer of the cervix uteri: a comparison of radiation therapy and radical surgery, Am. J. Roentgenol. **71**:501-508, 1954.

Vongtama, V., Piver, S. M., Yoshiaki, T., Barlow, J. J., and Webster, J.: Para-aortic node irradiation in carcinomas, Cancer **34**:169-174, 1974.

Waldrop, G. M., and Palmer, J. P.: Carcinoma of the cervix associated with pregnancy, Am. J. Obstet. Gynecol. **86**:202-212, 1963.

Way, S.: Response to irradiation of carcinoma of the cervix at the primary and secondary sites, Br. J. Radiol. **27**:651-655, 1954.

Weiner, S., and Wizenberg, M. J.: Treatment of primary adenocarcinoma of the cervix, Cancer **35**:1514-1516, 1975.

Werner, P., and Sederl, J.: Die Wertheimsche radikal Operation bei Carcinoma colli uteri, Wien and Innsbruck, 1952, Urban & Schwarzenberg. Quoted in Graham, J. B., and Graham, R. M.: The curability of regional lymph node metastases in cancer of the uterine cervix, Surg. Gynecol. Obstet. **100**:149-155, 1955.

Wildermuth, O., and Melhorn, G. I.: The management of adenocarcinoma of the cervix, Am. J. Roentgenol. **89**:78-83, 1963.

Zeitz, von H.: Positive Drusenbefunde bei der Wertheimschen Radikaloperation, Geburtsh. Frauenheilk **12**:804-809, 1952.

Zerne, R. M., and Morris, J. M.: Prognostic significance of cytologic response in radiation of gynecologic cancer, Obstet. Gynecol. **19**:145-155, 1962.

18
The endometrium

RESPONSE OF THE NORMAL UTERINE CORPUS TO IRRADIATION

The response of the uterine corpus to irradiation is similar to that described for the cervix. All of its tissues tolerate high doses of radiations. It is surprising how few changes are found after the high doses delivered during various radium procedures. Radiation necrosis of the surface epithelium may occur at points of high dose, but these are not usually clinically significant. Edema and vascular changes in the submucosa and myometrium that have been described for other organs occur but are not clinically significant. With these high uterine doses, the bowel and bladder, not the uterus, limit the dose. Secondary endometrial changes occur due to irradiation castration, a fact formerly used in the treatment of endometrial hyperplasia. For a discussion of the radiation sensitivity of surrounding organs, see Chapter 17.

As pointed out in Chapter 19, bleeding from the uterus is not peculiar to carcinoma of the endometrium. For this reason, abnormal vaginal bleeding and discharge demand careful evaluation and, frequently, curettage. In some institutions it was formerly the custom in near-menopausal patients with undiagnosed uterine bleeding to perform a dilatation and curettage and then, to avoid anesthetizing the patient a second time, to insert radium immediately. If the curettings showed adenocarcinoma, the radium was used for vigorous preoperative irradiation. If the curettings showed no tumor, the radium was removed after a dose thought sufficient to suppress ovarian activity.

However, this is not a good sequence to follow. If a focal carcinoma of the endometrium should be missed during the curettement, radium in doses used for suppression of ovarian activity may also temporarily suppress the growth of superficial cancer cells. The deeper cancer cells may have spread through the uterine wall by the time bleeding recurs to signal the need for more thorough study. When no cancer is present, the dose to the endometrium is several hundred times greater than that to the ovaries. This excessive endometrial dose is of little or no value in the treatment of endometrial hyperplasia. However, such an endometrial dose is unavoidable if radium is to be used to suppress ovarian activity. By external irradiation the required dose can easily be delivered to the ovaries. With this technique the uterus will get no more than the ovaries. Any adenocarcinoma that might have been missed will continue to bleed, and the necessity for another curettage will be evident. Thus the irradiation will not be responsible for a delay in making the correct diagnosis. Irradiation for this purpose is infrequently indicated in modern gynecology. In our experience cryostat-frozen sections of curettings are easily made, and their accuracy matches that of regular paraffin-embedded tissue. We now recommend that, when warranted, as for example in an occasional patient in whom a second anesthesia might be inadvisable, a quick diagnosis be obtained by this means and appropriate therapy initiated.

Radiation-induced malignant degeneration of uterine tissues undoubtedly occurs just as do such changes in other tissues. These are usually sarcomas but may be epithelial in origin. The incidence of this sequela must be low in view of the number of symptom-free survivors subsequent to irradiation for carcinoma of the cervix. If such a radiation-induced neoplasm is suspected of developing after *high* doses of radiations, it should be approached surgically.

The incidence of carcinoma of the endometrium is increased among those patients who received low-dose intracavitary radium for benign diseases. There is no reason to treat patients with such a history any differently from other patients with similar clinical stages.

CARCINOMA OF THE ENDOMETRIUM

Adenocarcinoma of the endometrium is by far the most common primary malignant tumor of the uterine corpus, and it is now the most common gynecologic cancer. Estrone is suspected of being an important etiologic agent in the increased incidence of this disease. This is true whether it is exogenous as sodium estrone or endogenously converted from androstenedione by the large volume of adipose tissue characteristic of many of these patients (Ziel and Finkle). A high proportion of patients with this cancer are obese, hypertensive, and diabetic. For this reason they are often greater operative risks and in addition demand special radiation therapy techniques to compensate for their large diameters. Adenoacanthoma is a common histologic variant composed of a mixture of apparently benign squamous metaplasia and adenocarcinoma. Such squamous metaplasia as well as mucin production are more commonly observed in the well-differentiated tumors. As far as treatment is concerned, adenoacanthoma is considered a well-differentiated adenocarcinoma. A mixture of adenocarcinoma and squamous cell carcinoma is termed adenosquamous carcinoma of the endometrium. Although Silverberg and associates and Ng and associates reported that this histologic type is more malignant than either adenocarcinoma or adenoacanthoma, Rubin and associates found no such difference in local controls or survivals. Regardless of the arguments relative to prognosis, we treat patients with this diagnosis as if they had high-grade carcinoma of the corpus.

Carcinosarcoma and mixed mesodermal tumors of the uterus are relatively rare, highly malignant neoplasms accounting for from 2% to 5% of all malignant tumors of the uterus. They are composed of epithelial components from the endometrial glands and mesodermal elements from the endometrial stroma. Heterologous components such as cartilage and skeletal muscle may be present in the mixed mesodermal but not in the carcinosarcoma. Inasmuch as no statistical differences in survival and clinicopathologic features have been found between the two groups, these are usually combined. In contrast to carcinoma of the cervix, carcinomas of the endometrium are usually postmenopausal. They may occasionally arise on polyps and may coexist with estrogen-secreting ovarian tumors. The etiologic importance of hyperplasia remains in doubt. The borderline between certain hyperplasias and adenocarcinoma is not clear, and errors in diagnosis on this point will naturally be reflected in survival rates.

The stage classification of carcinoma of the endometrium is based on the size of the uterine cavity, microscopic grade, and the clinical extent of the cancer. The American Joint Committee for Cancer Staging and End Results Reporting incorporated criteria of the International Federation of Gynecology and Obstetrics (FIGO) in the development of an almost identical stage classification.

TNM CLASSIFICATION*

T —Primary tumor

Stage 0	Preinvasive carcinoma (carcinoma in situ) (FIGO Stage 0)
Stage I	Carcinoma confined to the corpus
	Stage Ia The uterine cavity is not enlarged (8 cm or less).†
	Stage Ib The uterine cavity is enlarged (8 cm or more).
	Stage I patients are further subdivided with regard to degree of histologic differentiation into three grades—well-differentiated, differentiated with partly solid areas, and mostly solid or undifferentiated.
Stage II	Carcinoma involving the cervix
Stage III	Carcinoma extending outside the uterus, including spread to vagina, but remaining within the true pelvis
Stage IV	Carcinoma involving the mucosa of the bladder or the rectum or extending beyond the true pelvis (The presence of bullous edema is not sufficient evidence to classify the tumor as Stage IV.)
	Note: Stage IV may be subdivided into:
	Stage IVa Carcinoma involving the bladder or the rectum only and histologically proved
	Stage IVb Carcinoma extending beyond the true pelvis

N—Regional lymph nodes (used to clarify extent when available)

NX	When it is impossible to assess the regional lymph nodes the symbol NX is used, permitting eventual addition of histological information, thus: NX— or NX+
N0	No deformity of regional nodes as shown by available diagnostic methods
N1	Pelvic nodes distal to the bifurcation of the common iliac arteries deformed as shown by available diagnostic methods
N2	Intra-abdominal para-aortic nodes proximal to the bifurcation of the common iliac arteries deformed as shown by available diagnostic methods

M—Distant metastases

M0	No evidence of distant metastases
M1	Distant metastases present, including involved inguinal lymph nodes

---

*From the American Joint Committee for Cancer Staging and End Results Reporting: Manual for staging of cancer, Chicago, 1978, Whiting Press.

†Enlargement is judged on whether the sound passes more than 8 cm beyond the cervical os: the distance to be recorded.

When compared to carcinoma of the cervix, adenocarcinoma of the endometrium infiltrates and spreads slowly from its mucosal origin. Extension in any direction from its mucosal origin worsens prognosis. Invasion into the muscle, especially the deep muscle, extension to the cervix or fornices, metastases to the ovaries, or implants in the vaginal mucosa are characteristic of the higher histologic grades. Regardless of whether cancer is visible on the cervix, for the purpose of treatment, involvement of the cervix must be included in the treated volume.

Lymphatic drainage of the uterine corpus

Just as is the lymphatic system of the cervix, the lymphatic system of the corpus is formed as lymphatics of the endometrium unite with vessels of the myometrium to empty into an extensive subserosal plexus. This plexus is drained by four lymphatic trunks, which emerge from the lateral borders of the corpus (Fig. 18-1). The more superior trunks pass through the broad ligament paralleling the fallopian tube to nodes near the ovary, and from there they drain into the para-aortic nodes. Vessels from the inferior portion of the corpus pass through the broad ligament to nodes at the bifurcation of the common iliac artery. Subserosal lymphatics near the junction of the uterine tube and uterine body anastomose with lymphatics of the tube to drain into para-aortic nodes. Lymphatics pass from the corpus by way of the ovarian pedicle to anastomose with those of the uterine tube and empty into the para-aortic nodes. Finally, lymphatics near the root of the round ligament drain into vessels that follow the round ligament to the femoral region. There the lymphatics empty into the femoral nodes. Retrograde lymphatic permeation or metastases to the vaginal mucosa are not uncommon. Such pretreatment spread into the vagina is accepted as the cause of posthysterectomy recurrence of cancer in the vaginal vault. Iatrogenic

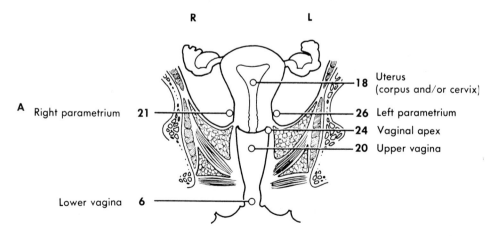

Continued.

Fig. 18-1. A, Number and site of recurrences in the genital organs of 124 patients with recurrent endometrial carcinoma. **B,** Lymph drainage and lymph node groups of the body of the uterus emphasizing the difference in drainage between the lower and upper uterine segments. (From Dede, J. A., Plentl, A. A., and Moore, J. G.: Surg. Gynecol. Obstet. **126:**536, 1968.)

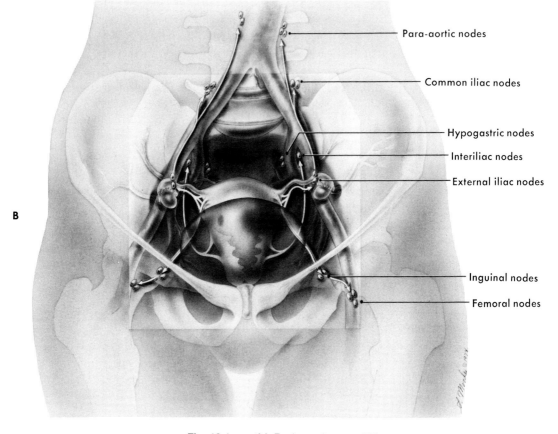

Para-aortic nodes

Common iliac nodes

Hypogastric nodes

Interiliac nodes

External iliac nodes

Inguinal nodes

Femoral nodes

B

Fig. 18-1, cont'd. For legend see p. 489.

seeding during the operative procedure is not thought to be a cause of such recurrence. Invasion through the myometrium to the serosa, the parametrium, or into the bladder or rectum is a late manifestation.

Metastases to regional nodes

It has been the impression of many oncologists for years that adenocarcinoma of the endometrium seldom metastasizes to regional nodes. The study of specimens removed during radical surgery for this disease reveals that this impression is wrong. Morrow and associates reviewed the literature and found that of 369 patients with Stage I carcinoma subjected to lymph node dissection, 39 (10.6%) showed node metastases. Creasman and associates collected data from three institutions and reported the incidence of metastases to pelvic nodes to be 11% of 140 patients with clinical Stage I lesions. In the same analysis of Stage I lesions 10% of 102 patients sampled had metastases to para-aortic nodes. Patients with Stage II carcinoma

Table 18-1. Incidence of metastasis to pelvic and para-aortic lymph nodes in Stage I carcinoma of the endometrium

Author	Total number of patients	Patients with positive pelvic nodes	Patients with positive para-aortic nodes
Stahlworthy	104	12 (11%)	—
Creasman			
1a	80	5 (6.2%)	3 (3.8%)
1b	60	11 (18.0%)	7 (11.7%)
Morrow and associates	369	(10.6%)	70% of those with positive pelvic nodes

develop metastases to pelvic nodes in 36.5% (Morrow and associates). The incidence of metastases to para-aortic nodes in this group is poorly defined, although De Saia found them present in about 70% of patients showing positive pelvic nodes. Table 18-1 illustrates the variation of the incidence of metastases within Stage I. The tumor is more likely to metastasize if it is near the cervix, but fundal lesions also metastasize. The more infiltrating lesions metastasize more frequently, but superficial lesions may also do so. An occasional patient with a positive node will live 5 or more years. In Schwartz and Brunschwig's series of ninety-three patients, thirteen had positive nodes and two lived 5 years free of disease. Both 5-year survivors received postoperative irradiation. A third patient was living and well after 2 years. In a review of the literature of Stage I lesions Morrow and associates identified thirty-two patients with positive pelvic nodes, ten of whom lived 5 years.

Treatment

There are two considerations that bear on the development of a rational irradiation therapy policy combining irradiation and surgery in the treatment of carcinoma of the endometrium. The first is the incidence of local (vault or upper vaginal) recurrence following hysterectomy alone. The second is the incidence of metastases to regional lymph nodes. Since the therapeutic measures necessary to diminish the incidence of vault recurrence include rather localized high-dose radium or transvaginal or external pelvic irradiation and those for nodal disease include external whole pelvis irradiation, it is important to identify patients at high risk for each of these two treatable causes of failure. The incidence of vault recurrence is shown in Table 18-2, and the factors associated with an increased incidence of vault recurrence are shown in Table 18-3. The incidence of the factors associated with increased metastases to regional nodes are shown in Table 18-4. It becomes clear from these tables that more often than not factors associated with an increased incidence of vault recurrence are also associated with an increased incidence of metastases to pelvic and para-aortic lymph nodes, that is, extension to the cervix, high histologic grade, and myometrial invasion. In patients thus identified we cannot specifically rule out either the vaginal vault or the draining lymph nodes as the site at increased risk for posthysterectomy persistent cancer.

Table 18-2. Incidence of vaginal persistence after treatment for adenocarcinoma of the endometrium

Hysterectomy alone		Preoperative irradiation and hysterectomy	
Author	Number and percent of persistences	Author	Number and percent of persistences
Rickford (1949)	23/160 (14.4%)	Dobbie (1953)	2/84 (2.4%)
Way (1951)	14/102 (13.7%)	Stander (1956)	1/103 (1%)
Dobbie (1953)	7/64 (11%)	Gusberg and associates (1960)	2/170 (1.1%)
Gusberg and associates (1960)	11/121 (9.1%)	Sala and del Regato (1960)	3/68 (4%)
Price and associates (1965)	6/41 (14%)	Price and associates (1965)	4/110 (3.6%)
Copenhaver and Barsamian (1967)	14/141 (10%)	Wade and associates (1967)	3/156 (1.9%)
Wade and associates (1967)	4/43 (9.3%)	Beiler and associates (1972)	1/64 (1.6%)
Beiler and associates (1972)	8/68 (12%)		
TOTAL	87/740 (11%)		16/755 (2.1%)

Table 18-3. Factors associated with increased incidence of vault recurrence in carcinoma of the endometrium in an analysis of 369 patients*

Factor	Number of patients with local recurrence	Percent patients with local recurrence
Grade		
Well differentiated	12/152	8
Poorly differentiated	27/61	44
Myometrial invasion		
Superficial	15/179	9
Deep	8/29	27
Cavity depth		
<8 cm	0/22	0
>8 cm	3/11	27
Clinical stage		
I	—	Low
II	—	High

*Modified from Morrow, C. P., Di Saia, P. J., and Townsend, D. E.: Am. J. Roentgenol. Radium Ther. Nucl. Med. **127:** 325-329, 1976.

During the pretreatment work-up we can determine histologic grade, length of uterine canal, and usually whether or not the cervix is involved. The depth of myometrial invasion cannot be determined prior to hysterectomy. However, there is a strong positive correlation between histologic grade and depth of myometrial invasion, prognosis being affected somewhat more by grade (Joelsson and associates). Occasionally curetted material contains an admixture of normal, or hyperplastic, endometrium and cancer. Since spread of endometrial carcinoma is usually circum-

Table 18-4. Factors associated with increased incidence of metastases to regional lymph nodes in an analysis of 369 patients*

Factor	Percent pelvic nodes involved
Grade	
Low	5.6
High	26.3
Myometrial invasion	
Minimal or superficial	0
Moderate	14.3
Deep	36.2
Clinical stage	
I	10.6
II (cervix involved)	36.5

*Modified from Morrow, C. P., Di Saia, P. J., and Townsend, D. E.: Am. J. Roentgenol. Radium Ther. Nucl. Med. **127:** 325-329, 1976.

ferential before it becomes invasive, this finding indicates localized and often not deeply invasive tumor. Also, the higher the grade, the more advanced the clinical stage and the more often the uterine cavity will be enlarged, that is, longer than 8 cm.

Therefore, when these factors indicative of higher risks of spread are present, it is necessary to consider preoperative treatment of *both the vaginal vault and the pelvic lymph nodes.* The recognition of this fact accounts for the increasing use of external pelvic irradiation with or without intracavitary sources whenever increased risks of central recurrence or metastases to pelvic nodes are identified.

Vaginal persistences are frequently small, nonulcerated, rather benign-appearing plaques. They are usually movable, and their treatment by simple excision or localized irradiation is highly tempting. In spite of the apparent limited nature of most vaginal recurrences, experience has shown that such lesions are usually just one manifestation of rather widespread persistence. This is especially true in lower vaginal lesions. Treatment by local means is rarely successful. Whether surgical or radiotherapeutic, treatment of recurrences must be radical and include whole pelvis irradiation combined with either transvaginal irradiation or radioactive sources placed in the vaginal vault.

From reports in the literature we might anticipate that 20% to 25% of such vault persistences can be subsequently controlled by irradiation. Death due to uncontrolled vaginal persistences may therefore be 8% to 10% of all lesions resected when no preoperative irradiation is used. The frequency with which irradiation can control nodal metastases in this disease is poorly defined, although there is every reason to believe that it is similar to that achieved in carcinoma of the cervix. For these reasons the selective use of adequate preoperative or immediate postoperative irradiation in the "high-risk" group is indicated.

PREOPERATIVE IRRADIATION. The aims of preoperative irradiation have been discussed in detail in Chapter 2. The aims as related to carcinoma of the corpus may be restated. The concept of rendering an inoperable lesion operable demands that that portion of the tumor producing inoperability be eradicated by irradiation, whereas it implies that a second part of the same tumor, incurable by irradiation, must be removed. This concept, then, assumes that a double standard of radiosensitivity exists in the inoperable primary tumor. Persistences presumably develop from transection of occult fingers of cancer or metastases in pelvic nodes. The destruction of these occult fingers and metastases is the major contribution of preoperative irradiation to the management of patients with carcinoma of the corpus.

Preoperative irradiation has also been recommended to render malignant cells that might later be implanted in the operative wound or circulatory system nonviable. There is ample experimental evidence to justify consideration of this view. However, such "inoculations" during surgery usually imply transection of cancer, and transection of cancer implies postoperative persistence of rather large pieces of cancer. The problem is one of destruction of potential implants plus destruction of a viable volume of cancer tissue.

The last aim of preoperative irradiation has something more definite to offer. If one method of therapy is more effective against limited cancer and another method is preferred if the lesion is advanced, a combination of both methods may be advantageous. If, before treatment, it is difficult to determine extent of spread and if the application of both modalities of treatment is not associated with a significant increase in morbidity or mortality, both modalities should be applied to most patients. To weigh the validity of this statement, the extent of spread as it affects success and failure reported by surgery and by irradiation will be examined later.

POSTOPERATIVE IRRADIATION. The theoretical and practical advantages of postoperative irradiation in comparison to preoperative irradiation were discussed in Chapter 2. The limitations of clinical staging in defining the true extent of carcinoma of the endometrium were brought into sharp focus by Morrow and associates. The most obvious differences in clinical and pathologic staging are in defining the depth of myometrial invasion, microscopic evidence of cervical involvement, ovarian or tubal involvement, and metastases to pelvic and para-aortic lymph nodes. The positive data acquired by the gynecologist at laparotomy and hysterectomy, combined with the description of the adequacy of excision and the histologic information obtained by the pathologist from the operative specimen, provide facts on which the radiation therapist can develop a rational plan for postoperative irradiation. This sequence has been used with considerable success in the management of advanced cancers of the head and neck. Whether or not these advantages of postoperative irradiation will outweigh the hazards of the transection and intra-abdominal dissemination of cancer and the risk of postoperative radiation-induced bowel damage is yet to be shown. However, it seems a logical sequence for Stage I, Grade I lesions. Morrow and associates have indicated the need for justification for clinical trials to define the role of such postoperative irradiation.

CAPABILITIES OF IRRADIATION. Irradiation, when applied as a preoperative

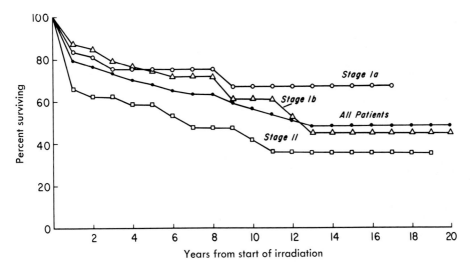

Fig. 18-2. Actuarial survival rates for patients irradiated for medically inoperable (unable to tolerate hysterectomy) carcinoma of the endometrium. (From Landgren, R. C., Fletcher, G. H., Delclos, L., and Wharton, J. T.: Am. J. Roentgenol. Radium Ther. Nucl. Med. **126:**148-154, 1976.)

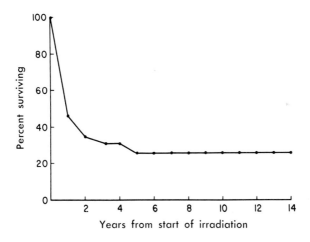

Fig. 18-3. Actuarial survival rates for patients irradiated for technically unresectable cancer of the endometrium. (From Landgren, R. C., Fletcher, G. H., Delclos, L., and Wharton, J. T.: Am. J. Roentgenol. Radium Ther. Nucl. Med. **126:**148-154, 1976.)

measure, can destroy all microscopic evidence of viable intrauterine cancer in at least 40% and perhaps 72% (Chau) of the surgically removed specimens. Strickland reported that thirty-one of forty-two patients (74%) were effectively cured by irradiation alone.

There is evidence from several institutions that adenocarcinoma of the corpus is relatively curable by radiation therapy alone; it responds to radiations as well as squamous cell carcinoma of the cervix. Chau reported a persistence rate of 27.4%

when radium was the sole treatment. Badib and associates reported a persistence rate of 21% Stage Ib patients with uterine depth of less than 8 cm, regardless of the technique of irradiation. If the uterine depth was greater than 8 cm, this low rate of persistence could be achieved only when external irradiation preceded radium placement. In their series of 285 patients treated by irradiation alone, 46% survived 5 years. Delclos and associates report a 57% 5-year survival for Stage Ib patients treated by irradiation alone. A summary of Landgren's experience is shown in Figs. 18-2 and 18-3 and Table 18-7.

Evaluation of the effectiveness of irradiation for the technically inoperable cancer is more difficult. If there is spread beyond the pelvis, there is little chance of cure. On the other hand, when the reason for inoperability is extrauterine but still localized extension, there is still a chance for cure by irradiation. This is demonstrated in Table 18-5 and Fig. 18-3.

These patients were recognized as inoperable during the pretreatment evaluation. Their irradiation was planned as their definitive treatment. The fact that some of these otherwise incurable patients can be cured by irradiation has thus been demonstrated.

From such data we can confidently predict an improved cure rate by administering vigorous irradiation to the apparently operable patient who has undetected or occult local extension beyond the limits of the proposed hysterectomy.

In planning preoperative irradiation, the concern is not so much with the intracavitary portion of the cancer as with local extension beyond the limits of the usual surgery. The classic treatment directed to the destruction of cancer in these

Table 18-5. Survival rate obtained by radiotherapy alone in patients technically inoperable (FIGO Stage III)

Author	Number and percent of inoperable patients surviving 5 years after irradiation only
Lampe (1963)	12/50 (24%)
Kottmeier (1959)	17/62 (27.4%)
Landgren (1976)	6/26 (26%)
TOTAL	35/138 (25.4%)

Fig. 18-6. Five-year survival rates using preoperative external pelvic irradiation followed by hysterectomy when possible

Author	Operable and had TAH*—preoperative irradiation plus surgery	Operable but no TAH*—irradiation only	Technically inoperable— irradiation only
Sala and del Regato (1962)	82/111 (74%)	6/30 (20%)	2/24 (4%)
Lampe (1963)	109/121 (90%)	53/97 (54%)	12/50 (24%)

*Total abdominal hysterectomy.

extrauterine tissues has been radium. Yet radium, with its rapid decrease in percentage of depth dose, is a second choice in the irradiation of extrauterine tissues. These tissues are best irradiated with external pelvic megavoltage or ^{60}Co therapy. Such external irradiation should be planned to include a long segment of the vagina and all tissues between the uterus and the lateral pelvic walls together with the commonly involved pelvic nodes (Fig. 18-1). The dose must be sufficiently high to be cancerocidal for a good proportion of these tumors. It is realized that this preoperative dose will not eradicate a sufficient proportion of the bulk of operable cancers to be the sole therapy. Sala and del Regato compared the results of preoperative external pelvic irradiation with those of preoperative radium. Their results, together with those of Lampe, confirm the effectiveness of external pelvic irradiation. Surgery must follow in 3 to 8 weeks. The results of preoperative external pelvic irradiation plus hysterectomy are shown in Table 18-6.

SUMMARY. The facts on which to base a decision to use preoperative or postoperative irradiation are as follows:

1. That this is a radiocurable cancer is proved by the fact that Kottmeier (1959) and Landgren (1976) were able to control the disease in over half the patients with irradiation alone.

2. When preoperative irradiation is used, no residual cancer will be found in 40% to 70% of the resected uteri.

3. Radiotherapy can control the cancer in well over a fourth of those patients in whom the nonresectable cancer is still confined to the pelvis.

4. After hysterectomy alone, adenocarcinoma of the corpus persists in the vaginal vault in 10% to 15% of the patients. The incidence of local persistence is reduced to a third of this number by preoperative irradiation.

5. We can identify a proportion of those apparently operable patients with a high risk for central recurrence and metastases to pelvic lymph nodes. This high-risk group should receive high-dose external pelvic irradiation preoperatively.

6. Patients with more advanced disease but with the cancer still confined to the pelvis should receive a curative attempt with radiation therapy.

7. Patients with none of the "high-risk" signs may not all require preoperative irradiation. This point is being studied.

8. There is a role for combined surgery and postoperative irradiation in the patient with clinical Stage I, Grade I cancer whose hysterectomy specimen shows unexpected extension of the cancer into the cervix, deep myometrium, or extrauterine structures such as the ovaries or lymph nodes.

9. Once postoperative persistence develops in the vaginal vault, the disease can be controlled by radiotherapy in at least 20% of the patients.

Preoperative irradiation probably does not alter the cure rate in the very limited or very advanced carcinomas of the endometrium. Surgery can easily control all lesions truly limited to the corpus, provided, of course, that the patient is a good operative risk. There is no question but that a few of these small lesions that are easily cured by surgery are resistant to currently employed radiation techniques. On the other hand, the more invasive lesions that remain confined to the pelvis may be controlled by radiations even if their lateral infiltration or vaginal spread should place them beyond the scope of the usual surgical approach. Thus, in the case of the corpus, there are some lesions curable by irradiation that would not be controlled by the usual surgery, and there are lesions curable by surgery that would not be controlled by the usual irradiation. When this is true and if the two methods of treatment are not associated with high morbidity or mortality, both methods can and should be applied. If the two methods are to be used, irradiation should usually precede surgery. The risk of cutting through and disseminating viable cancer is thus reduced.

TECHNIQUES. In keeping with the facts outlined previously, we believe there is a strong indication for preoperative irradiation aimed toward delivering maximal tolerated doses to extrauterine structures in a proportion of the operable patients. Should it be obvious from the beginning that surgery is not possible, vigorous irradiation of the corpus and cervix becomes paramount. However, *extrauterine* tissues should also be irradiated to the maximum tolerated dose. For the apparently limited cancer the use of radium alone as a competitor to surgery has been suggested by Bergsjo and Nilsen and by Strickland. For the elderly obese patient in poor general condition we have used radium alone, but it is doubtful that it should replace surgery or irradiation combined with surgery in an otherwise operable lesion.

Two intracavitary radium techniques, either alone or combined with external pelvic irradiation, are used in irradiating these patients.

1. Heyman's packing technique. In the original Heyman technique the uterine cavity is packed with 10 mg radium capsules. Currently in Stockholm, ^{137}Cs sources equivalent to 14 to 19 mg of radium are used (Joelsson and associates). The aim is to select a capsule size that permits about ten sources to be placed in the cavity. A special inserter is used to place each capsule accurately. A wire attached to each capsule is also attached to a numbered tag. This permits removal of the capsules in the proper order—the last placed capsule being removed first. A capsule of similar diameter must also be placed in the cervical canal to prevent it from contracting and thus preventing removal. For very limited lesions in a normal sized uterus when no external pelvic irradiation is given, three implants in the uterine cavity are made of 1500 mg-hrs each, which deliver doses to the uterine serosa varying from 800 rad to 2500 rad per implant (Joelsson and associates). To this is added vaginal sources to deliver 1500 mg-hrs during each of three applications instead of the high-intensity vaginal source of the classic Heyman technique. The above dose is low for most except very limited lesions. We increase the intrauterine dose by 500 mg-hrs for each of the three implants for the more advanced Stage I lesions, especially if the uterine cavity is enlarged.

Doses delivered to critical pelvic structures, that is, rectum and bladder, should be calculated using films to identify the location of radioactive sources. Maximum doses are similar to those used as guides in the treatment of cancer of the cervix. It is immediately obvious that there are several arrangements for the capsules. Cross

Table 18-7. Persistence rates in 285 patients treated by irradiation alone (Stage Ib) as related to depth of corpus and treatment technique*

Technique	Percent persistence†		5-year survival (%)
	<8 cm	>8 cm	
Manchester radium	22	65	39
External RT‡ plus Manchester radium	18	21	48
Heyman packing	22	30	46
External RT‡ plus Heyman packing	21	21	51

*Modified from Badib, A. O., Kurohara, S. S., Vongtama, V. Y., and Webster, J. H.: Radiology **93**:417-421, 1969.
†85% of all persistences in corpus with no major variation by technique.
‡Usually 4000 rad given prior to radium.

filtration, which cannot be ignored, will also vary. The dosimetry is therefore quite complex. Heyman's original tables do not fulfill the need, but they remain in use. Computer-aided dosimetry has been a valuable addition. When 60 to 80 mg of radium can be placed in the uterine cavity and 40 mg of radium can be placed in the vaginal vault, two implants 10 days to 2 weeks apart, each of 3500 to 4500 mg-hrs, approaches rectal tolerance. This has been used for some patients instead of the three implants used in the original Heyman technique.

At times a point has been made of stretching the walls of the corpus to permit insertion of yet another capsule. The aim is to thin the wall of the uterus and also to assure maximum contact between the radium and the uterine lining. We question the wisdom of this practice. It certainly is not a technique for improving irradiation of the tissues at the limits of the resection. It increases the risk of perforation and, because of the increased cross filtration, adds less than might be imagined to the endometrial dose. In fact, if regardless of the number of capsules, the same number of milligram-hours is given to each patient, the patient with the largest number of capsules will receive the smallest endometrial dose. This is because of cross filtration.

By the packing technique the entire endometrium is near the radium, and although the dose to the endometrium is relatively homogeneous, it is high compared to the dose reaching the parametrium or lateral pelvic wall.

2. If the aim of the radium application is to irradiate laterally, the intrauterine tandem is physically superior to the Heyman technique (Tod and Morris). In this technique, an afterloading differentially loaded uterine tandem is pushed into the uterine cavity. The fundal end of the tandem contains 20 to 25 mg of radium, and the remainder of the tandem is filled with enough 10 mg capsules to extend the length of the uterine cavity. A vaginal cylinder is used or, if the cervix shows malignant infiltration, the ovoids may be placed in the same fashion as for carcinoma of the cervix. A dose of 3800 rad 2 cm from the radium is usually given in each of two applications 1 week apart. When selecting radium dosages, the tolerances recognized in the treatment of carcinoma of the cervix are applicable, and a similar number of milligram-hours can be used if the Manchester recommendations are followed. By this technique, an uneven dose to the endometrium is the expense of improving the dose

Table 18-8. Sites of recurrence in 213 resected cases of carcinoma of the corpus*

Genital	37 cases
Vaginal apex	9
Vaginal wall	10
Urethra	3
Pelvis	15
Abdomen	9 cases
Pulmonary	5 cases
Bone	14 cases

*From Ingersoll, F. M., and Meigs, J. V.: Lymph node dissection for carcinoma of the endometrium, Proceedings of the Second National Cancer Conference, New York, 1954, American Cancer Society, Inc.

laterally. Yet in our opinion, radium by any technique is a poor approach to extra-uterine irradiation.

When the uterine cavity is small and cannot hold more than four Heyman's capsules, the afterloading tandem described before is used. Vaginal sources are distributed as described in the preceding technique.

There are three major clinical situations that warrant special radiation therapy technical considerations.

1. *Preoperative irradiation.* The indications for and aims of preoperative irradiation were presented previously. It is the extrauterine spread of this disease that leads to the surgical failures. This may present as implants on the ovaries or fallopian tubes, subclinical parametrial infiltration, spread to lymph nodes, or vaginal implant (Table 18-8). It is through the destruction of this extrauterine disease that radiotherapy may contribute most to the control of carcinoma of the endometrium. Intrauterine radium by any technique does not approach the efficacy of external pelvic irradiation in this regard. However, many of the patients are obese. Skin-midpelvis distances are great, and percentage depth doses are low. Before telecobalt or megavoltage beams became available, intracavitary radium was a valuable aid in raising the dose in the extrauterine tissues to effective levels. Currently, except in very obese patients, extrauterine tissues can be irradiated to optimum preoperative levels (4500 to 5500 rad in 5 to 7 weeks) using a four-port technique with ^{60}Co or megavoltage beams. For very obese patients, 10 to 25 mev photon beams are preferred. Pelvic nodes, including common iliac, hypogastric, and obturator nodes as well as the ovaries, tubes, and a generous segment of vagina, should be encompassed. Total hysterectomy with bilateral salpingo-oophorectomy should follow in 3 to 8 weeks. If this dose is not given faster than 900 rad per week, it is well tolerated and should rarely produce late sequelae of significance.

2. *Postoperative irradiation.* The indication for postoperative irradiation is the fact that prehysterectomy estimation of extent of the cancer is seriously limited by the inaccessibility of pelvic viscera and regional nodes. Thus postoperative irradiation is indicated when the surgeon or pathologist provides evidence that cancer may remain in the pelvis or regional or para-aortic nodes. Findings sufficient to warrant such irradiation are

a. Deep myometrial invasion in the resected uterus

b. Invasion of the cervix or vaginal vault in the resected specimen

c. Metastases to the ovary, tubes, or other pelvic viscera

d. Metastases to pelvic or para-aortic nodes

The technique must be tailored to the findings at hysterectomy and the findings in the resected specimen. If any of the first three indications are present, external pelvic irradiation is administered to encompass at least a generous segment of the vagina and the obturator, external, and common iliac nodes. A whole pelvic dose of no less than 5500 rad in 6 to 7 weeks is usually indicated. If cancer was known to have been transected in the vault, an additional 2100 rad are given in 7 fractions through a transvaginal cone. If common iliac or para-aortic nodes are involved, a midline port is extended to T11. A dose of 4500 to 5000 rad in 6 weeks is delivered to these nodes. Boosting doses are given through reduced ports to residual pelvic or para-aortic disease, which was marked with metal clips at the time of surgery.

3. *Irradiation alone for carcinoma of the endometrium.* Brief mention was made previously of using radium alone in the treatment of selected obese patients with Stage I carcinoma of the endometrium who, for medical reasons, could not tolerate a hysterectomy. This is a small proportion of patients and includes those with severe cardiac, diabetic, or renal problems who present with a reduced life expectancy.

In addition, radiation therapy is the major modality of treatment if the cancer has clinically extended beyond the uterus but is confined to the pelvis. This includes all patients with Stage III lesions and a proportion of those with more advanced Stage II lesions. The bulk of cancer in these patients is large, and doses should be raised to the maximum tolerated. Irradiation is initiated with external pelvic irradiation. The large diameter of most of these patients requires more than simple anterior and posterior pairs of opposed ports. A four-port box technique using the most energetic photon beams available is preferable. Since the volumes irradiated are large (16 cm wide and vertically from at least the midvagina to L4 if common iliac nodes are to be encompassed), the daily fractions are usually 160 to 180 rad. The total midpelvic dose from external pelvic irradiation is 5000 to 5500 rad in 28 to 30 fractions. An additional boosting dose of 1500 to 2000 rad should be delivered to the uterus and upper vagina using reduced ports or a rotational technique. An alternative to the boosting dose of external irradiation is intracavitary uterine and vaginal radium for a total of 4500 to 5000 mg-hrs divided equally between the uterus and the vagina. We prefer the Heyman technique when radium is used for this purpose. The justification for this sequence is found in the experience of Badib and associates in the treatment of patients by irradiation alone (Table 18-7). It is clear that the lowest persistence rate was seen in those patients given external whole pelvic irradiation prior to radium application. When the corpus is enlarged significantly, the Heyman packing technique appears superior to using an intrauterine tandem.

Prognosis and results

The 5-year survival rate of patients treated for adenocarcinoma of the endometrium is probably the best of any major malignancy. Yet Boronow emphasized the lethal potential of this disease and warned of complacency in its management. Adenocarcinoma of the endometrium must be treated aggressively with full appreciation of the hazards for local recurrence and metastases to regional lymph nodes. Some of the results are shown in Tables 18-5, 18-6, and 18-7. In weighing these results it is important to remember that control rates vary with clinical stage and histologic grade. Clinical Stage I, Grade 1 lesions are infrequently more advanced than their clinical staging implies (Green and associates). The 5-year disease-free survival rate of this highly favorable group will usually exceed 80% whether preoperative irradiation is administered or not (Wharam and associates; Lewis, 1977). However, as the histologic grade increases, the risks of local recurrence increase. Of fifty-six patients with Stage I, Grade 2 lesions administered preoperative radium, only 4% developed local recurrence. Of eighty-two patients given no preoperative irradiation, 18% developed recurrence. Finally, of twenty-two patients with Stage I, Grade 3 lesions given no preoperative irradiation, 41% were living and well at 5 years, whereas of thirteen patients given preoperative irradiation, eight (62%) were living and well at 5 years.

The high incidence of metastases to nodes (36.5%) and of vault recurrence in patients with clinical Stage II lesions justifies routine external pelvic irradiation. In some of these patients hysterectomy can follow the irradiation. Overall 5-year cancer-free survival rates in Stage II will average about 50% (Sall and associates).

Most Stage III lesions will be unresectable and should be treated with irradiation alone. The 5-year cancer-free survival rate will range from 20% to 30% (Figs. 18-2 and 18-3). As given previously, irradiation alone can control the disease in over 50% of all patients, including the inoperable group (Table 18-5).

Summary

Adenocarcinoma of the endometrium occurs predominantly in postmenopausal patients in whom vaginal bleeding is an alarming symptom. For this reason the diagnosis is frequently made relatively early and control rates are good. Regional lymph node metastases have been found to occur in a higher proportion of patients than previously suspected. They are much more frequent in those with advanced lesions nearer the cervix. Surgery alone fails not only because of the previously mentioned metastases, but also because of persistences in the vaginal vault and in the periurethral and parametrial regions. It is in this category of persistences that irradiation improves the results obtained by surgery alone. There is ample proof that such extensions can be controlled by irradiation procedures.

From the theoretical and practical viewpoints, irradiation is more effective if given before rather than after surgery. In our opinion, if treatment calls for preoperative irradiation, that technique will be most effective which irradiates those extra-uterine tissues in which postsurgical persistences are known to appear.

REFERENCES

American Joint Committee for Cancer Staging and End Results Reporting: clinical staging system for carcinoma of the corpus uteri, Chicago, 1972.

Badib, A. O., Kurohara, S. S., Vongtama, V. Y., and Webster, J. H.: Evaluation of primary radiation therapy in Stage I, Group 2 endometrial carcinoma, Radiology 93:417-421, 1969.

Beiler, D. D., Schmitz, D. A., and O'Rourke, T. L.: Carcinoma of the endometrium: radiation and surgery versus surgery alone, Radiology **102:** 159-164, 1972.

Bergsjo, P., and Nilsen, P. A.: Carcinoma of the endometrium: a study of 256 cases from the Norwegian Radium Hospital, Am. J. Obstet. Gynecol. **95:**496-507, 1966.

Boronow, R. C.: Endometrial cancer: not a benign disease, Obstet. Gynecol. **47:**630-634, 1976.

Chau, P. M.: Technic and evaluation of preoperative radium therapy in adenocarcinoma of the uterine corpus. In Anderson Hospital report: Carcinoma of the uterine cervix, endometrium, and ovary, Chicago, 1962, Year Book Medical Publishers, Inc.

Chuang, J. T., Van Velden, J. J., and Graham, J. B.: Carcinosarcoma and mixed mesodermal tumor of the uterine corpus, Obstet. Gynecol. **35:**769-780, 1970.

Copenhaver, E. H., and Barsamian, M.: Management of Stage I adenocarcinoma of the endometrium, Am. J. Obstet. Gynecol. **99:**864-868, 1967.

Creasman, W. T., Boronow, R. C., Morrow, C. P., Di Saia, P. J., and Blessing, J.: Adenocarcinoma of the endometrium: its metastatic lymph node potential, Gynecol. Oncol. **4:**239-243, 1976.

Dede, J. A., Plentl, A. A., and Moore, J. G.: Recurrent endometrial carcinoma, Surg. Gynecol. Obstet. **126:**533-542, 1968.

Delclos, L., Fletcher, G. H., Gutierrez, A. G., and Rutledge, F. N.: Adenocarcinoma of the uterus, Am. J. Roentgenol. **105:**603-608, 1969.

Di Saia, P. J.: Personal communication, Aug., 1977.

Dobbie, B. M.: Vaginal recurrences in carcinoma of body of uterus and their prevention by radium therapy, J. Obstet. Gynaecol. Brit. Emp. **60:** 702-705, 1953.

Green, N., Melbye, R. W., and Kernen, J.: Stage I well differentiated adenocarcinoma of the endometrium, Am. J. Roentgenol. **123:**563-566, 1975.

Gusberg, S. B., Jones, H. C., and Tovell, H. M.: Selection of treatment for corpus cancer, Am. J. Obstet. Gynecol. **80:**374-380, 1960.

Heyman, J., Reuterwall, O., and Benner, S.: Radiumhemmet experience with radiotherapy in cancer of corpus of uterus; classification, method of treatment and results, Acta Radiol. **22:**11-98, 1941.

Joelsson, I., Sandri, A., and Kottmeier, H. L.: Carcinoma of the corpus, Acta Radiol. (Suppl.) **334:** 1-63, 1973.

Kagan, A. R., Nussbaum, H., Ziel, H., and Gordon, J.: Adenocarcinoma of the endometrium, Am. J. Roentgenol. **123:**567-570, 1975.

Ingersoll, F. M., and Meigs, J. V.: Lymph node dissection for carcinoma of the endometrium, Proceedings of the Second National Cancer Conference, New York, 1954, American Cancer Society, Inc.

Kottmeier, H. L.: Carcinoma of the female genitalia, Baltimore, 1953, The Williams & Wilkins Co.

Kottmeier, H. L.: Carcinoma of the corpus uteri, diagnosis and therapy, Am. J. Obstet. Gynecol. **78:**1127-1140, 1959.

Lampe, I.: Combined surgical and radiological treatment for carcinoma, Proceedings of the Second National Cancer Conference, New York, 1954, American Cancer Society, Inc.

Lampe, I.: Endometrial carcinoma, Am. J. Roentgenol. **90:**1011-1015, 1963.

Landgren, R. C., Fletcher, G. H., Delclos, L., and Wharton, J. T.: Irradiation of endometrial cancer in patients with medical contraindication to surgery or with unresectable lesions, Am. J. Roentgenol. Radium Ther. Nucl. Med. **126:**148-154, 1976.

Lefevre, H.: Radical surgery in the treatment of carcinoma of the body of the uterus. In Meigs, J. V., and Sturgis, H. S., editors: Progress in gynecology, New York, 1957, Grune & Stratton, Inc.

Lewis, G. C., Rodrique, M., and Nelson, H. S.: Endometrial cancer: therapeutic decision and the staging process in early disease, Cancer **39:** 959-966, 1977.

Morrow, C. P., Di Saia, P. J., and Townsend, D. E.: Current management of endometrial carcinoma, Obstet. Gynecol. **42:**399-406, 1973.

Morrow, C. P., Di Saia, P. J., and Townsend, D. E.: The role of postoperative irradiation in the management of Stage I adenocarcinoma of the endometrium, Am. J. Roentgenol. Radium Ther. Nucl. Med. **127:**325-329, 1976.

Mortel, R., Koss, L. G., Lewis, J. L., and D'Urso, J. R.: Mesodermal mixed tumors of the uterine corpus, Obstet. Gynecol. **43:**246-252, 1974.

Moss, W. T.: Common peculiarities of patients

with adenocarcinoma of the endometrium, Am. J. Roentgenol. **58:**203-210, 1947.

Ng, A. B., Reagan, J. W., Storassli, J. P., and Wentz, W. B.: Mixed adenosquamous carcinoma of the endometrium, Am. J. Clin. Pathol. **59:** 765-781, 1973.

Price, J. J., Hahn, G. A., and Rominger, C. J.: Vaginal involvement in endometrial carcinoma, Am. J. Obstet. Gynecol. **91:**1060-1065, 1965.

Rubin, P., Salazar, O. M., DePapp, E., and Bonfiglio, T.: Adenosquamous carcinoma of the endometrium: an entity with an inherent poor prognosis? Cancer **40:**119-130, 1977.

Sala, J. M., and del Regato, J. A.: Treatment of carcinoma of the endometrium, Radiology **79:**12-17, 1962.

Sall, S., Sonnenblick, B., and Stone, M. L.: Factors affecting survival of patients with endometrial adenocarcinoma, Am. J. Obstet. Gynecol. **107:** 116-123, 1970.

Silverberg, S. B., Bolin, M. G., and DiGiorgi, L. S.: Adenocanthoma and mixed adenosquamous carcinoma of the endometrium: a clinical-pathologic study, Cancer **30:**1307-1314, 1972.

Stallworthy, J. A.: Surgery of endometrial cancer in the Bonney tradition, Ann. R. Coll. Surg. Engl. **48:**293-305, 1971.

Strickland, P.: Carcinoma corporis uteri: a radical intracavitary treatment, Br. J. Radiol. **16:**112-118, 1965.

Tod, M. C., and Morris, W. I. C.: Cancer of the uterus, cervix, and body. In Carling, E. R., Windeyer, B. W., and Smithers, D. W., editors: Practice in radiotherapy, St. Louis, 1955, The C. V. Mosby Co.

Wade, M. E., Kohorn, E. I., and Morris, J. M.: Adenocarcinoma of the endometrium, Am. J. Obstet. Gynecol. **99:**869-876, 1967.

Wharam, M. D., Phillips, T. L., Bagshaw, M. A.: The role of radiation therapy in clinical Stage I carcinoma of the endometrium, Int. J. Radiat. Oncol. Biol. Phys. **1:**1081-1089, 1976.

Williamson, E. O., and Christoperson, W. M.: Malignant mixed mullerian tumors of the uterus, Cancer **29:**585-592, 1972.

Ziel, H. K., and Finkle, W. D.: Increased risk of endometrial carcinoma among users of conjugated estrogens, N. Engl. J. Med. **293:**1167-1170, 1975.

19

The ovary

RESPONSE OF THE NORMAL OVARY TO IRRADIATION

Within the ovary not only do the various cell types respond differently to irradiation, but within a given cell type the response will vary strikingly according to the stage of maturation. It is impossible to make an overall statement about radiosensitivity of the ovary.

Among ovarian structures the follicle is the most important and has been studied the most. The ovum in the young follicle is more susceptible to direct radiation damage than the ovum of the mature follicle. In contrast, the granulosa cells become more sensitive as the follicle matures. For example, the primitive follicle consists of but a single layer of granulosa cells around the ovum. In the rabbit a single dose of 1200 rad to this structure produces early death of the ovum. The debris is phagocytized by the granular cells, which then themselves disintegrate (Lacassagne and Gricouroff). Three to 4 days may be required for complete disappearance of the follicle. A similar dose given to a graafian follicle produces early pycnotic changes and then death in the granulosa cells. Later, after a month or so, the ovum disintegrates. Even after the single dose of 1200 rad, some of the primitive follicles recover and later resume the process of maturation. The minimum dose required to arrest oogenesis permanently in human beings is uncertain but is known to depend on the age of the patient. A patient near the menopause requires a smaller dose than does a younger woman in her twenties or early thirties (Chapter 11). A single dose of the order of 200 rad to the ovaries of a young woman will usually produce temporary arrest of menses. It was formerly thought that a single dose of 400 to 500 rad delivered to the ovaries was sufficient to produce permanent arrest of menses. Although such a dose may be adequate in a woman in her late forties, a dose of 1200 to 2000 rad in 10 days to 2 weeks is now thought necessary in younger patients. With destruction of the ova and cessation of oogenesis, the hormonal changes produced by ovarian irradiation can be predicted. Secondary sex changes occur just as after surgical castration. Experience with irradiation of prepubertal girls or infants has been too limited to set guidelines of ovarian tolerance in childhood.

The interstitial gland cells originate from the cells of the corpora lutea, which in turn originate from the ruptured graafian follicles. It is to be expected, therefore, that

505

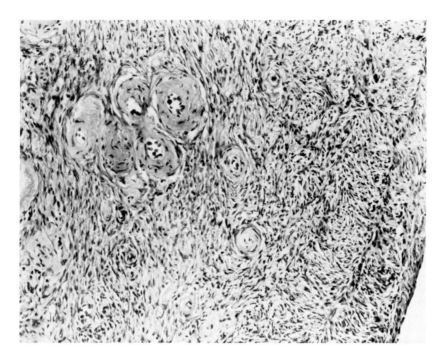

Fig. 19-1. Section of ovary from 30-year-old woman obtained 8 years after curative irradiation of an invasive squamous cell carcinoma of the cervix (combined intracavitary radium and external ^{60}Co). The ovaries were markedly shrunken. Histologically, there is total atrophy of the germinal epithelium. Markedly sclerotic vessels are present within a dense ovarian stroma. The picture resembles that seen in ovaries of elderly women.

even though the corpora lutea and interstitial cells are not particularly radiosensitive, they will disappear through lack of replacement when oogenesis is arrested (Fig. 19-1). Diczfalusy and associates irradiated the ovaries of seventeen premenopausal women with carcinoma of the breast and collected data on the preirradiation and postradiation levels of urinary estrogen excretion. Urinary estrogen levels are normally highest during the luteal phase of the cycle and lowest in the follicular phase. After three doses of 550 to 650 rad per day to the ovaries, urinary estrogens fell significantly below preirradiation follicular phase levels. Bilateral oophorectomy was performed 5 months after irradiation and did not further reduce urinary estrogen levels in these patients. Unfortunately, no information as to the duration of this radiation effect is available. Zuckerman published data supplied by Cole regarding the influence of age on the arrest of menses after a single dose of 400 to 500 rad to the ovaries. Menses resumed in ten of fifteen women 30 to 34 years of age but in only eleven of fifty-one 35 to 39 years of age. These patients were observed for up to 10 years after irradiation. We have seen several patients given doses of 2000 rad to pelvic lymph nodes during the teen years resume menses, and at least one of these girls became pregnant seven years after treatment for Hodgkin's disease. Other studies (Diczfalusy and associates) have shown that urinary estrogen excretion by postmenopausal women can be reduced by ovarian irradiation even 20 to 25 years after the onset of spontaneous menopause.

Doses producing the changes described undoubtedly produce extensive genetic changes. For this reason it is important, if possible, to avoid ovarian irradiation unless ovarian function is to be permanently arrested. The genetic effects of radiations were mentioned briefly in Chapter 16. The same general problems exist with ovarian irradiation. Damage to the developing embryo or fetus has been studied extensively by Hicks and D'Amato, by Rugh, and by W. L. Russell. Radiation-induced changes in an ovum or sperm may produce chromosomal alterations, resulting in grossly or subclinically changed offspring. Radiation-induced changes in selected totipotent cells of an embryo result in modifications of certain organs, areas, or systems, which, if not lethal, are not usually passed on to subsequent generations. However, the ability of developing tissues to compensate, the capacity for restitution of destroyed tissue, and the interdependence of organogenesis result in an exceedingly complex series of events. As just mentioned, these gross changes are not necessarily a result of simple arrest of growth of the organs recognized as abnormal. The excellent summary of Hicks and D'Amato should be consulted for an appreciation of the complexity of this important subject.

No significant data for human beings exist. However, Rugh pooled data from rodents and suggested that we may reasonably expect similar responses in the human embryo and fetus. It is possible that doses as small as 5 to 15 rad can kill a fertilized egg in the first 3 weeks. Injury of the human embryo during this stage rarely results in congenital anomalies, for damaged cells are eliminated and the remaining cells can produce a whole organism. The greatest sensitivity to anomalies occurs from the twentieth to the thirtieth day. During this period the organ-forming cells are undergoing rapid proliferation. They are highly sensitive, and the defective embryo often survives the injuries to produce an increased number of congenital anomalies. By the sixth week major organogenesis is completed. Individual cells, rather than whole organs or systems, are damaged by radiations. However, serious damage is still possible. For example, neuroblasts remain highly sensitive, and radiation injury may be manifested as serious psychologic or neurologic defects.

Griem and associates have analyzed illness in 3024 children, a third of whom received an exposure of 1.5 to 3 rad in utero during a trial period of routine pelvimetry in 1948. Categories of disease and malformation purportedly related to fetal irradiation were evaluated in their initial report. There was no increase in the frequency of leukemia, central nervous system anomalies, or anomalies of the eye. There was, however, a significant increase in the frequency of hemangiomas in children receiving this dose of radiations in utero.

No radiations should be given to the gonads, embryo, or fetus without firm medical justification. In the radiation therapy of malignant diseases, there is frequently little that can be done to protect the ovaries. The risk of genetic damage is then accepted as a part of the hazard of cure of cancer. In the irradiation of benign diseases, possible genetic damage is a major consideration, and the dangers are such that many procedures have been discontinued.

CARCINOMA OF THE OVARY

Malignant tumors of the ovary may arise from any of the cells composing this organ. However, nearly all the carcinomas arise from the germinal epithelium. A few may arise from misplaced blastomeres or embryonic cells. With this knowledge of their histogenesis, one might suspect that carcinomas of the ovary are highly radiosensitive; yet only the dysgerminomas fall into the highly radiosensitive category. The remaining ovarian carcinomas are actually rather poorly radiosensitive. For this reason radiotherapy assumes a secondary role in the treatment of these lesions.

The clinical characteristics of ovarian carcinomas vary rather widely, and their prognoses are correspondingly different. However, treatment for the resectable lesions remains the same—that is, radical removal of the carcinoma combined with hysterectomy and bilateral salpingo-oophorectomy. There is ample evidence that every palpable portion of the cancer should be resected surgically. Surgical debulking by itself clearly improves survival, and this improvement can be enhanced by the addition of irradiation or chemotherapy postoperatively.

At the time of surgery the subdiaphragmatic surface should be carefully explored, the para-aortic lymph nodes biopsied, and peritoneal and pelvic washings obtained for cytologic examination. The importance of such a systematic search was emphasized by Fisher and Young. Within 1 month of exploratory laparotomy, nine of sixteen patients (56%) previously assessed as having Stage I and II disease were found on peritoneoscopy to have, in fact, Stage III disease. Metastatic diaphragmatic involvement was common, that is, 61% of all patients studied. It should be specifically assessed in every patient. Such a high incidence of diaphragmatic involvement calls for a special arrangement of portals (Fuks). This high incidence also probably explains a proportion of radiation failures in patients thought to have disease limited to the pelvis. Prognosis is closely related to the gross extent of the tumor as revealed at surgery. We also use these gross findings to help us in determining the need for irradiation.

The following stage grouping for primary carcinoma of the ovary is based on findings at clinical examination and surgical exploration. The grouping originated from the International Federation of Gynecology and Obstetrics and has been adopted by the American Joint Committee.

STAGING CLASSIFICATION*

Stage I		Growth limited to the ovaries
	Stage Ia	Growth limited to one ovary; no ascites
	i	No tumor on the external surface; capsule intact
	ii	Tumor present on the external surface, or capsule(s) ruptured, or both
	Stage Ib	Growth limited to both ovaries; no ascites
	i	No tumor on the external surface; capsule intact
	ii	Tumor present on the external surface, or capsule(s) ruptured, or both
	Stage Ic	Tumor either Stage Ia or Ib, but with ascites present, or with positive peritoneal washings

*From the American Joint Committee for Cancer Staging and End Results Reporting: Manual for staging of cancer, Chicago, 1978, Whiting Press.

Stage II	Growth involving one or both ovaries with pelvic extension
	Stage IIa Extension and/or metastases to the uterus and/or tubes
	Stage IIb Extension to other pelvic tissues
	Stage IIc Tumor either Stage IIa or Stage IIb, but with ascites present, or with positive peritoneal washings
Stage III	Growth involving one or both ovaries with intraperitoneal metastases outside the pelvis, or positive retroperitoneal nodes, or both; tumor limited to the true pelvis with histologically proven malignant extension to small bowel or omentum
Stage IV	Growth involving one or both ovaries with distant metastases; if pleural effusion is present there must be positive cytology to allot a case to Stage IV; parenchymal liver metastases equals Stage IV
Special category	Unexplored cases that are thought to be ovarian carcinoma

The following histologic classification of the common tumors of the ovary has been proposed by the same committees.*

A. Serous cystomas
    1. Serous benign cystadenomas
    2. Serous cystadenomas with proliferating activity of the epithelial cells and nuclear abnormalities, but with no infiltrative destructive growth (low potential malignancy)
    3. Serous cystadenocarcinomas
B. Mucinous cystomas
    1. Mucinous benign cystadenomas
    2. Mucinous cystadenomas with proliferating activity of the epithelial cells and nuclear abnormalities, but with no infiltrative destructive growth (low potential malignancy)
    3. Mucinous cystadenocarcinomas
C. Endometrioid tumors (similar to adenocarcinomas in the endometrium)
    1. Endometrioid benign cysts
    2. Endometrioid tumors with proliferating activity of the epithelial cells and nuclear abnormalities, but with no infiltrative destructive growth (low potential malignancy)
    3. Endometrioid adenocarcinomas
D. Clear cell (mesonephroid) tumors
    1. Benign clear cell tumors
    2. Clear cell tumors with proliferating activity of the epithelial cells and nuclear abnormalities, but with no infiltrative destructive growth (low potential malignancy)
    3. Clear cell cystadenocarcinomas
E. Unclassified tumors that cannot be allotted to one of the groups A through D
F. No histology
G. Other malignant tumors

Malignant tumors other than those of the common epithelial types are not to be included with the categories listed. However, the more common ones such as granulosa cell tumor, immature teratoma, dysgerminoma, and endodermal sinus tumor may be collected and reported separately by institutions so desiring, particularly those with a pediatric population among their patients.

The clinical staging generally correlates with bulk of disease present at the time

---

*From the American Joint Committee for Cancer Staging and End Results Reporting: Manual for staging of cancer, Chicago, 1978, Whiting Press.

of surgery. The amount of residual disease coupled with the histologic grading of the tumor are the major determinants of prognosis (Griffiths).

In addition to hematogenous and lymphogenous metastases, carcinoma of the ovary may metastasize by seeding onto the peritoneum. This often occurs early. Fully half of all patients in most reported series present with locally advanced disease. If at all widespread, such disease cannot be successfully removed surgically and, because of the large volume, it cannot be irradiated curatively. Patients with such widespread disease, together with those showing distant metastases, may receive palliation after irradiation of the symptom-producing disease. However, their course is usually short and miserable. We believe we can do more for those patients who are thought to have limited, local, nonresectable, persistent disease. However, it is hard to justify postoperative irradiation where a radical operation has been performed on what has been proved both grossly and microscopically to be a limited lesion. In other words, we question the value of postoperative irradiation in patients with Stage Ia disease after apparently adequate surgery. For the remaining stages, recommended treatment is tailored to include the likelihood of diffuse abdominal seeding, the probability of primary pelvic regrowth, and the presence of nonresectable pelvic cancer. Thus a variety of situations arise, and we have chosen the following guidelines. At least 30% of the patients with Stages Ib, Ic, and IIa disease will already have occult extrapelvic spread. Thus the entire abdomen is irradiated, using the moving-strip technique. For patients with Stages IIb, IIc, and III disease, total abdominal irradiation is followed by a boosting pelvic dose to bring the total pelvic dose to about 5000 rad in an equivalent of about 6 weeks, depending on the extent of disease seen at surgery. In patients with Stage IV lesions, the symptom-producing disease should be irradiated with modest doses. It is important to note that between 15% and 25% of patients with endometrioid carcinoma of the ovary will have focal areas of hyperplastic change in the endometrium or superficial, well-differentiated adenocarcinoma. If the patient otherwise has disease limited to one ovary without ascites, irradiation would not be recommended.

As suggested, any value of postoperative irradiation should be most obvious in those patients with postoperatively residual cancer apparently confined to the pelvis. Certainly few of such a group would survive free of disease in the absence of further treatment, although 5-year survival with cancer of the ovary does occur. A high dose of radiations can be given to a volume encompassing the pelvis and including the known residual cancer. Unfortunately, a prospective statistically valid measurement of the difference in survival of these two groups has not been reported. Although results such as those summarized by Rubin and associates, by Kent and McKay, and by Fuks may encourage radiation oncologists to continue irradiating these patients, other equally meaningful results fail to suggest much improvement attributable to postoperative irradiation in any stage. Even though the curative value of postoperative irradiation in these patients is poorly defined, we will continue to recommend postoperative irradiation, with the view that palliative growth restraint is fully justified even when radiosensitivity of the cancer does not permit eradication.

Table 19-1. Published series (1960-1973) on treatment results in patients with carcinoma of the ovary*

Author	Surgery			Surgery and external irradiation		
	Stage I	Stage II	Stage III	Stage I	Stage II	Stage III
Kent (1960)	48/86 (56%)	9/32 (28%)	6/55 (11%)	45/66 (68%)	19/36 (53%)	6/52 (11%)
Rubin (1962)	15/17 (88%)	—	1/33 (3%)	20/25 (80%)	3/13 (69%)	8/52 (15%)
Van Orden (1966)	11/18 (61%)	2/8 (25%)	—	9/11 (82%)	8/22 (36%)	—
Ross (1966)	36/44 (81%)	1/9 (11%)	1/14 (7%)	18/32 (56%)	5/23 (22%)	0/12 (0%)
Munnell (1968)	92/118 (78%)	0/16 (0%)	1/84 (1%)	35/56 (62%)	9/29 (31%)	13/89 (15%)
Dalley (1969)	11/20 (55%)	0/5 (0%)	0/5 (0%)	37/92 (40%)	7/51 (13%)	1/20 (5%)
Barr (1970)	29/40 (72%)	9/27 (33%)	4/45 (9%)	11/17 (65%)	43/91 (47%)	14/80 (17%)
Kottmeier (1971)	—	—	—	29/64 (45%)	23/97 (24%)	8/146 (5%)
Aure (1971)	—	—	—	90/153 (59%)	32/122 (26%)	8/85 (9%)
Delclos (1973)	—	—	—	27/40 (67%)	20/72 (28%)	13/93 (14%)
Clark (1973)	28/46 (60%)	1/6 (17%)	1/44 (2%)	54/101 (53%)	16/51 (31%)	17/280 (6%)

*From Fuks, Z.: Semin. Oncol. **2:**253-266, 1975. By permission.

Interest in preoperative irradiation for patients found to have Stage II and Stage III disease at exploratory surgery arises from dissatisfaction with the results of incomplete surgery and postoperative irradiation. Long and Sala reported the results of preoperative irradiation in eight patients with Stage III locally advanced cancer. Seven of the eight patients survived 8 years, and the one death is attributed to intestinal obstruction. Vaeth has adopted a similar appraoch to Stage II and Stage III cancers. After operative staging he recommends a dose of 5500 rad to the entire pelvis and lower abdomen, and a lesser dose to the upper abdomen if it is involved. Tepper and associates treated seventeen patients in this category, using a dose of 3000 rad to large lower abdominal fields in combination with triethylenethiophosphoramide. At the time of the second operation, tumor regression was sufficient to permit gross total removal of the lesion in nine of the seventeen patients. No significant long-term results of this technique are yet available.

TECHNIQUE. The volume requiring irradiation in carcinoma of the ovary is invariably large. As mentioned previously, total abdominal irradiation with or without a boosting dose to the pelvis, depending on stage, is generally the aim of treatment. In view of the demanding nature of whole abdominal irradiation it should not be recommended lightly, particularly if its value is seriously questioned. However, when abdominal irradiation is indicated, we have found the moving-strip technique with the ^{60}Co or megavoltage beam superior to other methods (Delclos and associates) (Fig. 19-2). It seems to be tolerated better by the patient, and yet it delivers a suffi-

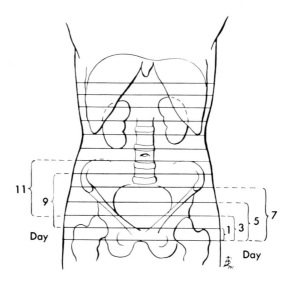

Fig. 19-2. Diagram of the moving-strip technique for irradiation of abdomen. Both anterior and posterior surfaces of abdomen are divided into 2.5 cm strips. On the first day, the most inferior anterior strip is irradiated. The opposing strip is irradiated the second day. A daily dose of 250 rad is delivered to the midplane. On the third day, a second 2.5 cm strip is added to the first. Each day thereafter the next superior strip is added to the port. After four strips are included, the most inferior strip is omitted each time a superior strip is added.

ciently high dose in a short period to be more effective biologically. The anterior and posterior aspects of the abdomen from the diaphragm to the floor of the pelvis are divided into transverse strips 2.5 cm wide. Alternating daily between the anterior and posterior positions, strips are irradiated, beginning at the pubis with the first 2.5 cm strip. A daily dose of 250 rad is given. Each day the next superior strip is added to the port until four strips have been irradiated. Each day thereafter one new strip is added superiorly, and the most inferior strip, which by then has been treated four times, is omitted. Smoron has evaluated the dose distribution of this technique, and we have adopted his suggested modifications. To avoid cold spots when using a 4 mev photon beam, the strips are purposely staggered so that the posterior surface line projects to the center of the anterior opposed strip. An additional exposure is given to the most cephalad and most caudad strips. Since the dose-time relationship with this technique may exceed renal tolerance in some cases, the kidneys should be shielded for part of the treatment. This can be done with simple lead blocks after proper localization. The white blood cell count usually remains above 4000/ml, and bothersome bowel or gastric upset is rarely encountered. If large masses remain in the pelvis, an additional 2000 to 3000 rad can be delivered through opposing tailored portals. The technique is flexible. A similar boost is given in Stage IIb and Stage III lesions, and, depending on the aim, a dose of 2500 to 4000 rad is added. Simple opposing portals may suffice for some cases, but when the dose of 4000 rad is added to the strip, this approaches tolerance of pelvic structures, and the use of an anterior and two posterior oblique ports may reduce the incidence of rectal complications.

In patients with rather widespread peritoneal extension or metastases, rapidly forming ascites may be bothersome. Control of ascites with external irradiation has been disappointing. In the past, colloidal [198]Au and ^{32}P were used with limited success, but disadvantages of this modality have largely led to its replacement by L-phenylalanine mustard.

A single alkylating agent is generally employed in patients with Stage III epithelial tumors when systemic chemotherapy is elected. Multidrug combinations with an alkylating agent have shown no significant superiority over the single drug, and side effects are greater. An excellent overview of the management of epithelial tumors by chemotherapy has been prepared by Tobias and Griffiths.

PROGNOSIS AND RESULTS. As implied before, it is impossible with available statistics to prove that there is an increased 5-year survival with the recommended combination of surgery and irradiation. Probably the best evidence that worthwhile results are obtained by radiotherapy is seen in those patients with palpable masses, ascites, pain, or vaginal bleeding from inoperable ovarian carcinoma. These symptoms can be controlled, sometimes permanently, with irradiation techniques described previously. The fact that the survival rate with ovarian carcinoma is highly variable makes any claims of increasing the 5-year survival rate open to question.

Griffiths and associates have pointed out that the survival time in patients with advanced carcinoma of the ovary is inversely proportional to the amount of residual

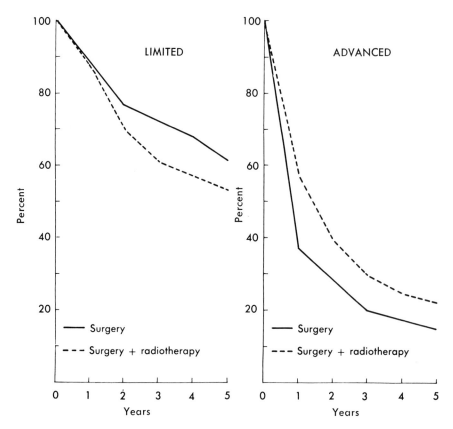

Fig. 19-3. Yearly survival of an initial group of 1722 women with ovarian carcinoma. Early cases (Stages I and II) showed no improvement when postoperative irradiation was employed. (From Maus, J. H., et al.: Am. J. Roentgenol. **102**:603-607, 1968.)

tumor remaining after surgery. In this context the benefits of postoperative irradiation or administration of alkylating agents may be to further reduce residual tumor volume after surgery. A similar observation has been made in Stage III cases by Buckler and associates. They categorized "favorable" cases as having a pelvic mass of less than 8 cm and extrapelvic nodules of less than 2 cm. "Unfavorable" cases had disease greater than this. In the favorable group median survival of patients treated either by postoperative irradiation or chemotherapy was approximately 23 months, whereas in the unfavorable group, median survival was 7 months with postoperative irradiation and 15 months with chemotherapy. We have accepted this difference in survival as significant and recommend treatment accordingly.

Data in Table 19-1 fail to reveal unquestioned increased cure rates attributable to irradiation. Data published by Rubin and associates, by Kent and McKay, and by Fuks suggest that cure rates are improved by radiotherapy. The composite data from 1722 patients in Ontario as presented by Maus and associates (Fig. 19-3) show an improved survival for all but Stage I cases when postoperative irradiation is given.

Table 19-2. Response to postoperative irradiation according to histologic classification*

Histology	Surgery only		Surgery and irradiation	
	Number of patients	5-year survival (%)	Number of patients	5-year survival (%)
Serous	101	32	100	46
Mucinous	33	49	20	50
Undifferentiated	16	13	12	42

*Modified from Kent, S. W., and McKay, D. G.: Am. J. Obstet. Gynecol. **80:**430-438, 1960.

The larger ports required to encompass more advanced disease cannot tolerate high doses. If whole abdominal irradiation is considered desirable, a midline depth dose of 2500 rad in 5 weeks is the upper limit. Except for dysgerminoma, we do not believe such a dose can produce more than temporary tumor regression and growth restraint. However, palliation may be worth the undesirable side effects. The moving-strip technique for whole abdominal irradiation is well tolerated, and results are at least comparable to wide-field whole abdominal irradiation (Burns and associates). As mentioned previously, the volume to be considered for irradiation is seldom less than the whole abdomen.

Stage for stage, endometrioid carcinoma has the best prognosis among the ovarian carcinomas. This is followed in order by the mucinous and serous carcinomas (Aure and associates; Kottmeier). Kent and McKay analyzed the response to postoperative irradiation according to histologic classification (Table 19-2). There was no improvement in the survival of patients with pseudomucinous cancers when postoperative irradiation was added. Long and associates reported a similar result for mucinous cancers.

Despite the questionable value of irradiation in the cure of carcinoma of the ovary, there is no question of its palliative usefulness. Large symptom-producing masses can be shrunk, ascites decreased, vaginal bleeding controlled, and the occasional osseous metastases arrested.

Dysgerminoma

Dysgerminoma is the female counterpart of seminoma. However, it is a rare tumor, and facts relative to its behavior and optimum treatment are uncertain. At laparotomy, 20% to 30% of the patients will have developed spread beyond the one ovary. The most common route of spread is by way of the retroperitoneal, mediastinal, and supraclavicular lymph nodes. Like seminoma, dysgerminoma is most frequent during the reproductive years.

The desire to preserve the function of reproduction has led to some practices that are unique in cancer therapy. For those patients with disease clinically limited to one ovary, Brody has recommended unilateral oophorectomy with postoperative irradiation of that half of the pelvis only. Thus function of the remaining ovary is preserved and childbearing is still possible. Patients with this selected group of early encapsulated dysgerminomas show an excellent survival rate of 95%. Yet irradiation of half the pelvis as he recommended to a minimum dose of 2000 rad in 3 weeks delivers substantial scattered radiations to the remaining ovary. Brody has estimated it to be from one to ten times the dose required to double the number of naturally occurring mutations.

Krepart and associates have defined their criteria for selecting patients for this type of limited surgery. They have not used irradiation in this selected group.

1. Unilateral encapsulated dysgerminoma, 10 cm or less in maximum diameter
2. No ascites
3. No visible or palpable evidence of metastases to any lymph nodes or abdominal viscera
4. Negative lymphangiogram

Is the retention of the function of reproduction worth the risk of limiting surgery and radiotherapy? There is now experience that seems to justify limiting surgery and omitting irradiation if the criteria mentioned before are respected. Thus all five patients Krepart treated in this manner were cured, and three subsequently had children. If disease remains, we believe irradiation of the full volume to the full dose as described in the discussion that follows is indicated.

Although it might seem desirable to tailor irradiated volume to the precise extent of the disease, this is seldom possible or advisable. Once the disease has exceeded the criteria for limited unilateral disease described before, the whole abdomen is at risk and should be irradiated. We have usually employed a moving-strip technique and given a dose of 2500 rad midabdomen. Additional boosting doses of 1500 rad are given to any involved retroperitonal nodes or pelvic masses. If the abdominal nodes were involved on lymphangiogram or known masses were present, the mediastinum and both supraclavicular areas were given 2500 rad in 2 to 3 weeks.

PROGNOSIS AND RESULTS. The infrequency of this disease, coupled with the variety of ways in which it has been treated, does not permit a clear-cut statement of survival rates as related to treatment. Pedowitz and associates reported a 5-year survival rate of 27.1% in seventy patients gathered from the literature. Thoeny and associates reported a 5-year survival rate of 70%. Brody reported a 95% 5-year survival if the cancer was unilateral, encapsulated, and mobile, 78% if the cancer was ruptured, adherent, or associated with ascites, and 33% when metastases were

Table 19-3. Survival of patients with dysgerminoma by stage*

Stage	Number of patients	Number surviving	Percent	Survival in months
I	14	14	100	36-212
II	2	2	100	102-133
III	13	10	77	36-273
IV	7	5	71	33-247
TOTAL	36	31	86	

*From Krepart, G., Smith, J. P., Rutledge, F., and Delclos, L.: Cancer **41**:986-990, 1978.

present. The more recent experience of Krepart and associates is shown in Table 19-3.

Summary

With the exception of dysgerminomas and perhaps some of the malignant granulosa cell tumors, malignant tumors of the ovary are not sufficiently radiosensitive to be frequently radiocurable. For this reason cure usually depends on a complete excision of the tumor. Removal of the carcinoma with salpingo-oophorectomy and hysterectomy should be done. If, on gross and microscopic examination, the carcinoma is confined to one ovary, postoperative irradiation has not been shown to improve results. If carcinoma is known or thought to have been left in the pelvis only, vigorous postoperative pelvic irradiation is mandatory. In view of the frequency of the seeding to the peritoneum, whole abdominal irradiation should be considered for Stages Ib through III. If widespread abdominal disease or distant metastases are present, one should direct palliative irradiation toward relieving symptoms. Dysgerminoma is sufficiently radiosensitive to warrant prophylactic irradiation not unlike that recommended for seminoma. Preoperative irradiation should be considered when locally advanced cancer is found on exploration.

REFERENCES

Aure, J. C., Høeg, K., and Kolstad, P.: Clinical and histologic studies of ovarian carcinoma: long-term follow-up of 990 cases, Obstet. Gynecol. 37:1-9, 1971.

Brody, S.: Clinical aspects of dysgerminoma of the ovary, Acta Radiol. 56:209-230, 1961.

Buckler, D. A., Kline, J. C., Davis, H. L., Ramirez, G., and Carr, W. F.: Stage III ovarian carcinoma: treatment and results, comparison of multiple drugs, and irradiation, Radiology 122: 469-472, 1977.

Burns, B. C., Rutledge, F. N., Smith, J. P., and Delclos, L.: Management of ovarian carcinoma, Am. J. Obstet. Gynecol. 98:374-383, 1967.

Delclos, L., Braun, E. J., Herrera, J. R., Jr., Sampiere, V. A., and Roosenbeek, E. V.: Whole abdominal irradiation by cobalt -60 moving-strip technic, Radiology 81:632-641, 1963.

Diczfalusy, E., Notter, G., and Nissen-Meyer, R.: Influence of ovarian irradiation on urinary estrogens in breast cancer patients. In Carlson, W. D., and Gassner, F. X., editors: Effects of ionizing radiation on the reproductive system, New York, 1964, The Macmillan Co.

Fisher, R. I., and Young, R. C.: Advances in the staging and treatment of ovarian cancer, Cancer 39:967-972, 1977.

Fuks, Z.: External radiotherapy of ovarian cancer: standard approaches and new frontiers, Semin. Oncol. 2:253-266, 1975.

Griem, M. L., Meier, P., and Dobben, G. D.: Analysis of the morbidity and mortality of children irradiated in fetal life, Radiology 88::347-349, 1967.

Griffiths, C. T.: Surgical resection of tumor bulk in the primary treatment of ovarian carcinoma, Natl. Cancer Inst. Monogr. 42:101-104, 1975.

Griffiths, C. T., Grogan, R. H., and Hall, T. C.: Advanced ovarian cancer: primary treatment with surgery, radiotherapy, and chemotherapy, Cancer 29:1-7, 1972.

Hicks, S. P., and D'Amato, J.: Effects of radiation on the developing embryo and fetus. In Meigs, J. V., and Sturgis, S. H., editors: Progress in gynecology, vol. 4, New York, 1963, Grune & Stratton, Inc.

Holmes, G. M.: Malignant ovarian tumours, J. Fac. Radiologists 8:394-402, 1957.

Kent, S. W., and McKay, D. G.: Primary cancer of ovary, Am. J. Obstet. Gynecol. 80:430-438, 1960.

Kottmeier, H. L.: Clinical staging in ovarian carcinoma. In Gentil, F., and Junqueira, A. C.: Ovarian cancer, UICC Monograph Series, vol. 11, New York, 1968, Springer-Verlag New York Inc.

Krepart, G., Smith, J. P., Rutledge, F., and Delclos, L.: The treatment of dysgerminoma of the ovary, Cancer 41:986-990, 1978.

Lacassagne, A., and Gricouroff, G.: Action des radiations ionisantes sur l'organisme, Paris, 1956, Masson et Cie.

Long, R. T. L., and Sala, J. M.: Radical surgery combined with radiotherapy in the treatment of advanced ovarian carcinoma, Surg. Gynecol. Obstet. 117:201-204, 1963.

Long, R. T. L., Johnson, R. E., and Sala, J. M.: Variations in survival among patients with carcinoma of the ovary, Cancer 20:1195-1202, 1967.

Maus, J. H., Mackay, E. N., and Sellers, A. H.: Cancer of the ovary, Am. J. Roentgenol. 102:603-607, 1968.

Pedowitz, P., Huffman, J. W., and Moss, W. T.: Dysgerminoma, Am. J. Obstet. Gynecol. 86:693-700, 1963.

Raventos, A., Lewis, G. C., and Chidiac, J.: Primary ovarian cancer: a twenty-year report, Am. J. Roentgenol. 89:524-532, 1963.

Rubin, P., Grise, J. W., and Terry, R.: Has postoperative irradiation proved itself? Am. J. Roentgenol. 88:849-866, 1962.

Rugh, R.: The impact of ionizing radiations on the embryo and fetus, Am. J. Roentgenol. 89:182-190, 1963.

Russell, W. L.: Genetic effects of radiation in mammals. In Hollaender, A., editor: Radiation biology, New York, 1954, McGraw-Hill Book Co.

Smoron, G. L.: Strip-staggering: elimination of inhomogeneity in the moving-strip technique of whole abdominal irradiation, Radiology 104:657-660, 1972.

Tepper, E., Sanfilippo, L. J., Gray, J., and Romney, S. L.: Second look surgery after radiation therapy for advanced stages of cancer of the ovary, Am. J. Roentgenol. 112:755-759, 1971.

Thoeny, R. H., Dockerty, M. B., Hunt, A. B., and Childs, D. S., Jr.: A study of ovarian dysgerminoma with emphasis on the role of radiation therapy, Surg. Gynecol. Obstet. 113:692-698, 1961.

Tobias, J. S., and Griffiths, C. T.: Medical progress, management of ovarian carcinoma, current concepts and future prospects. I. N. Engl. J. Med. 294:818-823, 1976.

Tobias, J. S., and Griffiths, C. T.: Medical progress, management of ovarian carcinoma, current concepts and future prospects. II. N. Engl. J. Med. 294:877-882, 1976.

Vaeth, J. M., and Buschke, F. J.: The role of preoperative irradiation in the treatment of carcinoma of the ovary, Am. J. Roentgenol. 105:614-617, 1969.

Zuckerman, S.: The sensitivity of the gonads to radiation, Clin. Radiol. 19:1-15, 1965.

20
The hemopoietic tissues

RESPONSE OF NORMAL HEMOPOIETIC TISSUES TO IRRADIATION

Total body irradiation produces early dramatic changes in the circulating blood. Similar doses delivered to whole blood in vitro produce few significant immediate or delayed blood modifications. The changes in the circulating blood after total body irradiation by sublethal doses are chiefly a result of damage to the blood-forming organs and are not a direct effect on the circulating blood. Although the effects of radiations on hemopoietic tissues account for most of the changes appearing in the formed elements of the blood, plasma changes reflect the combined radiation damage and reaction of all body tissue, since all contribute to the plasma contents. The voluminous literature on this subject cannot be reviewed here. This discussion will be confined to the clinically important changes produced by doses near the therapeutic range.

BONE MARROW. A short, single dose of total body irradiation is rarely practiced in radiotherapy, but the results of such doses in laboratory animals have clarified many problems arising in therapy subsequent to the inclusion of extensive hemopoietic tissue in the irradiated volume. These data could not be obtained in normal human beings, but similar reactions may reasonably be expected in man, with variations only in degree, time of onset, and duration. A single total body irradiation, lethal in 30 days to 50% of a group of animals, is termed the $LD_{50/30}$. For man this is usually given as about 450 R (air). Some workers suggest that this value may be high (Cronkite and Bond). Probably a dose of 350 rad uniformly distributed throughout the tissues and given at a fairly rapid dose rate is a more nearly correct value.

Bloom has made a careful study of changes in the rabbit's marrow after the administration of this dose. A half hour after such a dose, there is a cessation of mitosis in bone marrow. By this time, the nucleated red cell count has already started to decrease and the more mature forms predominate. Progressively, the number of dead cells in the marrow increases, primarily at the expense of the erythrocytic series. The granulocyte count decreases but to a lesser degree. During these first hours, the megakaryocytes remain normal in number and appearance, but will have disappeared in 2 days. Filling the spaces left by the destroyed cells is a gelatinous

519

marrow that forms in increasing quantity. The nucleated red cell count drops to a minimum in 24 hours, whereas the myelocyte count continues to decrease for 9 days. Repopulation of the marrow begins 10 to 14 days after irradiation. Erythropoiesis becomes active at this time and granulocytopoiesis begins a few days later. In 41 days the marrow appears completely repopulated with apparently normal cells.

The radiosensitivity of marrow varies with its position in the bones. Cells in the metaphysis are more radiosensitive than those of the shaft. The shaft marrow recovers more rapidly. Some workers ascribe greater radiosensitivity to the granulocytic series, but such conclusions may be colored by the peripheral blood counts to be described. We would agree with Lacassagne and Lavedan that this difference in sensitivity is probably not of great importance. Valentine and Pearce bled cats vigorously and then compared recovery times with and without 200 R total body irradiation. Erythrocyte counts reached normal levels only slightly less rapidly in the irradiated group than in the controls. Granulopoiesis, measured by peripheral leukocyte counts, required 30 days to reach the level seen in nonirradiated animals. Functional impairment is recognized as being greater in granulopoiesis. Similarly, chronic total body irradiation of 50 rad per day given to the rat for 130 days has little effect on the response of erythropoietic tissues but a moderate effect on the ability to produce a leukocytosis (Lamerton). Lower doses produce proportionately less bone marrow damage, and recovery is more rapid.

Locally irradiated marrow recovers more quickly than the marrow of animals given total body irradiation. Knospe and associates gave single doses of 2000, 4000, 6000, or 10,000 rad to the hind limbs of rats and examined the marrow at intervals up to 1 year. Initial hemopoietic regeneration began 7 to 14 days after irradiation regardless of the dose, although the degree of cellularity at any time was dose-dependent. During the second and third month after irradiation there was sinusoidal disruption and disappearance of sinusoids in all irradiated marrow specimens. This correlated with maximum decrease in marrow cellularity. After 6 months, marrow regeneration was evident only in those animals receiving 2000 rad, and this recovery followed regeneration of the sinusoidal structures. This suggests the dependence of hemopoietic recovery on regeneration of the sinusoidal microcirculation. Fishburn and associates demonstrated that the juvenile rat marrow was able to repopulate with higher levels of cellularity and after higher doses of radiations than did the adult rodent marrow. In man, locally irradiated marrow shows a marked decrease in early cell types after a dose of 400 rad in 3 days (Lehar and associates). After 1000 rad in 8 days there is complete disappearance of normoblasts and early granulocytes, as well as a significant reduction of marrow cellularity. Some mature granulocytes persist after a dose of 2000 rad in 16 days, but megakaryocytes are absent; few are present at the 1000 rad sampling. There are no significant changes in the unirradiated marrow of these patients.

Knowledge of the distribution of active marrow is useful in anticipating the magnitude of the effect of irradiating various local sites in clinical practice. The best available information in this regard is the work of Ellis. Approximately 40% of the active adult marrow is in the pelvis, and 25% is in the thoracic and lumbar vertebrae. The significance of this distribution in the treatment of Hodgkin's disease is illustrated in Fig. 20-10. In children a significant amount of marrow is in the long bones (45% at age 5 years), but this rapidly diminishes in adolescence, and after the age of 20 years negligible amounts of active marrow are present in the long bones (Atkinson; Ellis).

High local doses, as are administered in clinical radiotherapy, may produce such severe marrow injury that repopulation will never occur. Sykes and associates found that in the sternal marrow this dose began at 3000 rad. Regeneration occurred regularly within 1 month after doses up to 2500 rad. When the bone marrow is not repopulated, the predominant picture is of fatty replacement. Despite the inability of the marrow to repopulate, it can support the growth of metastatic cancer cells (Sykes and associates).

The study of bone marrow regeneration following total nodal irradiation for Hodgkin's disease indicates that after 4000 rad to this large volume of bone marrow there is prolonged suppression, which continues for at least 1 year (Rubin and associates). In the twenty-seven patients they studied with bone marrow scanning agents, 50% showed evidence of partial or complete regeneration at 1 year, and this increased to 80% by 2 to 3 years. There was redistribution of bone marrow activity in half of the patients studied.

LYMPH NODES. The cells composing lymphopoietic tissues also vary tremendously in their radiosensitivity. Lymphocytes and lymphoblasts are supported by a fibrous framework transporting blood vessels. Lymph passes into the node through lymph sinuses and then between the lymphocytes, phagocytic reticulum, and macrophages. Lymph is collected by a similar efferent system. Each of these elements (lymphocytes, fibrous framework, and macrophages) exhibits different radiosensitivity.

De Bruyn reviewed the literature and described his own findings on this subject. His observation of the response of lymphoid tissue in the rabbit is presented as typical, with the same qualifications as mentioned in the discussion of bone marrow. Within half an hour of delivering 800 R (air) total body irradiation ($LD_{50/30}$, 200 kv radiations filtered with 0.5 mm Cu and 1 mm Al at 70 to 90 cm TSD) to rabbits, nuclear debris is apparent in the node. This rapidly increases in amount and reaches a maximum in 8 hours. With this dose, macrophages are not noticeably altered directly but become phagocytically active as the debris appears. Most of the debris is phagocytized in 20 hours (Fig. 20-1). By then the fibrous framework and macrophages dominate the picture. Plasma cells may be seen beginning 9 days after irradiation but are less numerous in 5 to 6 weeks. Intranodal hemorrhage and perivascular edema are seen irregularly.

In addition to the alteration of lymphopoietic function, the functions of reticuloendothelial elements are altered by higher doses. With 2000 to 3000 rad their functions are decreased, and with 6500 rad they are abolished (Teneff and Stoppani). At the same time, Teneff and Stoppani found that this dose produced no obstruction

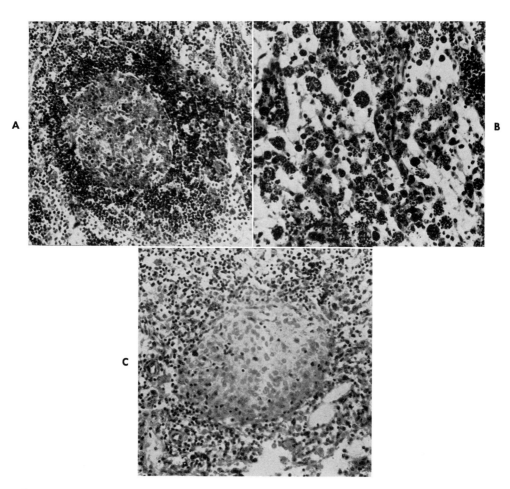

Fig. 20-1. Response of mesenteric lymph node of the rabbit to irradiation. **A,** Normal nodule with active germinal center (magnification ×245). **B,** Seventeen hours after a single dose of 800 R (magnification ×245). **C,** Twenty-four hours after a single dose of 800 R (magnification ×245). (Courtesy United States Atomic Energy Commission; from De Bruyn, P. P. H.: Lymph node and intestinal lymphatic tissue. In Bloom, W., editor: Histopathology of irradiation, New York, 1948, McGraw-Hill Book Co.)

of lymph flow through the nodes. As will be seen later, the composition of the lymph is altered.

About 5 days after the $LD_{50/30}$ dose, lymphocytes begin to reappear in the denuded node. The process by which this is achieved is not known. About 3 weeks after irradiation, lymphopoiesis in cortical areas starts, and by 4 months the node appears normal.

With smaller doses, destruction is less severe and the return to normal is much more rapid. Thus, after 50 rad, the node will appear normal in 27 hours. Smaller, repeated daily doses of 5 to 10 R (air) as used in therapy of leukemic patients produce cell death at such a slow rate and phagocytosis is so efficient that lymph node damage is sometimes difficult to detect microscopically. Clinically, the nodes are seen to shrink.

Engeset described the effects of locally administered doses of 3000 rad on the popliteal lymph nodes of rats. At 12 hours there was marked degeneration of lymphocytes and disruption of follicles. Nuclear debris was abundant. Lymphocyte repopulation was evident at 24 hours, and by 48 hours the nuclear debris was gone. At that time follicles were increasing in number. Although early recovery was nearly complete in the first week after irradiation, chronic changes began after 2 weeks. There was a gradual increase in connective tissue and a progressive decrease of cortical lymphocytes and germinal centers. Nine to 12 months after irradiation there was nearly complete disruption of normal lymph node structures. In addition to these histologic alterations, there were functional changes in the irradiated lymph nodes. In view of the clinical implications of these changes, the interested reader should review Engeset's original paper.

A number of investigators, including Engeset, have devised experiments to evaluate the ability of locally irradiated lymph nodes to remove and retain particulate material, such as animal tumor cell suspensions, erythrocytes, charcoal particles, and radioactive colloidal gold, infused into the afferent lymphatics. High-increment doses in single or few fractions were generally given, and most experiments were concerned with immediate effects. In view of the histologic disruption of irradiated lymph nodes under these conditions, it is not surprising that most such studies indicate that irradiation significantly reduces the "barrier function" of nodes (Engeset; Dettman and associates; Fisher and Fisher; O'Brien and associates). Attempts to correlate such changes with those expected in the clinical setting are difficult. Transient suppression of lymph node function may indeed occur, but with conventional fractionation lymph nodes appear to recover after modest or even high doses (Fig. 20-2).

Lymphatic vessels are resistant to doses of radiations sufficient to produce skin slough and necrosis in the hind limb of dogs (Sherman and O'Brien). Nineteen months after a dose of 3600 rad skin (1200 rad given three times in 14 days; 280 kvp; hvl, 1.3 mm Cu; TSD 50 cm), those authors demonstrated normal lymphatics in the irradiated zone of animals that had developed extensive soft tissue necroses. Similar evidence of the resistance of these vessels to irradiation was presented by Engeset and by Lenzi and Bassani. Although irradiation has frequently been implicated as a direct cause of lymphatic obstruction, it is more likely that radiation-induced connective tissue fibrosis impairs the patency of both lymphatic and venous channels and gives rise to the picture of combined lymphatic and venous obstruction. In such instances, the development of lymphedema is hastened by the functional loss of lymphaticovenous shunts. Once extrinsic venous obstruction is established and edema ensues, phlebography will show changes of chronic thrombophlebitis.

SPLEEN. The radioresponsiveness of the spleen is comparable to that described for lymph nodes. This is as expected, since the white pulp is in fact similar in struc-

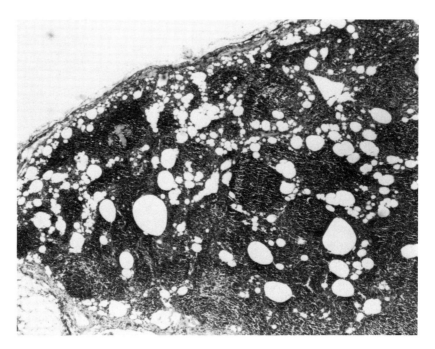

Fig. 20-2. Para-aortic lymph node 3 years after dose of 3500 rad in 4 weeks for metastatic seminoma. The anatomy of node appears well preserved. The capsular and medullary sinusoids contain lipid droplets from a recent lymphangiogram. An embryonal carcinoma was discovered in remaining testicle. (magnification × 160.)

ture to the lymph nodes. Its close relationship to arteries and the fact that it, like the red pulp, is inserted in the blood circulatory system do not seem to alter significantly the response of this lymphoid tissue to irradiation. The white pulp gradually merges into the red pulp, which has a fibrous framework and phagocytic reticular cells not unlike those of lymph nodes. In this framework are found all the formed elements of whole blood, in addition to free macrophages. In man, lymphocytes only are normally formed in the white pulp. In certain pathologic conditions, granulopoiesis may occur in the red pulp. In rabbits, rats, and mice, granulopoiesis is normally found in the spleen, and such animals provide the opportunity of studying the relative radiosensitivity of lymphopoiesis and granulopoiesis side by side.

Murray has described the morphologic splenic changes subsequent to 800 R (air) total body irradiation of rabbits. As stated previously, in the rabbit this dose constitutes the $LD_{50/30}$. Within half an hour cessation of mitosis is seen. In 3 hours the white pulp retains but a few large and small lymphocytes. In 8 hours the reticular cells show clumping of nuclear chromatin but do not die. During this same period there is rapid destruction of all elements of the red pulp except the reticular cells and the circulating blood. Despite sporadic lymphopoiesis, no real increase in lymphocytes occurs for about 9 days. Erythroblasts and myeloblasts reappear in 14 days, and after 21 days myelopoiesis becomes hyperactive.

As a consequence of this massive cell destruction, the spleen shrinks rapidly. Within 24 hours it is half its normal weight. The more radioresistant cells of the fibrous framework are pushed together to give the false impression of reticuloendo-thelial hyperplasia. Regeneration is thought to occur after the conversion of reticular cells to lymphoblasts, erythroblasts, and myeloblasts. After such a large dose as 800 R (air), lymphopoiesis is always resumed prior to myelopoiesis, but the lymphocyte count in the peripheral blood is slower in returning to a normal level than the erythrocyte count. Total body irradiation of various species with equal doses produces comparable splenic injury irrespective of the differences in $LD_{50/30}$ for these species. Some of the effects of splenic irradiation on splenic function can be deduced from the numerous spleen-shielding experiments reported by Jacobson. The ability of the spleen to store red blood cells, the variation in rate of blood flow through the spleen, its erythrocytolytic activity, the capacity of the spleen for storing iron-con-taining pigment, and its production of antibodies are probably altered. However, the directions and magnitudes of any such changes have not been reported.

Splenic irradiation in patients with chronic myelogenous leukemia produces not only massive death of leukemic cells in the spleen but produces profound change in hemopoietic tissues remote from the spleen (Hotchkiss and Block). The elevated leukocyte count drops, the hemoglobin increases, and sternal marrow biopsies show improvement. A suggested explanation is that not only does the spleen act as a source of supply for a large proportion of the leukemic cells but it also acts as a "trap" for normal and abnormal leukocytes. Studies with ^{51}Cr indicate red cell survival in-creases and red cell production increases with the improvement of the marrow. The therapeutic effects are similar to those obtained from total body irradiation or admin-istration of some of the cytotoxic agents.

Changes in circulating blood subsequent to large field or total body irradiation

As stated previously, total body irradiation produces early dramatic changes in the circulating blood. Most of these changes in blood cell counts and ratios are secondary to damage of the hemopoietic tissues. The response in all tissues con-tributes to plasma changes.

FORMED ELEMENTS

There is normally a delicate balance between the circulating lives of blood cells, the rates of replacement of these cells, and the body's demand for them. Radiation damage of the hemopoietic tissues upsets this balance by reducing or interrupting the supply of blood cells. Leukopenia, erythrocytopenia, and thrombocytopenia develop at rates in keeping with the severity of the damage and the circulating lives of the already developed cells.

LEUKOCYTES. The postirradiation fluctuations of leukocyte counts and the percentages of granulocytes and mononucleated cells are shown graphically in Fig. 20-3. The response varies widely with the dose of radiations. After a large nonlethal

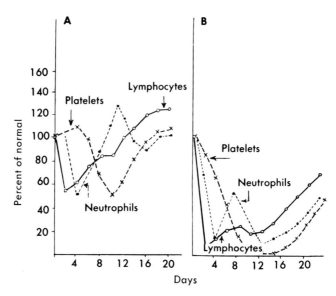

Fig. 20-3. Effect of various doses of total body irradiation on blood cell counts in the rat. **A,** After 100 R single-dose total body irradiation. **B,** After 400 R single-dose total body irradiation. (Modified from Elson, L. A.: In Hevesey, G., et al., editors: Advances in radiobiology, Edinburgh, 1957, Oliver & Boyd, Ltd.)

dose there is immediate but transient leukopenia, changing in a few hours to a leuko-cytosis. This early leukopenia has not been frequently recognized or described. It has been attributed to alterations in the repair of leukocytes effected in vascular beds. The subsequent leukocytosis is likewise brief, for by the second day a severe increasing leukopenia is in progress. If the dose has not been too great, a minimum total white cell count is obtained about the third day, and the total count begins to increase soon thereafter. A normal count may be obtained in 8 to 10 days or it may require 1 to 3 months, depending on the dose and method of administration. In the Marshallese exposed to fallout radiations, recovery of leukocytes was incomplete at 10 years (Conrad and Hicking).

Within the leukocytic series, all cells do not respond alike. The normal life-span of most circulating lymphocytes appears to be short. Lawrence and associates (1945) found it to be less than 24 hours. However, their life-span may be 3 to 4 days or occasionally even 100 to 200 days (Brecher and associates, 1962). Recirculation of lymphocytes through lymphoid tissues has made the circulating life-span appear shorter than it actually is. Regardless of which figure may be correct, the extreme radiosensitivity of the lymphopoietic tissues is manifested early as relative lympho-penia. Both clinically and microscopically, lymph nodes seem to recover early, whereas the lymphocyte count is slow in returning to a normal level. Unlike the other circulating formed elements, the circulating lymphocyte is sufficiently sensitive to be seriously damaged by total body irradiation. Circulating leukemic lymphocytes are more radiosensitive than are circulating normal lymphocytes (Jage). Following

total nodal irradiation in Hodgkin's disease there is significant decrease in lymphocyte function. This effect on lymphocyte function is gradually reversed so that by 5
years following irradiation, the lymphocytes of such patients function normally (Kun
and Johnson; Hoppe and associates).

The early leukocytosis is due almost entirely to rapid granulocytosis occurring
within the first 24 hours. This is probably a reaction to injury mediated through a
mobilization rather than a new production of granulocytes (Bloom and Jacobson). A
day or so later, the migration of leukocytes seems impaired (Shechmeister and Fishman). The major function of the granulocytes is extravascular. These cells appear in
the circulating blood briefly en route to the tissues. Since granulopoietic tissues are
easily damaged by radiations, a neutropenia is observed soon after the onset of the
lymphopenia described. Maximum neutropenia occurs in 3 or 4 days. The return to a
normal count usually precedes that of the lymphocyte count. There are functional
changes in the circulating granulocytes as well as in the numerical decrease. Thus
early postirradiation granulocytes possess fewer bactericidal capabilities than do
nonirradiated granulocytes (Fishman and Shechmeister).

PLATELETS. Platelets have their origin from megakaryocytes in the marrow or
in the lungs, and as was seen previously, megakaryocytes are the least radiosensitive
of the myeloid elements. They are nevertheless sufficiently sensitive to be damaged
by even moderate doses of radiations. Platelets have a maximum circulating life of
8 to 11 days. Radiation damage of megakaryocytes is soon reflected in the circulating
blood as an alteration in platelet counts. For 2 to 3 days after a single total body dose
of 150 to 400 R (air), a slight increase in platelet count may occur (Cronkite and
Brecher). Then the thrombocytopenia begins. Subsequent to total body doses of this
level, the decrease in platelets is a function of the dose. However, with doses above
400 R (air) the depression in the count becomes maximal, whereas below 150 R (air)
the changes are relatively minor. With intermediate doses permitting survival, the
maximum depression is reached in 10 to 12 days and recovery may begin after the
twentieth day. Cronkite and Brecher have made excellent detailed studies of these
changes in the dog. Normal platelet counts may be obtained 7 to 8 weeks after exposure. When high doses have been given, death may occur before any decrease in
count is detected, or with lower but still lethal doses death may occur despite partial
recovery of the platelet count. The recognized functions of platelets disappear as
the thrombocytopenia progresses.

A serious defect in hemostasis is expected, and thrombocytopenia is the most
important factor in its development. Other than platelet transfusions, there is no
treatment for radiation-induced thrombocytopenia or the resulting defect in hemostasis. Whole blood transfusions are of little value in correcting this defect. However,
death from excessive irradiation of the $LD_{50/30}$ level is not frequently attributable to
thrombocytopenic hemorrhages, although they are often present (Bond and associates).

Unlike their precursors, circulating platelets are resistant to high doses of radiations (7500 rad in vitro) (Greenberg and associates).

RED BLOOD CELLS. Circulating red blood cells, like most other circulating formed elements, are resistant to direct damage by irradiation. Irradiation of rats (single-dose total body irradiation of 500 to 600 R [air]; 250 kv; filter, 0.6 mm Cu; dose rate, 25 R [air] per minute) increases the thermal fragility of circulating red cells. The fragility returns to normal in 24 hours (Goldschmidt and associates). The normal red cell has an average circulating life-span of 120 days. The rate of erythrocyte turnover in man and dog is normally about 0.83% of the erythrocytes daily, or the erythrocytes in about 50 ml of normal blood. With doses of radiations employed clinically, the red cell count decreases slowly. Several weeks of poorly functioning bone marrow are required to produce a clinically noticeable decrease in the total red count. But the easily damaged erythropoietic tissues recover rapidly after a single moderate dose of radiations, and normal functions may be reestablished before an anemia becomes clinically obvious. A second explanation for an earlier anemia seen in laboratory animals is that of Kahn and Furth. Doses of radiations much above clinical levels increase the permeability of capillaries, permitting an exit of erythrocytes from the circulation. The destruction of these cells is presumably related to their extravasation and not to direct radiation injury. However, in clinical radiotherapy this is probably not an important cause of anemia. The precursor of the erythrocyte, the reticulocyte, disappears from the circulating blood almost as quickly as the lymphocyte. A dose of about 400 R (air) total body dose in man reduces the reticulocyte count to zero in 10 to 15 days. It may not be restored to normal levels for months.

When low-dose total body irradiation is given over a period of many months, an entirely different blood picture is produced. The highly radiosensitive erythropoietic tissues are not allowed to recover, and an anemia develops in addition to the previously described leukopenia. The marrow may become aplastic. The exact dose levels producing these changes in man are not known. In mice, a daily dose as great as 1.1 rad every 8 hours from maturity to death does not produce a significant change in red cell count (Lorenz). The former permissible dose for radiologists (0.3 rad per week) did not produce detectable hematologic changes in man. In fact doses otherwise harmful and larger than 0.3 rad per week do not produce consistent changes in blood counts. For this reason, blood counts are not a safe guide to radiation protection but are rather a measure of the severity of considerable overdosage.

Effects of irradiation on blood plasma, lymph, and tissue fluids

In balance and electrolyte studies, the effects produced by irradiation such as anorexia, nausea, vomiting, diarrhea, infection, and fever are difficult to separate from possible direct radiation-induced tissue effects. This has led to many conflicting reports in the literature. Bane and associates described the significance of radiation-induced vomiting, diarrhea, and inanition in the production of hypochloremic alkalosis, acidosis, and potassium depletion alkalosis, respectively. The following findings were taken from a carefully conducted study in which both direct and remote effects were considered (McDonald and associates).

After whole body irradiation of 450 to 500 R (air) (250 kv; TSD, 125 cm) to dogs, water intake is decreased, yet water losses remain normal. However, the resulting decrease in total body water is small except terminally. Blood volume decreases only slightly, since the progressive anemia is compensated for by a plasma volume increase in spite of the previously mentioned dehydration. There is a negative sodium and potassium balance from the beginning, whereas a negative chloride balance becomes obvious only after the onset of anorexia. The potassium-nitrogen balance ratio increases after irradiation and increases still more after the onset of anorexia. The digestion, absorption, and metabolism of nitrogen remain apparently normal until anorexia begins. From these studies, McDonald and associates found no indication of acid-base disturbances. There is no significant depletion or internal shifting of sodium, potassium, or chloride. Tissue contents of water and electrolytes in the postirradiation period were also studied (McDonald and associates). In highly radiosensitive tissues such as lymph nodes, potassium decreases, whereas sodium and chloride increase. Thus, as the cells are destroyed and intracellular contents removed, extracellular fluid increases locally. The more radioresistant tissues show no such changes.

By a variety of techniques, irradiation of the level described previously has been shown to increase capillary wall permeability for certain dyes (Clemente and Holst) and for red blood cells (Kahn and Furth). In addition, the rate of lymph flow from the thoracic duct increases considerably. Fluid leaves the blood vascular system more readily, but it also returns to that system more rapidly. Undoubtedly, certain products of tissue radiation injury are circulating in the blood. In leukemic patients, irradiation of the spleen alone may produce depression of bone marrow (Parsons and associates). The same type of irradiation or total body irradiation in leukemic patients may be followed by renal failure secondary to the deposit of uric acid crystals in the renal tubules.

These well-recognized, acute, nonspecific, indirect effects of irradiation are the consequence of massive cellular destruction in the beam of radiations. The breakdown products circulate in the blood plasma and lymph, producing a variety of effects on many tissues. Muntz and associates studied the dog's plasma proteins electrophoretically after 350 to 400 R single-dose total body irradiation (200 kv; filter, 0.5 mm Cu and 1 mm Al). No significant change occurred during the first 7 days. Thereafter until death, the albumins diminished steadily. With the onset of the terminal fever, $alpha_3$-globulin, beta-globulin, fibrinogen, and total proteins increased. Changes in the A/G ratio are variable, for it has been reported both increased and decreased. These changes have also been reported in dogs with distemper; therefore they do not appear peculiar to the irradiation response. Only minor changes in plasma proteins have been reported in patients receiving conventional radiation therapy (Snavely and associates).

The thoracic duct lymph of the dog shows additional minor changes after a single body irradiation of 500 R (air) (2000 kv; unfiltered; TSD, 200 cm) (Brown and associates). Lymph uric acid and blood uric acid reach maximum levels coincident with maximum lymphoid tissue destruction. Lymph total protein decreases slightly as does lymph creatinine. Sugar and chloride levels remain unchanged. No change in lymph bacteria occurs during the first 11 days—the duration of Brown and associates' experiment. The erythrocyte count found in the lymph during this postirradiation period has been previously discussed. It may reach one million cells per milliliter after large total body doses in dogs (Ross and associates). As expected, the lymphocyte count in thoracic duct lymph simultaneously drops.

Leukemogenic effects of radiations

Furth and Upton pointed out that all ionizing electromagnetic and corpuscular radiations are leukemogenic in certain mice. However, marked differences in susceptibility exist between various species and strains. Man and mouse are susceptible, whereas the rat, rabbit, and guinea pig seem relatively resistant. With man and mouse, it appears that the higher the otherwise sublethal dose of total body irradiation, the greater the incidence of leukemia. In addition, it has been shown in mice that the younger the animal, the greater the susceptibility, and that irradiation decreases the average age of onset of the disease (Lorenz and associates; Lorenz). These factors cannot be determined for man from data now available. In man there are three population groups subjected to radiations who have been shown to develop an increased incidence of leukemia:

1. The Japanese who were exposed to a single acutely administered dose of mixed radiations from the atomic bombs
2. Physicians who were exposed to highly fractionated doses over their lifetimes during their use of x rays
3. Patients with benign diseases, usually ankylosing spondylitis, and long life expectancy given substantial therapeutic radiations over several weeks to a large proportion of their marrow.

Among the atomic bomb survivors, granulocytic leukemia was much more frequent than lymphocytic leukemia, but a somewhat similar ratio may exist in the unirradiated Japanese population (Lange and Moloney) (Fig. 20-4). The relative risk of leukemia increases with increasing dose (Table 20-1). The acute form predominated. No difference in susceptibility between sexes could be detected. In man there appears to be a short latent period after a single total body exposure. The maximum annual incidence appeared 5 years after the blast (Fig. 20-4, *B*).

An increased incidence of leukemia in radiologic workers was suspected in 1911 (von Jagic and associates) and has been confirmed repeatedly since. March (1950) found that from 1928 through 1948 there were 65,922 deaths among nonradiologic physicians. Of these deaths, 334 or 0.51% were from leukemia. During the same period, 299 radiologists died, fourteen, or 4.68%, of whom died from leukemia. In this study the incidence of leukemia in radiologists is nine times that of nonradiologic physicians. In a more recent review March (1961) found this incidence had dropped so that from 1949 to 1958 the incidence of leukemia in radiologists was four or five times as great as in nonradiologic physicians. Thus, of 361 radiologists, eleven

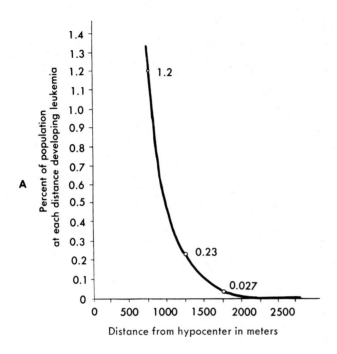

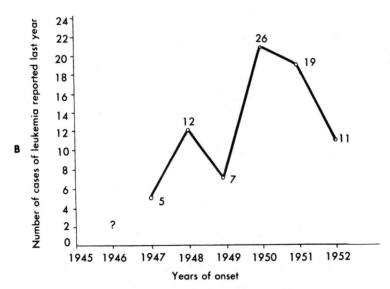

Fig. 20-4. Incidence of leukemia in atomic bomb blast survivors. **A** shows the percentage of survivors developing leukemia at various distances from the blast. **B** suggests that the peak incidence of leukemia occurred about 5 years after blasts. (**A** based on data from Moloney, W. C., and Kastenbaum, M. A.: Science **121**:308-309, 1955; **B** based on data from Moloney, W. C.: N. Engl. J. Med. **253**:88-90, 1955.)

Table 20-1. Average incidence of leukemia in atomic bomb survivors at Hiroshima (1950-1958) (survivors partially shielded and dose estimated from hypocenter)*

Dose in rad†	Man-years 1950-1958	Leukemia cases	Rate per million man-years 1950-1958
Over 1281	3204	5	1561
641-1280	9999	10	1000
321-640	7623	5	656
161-320	21,888	7	320
81-160	37,278	7	188
41-80	48,798	3	61
21-40	48,402	2	41
0-20	547,839	12	22

*Modified from Brill, A. B., Tomonaga, M., and Heyssel, R. M.: Ann. Intern. Med. **56**:590-609, 1962.
†Dose must be regarded as relative and may be high by a factor of 2.

(3.05%) died of leukemia. Of nonradiologists, 0.51% died of leukemia. Many early workers disregarded protective measures while using both x rays and radium. Doses received were undoubtedly high by present standards. With 8.8 R every 8 hours daily, the incidence of leukemia in a susceptible strain of mice increased from 45% to 70% (Lorenz and associates). As a result of such work, the permissible dose for radiologists was decreased first from 0.1 R per day to 0.3 R per week and finally to 0.1 R per week. Many years will be required to determine the effectiveness of this measure in man. It is expected that the decreasing incidence of leukemia will continue as current precautions against overexposure bear fruit. However, the increased incidence is not expected to disappear entirely.

Court-Brown and Abbatt reviewed the data on 9364 patients irradiated for ankylosing spondylitis between 1940 and 1954. The death from subsequent leukemia in this group was five to ten times higher than in a normal nonirradiated group. The majority of cases are myelogenous leukemia, and mortality from leukemia is highest between 3 and 5 years after irradiation. The work of Court-Brown and Doll suggests the existence of a linear dose-response relationship in radiation leukemogenesis, although all findings cannot be explained on this basis. It is obvious that a single large exposure, as occurred with the atomic blasts, produced a greater incidence of leukemia than the same dose given over a period of years. Currently available data do not permit one to determine if there is a threshold of dose necessary for the production of leukemia, primarily because of the scarcity of information in the low dose range.

It is becoming apparent that in addition to irradiation, alkylating agents employed in the treatment of ovarian carcinoma and Hodgkin's disease are associated with an increased incidence of acute myelogenous leukemia. Reimer and associates reported a review of 5455 women treated for advanced ovarian cancer with alkylating agents. Thirteen developed acute leukemia when 0.62 cases would have been expected. Nine of the thirteen women received some irradiation in addition to alkylating agents. They compared these results to an historic control of 13,309 women in the National Cancer Institute End Results Program. No excessive leukemia was noted in that group even though half of the women had received radiation. Coleman and associates and Cadman and associates have reported an increased incidence of acute nonlymphocytic leukemia in patients with Hodgkin's disease treated by combinations of irradiation and chemotherapy. In Coleman's report none of the patients treated with irradiation alone developed leukemia, neither did the small number treated with chemotherapy alone. However, six cases occurred of 330 patients treated with combination therapy. The leukemias are characteristically nonlymphocytic and are usually preceded by a variable period of pancytopenia. The response of these leukemias to the therapy has been extremely poor, and survival has been short. The latent interval before the diagnosis of leukemia is variable, but in general the more intensive therapies are associated with the shorter interval.

TREATMENT OF LEUKEMIA

In the past the natural history of the different types of leukemia determined the appropriate designation of acute or chronic. Thus, before the development of an effective therapeutic regimen, the child with acute lymphoblastic leukemia had a survival measured in weeks, whereas the adult with a chronic lymphocytic leukemia could be expected to survive for several years. With the drug combinations employing prednisone and sanctuary irradiation, about half the children with acute lymphoblastic leukemia (ALL) now survive 5 years. This median survival for children with ALL now clearly exceeds that of the adult with chronic lymphocytic leukemia (CLL). The acute nonlymphoblastic leukemias (myeloblastic, myelomonocytic, and erythroleukemia) are less frequent and as yet do not respond as well to multiagent drug therapies. The chronic form of myeloid leukemias are managed with busulfan therapy, but irradiation may play a role in the treatment of this leukemia as well.

Acute leukemia

In the current management of acute lymphoblastic leukemia of childhood, approximately 50% of the children will survive 5 years. What number of these are truly cured is not yet apparent from the results of the various clinical trials. There are now bold efforts to take children in continuous remission for 3 years or longer off all therapeutic agents. There are a variety of prognostic factors that have been employed in judging the intensity of therapy and the duration of total treatment time. The recognized bad prognostic factors include increased age, with the exception of children under the age of 1 year, initial white counts greater than 30,000/ml, and presentation in sanctuary sites. Lee and associates have proposed that these bad prognostic factors are encompassed in cytomorphologic determinants that include periodic acid-Schiff (PAS) reactivity, cell size and number, and prominence of nucleoli. Mauer and Simone have beautifully summarized the current status of the management of ALL in childhood, and their work should be reviewed for an appreciation of the management strategies employed.

Induction of remission can be achieved in as many as 95% of all cases of ALL, but continued remission can only be achieved by employing maintenance therapies and "prophylactic" treatment of the central nervous system. As median survival improved in the 1960s, it became apparent that certain sites of the body could harbor leukemic cells and emerge as an extramedullary focus of relapse. Commonly, after relapse in these sites, bone marrow relapse follows. The most important of these sanctuary sites is the central nervous system. Without prophylactic treatment at least 50% of children in clinical bone marrow remission will have relapse in the central nervous system. Relapse is usually associated with signs and symptoms of increased intracranial pressure, although occasionally back pain may signal the relapse. Other sites of extramedullary relapse include the kidneys, testicle, liver, and spleen, but of these only the testicle is of particular clinical importance. To prevent failures in the central nervous system children are now given prophylactic treatment to the central nervous system at the time remission is first achieved. Although irradiation alone and intrathecal methotrexate alone have been employed, the most successful prophylaxis involves a combination of cranial irradiation with intrathecal methotrexate. A dose of 1800 to 2400 rad is delivered to the center of the brain using opposing lateral portals and daily fractions of 200 rad. Intrathecal methotrexate is given concomitantly. The acute and late sequelae of such treatment are discussed in Chapter 22. There is ample evidence that such prophylactic treatment of the brain at the time of initial induction of remission not only significantly reduces the subsequent onset of central nervous system relapse, but also improves survival. In children who have remained in continuous remission for sufficiently long periods who have not had prophylactic treatment of the CNS, such treatment should be given before any consideration of discontinuing maintenance drug therapy.

There is increasing evidence that boys who discontinue maintenance therapy are at significant risk for relapse in the testicles. Whether or not this risk is sufficient to lead to the recommendation of testicular irradiation in all boys is not known. When relapse in the testicle does occur, doses of 1800 to 2400 rad should be administered to both testicles. This is true even if testicular swelling subsides prior to irradiation secondary to drug therapy. We believe CNS relapses are best treated by administration of intrathecal methotrexate until the cell count in the cerebrospinal fluid is normal. This is followed by cranial-spinal irradiation to the doses mentioned before. In those children who fail to respond to drug therapy and have symptomatic lesions at other sites, doses in the range of 1000 rad or less are usually sufficient for palliation.

The value of prophylactic CNS irradiation in acute nonlymphoblastic leukemias is not clearly established. The advantage may be obscured by the lessened chance of induction of remission and shorter duration of survival. It should be recalled that until median survivals approached 2 years in children with ALL, the benefits of prophylactic treatment of the central nervous system were not apparent. Law and Bloom reported the incidence of CNS relapses in adults with acute leukemia. Twelve of twenty-four with acute lymphoblastic leukemia and four of twenty with non-

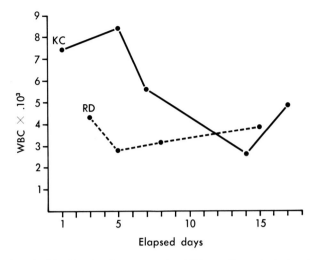

Fig. 20-5. Examples of white blood cell response in children with acute leukemia given a dose of 2400 rad to cranial-spinal axis at time of first remission.

lymphoblastic leukemias had CNS relapses. Although they do not recommend it, any incidence of 15% to 20% of CNS relapse in patients with ALL would seem to justify some form of prophylactic treatment of the central nervous system for these types of leukemias. Examples of the peripheral white blood response to prophylactic CNS irradiation are shown in Fig. 20-5.

Chronic leukemia

CHRONIC LYMPHOCYTIC LEUKEMIA (CLL). The traditional view that chronic lymphocytic leukemia is associated with long survival in spite of an unimpressive response to chemotherapeutic agents and palliative irradiation of both peripheral masses and the spleen is being challenged. It is now recognized that there are both indolent (preclinical) and active phases of this disease, which differ by the presence or absence of significant anemia, thrombocytopenia, infection, and constitutional symptoms. Once the disease is in the active phase, median survivals rarely exceed 2 years. Complete response to chemotherapeutic agents is at best expected less than one third of the time (Bennett). Splenic irradiation has been successful in reducing the peripheral lymphocyte count, reducing the anemia and thrombocytopenia present, and relieving symptoms from an enlarged spleen. The role of total body irradiation in the treatment of CLL has been reviewed by del Regato.

Johnson and Ruhl reported the results of a prospective randomized trial of total body irradiation (TBI) versus conventional chemotherapy. Of sixty evaluable patients, forty-two received total body irradiation and eighteen received chemotherapy. The median survival from onset of treatment was 27 months for the patients treated with chemotherapy and 57 months for those given TBI. Fourteen of the forty-two TBI patients had complete remissions versus one of eighteen patients given conventional therapy. Six patients had recovery of immunoglobulins to normal levels following TBI. Such recovery has not previously been noted in patients treated with chemotherapeutic agents. In view of this report we believe that TBI should become standard treatment for patients in the active phase of CLL. With daily doses of 5 to 10 rad and total doses of 100 to 150 rad, treatment is well tolerated and side effects are extremely rare. Relapse after TBI does not preclude retreatment with the same modality or supplementary local irradiation when necessary.

CHRONIC MYELOGENOUS LEUKEMIA (CML). Splenic irradiation produces an effect in the unirradiated bone marrow. This indirect effect has been studied by taking serial sternal marrow biopsies during splenic irradiation of patients with myelogenous leukemia (Parsons and associates; Hotchkiss and Block). All cells of the myeloid series decrease, but the differential white cell count shows a percentage increase in mature neutrophils. Erythropoiesis appears less affected. Parsons and associates found marrow changes a better indication of the response to treatment than peripheral blood counts. These remote changes are highly significant in explaining the effectiveness of localized splenic irradiation in myelogenous leukemia. Splenectomy produces relatively little or no such effect in the usual leukemic patient. In contrast excessive splenic irradiation may produce profound depressions in all lymphopoietic and hemopoietic tissues. Wilson and Johnson pointed out the hazards of splenic irradiation in patients with blastic crises of CML. Those patients showed prompt serious hematologic complications. The mechanism of such indirect effects is poorly understood. The spleen acts as a source of supply for a large proportion of leukemic cells and also acts as a trap for normal and abnormal leukocytes. Splenic irradiation with a series of daily fractions can thus produce a profound systemic effect.

The anemias in many debilitated patients are associated with an increased rate of red cell destruction and splenic sequestration. Erythropoiesis may be normal or increased but is inadequate to compensate for the increased destruction. After splenic irradiation the increased erythroclastic activity of this organ returns to normal as does the red cell survival time (Awwad and associates).

Barrett and associates have presented evidence to suggest that splenic irradiation is effective in CML because of its lethal effect on colony-forming cells. This would mean that the colony-forming cells, if not true myeloblasts, circulate freely between the blood, spleen, and possibly bone marrow.

Splenic irradiation is widely administered. In the usual practice it carries less risk of severe marrow damage than total body irradiation. The larger the port, the smaller the recommended daily dose. For a large spleen 25 to 50 rad (surface) daily may be sufficient, whereas 100 rad may be tolerated for minimal splenomegaly. Either of these dose rates should be modified according to the spleen size. The ports should be decreased in size as the spleen shrinks. The total dose can never be predetermined from pretreatment clinical and laboratory data. Dose rate, symptomatic and physical changes in the patient, and blood counts must all be weighed in determining total dose. Newall has pointed out the constancy of total dose for repeated treatment in the individual patient. When the disease accelerates the so-called blastic phase, irradiation has little to offer. Approximately 60% to 90% of patients will die in this blastic phase (Boggs).

THE MALIGNANT LYMPHOMAS
Hodgkin's disease

Hodgkin's disease is generally regarded as a special form of malignant lymphoma in which atypical reticulum cells and Sternberg-Reed cells constitute the neoplastic element. These in turn elicit a variable host response made up of various types of nonneoplastic cells, for example, lymphocytes, histiocytes, plasma cells, eosinophils, and polymorphonuclear leukocytes. Necrosis and tissue fibrosis are also seen in some forms. It was recognized that the various proportions of reactive cellular elements and neoplastic cells had prognostic significance. Early attempts at classification were based on this observation and culminated in the widely used Rye classification (listed in order of decreasing 5-year survival), which has made all previous classifications obsolete:

Lymphocytic predominance (LP)
Nodular sclerosing (NS)
Mixed cellularity (MC)
Lymphocytic depletion (LD)

This classification is based on the relative proportions of lymphocytes and histiocytes and distinguishes nodular sclerosis as a unique form of Hodgkin's disease with distinctive clinical and morphologic manifestations. The relative frequencies of the four subtypes are shown in Table 20-2. The relatively high proportion of nodular sclerosing types reported by Kadin and associates and the absence of any cases of lymphocytic depletion are not representative of the general distribution. Their data are based on 117 cases selected for exploratory laparotomy at Stanford University Medical Center. Table 20-3 shows the relationship of clinical stage at the time of diagnosis to histologic type. Prognosis and therapy do vary with the clinical extent of the disease. For this reason, clinical staging is useful even though one may believe all lymphomas are multicentric in origin and are incurable.

Almost all staging of lymphoma is based on some modification of the system proposed by Peters. The Committee on the Staging of Hodgkin's Disease recommended the following:

Stage I_1 Disease limited to one anatomic region
Stage I_2 Disease limited to two contiguous anatomic regions, on the same side of the diaphragm
Stage II   Disease in more than two anatomic regions or in two noncontiguous regions on the same side of the diaphragm
Stage III   Disease on both sides of the diaphragm, but not extending beyond the involvement of lymph nodes, spleen, and/or Waldeyer's ring
Stage IV   Involvement of the bone marrow, lung parenchyma, pleura, liver, bone, skin, kidneys, gastrointestinal tract, or any tissue or organ in addition to lymph nodes, spleen, or Waldeyer's ring

Table 20-2. Reported incidence of Hodgkin's disease (histologic types)

Author	Lymphocytic predominance	Nodular sclerosing	Mixed cellularity	Lymphocytic depletion
Lukes and associates (1966)	63 (17%)	149 (40%)	97 (26%)	68 (18%)
Keller and associates (1968)	9 (5%)	92 (52%)	65 (37%)	10 (6%)
Coppleson and associates (1970)	41 (13%)	124 (40%)	112 (36%)	35 (11%)
Kadin and associates (1971)	13 (11%)	85 (73%)	19 (16%)	—
Fuller and associates (1971)	13 (10%)	71 (54%)	43 (33%)	5 (3%)
Selzer and associates (1972)	17 (14%)	32 (27%)	43 (36%)	28 (23%)
Axtell and associates (1972)	45 (17%)	96 (35%)	92 (34%)	37 (13%)
AVERAGE	12%	46%	31%	10%

Table 20-3. Relationship of clinical stage and histologic types in 277 patients*

Stage	Lymphocytic predominance (%)	Nodular sclerosing (%)	Mixed cellularity (%)	Lymphocytic depletion (%)
I	38	10	22	13
II	33	68	36	33
III	18	10	29	13
IV	11	12	13	41

*Modified from Berard, C. W., Thomas, L. B., Axtell, L. M., Kruse, M., Newell, G., and Kagan, R.: Symposium by the American Cancer Society and the National Cancer Institute, Ann Arbor, Mich., April 26-28, 1971.

All stages are subclassified as A or B to indicate the absence or presence of systemic symptoms. Symptoms of weight loss of more than 10% of the body weight 6 months prior to diagnosis, fever with temperatures above 38° C, and night sweats otherwise unexplained are the recognized systemic symptoms. In 1971 the Committee on Hodgkin's Disease Staging Classification recommended a pathologic staging to supplement the clinical staging that takes into account the (1) favorable prognosis of localized extralymphatic disease and (2) the necessity of designating those patients staged by laparotomy compared to those staged without the help of this procedure (Carbone and associates). The original Rye staging as previously shown has gained widespread acceptance, as has the careful prestaging work-up of patients with Hodgkin's disease. The newer modifications are based on findings at laparotomy and form a pathologic stage (PS) that may be appended to the clinical stage (CS). Thus a patient with Hodgkin's disease in a single cervical lymph node without systemic symptoms who at laparotomy has a histologically normal liver and spleen but biopsy-proved para-aortic lymph nodes not recognized by lymphangiography would be classified CSIA PSIII$_{S-H-N+}$.

Recently Desser and associates have proposed a modification of pathologic Stage III. In their Stage III patients with abdominal disease limited to the spleen, splenic, celiac, or portal nodes, a 93% 5-year survival rate was obtained after a total nodal irradiation. This is in contrast to a 57% 5-year survival rate when the abdominal disease included para-aortic, iliac, or mesenteric nodes. In the unfavorable group treated by irradiation alone, fourteen of seventeen patients relapsed. Twelve of these relapses were in extralymphatic sites.

This staging system is primarily intended for use in Hodgkin's disease, but it can be adapted to the other malignant lymphomas.

In the past, considerable emphasis has been placed on whether Hodgkin's disease was unicentric in origin. Support for this concept has been the frequent observation that the site of next clinical appearance in locally treated disease is more often than not in a contiguous group of lymph nodes. Sheer found that the first manifestation of regrowth appeared immediately adjacent to the previously irradiated zone in thirty-one of sixty-eight patients (45%) with Hodgkin's disease. For lymphosarcoma, the incidence was six of thirty-one patients (20%), and a similar incidence was found for reticulum cell sarcoma. Han and Stutzman found contiguous involvement in 68% of 106 patients with Hodgkin's disease and in 36% of 103 patients with lymphosarcoma or reticulum cell sarcoma. Kaplan (1973), in a review of 100 previously untreated patients with Hodgkin's disease, reported twenty-six patients who developed extension to other sites after initial local therapy. In twenty-two of the twenty-six, extension was to contiguous node areas. Lee and associates performed lymphangiograms in 186 patients. Of sixty-three patients with apparently localized Hodgkin's disease, twenty-eight had occult involvement of the retroperitoneal nodes, whereas thirty-nine of forty patients with apparently localized non-Hodgkin's lymphoma had occult retroperitoneal nodes. Such clinical evidence supports the notion of a unicentric origin of Hodgkin's disease, but Smithers has suggested that such spread is only a manifestation of the multicentric origin of Hodgkin's disease rather than conclusive evidence of its unicentric origin. His criticism of the unicentric theory should be read by all.

Regardless of the exact mechanism of spread, it is obvious that Hodgkin's disease and other malignant lymphomas that appear clinically localized are best treated when every effort has been made with clinical and surgical staging techniques to define precisely the extent of disease.

STAGING PROCEDURES IN MALIGNANT LYMPHOMA. In the past, for patients with systemic symptoms but no proof of retroperitoneal node involvement, irradiation of the retroperitoneal nodes was recommended and produced symptomatic relief in a modest percentage of patients. In the late 1950s the technique of lymphangiography became available, and the empiric observation just cited gave way to a diagnostic procedure for demonstrating retroperitonal node disease. For the first time the clinician was able to evaluate the lymph node regions that he could not palpate or properly study by the simpler procedure of intravenous pyelography. Lymphangiography remains the single most important procedure in the pretreatment evaluation of the retroperitoneal lymph nodes. If a diagnostic laparotomy follows the procedure, the surgeon may be guided to a suspicious area not otherwise sampled by biopsy. In addition, opacification of the retroperitoneal lymph nodes facilitates portal arrangements in those patients selected for primary irradiation. Supplemental radiographic procedures should include a chest x-ray film, intravenous pyelogram, and, if the lymphangiogram was interpreted as normal, a computed tomographic scan of the abdomen. The combination of these procedures permits evaluation of the axial skeleton. The laboratory tests should include adequate studies of the hemopoietic system, serum alkaline phosphatase, tests of liver and kidney function, and bone marrow biopsy.

EXPLORATORY LAPAROTOMY. In a further effort to define the pretreatment extent of involvement in Hodgkin's disease, interest has focused on exploratory laparotomy in patients with apparent localized disease. This has been employed in patients with Hodgkin's disease as well as with other malignant lymphomas. The Committee on Hodgkin's Disease Staging Procedures defines the primary purpose of exploratory laparotomy as being to evaluate the presence or absence of disease in the spleen (Rosenberg and associates). Gladstein and associates reported their results of fifty diagnostic laparotomies in unselected, untreated patients. Twenty-two of the fifty patients had systemic symptoms. Seven of twelve patients with clinical evidence of splenic enlargement had histologic evidence of disease in the spleen, and ten of thirty-eight patients without clinical suspected splenic involvement had histologic evidence of Hodgkin's disease in the spleen. Only one of this group of twenty-eight patients had a positive liver biopsy. There was no mortality from the operative procedure, but three postoperative infections and one colonic cutaneous fistula developed. One third of the patients with nodular sclerosing forms and two thirds with either lymphocytic predominance or mixed cellularity were found to have intra-abdominal disease. In addition to splenectomy, the surgical procedure involves liver, lymph node, and bone marrow biopsies.

Serious complications following laparotomy and splenectomy occur in 9% of children with Hodgkin's disease. In a review of 200 children entered in Children's Cancer Study Group protocols, there were eighteen who developed postoperative septicemia and meningitis, and eight of these children died as a result of infectious complications (Chilcote and associates). The most common organisms isolated were pneumococcus and streptococcus. As a result of this observation it is now recommended that children undergoing splenectomy be given penicillin prophylactically.

Kadin and associates reviewed the clinical pathologic findings in 117 patients subjected to laparotomy in the pretreatment evaluation of Hodgkin's disease. Seventy-three percent were of the nodular sclerosing type, 16% of mixed cellularity, and 11% had lymphocytic predominance on the initial biopsy. Of the eighty-five patients with nodular sclerosing Hodgkin's disease, sixty-nine had involvement of the mediastinum and thirty-three had confirmed disease in the abdomen. The mediastinal involvement without intra-abdominal disease was four times as frequent as intra-abdominal disease without mediastinal involvement (forty-eight vs twelve patients). Of sixty-three patients without systemic symptoms only one had histologically proved disease in the liver. One other interesting observation was in the difference of intra-abdominal involvement according to the side of involved cervical lymph nodes. In only one of fifteen patients with right cervical lymph node involvement only was abdominal disease proved, whereas in patients with either bilateral or left-sided cervical lymph nodes only, 50% had intra-abdominal disease. Zarembok and associates confirmed the inaccuracy of clinical evaluation of the spleen compared to laparotomy with splenectomy. In a series of thirty patients, six of seven spleens judged preoperatively to be positive either by palpation or spleen scan were histologically confirmed positive, and nine of twenty-three spleens judged negative were found to be involved. The combined error in preoperative evaluation of splenic involvement is approximately 33%.

Although some workers would prefer splenic irradiation without proceeding to exploratory laparotomy and splenectomy, we prefer the latter approach because it permits a reduction of the irradiated volume and a sparing of the left kidney. We do not believe that the leukocytosis associated with splenectomy is of itself an adequate reason to recommend the procedure.

Approximately one third of patients with clinical Stages I and II disease will be found at laparotomy to have intra-abdominal disease. Gamble and associates reviewed the results of laparotomy in 139 patients with Stages I and II disease and found abdominal involvement in 34.5% and 31.2%, respectively. The clinical significance of this was substantiated in the report of Baldetorp and associates. They had thirty-nine patients with disease clinically limited to supradiaphragmatic sites and irradiated through a mantle-shaped portal only. Twelve of these patients (31%) subsequently had relapses in abdominal sites. The majority of the relapses were in lymph node sites. Griffin and associates argue that laparotomy is not necessary for patients with clinical Stages IA and IIA if, in addition to the mantle-shaped portals, the spleen and para-aortic lymph nodes are irradiated. Only three of thirty-nine patients treated in this fashion developed relapse, and none of the relapses occurred in pelvic lymph nodes. Two failures were in previously irradiated sites, and one was a recurrence in the occipital area not included in the original field. Their 5-year relapse-free survival was 92%.

There are fewer reports and less certainty as to the role of exploratory laparotomy and splenectomy in the staging of non-Hodgkin's malignant lymphoma. Hanks and associates reported an experience with fifteen patients staged by laparotomy. In ten of the fifteen, mesenteric lymph nodes were biopsied and seven of the ten were histologically positive. This is in sharp contrast to the findings in Hodgkin's disease in which mesenteric lymph nodes are rarely involved. Hass and associates reported their findings in twenty-five patients with non-Hodgkin's malignant lymphoma. In twelve cases the spleen was histologically positive, and in five of twenty-three cases liver biopsies were also positive. For the present we do not believe that the indications for exploratory laparotomy in non-Hodgkin's malignant lymphoma have been defined.

It should be emphasized that no single procedure precludes the benefits to be gained from the other procedures. This is to say that exploratory laparotomy does not eliminate the need for a lymphangiogram or does gallium scanning replace any of the other diagnostic procedures.

TREATMENT OF HODGKIN'S DISEASE. It is now generally accepted that irradiation is the treatment of choice for Stages I, II, and IIIA Hodgkin's disease. The aggressive approach at pretreatment staging employed in recent years provides us with some indication of the anticipated clinical behavior of each subtype. This is especially true in nodular sclerosing Hodgkin's disease. Three approaches to therapy are possible:

1. Local irradiation to the proved local limits of disease
2. Extended field irradiation to include the contiguous or regional uninvolved lymph nodes
3. Total nodal irradiation to include in continuity all lymph nodes of the inguinal, iliac, para-aortic, mediastinal, cervical, and axillary areas

For Stages I and II disease, Peters and associates advocate either the local or extended field technique, with ports tailored to the anticipated behavior of the histologic type being irradiated. For nodular sclerosing disease they have always treated the mediastinum, but in view of less frequent mediastinal involvement in patients with mixed cellularity type, they have not treated the mediastinum electively. Similarly, advocates of extended field therapy may justify portal arrangements based on the presence of only right-sided cervical disease with its infrequent association with intra-abdominal disease. This is compared to the 50% probability of left-sided cervical nodes having concomitant intra-abdominal disease. Kaplan (1973) advocates total lymph node irradiation employing large shaped fields to encompass all major lymph node groups. He recommends this procedure for all patients in Stages I through IIIA, including those with a single extranodal focus. Both Peters and associates and Kaplan agree that all patients with Stage IV and probably those with Stage IIIB are best treated by chemotherapeutic agents.

Goodman and associates treated eighty-one consecutive patients with Stages IA and IIA (laparotomies performed on all) with mantle-shaped portals and para-aortic nodal irradiation only. The disease recurred in three patients in irradiated sites, two had disease in unirradiated lymph nodes, and one patient developed extranodal extension. There were no instances of failure in pelvic nodes. The disease-free survival rate for patients with Stages IA and IIA were 95% and 86%, respectively. This report and that of Griffin and associates leads us to recommend the omission of pelvic nodal irradiation in patients surgically staged as having Ia and IIa disease. The ability to eliminate pelvic irradiation in this group of patients significantly reduces both hemopoietic and gonadal morbidity. A second category of patients in whom omission of pelvic irradiation could be considered are the patients with Stage IIIA S+n−. In our own experience this is perhaps the most common stage seen, particularly in the pediatric age group. Desser and associates have pointed out the better survival rate in this group as compared to those with Stage IIIA S+n+ (93% vs 57%). The favorable survival of such patients with Stage III lesions (treated with mantle-shaped ports and irradiation of para-aortic nodes only) was reported by Levi and Wiernik. Unfortunately the numbers are small, but the observations by both groups suggest the possible omission of the pelvic field in patients with Stage IIIA S+n−. This is particularly tempting in teenage and young adult females in whom preservation of ovarian function is desirable. Other than those mentioned, we recommend total nodal treatment for patients who are selected for primary irradiation. For patients with particularly large mediastinal masses, we favor preirradiation administration of three courses of MOPP. Based on the observation by Desser and associates we recommend the same approach for patients with extensive intra-abdominal lymph node involvement. In patients with Stages IIIB and IV who are initially selected for chemotherapy, we attempt the use of mantle-shaped ports and para-aortic node irradiation following six cycles of MOPP. In our experience hemopoietic tolerance has not permitted routine irradiation of pelvic lymph node sites after such chemotherapy.

TECHNIQUE OF IRRADIATION. The major aim in the irradiation of Hodgkin's disease is the delivery of a homogeneous dose of radiations to the major lymphatic chains of the torso using as few field junctions as possible. To accomplish this, large anterior and posterior shaped ports are used. The total dose necessary to control a given node group in a high proportion is between 3500 and 4000 rad (Fig. 20-6) with

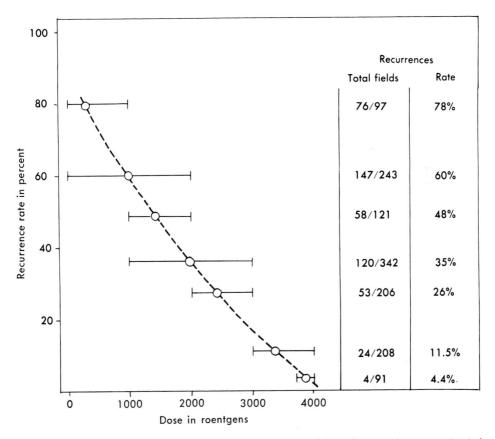

Fig. 20-6. Recurrence rate of Hodgkin's disease as a function of dose. This graph was constructed from pooled data. (From Kaplan, H. S.: Cancer Res. **26:**1221-1224, 1966.)

megavoltage beams given at a rate of 850 to 900 rad a week. Fletcher and Shukovsky have criticized the data Kaplan employed in developing the dose-response curve. In their own review they conclude that 3500 rad given in as long as 6 weeks will yield control rates of 95% and that doses as high as 6000 rad will not prevent some recurrences. There is rather widespread acceptance of these figures. Multiple small ports are not acceptable in view of the hazards of overlap and gaps. A variety of techniques are available for shaping large fields for the volumes desired, but they will not be discussed here. In a typical patient, irradiation may be initiated with a so-called "mantle"-shaped field. This is tailored to encompass the lymph nodes from both

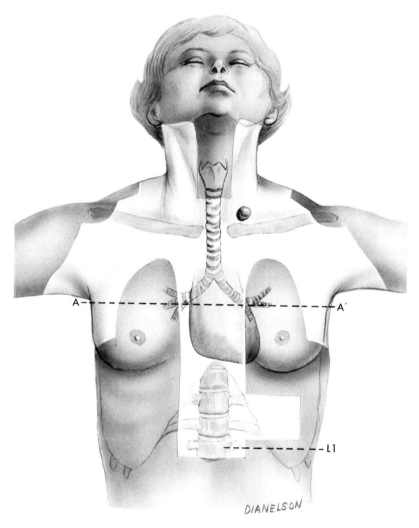

DIANELSON

Fig. 20-7. Diagram to illustrate lymph node volume irradiated with the mantle technique. The splenic pedicle is easily included in shaping this single large field. The mediastinal beams should be tailored to encompass the hila of the lungs.

mastoid tips down to the level of L2 and laterally to include both axillae (Fig. 20-7). This field can be simply modified to include the splenic pedicle. Care should be taken to include the low axillary and pectoral node chains lest a geographic miss be regarded as a late failure of the technique. Although much is said of the total dose necessary, there is no evidence that the total dose must be delivered in 4 weeks. When treating the mantle we prefer dose rates of 900 rad or less in 5 fractions per week. With this fractionation, not a single case of pericardial or spinal cord damage has been observed.

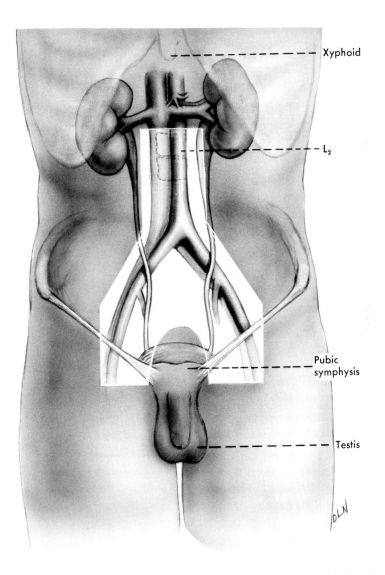

Fig. 20-8. Inverted Y field shaped to encompass major lymph node areas below the diaphragm. When used in conjunction with the mantle field (Fig. 20-7), the junction of the fields must not overlap.

After completion of irradiation through mantle-shaped ports, the inverted Y field is used, and the gap at the junction is carefully calculated to avoid hot spots in depth. The inverted Y field encompasses the retroperitoneal and pelvic lymph nodes but does not extend to include the femoral nodes, since they are rarely involved in Hodgkin's disease (Fig. 20-8). If this technique is employed for non-Hodgkin's malignant lymphoma, the femoral nodes should be included. Although the total dose through this volume is the same as that for the mantle, weekly doses may be reduced to 750 rad, depending on the general status of the patient and peripheral blood counts. It is in the planning of this field that the pretreatment lymphangiogram may provide its greatest benefit. The lymphangiogram permits greater shielding of the pelvic bone marrow by providing an opportunity for better definition of the position of the lymph nodes. It has been our experience that, in those patients without a lymphangiogram, greater amounts of the pelvic bone marrow have been encompassed because of our uncertainties, and these patients generally show greater hemopoietic depression. During treatment of the inverted Y, white blood counts are obtained three times a week unless the count falls below 2000, at which time daily platelet and white blood cell counts are obtained. If significant white blood cell count depression is present but platelets are adequate, the pelvic portion of the inverted Y may be blocked out without altering the geometry of the entire field until the counts recover sufficiently to permit continuation of the pelvic portion. Examples of peripheral white counts during total nodal irradiation are shown in Figs. 20-9 and 20-10. The peripheral white count usually remains depressed for a number of months after treatment and a transient anemia develops (see p. 521). Techniques of dose calculation for both mantle and inverted Y fields have been described by Page and associates. When pelvic lymph node irradiation is to be omitted, a simple rectangular field is sufficient to encompass the para-aortic lymph nodes down to the bifurcation of the aorta.

PROGNOSIS AND RESULTS. The variation in clinical stage and histologic type makes a single statement regarding prognosis relatively meaningless. As noted previously, recent staging techniques and histologic classifications coupled with consistent delivery of an adequate dose not only to the known disease but also to generous segments of apparently uninvolved node areas make comparison with older data impossible. As Peters and associates have pointed out from their own experience, survival rates have improved over the past four decades with each advance in technique. The overall 5-year survival in the period of 1931 to 1941 was 37%, whereas in the period between 1965 and 1969, overall survival improved to 59%. Kaplan (1973) has stated that we can expect disease-free 5-year survival rates of as high as 90% in Stages I and II and 70% in Stage III patients if careful staging is done and adequate treatment given. Recognizing the two subgroups of patients within Stage III, the survival rate of 90% for patients with favorable Stage IIIA S+n−, and the addition of adjuvant chemotherapy to the less favorable Stage IIIA S+n+, we anticipate an improved survival for all patients with Stage III lesions. The influence of adequate staging on end result reporting is demonstrated in the review of ninety-four Stage IA patients seen at the M. D. Anderson Hospital between 1947 and 1969

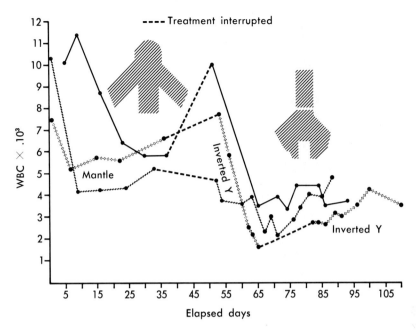

Fig. 20-9. Typical response of peripheral white blood cell counts to doses of 4000 rad total nodal irradiation. A 2-week rest period is given after mantle field irradiation. Weekly doses are generally reduced during treatment of the inverted Y field.

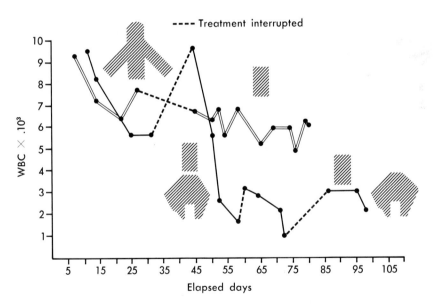

Fig. 20-10. Influence of pelvic bone marrow irradiation on peripheral white blood cell counts is clearly shown in these two cases. In both instances counts were in the normal range after mantle field irradiation. One patient (•═•) was selected for para-aortic irradiation only, and the other patient (•─•) was treated with an inverted Y field. After several treatment interruptions because of leukopenia, the pelvis portion of the inverted Y was shielded and treatment of the para-aortic nodes continued to 4000 rad. Treatment of the pelvic nodes was then resumed.

(Ibrahim and associates). The 5-year survival for those staged clinically was 72%, whereas the patients staged since the incorporation of lymphangiography had a 91% 5-year survival. The effect of patient selection is obvious.

We believe the preliminary results of the techniques recommended justify their continuation.

Non-Hodgkin's malignant lymphoma

CLASSIFICATION. The Rappaport classification of non-Hodgkin's lymphomas is the most widely accepted by pathologists and clinicians in this country. It is based on two principal parameters. The first and most important is the presence or absence of a nodular (follicular) pattern of growth. The second is based on cytomorphologic features. The clinical relevance of Rappaport's classification has been supported by clinical studies (Byrne, 1977; Nathwani, 1978). The nodular pattern carries a better prognosis than the diffuse pattern in patients with lymphomas. On the other hand, with exception of the rare well-differentiated lymphocytic lymphoma, the cell type has less prognostic significance.

In recent years the acquisition of new knowledge based on ultrastructural, cytochemical, and immunologic studies has challenged some of the concepts involved in the Rappaport classification.

As a result there has been a plethora of new classifications purporting to possess a more meaningful "functional" significance than Rappaport's scheme.

Clinicians and statisticians, not to mention pathologists, have been thrown into a state of confusion by this state of affairs. For a review of the various classifications see Dorfman (1977).

An effort to develop a compromise classification such as resulted at the Rye meeting for Hodgkin's disease took place at Airlie House, Warrenton, Virginia in 1975. This, however, was unsuccessful.

Under the auspices of the National Cancer Institute a retrospective review of 1000 cases of non-Hodgkin's lymphoma using the various histopathologic classifications is being conducted by a panel of experts. After comparative statistical analysis of the data, it is hoped that a clinically useful and practical classification will be adopted. In the interim we prefer, as do most pathologists and clinicians in this country, to use the time-honored Rappaport classification, albeit with some minor modifications.

Modified Rappaport classification of non-Hodgkin's lymphoma

Nodular lymphomas
  Poorly differentiated, lymphocytic
  Mixed
  Histiocytic
Diffuse lymphomas
  Well-differentiated lymphocytic
  Poorly differentiated lymphocytic

Mixed
Histiocytic
Lymphoblastic
  Convoluted
  Nonconvoluted
Undifferentiated
  Burkitt
  Non-Burkitt

TREATMENT. As mentioned previously, both the staging system employed for Hodgkin's disease and the staging procedures recommended may be applied to the other malignant lymphomas. The histologic classification recommended by Rappaport and associates has prognostic significance.

In most large series patients are equally divided between nodular and diffuse histologic patterns. The poorly differentiated lymphocytic, mixed histiocytic and lymphocytic, and histiocytic patterns account for about 90% of all cell types. Liver involvement was present in forty of 100 consecutive patients who underwent percutaneous liver biopsy or laparotomy (Lotz and associates). Overall, abdominal disease is present in about 60% of patients and includes involvement of a large proportion of mesenteric and hepatic portal nodes. Such findings emphasize the inappropriateness of employing Hodgkin's disease techniques for the treatment of abdominal disease in non-Hodgkin's lymphoma. Localized Stages I and II non-Hodgkin's lymphoma varies in frequency from 11% reported by Hellman and associates to 32% reported by Reddy and associates. Because of the systemic nature of involvement in this disease, chemotherapy has become the more favored mode of treatment. The drugs selected usually include cyclophosphamide, vincristine, and prednisone or some variation of that combination. Five approaches to therapy are possible:

1. Local irradiation to the proved local limits of the disease
2. Total nodal irradiation including the whole abdomen
3. Total body irradiation
4. Chemotherapy
5. Combinations of irradiation and chemotherapy

For patients with Stages I and II disease, irradiation of either involved fields or extended fields yields good survival, particularly for the nodular types. Reddy and associates reported an actuarial 5-year survival rate of 90% for nodular lymphoma and a 55% survival rate for patients with diffuse lymphoma. In patients who had relapses, 70% had relapses in node sites. Few of their patients had elective laparotomies. Similar results are reported by Hellman and associates with sixty-five previously untreated patients. The survival rate at 5 years was 82% for the entire group but generally better for the nonhistiocytic lymphomas and those with nodular morphology. Both groups were treated with doses of 3500 to 4000 rad.

In patients with Stages III and IV non-Hodgkin's lymphoma, local field irradiation would be used only as an adjunct to systemic chemotherapy. The results of total body irradiation have been reported both by Johnson and by Hellman and associates. Doses employed were 5 to 10 rad daily, 5 days a week for a total of 100 to 150 rad or 15 rad twice weekly to the same total dose. Hellman and associates reported a doubling of the 5-year survival rate for these patients treated with total body irradiation compared to chemotherapy regimens that included cyclophosphamide, vincristine, and prednisone. These reports emphasize the role of radiation therapy in advanced non-Hodgkin's lymphomas.

We do not know the long-term results from total nodal irradiation coupled with whole abdominal irradiation after careful staging in patients with limited non-Hodgkin's lymphoma. However, we believe that selected patients will benefit from this procedure.

REFERENCES

Allen, J. G., and Jacobson, L. O.: Hyperheparinemia; the cause of hemorrhagic syndrome associated with total body exposure to ionizing radiation, Science **105**:388-389, 1947.

Allen, J. G.: The pathogenesis of irradiation hemorrhage; blood clotting and allied problems. In Flynn, J. E., editor: Transactions of the Fifth Conference of the Josiah Macy Jr. Foundation, New York, 1952.

Atkinson, H. R.: Bone marrow distribution as a factor in estimating radiation to the blood-forming organs: a survey of present knowledge, J. Coll. Radiol. Aust. **6**:149-154, 1962.

Awwad, H. K., Badeeb, A. D., Massoud, G. E., and Salah, M.: The effects of splenic x-irradiation on the ferrokinetics of chronic leukemia with a clinical study, Blood **29**:242-256, 1967.

Axtell, L. M., Myers, M. H., Thomas, L. H., Berard, C. W., Kagan, A. R., and Newell, G. R.: Prognostic indicators in Hodgkin's disease, Cancer **29**:1481-1488, 1972.

Baldetorp, L., Landberg, T., and Svahn-Tapper, G.: Clinical course after mantle treatment of non-laparotomized patients with Hodgkin's disease, Acta Radiol. (Ther.) (Stockh.) **15**:193-200, 1976.

Bane, H. N., Glicksman, A. S., and Nickson, J. J.: Common electrolyte disturbances in the radiation therapy patient, Am. J. Roentgenol. **79**:465-471, 1958.

Barrett, A. J., Longhurst, P., Humble, J. G., and Newton, K. A.: Effect of splenic irradiation on circulating colony-forming cells in chronic granulocytic leukaemia, Br. Med. J. **1**:1259, 1977.

Bennett, J. M.: Chronic lymphocytic leukemia; therapeutic options, Int. J. Radiat. Oncol. Biol. Phys. **1**:559-560, 1976.

Berard, C. W., Thomas, L. B., Axtell, L. M., Kruse, M., Newell, G., and Kagan, R.: The rela-

tionship of histopathological subtype to clinical stage of Hodgkins' disease at diagnosis, Cancer Res. **31**:1776-1785, 1971.

Bisgard, J. D., Hunt, H. B., Neely, O. A., and Scott, J.: Experimental studies of the mechanism of action of x-ray therapy upon infection, Radiology **39**:691-696, 1942.

Bloom, W.: Histopathology of irradiation from external and internal sources, New York, 1948, McGraw-Hill Book Co.

Bloom, W., and Jacobson, L. O.: Some hematologic effects of irradiation, Blood **3**:586-592, 1948.

Boggs, D. R.: The pathogenesis and clinical patterns of blastic crisis of chronic myeloid leukemia, Semin. Oncol. **3**:289, 1976.

Bond, V. P., Silverman, M. S., and Cronkite, E. P.: Pathogenesis and pathology of post-irradiation infection, Radiat. Res. **1**:389-400, 1954.

Brecher, G., von Foerster, H., and Cronkite, E. P.: Production, differentiation, and life-span of leukocytes. In Braunsteiner, H., and Zucker-Franklin, D., editors: The physiology and pathology of the leukocytes, New York, 1962, Grune & Stratton, Inc.

Brown, C. S., Hardenbergh, E., and Tullis, J. L.: Biochemical, cellular, and bacteriologic changes in thoracic duct lymph of dogs exposed to total body irradiation, Am. J. Physiol. **163**:668-675, 1950.

Byrne, G. E.: Rappaport's classification of non-Hodgkin's lymphoma: histologic features and clinical significance, Cancer Treat. Rep. **61**:935-944, 1977.

Cadman, E. C., Capizzi, R. L., and Bertino, J. R.: Acute non-lymphocytic leukemia: a delayed complication of Hodgkin's disease therapy: analysis of 109 cases, Cancer **40**:1280-1296, 1977.

Carbone, P. P., Kaplan, H. S., Musshoff, K.,

Smithers, D. W., and Tubiana, M.: Report of the Committee on Hodgkin's Disease Staging Classification, Cancer Res. **31:**1860-1861, 1971.

Chilcote, R. R., Baehner, R. L., Hammond, D., and the Investigators and Special Studies Committee of the Children's Cancer Study Group: Septicemia and meningitis in children splenectomized for Hodgkin's disease, N. Engl. J. Med. **295:**798-800, 1976.

Clemente, C. D., and Holst, E. A.: Pathological changes in neurons, neuroglia and blood-brain barrier induced by x-irradiation of heads of monkeys, Arch. Neurol. & Psychiat. **71:**66-79, 1954.

Coleman, C. N., Williams, C. J., Flint, A., Glatstein, E. J., Rosenberg, S. A., and Kaplan, H. S.: Hematologic neoplasia in patients treated for Hodgkin's disease, N. Engl. J. Med. **297:**1249-1252, 1977.

Conrad, R. A., and Hicking, A.: Medical findings in Marshallese people exposed to fallout radiation, J.A.M.A. **192:**457-459, 1965.

Coppleson, L. W., Factor, R. M., Strum, S. B., Graff, P. W., and Rappaport, H.: Observer disagreement in the classification and histology of Hodgkin's disease, J. Natl. Cancer Inst. **45:**731-740, 1970.

Court-Brown, W. M. C., and Abbatt, J. D.: The incidence of leukemia in ankylosing spondylitis treated with x-ray: a preliminary report, Lancet **1:**1283-1285, 1955.

Court-Brown, W. M. C., and Doll, R.: Leukemia and aplastic anemia in patients irradiated for ankylosing spondylitis, M. Res. Counc. Spec. Rep. Ser. (Lond.), No. 295, 1957.

Cronkite, E. P., and Brecher, G.: Defects in hemostasis produced by whole body irradiation. In Flynn, J. E., editor: Blood clotting and allied problems, Transactions of the Fifth Conference of the Josiah Macy, Jr. Foundation, New York, 1952.

Cronkite, E. P., and Bond, V. P.: Diagnosis of radiation injury and analysis of the human lethal dose of radiation, U.S. Armed Forces M. J. **11:**249-260, 1960.

De Bruyn, P. P. H.: Lymph node and intestinal lymphatic tissue. In Bloom, W., editor: Histopathology of irradiation, New York, 1948, McGraw-Hill Book Co.

del Regato, J. A.: Total body irradiation in the treatment of chronic lymphogenous leukemia, Janeway Lectures, Colorado Springs, Colo., 1973, American Radium Society.

Desser, R. K., Golomb, H. M., Ultmann, J. E., Ferguson, D. J., Moran, E. M., Griem, M. L., Vardiman, J., Miller, B., Oetzel, N., Sweet, D., Lester, E. P., Kinzie, J. J., and Blugh, R.: Prognostic classification of Hodgkin's disease in pathologic Stage III, based on anatomic considerations, Blood **49:**883, 1977.

Dettman, P. M., King, E. R., and Zimberg, Y. H.: Evaluation of lymph node function following irradiation or surgery, Am. J. Roentgenol. **96:**711-718, 1966.

Dorfman, R. F.: Pathology of the non-Hodgkin's lymphoma: new classifications, Cancer Treat. Rep. **61:**945-951, 1977.

Ellis, R. E.: The distribution of active bone marrow in the adult, Phys. Med. Biol. **5:**255-258, 1961.

Engeset, A.: Irradiation of lymph nodes and vessels, Acta Radiol., suppl. 229, 1964.

Fishburn, R. I., Dobelbower, R. R., Patchefsky, A. S., Leeper, D. B., and Kramer, S.: The effect of age on the long-term response of bone marrow to local fractionated irradiation, Cancer **35:**1685-1691, 1975.

Fisher, B., and Fisher, E. R.: Barrier functions of lymph node to tumor cells and erythrocytes. I. Normal nodes, Cancer **20:**1907-1913, 1967.

Fisher, B., and Fisher, E. R.: Barrier function of lymph node to tumor cells and erythrocytes. II. Effect of x-ray, inflammation, sensitization and tumor growth, Cancer **20:**1914-1919, 1967.

Fishman, M., and Shechmeister, I. L.: The effect of ionizing radiation on phagocytosis and the bactericidal power of blood. II. The effect of radiation on ingestion and digestion of bacteria, J. Exp. Med. **101:**275-290, 1955.

Fletcher, G. H., and Shukovsky, L. J.: The interplay of radiocurability and tolerance in the irradiation of human cancers, J. Radiol. Electrol. **50:**383-400, 1975.

Fuller, L. M., Gamble, J. F., Shullenberger, C. C., Butler, J. J., and Gehand, E. A.: Prognostic factors in localized Hodgkin's disease treated with regional radiation, Radiology **98:**641-654, 1971.

Furth, J., and Upton, A. C.: Induction of leukemia by ionizing irradiation. In Wolstenholme, G. E. W., and Cameron, M. P., editors: Ciba Foundation symposium on leukemia research, Boston, 1954, Little, Brown & Co.

Gamble, J. F., Fuller, L. M., Martin, R. G., Sullivan, M. P., Jing, B., Butler, J. J., and Shullenberger, C. C.: Influence of staging celiotomy in localized presentations of Hodgkin's disease, Cancer **35:**817-825, 1975.

Glatstein, E., Trueblood, H. W., Enright, L. P., Rosenberg, S. A., and Kaplan, H. S.: Surgical staging of abdominal involvement in unselected patients with Hodgkin's disease, Radiology **97:**425-432, 1970.

Goldschmidt, L., Rosenthal, R. L., Bond, V. P.,

and Fishler, M. C.: Alterations in thermal fragility of rat erythrocytes following total body x-irradiation, Am. J. Physiol. **164**:202-206, 1951.

Goodman, R. L., Piro, A. J., and Hellman, S.: Can pelvic irradiation be omitted in patients with pathologic Stages IA and IIA Hodgkin's disease, Cancer **37**:2834-2839, 1976.

Greenberg, M. L., Chanana, A. D., Cronkite, E. P., Schiffer, L. M., and Stryckmans, P. A.: Extracorporeal irradiation of blood in man: radiation resistance of circulating platelets, Radiat. Res. **35**:147-154, 1968.

Griffin, T., Gerdes, A., Parker, R., Taylor, E., Hafermann, M., Taylor, W., and Tesh, D.: Are pelvic irradiation and routine staging laparotomy necessary in clinical stages IA and IIA Hodgkin's disease, Cancer **40**:2914-2916, 1977.

Han, T., and Stutzman, L.: Mode of spread in patients with malignant lymphoma, Arch. Intern. Med. **120**:1-7, 1967.

Hass, A. C., Brunk, S. F., Gulesserian, H. P., and Givler, R. L.: The value of exploratory laparotomy in malignant lymphoma, Radiology **101**:157-165, 1971.

Hellman, S., Chaffey, J. T., Rosenthal, D. S., Moloney, W. C., Canellos, G. P., and Skarin, A. T.: The place of radiation therapy in the treatment of non-Hodgkin's lymphomas, Cancer **39**:843-851, 1977.

Hersh, E. M., and Oppenheim, J. J.: Impaired in vitro lymphocyte transformation in Hodgkin's disease, N. Engl. J. Med. **273**:1006-1012, 1965.

Hoppe, R. T., Fuks, Z. Y., Strober, S., and Kaplan, H. S.: The long-term effects of radiation on T and B lymphocytes in the peripheral blood after regional irradiation, Cancer **40**:2071-2078, 1977.

Hotchkiss, D. J., and Block, M. H.: Effect of splenic irradiation on systemic hemopoiesis, Arch. Intern. Med. **109**:695-711, 1962.

Hurst, D. W., and Meyer, O. O.: Giant follicular lymphoblastoma, Cancer **14**:753-778, 1961.

Ibrahim, E., Fuller, L. M., Gamble, J. F., Jing, B. S., Butler, J. J., and Gehan, E. A.: Stage I Hodgkin's disease: comparison of surgical staging with incidence of new manifestations in lymphogram- and prelymphogram-studied patients, Radiology **104**:145-151, 1972.

Jacobson, L. O.: Hematologic effects of ionizing radiation. In Hollaender, A., editor: Radiation biology, New York, 1954, McGraw-Hill Book Co.

Jage, M.: The radiosensitivity of normal leukaemic human blood lymphocytes, Clin. Radiol. **12**:59-65, 1961.

Johnson, R. E.: Total body irradiation (TBI) as primary therapy for advanced lymphosarcoma, Cancer **35**:242-246, 1975.

Johnson, R. E., and Ruhl, U.: Treatment of chronic lymphocytic leukemia with emphasis on total body irradiation, Int. J. Radiat. Oncol. Biol. Phys. **1**:387-397, 1976.

Kadin, M. E., Glatstein, E., and Dorfman, R. F.: Clinicopathologic studies of 117 untreated patients subjected to laparotomy for the staging of Hodgkin's disease, Cancer **27**:1277-1294, 1971.

Kahn, J. B., and Furth, J.: Pathogenesis of postirradiation anemia, Blood **7**:404-416, 1952.

Kaplan, H. S.: Radiotherapy of regionally localized Hodgkin's disease, Radiology **78**:553-561, 1962.

Kaplan, H. S.: Evidence for a tumoricidal dose level in the radiotherapy of Hodgkins disease, Cancer Res. **26**:1221-1224, 1966.

Kaplan, H. S.: Radiotherapy of advanced Hodgkin's disease with a curative intent, J.A.M.A. **223**:50-53, 1973.

Keller, A. R., Kaplan, H. S., Lukes, R. J., and Rappaport, H.: Correlation of histopathology with other prognostic indicators in Hodgkin's disease, Cancer **22**:487-499, 1968.

Knospe, W. H., Blom, J., and Crosby, W. H.: Regeneration of locally irradiated bone marrow, Blood **28**:398-415, 1966.

Kun, L. E., and Johnson, R. E.: Hematologic and immunologic status in Hodgkin's disease 5 years after radical radiotherapy, Cancer **36**:1912-1916, 1975.

Lacassagne, A., and Lavedan, J.: Cited in Lacassagne, A., and Gricouroff, G.: Action des radiations sur les tissues, Paris, 1941, Masson et Cie.

Lamerton, L. F.: Late effects of continuous irradiation. In Symposium on radiosensitivity, Quebec, 1963, Laval Medical, Inc.

Lange, R. D., and Moloney, W. C.: Leukemia in atomic bomb survivors. I. General observations, Blood **9**:574-585, 1954.

Law, I. P., and Bloom, J.: Adult acute leukemia, frequency of central nervous system involvement in long-term survivors, Cancer **40**:1304-1306, 1977.

Lawrence, J. S., Ervin, D. M., and Wetrich, R. M.: Life cycle of white blood cells, Am. J. Physiol. **144**:284-296, 1945.

Lawrence, J. S., and Valentine, W. N.: The blood platelets: the rate of their utilization in the cat, Blood **2**:40-49, 1947.

Lawrence, J. S., Dowdy, A. H., and Valentine, W. N.: Effects of radiations on hemopoiesis, Radiology **51**:400-413, 1948.

Lee, S. L., Kopel, S., and Glidewell, O.: Cytomorphological determinants of prognosis in acute lymphoblastic leukemia in children, Semin. Oncol. **3:**209-217, 1976.

Lehar, T. J., Kiely, J. M., Pease, G. L., and Scanlon, P. W.: Effect of local irradiation on human bone marrow, Am. J. Roentgenol. **96:**183-190, 1966.

Lenzi, M., and Bassani, G.: The effect of radiation on the lymph and on the lymph vessels, Radiology **80:**814-817, 1963.

Levi, J. A., and Wiernik, P. H.: The therapeutic implications of splenic involvement in Stage IIIA Hodgkin's disease, Cancer **39:**2158-2165, 1977.

Lorenz, E., Heston, W. E., Eschenbrenner, A. B., and Deringer, M. K.: Biological studies in the tolerance range, Radiology **49:**274-285, 1947.

Lorenz, E.: Some biologic effects of long-continued irradiation, Am. J. Roentgenol. **63:**176-185, 1950.

Lotz, M. J., Chabner, B., DeVita, V. T., Jr., Johnson, R. E., and Berard, C. W.: Pathological staging of 100 consecutive untreated patients with non-Hodgkin's lymphomas, extramedullary sites of disease, Cancer **37:**266-270, 1976.

Lukes, R. J., Craver, L. F., Hall, T. C., Rappaport, H., and Ruben, P.: Report of the nomenclature committee, Cancer **26:**311, 1966.

McDonald, R. E., Jensen, R. E., Urry, H. C., Bolin, V. S., and Price, P. B.: A study of the irradiation syndrome. I. Water, electrolyte and nitrogen balances, Am. J. Roentgenol. **74:**701-710, 1955.

McDonald, R. E., Jensen, R. E., Urry, H. C., Bolin, V. S., and Price, P. B.: A study of the irradiation syndrome. II. Tissue water and tissue electrolytes, Am. J. Roentgenol. **74:**889-897, 1955.

March, H. C.: Leukemia in radiologists in a 20 year period, Am. J. Med. Sci. **220:**282-286, 1950.

March, H. C.: Leukemia in radiologists, ten years later, Am. J. Med. Sci. **242:**137-149, 1961.

Mauer, A. M., and Simone, J. V.: The current status of the treatment of childhood acute lymphoblastic leukemia, Cancer Treat. Rev. **3:**17-41, 1976.

Moloney, W. C.: Leukemia in survivors of atomic bombing, N. Engl. J. Med. **253:**88-90, 1955.

Moloney, W. C., and Kastenbaum, M. A.: Leukemogenic effects of ionizing radiation on atomic bomb survivors in Hiroshima city, Science **121:**308-309, 1955.

Muntz, J. A., Barron, E. S. G., and Prosser, C. L.: Studies on the mechanism of action of ionizing radiations. III. The plasma protein of dogs after x-ray irradiation, Arch. Biochem. **23:**434-445, 1949.

Murray, R. G.: The spleen. In Bloom, W., editor: Histopathology of irradiation, New York, 1948, McGraw-Hill Book Co.

Nathwani, B. N., Kim, H., Rappaport, H., Solomon, J., and Fox, M.: Non-Hodgkin's lymphomas. A clinicopathologic study comparing two classifications, Cancer **41:**303-325, 1976.

Newall, J.: Splenic irradiation, Clin. Radiol. **14:**20-27, 1963.

O'Brien, P. H., Moss, W. T., Ujiki, G. T., Putong, P., and Towne, W.: Effect of irradiation on tumor-infused lymph nodes, Radiology **94:**407-411, 1970.

Page, V., Gardner, A., and Karzmark, C. J.: Physical and dosimetric aspects of the radiotherapy of malignant lymphomas. I. The mantle technique, Radiology **96:**609-618, 1970.

Page, V., Gardner, A., and Karzmark, C. J.: Physical and dosimetric aspects of the radiotherapy of malignant lymphomas. II. The inverted Y technique, Radiology **96:**619-626, 1970.

Parsons, W. P., Watkins, C. H., Pease, G. L., and Childs, D. S., Jr.: Changes in sternal marrow following roentgen-ray therapy to the spleen in chronic granulocytic leukemia, Cancer **7:**179-189, 1954.

Peters, M. V., Brown, T. C., and Rideout, D. F.: Prognostic influences and radiation therapy according to pattern of disease, J.A.M.A. **223:**53-59, 1973.

Rappaport, H., Winter, W. J., and Hicks, E. B.: Follicular lymphoma: a re-evaluation of its position in the scheme of malignant lymphomas, based on a survey of 253 cases, Cancer **9:**792-821, 1956.

Reddy, S., Saxena, V. S., Pellettiere, E. V., and Hendrickson, F. R.: Early nodal and extra-nodal non-Hodgkin's lymphomas, Cancer **40:**98-104, 1977.

Reimer, R. R., Hoover, R., Fraumeni, J. F., and Young, R. C.: Acute leukemia after alkylating-agent therapy of ovarian cancer, N. Engl. J. Med. **297:**177-181, 1977.

Rosenberg, S. A., Boiron, M., DeVita, V. T., Jr., Johnson, R. E., Lee, B. J., Ultmann, J. E., and Viamonte, M., Jr.: Report of the Committee on Hodgkin's Disease Staging Procedures, Cancer Res. **31:**1862-1863, 1971.

Ross, M. H., Furth, J., and Bigelo, R. R.: Changes in cellular composition of the lymph caused by radiations, Blood **7:**417-428, 1952.

Rubin, P., Landman, S., Mayer, E., Keller, B., and Ciccio, S.: Bone marrow regeneration and extension after extended field irradiation in Hodgkin's disease, Cancer **32:**699-711, 1973.

Selzer, G., Kahn, L. B., and Sealy, R.: Hodgkin's

disease: a clinicopathologic study of 122 cases, Cancer **29**:1090-1100, 1972.

Schechmeister, I. L., and Fishman, M.: The effect of ionizing radiation on phagocytoses and the bactericidal power of the blood. I. The effect of radiation on migration of the leukocytes, J. Exp. Med. **101**:259-274, 1955.

Sheer, A. C.: The course of Stage I malignant lymphomas following local treatment, Am. J. Roentgenol. **90**:939-943, 1963.

Sherman, J. O., and O'Brien, P. H.: Effects of ionizing irradiation on normal lymphatic vessels and lymph nodes, Cancer **20**:1851-1858, 1967.

Smithers, D. W.: Spread of Hodgkin's disease, Lancet **1**:1262-1267, 1970.

Snavely, J. R., Bullington, R. H., and Schlosser, J. V.: Effect of therapeutic irradiation of carcinoma of cervix on liver function, Arch. Intern. Med. **92**:195-203, 1953.

Sykes, M. P., Chu, F. C., Savel, H., Bonadonna, G., and Mathis, H.: The effects of varying dosages of irradiation upon sternal marrow regeneration, Radiology **83**:1084-1088, 1964.

Sykes, M. P., Savel, H., Chu, F. C., Bonadonna, G., Farrow, J., and Mathis, H.: Long-term ef-

fects of therapeutic irradiation upon bone marrow, Cancer **17**:1144-1148, 1964.

Teneff, S., and Stoppani, F.: L'influenza delle irradiazioni sulle linfoghiandole e sulla circolazione linfatica, Radiol. Med. **22**:768-787, 1935.

Valentine, W. N., and Pearce, M. L.: The relative sensitivity of erythroid and myeloid elements, Blood **7**:1-13, 1952.

von Jagic, N., Schwarz, G., and von Siebenrock, L.: Blutefunde bei Röntgenologen, Berl. Klin. Wchnschr. **48**:1220-1222, 1911.

West, R. J., Graham-Pole, J., Hardisty, R. M., and Pike, M. C.: Factors in pathogenesis of central-nervous-system leukaemia, Br. Med. J. **3**:311-314, 1972.

Wilson, J. F., and Johnson, R. E.: Splenic irradiation following chemotherapy in chronic myelogenous leukemia, Radiology **101**:657-661, 1971.

Wintrobe, M.: Clinical hematology, Philadelphia, 1956, Lea & Febiger.

Zarembok, I., Ramsey, H. E., Sutherland, J., and Serpick, A. A.: Laparotomy and splenectomy in the staging of untreated patients with Hodgkin's disease, Radiology **102**:673-678, 1972.

21

The bone*

RESPONSE OF NORMAL BONE TO IRRADIATION

ENERGY ABSORPTION IN BONE. Low- and medium-energy radiations (100 to 200 kv) are absorbed chiefly by the photoelectric process. Photoelectric absorption of a given wavelength varies directly as the fourth power of the atomic number of the absorber. Bone has an effective atomic number of 13.8 (Spiers, 1946) and is 1.8 times as heavy as soft tissue. For these reasons at these low energies bone absorbs a much larger proportion of such radiations than does a comparable volume of soft tissue. Regaud described the bone as "burning itself" because of these facts. With higher energy photons (400 to 4000 kv), the proportion of absorption occurring by the photoelectric process is less, whereas the proportion occurring by the Compton process increases. Since Compton absorption is practically independent of the atomic number of the absorber, the theoretical clinical advantage of higher energy radiations is obvious. For a given dose in soft tissues, bone will absorb fewer radiations produced in the megavoltage range than in the medium-voltage range. This physical fact was confirmed biochemically by Woodward and Spiers and histologically by Rosenthal and Marvin.

Woodward and Spiers found that alkaline phosphatase activity was depressed less with 1000 kv radiations than with 100 kv radiations, despite the fact that tissue doses calculated in the usual manner were equal. The energy absorbed by the soft tissue elements in bone—that is, osteocytes and vascular structures—varies with the wavelength of the radiations and with the size of the cavity occupied by these structures. In larger cavities (50 μ in diameter), the average energy absorbed will be less than in smaller cavities (10 μ in diameter). Aspin and Johns made theoretical calculations of the dose to small cavities in bone with a variety of wavelengths. Then they verified their calculations by measuring the viability of bacteriophage irradiated in capillary tubing of various diameters. The tubing was made of leaded glass to simulate bone. There are differences in energy absorbed by osteocytes and the vascular structures. There are also differences in absorption between megavoltage beams and

---

*Doses are given in rad when possible. However, in the literature the failure to specify quality of beam used makes it impossible to accurately convert roentgens to rad for bone. We have, therefore, usually given doses as they have been reported.

555

medium-voltage beams. Rosenthal and Marvin found no quality difference when longitudinal growth was measured. The cartilage of the epiphyseal plate has about the same density as soft tissues. However, x rays of an hvl of 0.4 mm Cu produce twice the damage in cortical bone as do x rays of an hvl of 2.4 mm Cu. The variation in rad delivered to the haversian canal system with changes in wavelength is illustrated in Fig. 21-1.

For a given dose to soft tissue adjacent to bone, the intraosseous cellular structures will always receive a higher dose with medium-voltage beams than with megavoltage beams. Longheed and Brown showed that the stunting of bone growth was much more marked for 2000 R (surface) given with 250 kv beams than with ^{60}Co beams.

The relative radiosensitivities of the normal cellular components of bone vary

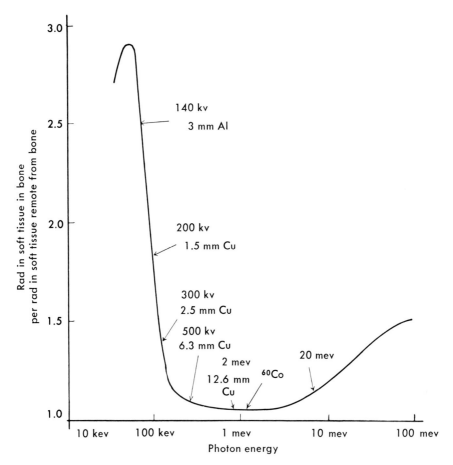

Fig. 21-1. Variation in energy in rad delivered to the haversian canal system with changes in wavelength. It is obvious also that the conversion of roentgens to rad for bone in the region of 100 kv requires great knowledge of the beam in question. Small differences in kilovoltage make a large difference in conversion factor. (From Meredith, W. J.: Am. J. Roentgenol. **79:**57-63, 1958.)

according to the cell in question and the growth rate of the bone. Although all phases of bone development may be disturbed by appropriate doses of radiations, bone is most easily affected during those periods of rapid growth. The following discussion is therefore divided according to types of bone growth.

EFFECTS OF RADIATIONS ON INTRACARTILAGINOUS OSSIFICATION. The intracartilaginous ossification type of bone formation is exemplified in the development of long bones. Growth in length occurs through the production of, and changes in, the hyaline cartilage of the epiphyseal plate. As the bone increases in length, the epiphyseal plate maintains its thickness. Those cartilage cells near the epiphyseal surface of the epiphyseal plate are flat, undergo frequent mitosis, and represent the source of the larger mature cartilage cells nearer the metaphysis. Normally the cartilage cells are in neat columns. The length of each column is maintained by the multiplication of the flat cells toward one surface of the cartilage, whereas at the other surface, mature cells degenerate coincidentally with the dissolution of cartilage and its replacement by spongy bone. This process occurs as the blood vessels and connective tissues of the marrow cavity penetrate the epiphyseal plate. The newly formed spongy bone later undergoes reconstruction and may form compact bone.

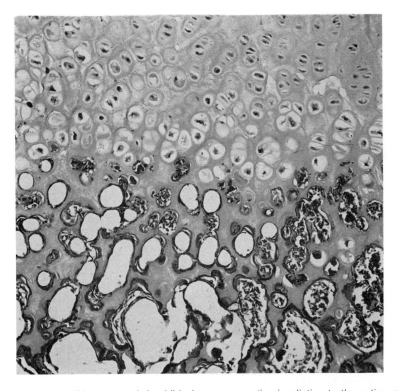

Fig. 21-2. Disruption of bone growth in child given preoperative irradiation to the entire radius for Ewing's tumor of bone. No tumor involved the epiphyseal plate. Bone was removed 4 weeks after an estimated 2400 rad (surface) had been given in 3 weeks with orthovoltage radiations. (W. U. neg. 47-4649A; courtesy Dr. L. V. Ackerman.)

Radiations affect these steps in bone development at several points. Sissons found that in young rats the rate of cartilage cell mitosis is reduced a few hours after a single dose of 400 R (air) (190 kv, 0.5 mm Cu filter). Within 8 days the rate is 50% of normal. Since with this dose proportionate narrowing of the epiphyseal plate does not occur, the process of vascular invasion and subsequent ossification must be similarly suppressed. Two days after a dose of 1500 R (air) changes in cellular nuclei and cytoplasm are detectable, and within 6 days the neat columns of cartilage cells have become severely disrupted (Fig. 21-2). Such high doses narrow the epiphyseal plate, suggesting that at this level mitosis may be more severely affected than the process of ossification. In 100 days the plate is less than half its expected width (Sissons) (Fig. 21-3).

In addition to those changes in the epiphyseal plate, radiation-induced changes in the metaphysis are early and severe. Three days after a dose of 600 R (factors as given previously) the mature cartilage cells adjacent to the ossification process have become swollen, and by 9 days the normal interdigitation of cartilage and newly formed spongy bone of the metaphysis has disappeared (Heller). Heller termed this destruction process "severance." Whether these changes are secondary to radiation-induced damage of the vascular connective tissues in the metaphysis, direct injury to osteoblasts, or changes in cartilage cells is not known. However, 75 days after a dose of 2300 rad, the microvascular supply of growth cartilage in rats is essentially intact

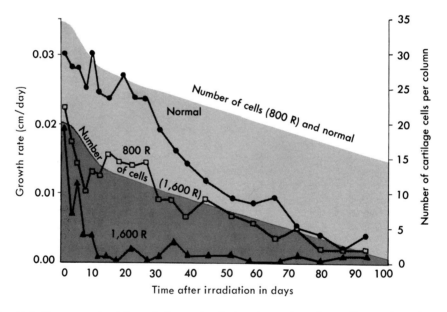

Fig. 21-3. Response of epiphyseal plate to irradiation after various doses. The number of cells in cartilaginous columns is shown by edges of the light gray and dark gray zones. Scale at right is in terms of number of cells per column. Growth rates of plates with various doses are plotted by solid black lines, and scale at left is in terms of centimeters per day. (Modified from Sissons, H. A.: Experimental study of the effect of local irradiation on bone growth. In Mitchell, J. S., et al., editors: Progress in radiobiology, Edinburgh, 1956, Oliver & Boyd, Ltd.)

(Kember). The osteocytes of the newly formed bone frequently die after irradiation, and resorption of the "dead" bone follows the appearance of an increased number of osteoclasts. If the dose has not been too high, recovery of bone growth occurs. However, single doses as low as 400 rad may produce a permanent shortening of a growing bone. A still lower dose in a young animal may produce no significant retardation of growth in length but may produce detectable changes in epiphyseal morphology. Single doses of 1700 rad or greater or their biologic equivalent will usually permanently arrest this type of bone growth (Woodward and Spiers). An extensive review of the relative effectiveness of various doses of radiations, the significance of the age of the animal at the time of irradiation, and the contributions of the various portions of the bone to its growth (distal and proximal epiphyseal plates and the shaft) have been presented by Hinkel (1942).

Growth in bone thickness and in total diameter is likewise retarded or arrested by irradiation, but changes in these measurements are less striking. Bowing of a limb, spontaneous fracture, or atrophy of muscles may follow months or years later (Lacassagne and Gricouroff). For more detailed accounts of these radiation-induced

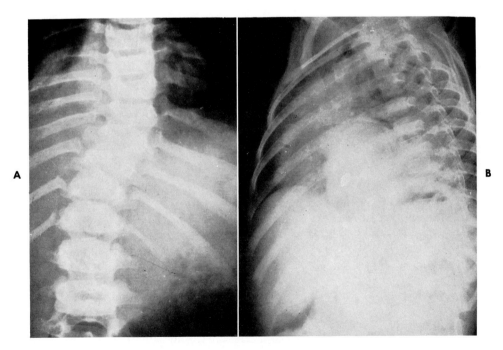

Fig. 21-4. The patient had irradiation of right lower chest field and adjacent right half of spine through 10 × 10 cm anteroposterior, posteroanterior, and lateral ports. Dose to each field was approximately 2200 rad (skin) in 33 days. Calculated midchest dose was 2900 rad in 33 days (200 kv; hvl, 1 mm Cu; TSD, 50 cm). The patient was then 2 years old. **A** shows the subsequent asymmetry of the vertebral bodies (small facets on right) and scoliosis. **B,** Lateral view of same patient. (Courtesy Dr. W. E. Powers.)

dysplasias, consult the work of Rubin and associates and the beautiful study of Barnhard and Geyer.

As might be anticipated from the discussion on growth disturbances, alkaline phosphatase activity, the uptake of ^{90}Sr and ^{32}P, and the ability to calcify under stimulation by estrogen are all decreased after irradiation (Woodward; Wilson). The severity of these disturbances is proportionate to the energy absorbed.

There are many clinical reports of radiation-induced bone deformities in children. Neuhauser and associates found that doses of 2000 R (200 kv or above in 4 to 6 weeks to the spine of children under 9 years of age inevitably produced late radiographic abnormalities in the vertebral bodies. The bodies are flattened, and their anterior margins are rounded off both superiorly and inferiorly. Doses below 1000 rad (skin) rarely produce such changes. Whitehouse and Lampe reported the occurrence of late scoliosis after unilateral radiation damage of the spine of children (Fig. 21-4). Neuhauser and associates suggested that such scoliosis might be prevented by treating the entire width of the spine when it is necessary to irradiate any portion of the vertebrae. Unfortunately, the routine inclusion of the entire width of the vertebrae does not ensure the avoidance of scoliosis, thus indicating the significance of unilateral soft tissue irradiation.

The younger the child, the more radiosensitive are his bones; at a given age, the more active the epiphyseal plate, the more dramatic are the effects of growth suppression; and, finally, the greater the proportion of anticipated growth, the more amplified are the effects of growth arrest (Fig. 21-5). No single dose can be regarded as safe for all circumstances. We have seen arrested bone growth from childhood irradiation of benign soft tissue or bone lesions. Such damage to bone and other organs demands exclusion of radiations as a useful modality in the treatment of benign disease of childhood (Fig. 11-2). After the necessary irradiation of bones during the treatment of malignant diseases in children, one must accept damage to bone growth as an unavoidable sequela. (See Chapter 24.)

The entire skull of a child may be given doses that vary from 2000 to 5000 rad in the irradiation of intracranial neoplasms. The effects of these doses of radiation on the skull have not been documented. However, they should be of concern, especially in the treatment of infants (Fig. 22-6). Although there is little knowledge of the effect of radiation on the growth of the membranous bones of the skull, the bones of the base of the skull are preformed in cartilage, and we would expect an effect similar to that seen on growing cartilage elsewhere. We do know that the mandible, which is a membranous bone, undergoes growth arrest when given doses of the order just mentioned.

EFFECTS OF RADIATIONS ON ADULT BONE. Hardly an area or volume in the body can be irradiated without irradiating bone. This may be an important weight-bearing bone or bone subject to frequent trauma, in which case even minor changes in the bone significantly increase the risk of serious disruption of function. The effects of irradiation on adult bone are a consequence of injury to its cellular and vascular components.

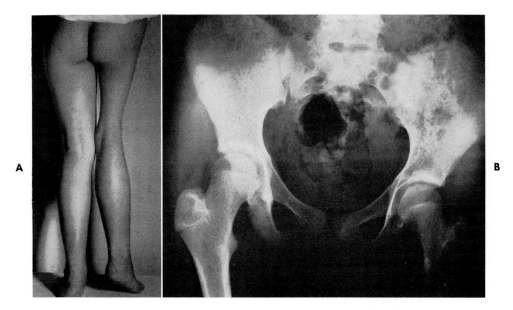

Fig. 21-5. A, Atrophy of muscles of right thigh with bone shortening secondary to irradiation of thigh for Ewing's tumor in an infant 4 months of age (11 years previously). Calculated dose to center of femur was 4200 R in 23 days. Calculated dose to distal epiphysis was 1800 R in 23 days. The factors were 200 kv; hvl, 0.9 mm Cu; TSD, 40 cm; 8 × 10 cm ports. **B,** Film of pelvis showing bone changes associated with arrest of growth described. (From Murphy, W. T., and Berens, D. L.: Radiology **58:**35-42, 1952.)

1. The periosteum of adult bone consists of a laminated membrane adherent to the surface of the bone. Numerous blood vessels, nerves, and the perforating fibers of Sharpey pass between the periosteum and the bony surface. The endosteum has a similar structure. Apparently, osteoblasts develop from the periosteum in response to injury or fracture. If the periosteum is separated from the bone, the denuded bone will frequently die from a lack of blood supply. Similarly, damage to the periosteum by disease or by high doses of radiations may result in bone death.

2. The radiation injury of other cellular components of adult bone is of equal importance. Adult bone is continuously changing by the destruction of certain areas and the reconstruction of new layers. In some unknown way osteoclasts dissolve bone and then disappear. Osteoblasts reappear to reconstruct the bone in accordance with Wolff's law. This well-balanced process of destruction and reconstruction is upset by high doses of radiations. Dahl demonstrated osteoblasts to be more easily injured than osteoclasts after a given dose, but both are injured. Stampfli and Kerr concluded that damage to these cellular structures was largely responsible for changes in adult bone, since they could detect no vascular changes in their patients. Whether the damage is directly to the osteocytes or the osteoblasts or secondary to vascular damage is unknown, but the result, osteoporosis leading to osteonecrosis, is an expected sequela of high doses, poor fractionation, or repeated courses of low-energy irradiation (Fig. 21-6).

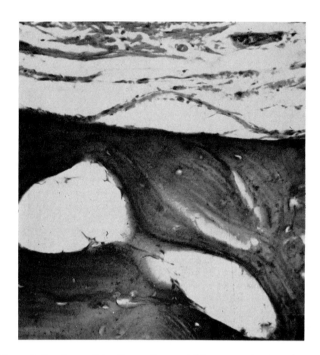

Fig. 21-6. Radiation osteitis of mandible after radium mold therapy and external roentgenotherapy for squamous cell carcinoma of lower gingiva. Six months before jaw resection the patient was given a calculated dose of 2900 rad in 5 days to surface of bone by the mold. This was followed immediately by an additional 3900 rad (muscle) delivered in 1 months, using external roentgenotherapy (1000 kv; hvl, 3 mm Pb; TSD, 70 cm). Note elevation of periosteum, empty lacunae, and absence of marrow.

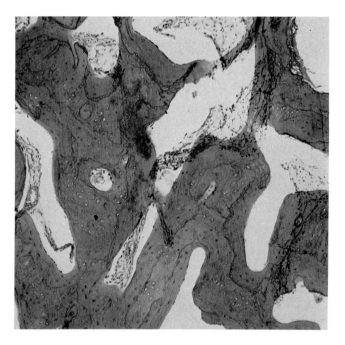

Fig. 21-7. Heavily irradiated trabeculae with empty lacunae and absence of marrow. (W. U. neg. 57-4645A; courtesy Dr. L. V. Ackerman.)

Radiation-induced osteitis or bone death may be of little significance if the bone does not become infected or if the bone is not subjected to great stress or trauma. Radiation damage of the mandible is frequently serious because of the ease of infection, and that of the femoral neck may be serious because of the increased brittleness. Pain is usually the first symptom of radiation bone damage. This may be 4 months to several years in developing. Soon thereafter the radiograph will show osteoporosis and bone condensation. Biopsy at this point shows striking osteoporosis with thinner trabeculae and rare osteocytes (Stampfli and Kerr; Stephenson and Cohen) (Fig. 21-7). In a weight-bearing bone such as the femoral neck, fracture may occur if the dose has been high—5000 rad in 1 month (200 kv; hvl, 1 mm Cu) or its biologic equivalent. At first this may appear as a molecular fracture. Displacement later occurs. The joint space is usually narrowed. Barr and associates have pointed out, however, that structures associated with joints—synovia and articular cartilage—are not apparently affected until many months after high doses. Such joint changes can be seen in the amputated fingers of physicians with chronic radiodermatitis. Radiographically, there are degenerative arthropathies in the interphalangeal joints. Microscopically,

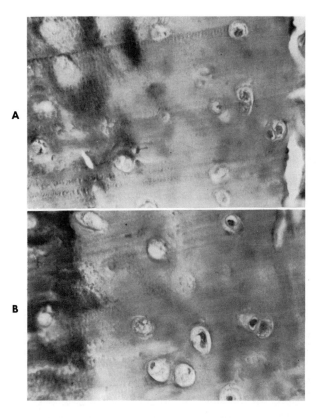

Fig. 21-8. Photomicrographs of articular cartilage from amputated finger of a distinguished radiologist. There is uneven calcification in the cartilage, **A,** and cytoplasmic vacuolization of chondrocytes with chondrocyte degeneration, **B.** (Courtesy Dr. Paul Putong.)

the articular cartilage is thinned, and there are atrophy and fibrosis of the synovial lining of the joint capsule. Near the surface, chondrocytes are flattened, and the deeper layers show irregular organization with vacuolization and some degeneration (Fig. 21-8). The cartilaginous matrix contains focal areas of calcification. The trabeculae are osteoporotic, and osteoblasts are diminished in number. As would be expected, the capsular connective tissue is partially hyalinized, and arteriolar narrowing with subendothelial hyalinization and thickening occurs. Ankylosis may result (Kolar and associates). In addition to this group with chronic exposure to ionizing radiations, Kolar and associates also described arthritic changes in thirty-six patients irradiated for extraosseous malignancies. Estimated doses to the joints were greater than 2800 R (140 to 200 kv). The average latent period was 9 years, and symptoms consisted of pain, limitation of motion, and swelling. Radiographically, degenerative changes were noted with prominent joint space narrowing. In some of these patients, fracture through the irradiated femoral neck occurred. In the earlier days of radiotherapy a certain number of these fractures of the femoral neck were acceptable as the price of curative irradiation. With current techniques using pelvic ports tailored to encompass only the contents of the pelvis and using megavoltage beams, radiation-induced fractures of the femoral neck belong to history.

Naturally, when the fracture appears in a patient whose femoral neck has been irradiated, biopsy should be made to eliminate the chance that one is confronted with a metastasis. Internal fixation has given good results.

Effect of radiations on selected bone abnormalities

Following is a discussion of the effects of radiations on the rate of healing of fractures, osseous metastases, production of bone sarcoma, ankylosing spondylitis, and bursitis.

EFFECTS OF RADIATIONS ON THE RATE OF HEALING OF FRACTURES. As might be expected from the preceding discussion, radiations have a deleterious effect on the healing of fractures. In the rabbit, local irradiation of 1000 to 1600 R (air) (200 kv; hvl, 0.5 to 1.0 mm Cu) given 10 to 14 days before fracture inhibits callus formation. The callus is not only smaller in volume, but is also weaker, and nonunion is more frequent. Phosphatase activity is much below that measured at the fracture site in nonirradiated control animals (Regen and Wilkins). A similar suppression of callus formation may occur as long as 2 months after irradiation (Lovisatti). In rats, 2000 R given in 10 fractions of 200 R each (280 kv, hvl 1.0 mm Cu), after manual fracture of a long bone, inhibits effective callus formation and results in nonunion of the fracture. Hayashi and Suit, in a study of callus formation in the fractured femur of mice, found that total dose for a specific degree of inhibition increased with increasing number of fractions and that the overall time between fractions was unimportant. This implies that there is little or no proliferative response by the persistent cells surviving the initial dose.

Bonarigo and Rubin implanted tumor cells into fractured long bones of rats and observed absence of callus and nonunion. When these "pathologic fractures" were irradiated (2000 R, as before), tumor growth was arrested, but the fracture did not heal. If the "pathologic fracture" was immobilized with an intramedullary pin and irradiated, healing of the fracture took place despite the absence of significant callus formation. Since both growing tumor and irradiation prevent callus formation and fracture healing unless the bone is internally immobilized, they recommend internal fixation of the pathologic fracture after arrest of the tumor with a sufficient dose of radiations. A similar course is recommended in those patients in whom fracture appears imminent. Patients developing fractures in previously irradiated femoral necks may show slow healing and, in our experience, have shown frequent nonunion. Bonfiglio and Stephenson and Cohen pointed out, however, that healing may be nearly normal. Lynch and associates reported fifteen cases of femoral neck fracture occurring spontaneously after irradiation of the hips coincident to treatment of pelvic malignancies. The average healing time was 6.7 months in the ten patients in whom this could be evaluated. Eleven of the fifteen patients recovered full weight-bearing function without the aid of crutches or canes.

Single-dose total body irradiation of the $LD_{50/30}$ level in rats also severely inhibits fracture healing. This is particularly striking for 3 weeks after such irradiation (Spittler and associates).

EFFECTS OF RADIATIONS ON OSSEOUS METASTASES. Tumor metastatic to bone may result in bone deposition or destruction. This may or may not be evident radiographically. Baker has pointed out that metastatic tumor cells do not destroy bone directly but they stimulate osteoclasts to absorb bone. Tumor cells act through local changes in pressure, blood supply, or enzymes. Similarly, tumor cells do not deposit bone but stimulate the normal bone-forming cells into activity. Radiations destroy or inhibit the growth of osseous metastases, permitting partial restoration of the normal balance of bone absorption and deposition. However, as described earlier, high doses of radiations will also disrupt the normal process of bone deposition and absorption. It is to be expected, therefore, that normal repair of bone almost never follows irradiation of osseous metastases (Fig. 21-11).

PRODUCTION OF BONE SARCOMA BY RADIATIONS. Under certain circumstances, external irradiation may produce malignant degeneration in osteoblasts. This is not surprising, since radiation-induced malignant tumors in various other connective tissues, epithelia, and the hemopoietic tissues have already been discussed. Normal bone such as may be irradiated during the treatment of carcinoma of the cervix or breast only rarely becomes sarcomatous, although six such cases were reported by Cruz and associates. The malignant change takes place more readily if, at the time of irradiation, there is an associated osteomyelitis or benign bone neoplasm stimulating osteoblastic activity. Many reported cases have occurred after irradiation of tuberculous joints or benign bone tumors. Baserga and associates found that more bone tumors were produced if the radiations were given when the growth rate was high than when it was low.

Hatcher, Cahan and associates, and Cruz and associates have reviewed the literature on this subject. Just as in the cases of other radiation-induced malignant tumors, treatment was usually, although not invariably, given in repeated small doses over long periods of time. The total dose to the bone calculated by conventional isodose curves was 1550 to 16000 rad. The latent period between the end of irradiation and the first signs of malignant change varied from 3 to 22 years. The median latent period in Hatcher's series was 6 years. He also pointed out that chondrosarcoma seems to compose a larger proportion of radiation-induced malignant bone tumors than occurs naturally, but many tumor types are represented. In Cruz and associates' series of eleven patients, five had tumors diagnosed histologically as fibrosarcoma and six had osteoid and cartilage-producing osteosarcomas. In Dahlin's series of forty-three radiation-induced sarcomas, there were twenty-three osteogenic sarcomas, eighteen fibrosarcomas, one chondrosarcoma, and one Ewing's tumor. In only six of the forty-three patients had the radiations been given for a nonosseous histologically verified malignancy. Of twelve cases reported by Steiner, one patient had been treated for carcinoma of the cervix and nine had been treated for benign bone lesions. Similar malignant changes have been produced in irradiated animals previously chronically infected locally with bacteria (Lacassagne and Vinzent). Phillips and Sheline reported two patients who developed osteosarcoma in bone previously irradiated while treating a sarcoma of the cervix and a carcinoma of the breast. The doses (uncorrected for increased absorbed dose in bone) were 6000 R in 5 weeks (hvl, 9.5 mm Cu) and 4800 R in 39 days (hvl, 1.4 mm Cu). This is a rare occurrence—that is, two cases in 6000 patients treated or 0.1% of the 5-year survivors.

Perhaps the best data on radiation-induced bone sarcomas were reported by Sagerman and associates in a review of 243 children treated at the Retinoblastoma Clinic of the Columbia-Presbyterian Medical Center, New York, between 1930 and 1963. All the children were 4 years or younger when treated and had been followed for 5 or more years at the time of the report. Nineteen neoplasms arose in the irradiated tissues of this group of patients. Fifteen of the nineteen tumors were sarcomas and nine of these were osteosarcomas. The relationship between dose and incidence of tumor in the irradiated tissues is shown in Table 21-1. Most of these children were treated with orthovoltage techniques, and the doses shown are not corrected for increased absorption in bone. During the period of observation, osteosarcoma was not seen when doses under 8000 R had been given. The latent period varied between 4 and 30 years, with a peak incidence between 4 and 5 years after

Table 21-1. Incidence of neoplasia in orbital tissues irradiated for treatment of retinoblastoma in 232 patients followed 5 years or more*

Calculated dose	Incidence radiation-induced neoplasia
6000 R or less	3/121 (2.5%)
6000 R to 10,999 R	4/73 (5.5%)
11,000 R to 15,000 R	12/38 (32%)

*Modified from Sagerman, R. H., Cassady, J. R., Tretter, P., and Ellsworth, R. M.: Am. J. Roentgenol. **105:**529-535, 1969.

irradiation. This report is especially valuable because the group of patients treated for retinoblastoma had no known or suspected coexistent disease of the orbital tissues.

Similar malignant degeneration of osteoblasts may occur after the administration either orally or intravenously of various radioactive "bone-seekers." Radium was the first to be incriminated (Martland; Looney and associates; Looney and Colodzin) (Figs. 21-9 and 21-10). Radium doses sufficient to produce osteosarcoma do not necessarily produce clinically serious hematologic changes. More recently, many artificially produced radioactive isotopes such as ^{32}P, plutonium, ^{89}Sr, and ^{91}Y have produced malignant bone tumors in laboratory animals. The latent period in man may be from 10 to 30 years, with an average of 25 years (Looney and Colodzin).

Bone irradiated by either external or internal sources shows characteristic radiographic and microscopic changes described previously. The transition from radiation osteitis to frank cancer is apparently preceded by accelerated osteoblastic activity, but the details are otherwise unknown.

Osteochondromas have been reported arising in bone irradiated coincident to treatment of benign childhood disease (Saenger and associates; Pifer and associates). Relatively low doses were given.

ANKYLOSING SPONDYLITIS. Ankylosing spondylitis is a benign disease that usually begins as pain and ankylosis first in the sacroiliac region and in turn involves

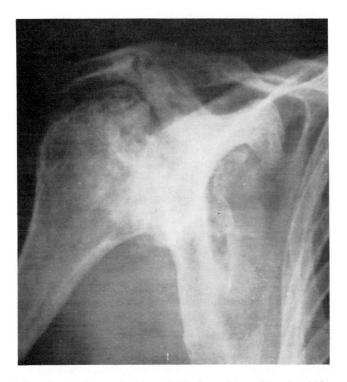

Fig. 21-9. Film of shoulder showing marked loss of articular surfaces of the glenoid fossa and humerus after aseptic necrosis of bone produced by radium poisoning. (Courtesy Dr. A. Cannon.)

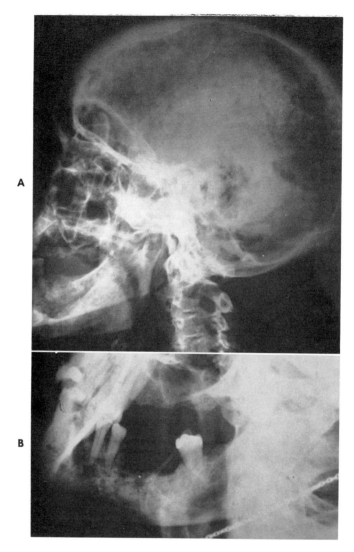

Fig. 21-10. A, Marked hyperemic absorption of bone in occipital and posterior parietal areas produced by radium intoxication. Also note residues of osteomyelitis in mandible. **B,** Resorption of bone in mandible due to osteomyelitis associated with radium poisoning. There is a sequestrum in midpart of the body of mandible. (Courtesy Dr. A. Cannon.)

the lumbar, dorsal, and cervical spines. The classic irradiation has been to give skin doses of about 1500 rad over the painful areas. Pain is invariably decreased, and probably as a result of decrease in pain there is usually objective improvement in function. It is questionable, however, if the process is arrested or reversed by irradiation. Radiations are rarely given for this disease since the association of treatment with leukemia was described (p. 530).

BURSITIS. Irradiation has frequently been recommended for subacromial and other types of bursitis, particularly when acute or subacute. Several studies have been made in which patients selected at random were irradiated and compared with

Table 21-2. Classification of primary benign and malignant neoplasms of bone*

Tissue of origin	Benign	Malignant
Bone forming	Osteoma Osteoid osteoma and osteoblastoma	Osteosarcoma Juxtacortical (parosteal) osteosarcoma
Cartilage forming	Chondroma Osteochondroma Chondroblastoma Chondromyxoid fibroma	Chondrosarcoma Juxtacortical chondrosarcoma Mesenchymal chondrosarcoma
Osteoclast	Giant cell tumor (osteoclastoma)	Giant cell tumor (osteoclastoma)
Marrow	—	Ewing's sarcoma Malignant lymphoma Myeloma
Vascular	Hemangioma Lymphangioma Glomus tumor	Angiosarcoma (low and high grade)
Connective tissue	Lipoma Desmoplastic fibroma	Liposarcoma Fibrosarcoma Malignant mesenchymoma Undifferentiated sarcoma
Other	Schwannoma Neurofibroma	Chordoma Adamantinoma of long bones
Tumor-like lesions	Solitary bone cyst (unicameral bone cyst) Aneurysmal bone cyst Juxta-articular bone cyst (intraosseous ganglion) Metaphyseal fibrous defect (nonossifying fibroma) Eosinophilic granuloma Fibrous dysplasia "Myositis ossificans" "Brown tumor" of hyperparathyroidism	

*Modified from Schajowicz, F., Ackerman, L. V., and Sissons, H. A.: Histological typing of bone tumors. International histological classification of tumours, No. 6, Geneva, 1972, World Health Organization.

unirradiated patients. Almost without exception, no difference could be detected between the irradiated and unirradiated patients. For this reason we do not encourage the use of radiotherapy for bursitis.

RADIOTHERAPY FOR BONE TUMORS

One can make reasonably accurate predictions of the relative radiosensitivity of bone tumors if one recalls the radiosensitivity of their cells of origin. The radiosensitivities of the normal constituents of bone have been discussed in the first part of this chapter and in Chapter 20. The histologic classification of bone tumors that we employ is reproduced in Table 21-2. It is adapted with minor changes from the World Health Organization classification.

In general, tumors originating from cells of the myeloid series and their support-ing structures are radiosensitive, just as are most elements of their normal counter-parts. Plasma cell myeloma, malignant lymphoma, and Ewing's tumor usually respond well to irradiation. In contrast, tumors arising from cartilage or bone-form-ing cells usually respond poorly, as is suggested by the radiation tolerance of normal adult cartilage cells and osteocytes.

There are other radiographic and microscopic findings that assist us in predicting radiosensitivity. Highly cellular bone tumors are usually more radiosensitive than the relatively noncellular tumors containing large amounts of intercellular substance—that is, cartilage, or osseous or myxomatous substances. Other factors such as vascularity, location within the body, and growth rate, when considered indepen-dently of the previously mentioned factors, play an unknown role in determining radiosensitivity.

Giant cell tumor of bone

Many lesions of bone contain giant cells. Less than half of these lesions will be true giant cell tumors of bone. The radiographic and microscopic findings that distinguish giant cell tumor of bone from the many variants are discussed admirably elsewhere (Jaffe and associates; Lichtenstein, 1972) and will not be reviewed here. Walter found that less than half of those lesions originally irradiated as giant cell tumors of bone actually were giant cell tumors. Such errors account for some of the conflicting views on treatment. If a good history, radiographs, and biopsy are systematically obtained in each patient and the criteria as established by Jaffe and associates are adhered to, much of the confusion can be avoided.

It is the consensus that giant cell tumor of bone originates from the relatively radioresistant, nonbone-forming connective tissue of marrow. As the tumor expands, it exerts pressure on the normal trabeculae, cortical bone, and periosteum. We mentioned previously that such pressure changes stimulate local bone absorption and at times bone deposition. The resulting variations in bone density seen on the radiograph are characteristic of giant cell tumor of bone. Irradiation will suppress growth of the soft tissue tumor, and, indeed, if irradiation is sufficiently vigorous, the tumor may be eradicated. The same irradiation alters periosteum and cortical bone included in the treated volume. With high doses, periosteum may be severely injured or even killed, and the osteocytes and vascular structures of bone may be damaged irreparably. Radiation injury of normal adult bone has been discussed previously. When the radiosensitivity of a giant cell tumor permits eradication, the process of repair may be delayed 6 months or more; it may continue over a period of years.

The indications for radiotherapy or for surgery of giant cell tumors of bone are not well established. Opinion varies from that denying radiotherapy any part in the treat-ment of these lesions to that recommending radiotherapy for all but a few. In justify-ing the surgical approach, Compere and Williams and associates questioned the curability of large lesions by irradiation and denied the necessity of irradiating small giant cell tumors when curettement is so simple. Johnson and Dahlin reported that in their series thirteen giant cell tumors of bone were irradiated (technique not given) and none was controlled by the irradiation alone. Walter, on the other hand, irradiated fifteen such tumors and had control in nine patients for 2 to 20 years. Lichtenstein (1977) has written a spirited analysis of the problems of therapy that should be read by any physician concerned with the management of these patients. There is ample evidence, however, that a proportion of lesions in surgically inaccessible sites can be controlled by irradiation. There is also evidence that some lesions, although resectable, may be controlled with less deformity by irradiation. With this knowledge in mind, Cade asked the question, "If irradiation is successful in inaccessible and deeply situated tumors, why should it be denied to patients with accessible and superficial lesions?"* Some radiation oncologists, particularly those in England (Windeyer and Woodyatt; Ellis) advocated radiotherapy for the majority of giant cell tumors of bone. They argued that curettement weakens the bone and permits fracture. Also, the difficulty in curetting all tumor tissue has led to frequent postoperative recurrences (Cade). They believe that radiotherapy can not only control a higher percentage of these lesions but that it can also do so with less risk of deformity and usually without admitting the patient to the hospital except for biopsy.

Because of their nonresectability, special attention has been given to the irradiation of giant cell tumors of the vertebrae. This rare disease comprises 7.4% of all giant cell tumors of bone (Berman). Their location and the consequences of their continued growth make early treatment imperative. If cord pressure is present, decompression and biopsy should be performed. Irradiation should follow. Berman used doses of 4500 to 5000 rad in 4 to 5 weeks. Of his five patients, two were alive and well at 4 and 12 years and one was alive at 17 years but with paralysis. One died from malignant transformation of the tumor and one from complications of progression of the tumor. Cohen and associates reported three of their sixteen true giant cell tumors of vertebrae were controlled by irradiation.

Giant cell tumor of bone is not a very radiosensitive lesion. We believe relatively high doses of radiations are required and that at least some of the disappointing results have occurred after the administration of small doses. The fact that high doses are required to eradicate a benign tumor, together with the fact that healing requires many months, has justifiably shifted some of the emphasis of treatment from irradiation to surgery for the more accessible lesions.

The oncogenic effects of radiations on bone have been discussed previously. It would not be surprising if the irradiation of giant cell tumors occasionally produced malignant changes in "normal" bone. However, the fact that 10% to 15% of giant cell tumors follow a malignant course even if no irradiation is performed obscures the contribution of irradiation to this complication. We agree with Buschke and Cantril that the chances of adequate irradiation producing cancer are small and should not significantly influence the decision of method of treatment. Lichtenstein (1977)

---

*From Cade, S.: J. Bone Joint Surg. **31-B:**158-160, 1949.

concludes that about half of all giant cell tumors of bone are likely to have a favorable outcome if properly treated by whatever method. Another third are sufficiently aggressive to recur after the usual treatment, and about 15% are frankly malignant or soon to become so. It is to be expected that the frankly malignant lesions or those potentially malignant aggressive lesions will be the ones to recur more often. If radiotherapy is given to the surgical failures only, there will, of course, be this higher proportion of malignant lesions or potentially malignant lesions in the irradiated group from the start. This bias voids any possible conclusion that radiotherapy converts a sizable proportion of benign giant cell tumors of bone to malignant tumors of bone.

TECHNIQUE. The optimum time-dose relationship for irradiating giant cell tumor of bone is unknown. This information is particularly difficult to collect due to the sparsity of well-documented data on patients treated by various irradiation techniques, the extremely delayed response, and the limited means for measuring the adequacy of irradiation. In the small series reported by Woodward and Coley, no patient who received a dose of 3000 R (orthovoltage) or more at the center of the lesion in 3 to 4 weeks had recurrence, although skin changes were sometimes serious and bone regeneration delayed. Baclesse believed that a dose of 4000 R (orthovoltage) in 6 weeks was optimum. We have used doses of 4000 to 5000 rad in 5 to 6 weeks delivered to vertebral lesions using megavoltage techniques.

PROGNOSIS AND RESULTS. As indicated previously, results of radiotherapy are fragmentary and difficult to evaluate. Windeyer and Woodyatt summarized the treatment and results in thirty-eight patients. Only sixteen were treated by irradiation alone. Of these, one was lost to follow-up, two were treated so recently that results were not known, and one died of intercurrent disease. One patient's lesion showed a malignant course and the leg was amputated. The remaining eleven patients had been observed for 1 to 10 years. All were well, none showed signs of tumor growth, and all showed sclerosis of the lesion.

Ellis reported on twenty-one patients, only five of whom had biopsies and were treated by irradiation alone. Three were well 2½, 3, and 4 years, respectively, after irradiation, one had a permanent deformity, and one died of apparently unrelated uremia in 5 months. Buschke and Cantril reported control of growth for 5 years or more in five or six patients who had been observed for at least 5 years. Bradshaw reported the results with Paterson's technique. In view of the rarity of true giant cell tumor before closure of the physis, he tabulated patients over 20 years of age separately. Of those treated by radiations alone, twelve of fourteen were without clinical or radiographic signs of active tumor at 5 years, ten of twelve at 10 years, and five of eight at 15 years. If those who received postoperative irradiation are included, a good result is seen in twenty-one of twenty-five at 5 years, seventeen of twenty at 10 years, and nine of thirteen at 15 years.

These results far from settle the question of the efficacy of irradiation in controlling giant cell tumor of bone. They are representative, however, and, although inadequate, they are the best we have to formulate our policies.

Osteosarcoma

Osteosarcoma is characterized by anaplastic, osteoid, and bone-forming malignant tumor cells. The tumor nearly always involves the medullary cavity and extends through the cortex to involve the periosteum either by elevating or perforating it. Early hematogenous spread is the rule. Regional nodes are rarely involved. Osteosarcoma is one of the most radioresistant tumors. It usually continues to grow even after doses that severely damage associated normal tissues. Radical surgery will often control peripheral primary lesions only to have the patient die from the hematogenous metastases. In those patients who develop pulmonary metastasis, the mean interval from diagnosis of the primary tumor is 5 to 7 months (Jenkin and associates, 1972; Royster and associates). Pratt and associates noted the same disease-free interval of 5 months for a group of fourteen children given adjuvant chemotherapy with vincristine and cyclophosphamide, but noted a disease-free interval of 15 months for a group of twenty children treated adjuvantly with doxorubicin (Adriamycin), cyclophosphamide, and high-dose methotrexate and citrovorum factor (Leucovorin) rescue.

In view of the frequent failures following amputation of a limb for the treatment of osteosarcoma, there have been over the years numerous proponents of preoperative irradiation. Francis and associates suggested that the mass of tumor breakdown after high doses of radiations may increase the body's resistance to hematogenous metastases. Lee and Mackenzie advocated preoperative irradiation as a means of delaying amputation so that those patients who already had pulmonary metastases may be recognized and spared a needless amputation. We believe that neither argument justifies attempts at preoperative irradiation. There is nothing to suggest that the results of these authors or those of Tudway or Shanks are superior to those obtained by radical surgery alone. Reported experience with preoperative irradiation (Jenkin and associates, 1970; Royster and associates; Caceres and Zaharia) provides no new support for the continued use of this modality. Caceres and Zaharia employed a massive dose technique (8000 rad in 8 days to 12,000 rad in 10 days in thirty-four patients). In thirty-two of the thirty-four, histologic preparations of the tumor were compared before and after irradiation. In five of the thirty-two patients, the post-treatment specimen showed persistent areas of tumor resembling the original biopsy specimen. In nine of the thirty-two patients, there was no evidence of residual tumor in the amputated specimen. These changes were neither dose-specific nor of any prognostic value. Jenkin and associates (1972) employed doses of 4500 to 6500 rad with conventional fractionation and delayed amputation in twenty-two patients under 30 years of age with a primary tumor in a limb. In all cases local recurrence, pulmonary metastases, or both were present before the 6-month interval had been reached. With the doses employed, they found the mean duration of tumor control to be only 3.6 months. Royster and associates used preoperative doses of 6000 to 8600 rad given in 21 to 82 days (average of 50 days) in seventeen patients. At the time of their review, four of twelve eligible patients had survived 5 years. It can thus be seen that a variety of techniques and rationales for preoperative irradiation have been employed without clearly demonstrating an improvement in survival. They do, however, give some guidelines to the doses necessary for either palliation of a primary nonresectable lesion or in the patient who refuses amputation.

There are rare cases that have been controlled by irradiation alone. Tudway irradiated nine patients for osteosarcoma. Five of the nine were alive 3 to 4 years after treatment. Doses of 5500 to 8000 rad (bone) were given over periods of 5 weeks to 3 months. Four of these patients showed no local recurrence or metastases, and the fifth showed no local recurrence but did develop pulmonary metastasis. These occasional long-term controls are not an argument for either preoperative irradiation or irradiation alone in operable patients. They are, however, a valid argument for vigorous irradiation of localized lesions in surgically inaccessible sites. Beck and associates dispute this point in a review of seventy patients treated between 1950 and 1974. They concluded that irradiation without some adjuvant chemotherapy offers little in terms of palliation or enhanced survival in patients who are not treated by radical surgery.

As noted before, Pratt and associates found a prolongation of disease-free survival in a group of twenty patients treated with intensive chemotherapy. A unique approach to combination therapy has been reported by Rosen and associates in which pretreatment with intensive chemotherapy followed by resection of the primary tumor and replacement with a prosthesis have resulted in no evidence of local recurrence in a follow-up period of 2 to 15 months. In addition of the thirteen patients who did not have pulmonary metastases, none have developed them in a period of observation of 7 to 21 months. These reports of improvement in disease-free survival with the use of adjuvant chemotherapy and the possibility of tumor resection without amputation hold the hope for improved survival while maintaining function of the involved limb.

Palliative irradiation of the primary lesion in a patient with distant metastases may be indicated. If a minimum dose to the tumor of 4000 rad in approximately 4 weeks can be tolerated, some palliation can be expected. Eleven of twelve patients so treated responded with temporary relief of pain or cessation of tumor growth. This lasts from 1 to 24 months (Woodward and Coley).

Chondrosarcomas

The radiotherapy of chondrosarcomas has the same indications and contraindications as radiotherapy for osteosarcomas. The fact that these tumors may at times run a less malignant course than osteosarcomas does not alter the limited role of radiotherapy. Of all sarcomas, this tumor is the least likely to respond significantly to irradiation. Evans and associates in a clinical pathologic analysis of eighty-one patients with chondrosarcoma found no instance in which clinical improvement or prolongation of survival was attributed to irradiation in those few patients in whom it was used. We do have one recent patient in whom high LET irradiation resulted in significant tumor reduction and relief of pain. Consideration of this form of irradiation should be given patients with primary inoperable tumors or locally recurrent symptomatic lesions.

Ewing's sarcoma of bone

Ewing's sarcoma of bone is most common in adolescents and young adults. The lesion usually begins in the medullary cavity of the shaft of a long bone, but almost any part of any bone may be the primary site. Radiographically, the findings are those of an expanding destructive lesion of the medullary cavity. Extension is usually far beyond the radiographic defect. Periosteum is often stimulated to produce new bone. This may occur as multiple parallel layers to present an onionskin appearance, or bone may be deposited at right angles to the cortex and appear as radiating spicules. Since these classic findings are not pathognomonic of Ewing's sarcoma and are present in only a fraction of all cases, biopsy is essential.

The cell of origin of this lesion has been a subject of much debate. The present consensus is that Ewing's tumor arises from the reticular cells of the marrow. Differentiation from malignant lymphoma is possible microscopically and is justified clinically. The same can be said of neuroblastoma, metastatic carcinoma, and osteosarcoma. In its usual clinical course, early hematogenous metastases occur to other bones and to the lungs. Regional lymph node metastases also occur, but the frequency of such spread is not well documented. In the past the average interval between diagnosis of primary and first metastases has been reported to be 7 to 8 months (Jenkin and associates, 1970; Freeman and associates).

Ewing's sarcoma usually extends well beyond the limits of the radiographic defect. Similarly, the tumor generally infiltrates surrounding soft tissues to an extent and in a fashion that cannot be appreciated by palpation. Therefore, in planning irradiation of this tumor, the entire bone and a generous margin of adjacent soft tissues should be routinely included in the field. The entire shaft of an involved long bone should be irradiated. The use of computed tomography in lesions arising in pelvic bones is extremely helpful in defining the hitherto often unappreciated soft tissue extension of tumors arising in this location.

Ewing's tumor of bone is a moderately radiosensitive tumor and is frequently locally radiocurable. In many patients the local lesion was controlled but the patients died from metastases. Just as was the case in rhabdomyosarcoma, these facts led to a search for effective adjuvant chemotherapy regimens in apparently localized Ewing's tumor. The earliest forms of systemic therapy employed were either total body irradiation or cyclophosphamide.

Jenkin and associates (1970) reported twenty-six patients whose primary lesions were treated with doses of 4500 to 6000 rad, and in only six patients did recurrence of the primary site occur prior to or simultaneously with metastasis. Ten of their twenty-six patients were given 300 rad total body irradiation after treatment of the primary site. Two of the ten patients lived more than 4 years, whereas none of the sixteen patients with treatment of only the primary site survived beyond 21 months. Freeman and associates elected the use of chemotherapeutic agents as a method of systemic treatment and reported two of nine patients so treated surviving more than 3 years. Hustu and associates reported an early experience in fifteen patients primarily treated with radiation and given vincristine and cyclophosphamide as systemic agents for 1 to 2 years. Only one of fifteen patients had recurrence at the primary site during the period of observation, and eight of the fifteen patients survived 1 year or more. These preliminary results encouraged the formation of a clinical trial employing both chemotherapy and pulmonary radiation as adjunctive systemic measures in the primary treatment of Ewing's tumor.

The volume to be irradiated is usually large and, after an initial dose of 4500 rad, should be reduced by all available imaging procedures for a final boosting dose of 1000 to 1500 rad. If the tumor arises in an extremity, an effort should be made to spare a strip of skin and connective tissue during the latter part of treatment to avoid serious damage and preserve function of the extremity. For further information on the problem of irradiation of an entire limb, Cohen's discussion of the treatment of Kaposi's sarcoma should be reviewed.

In the present management of Ewing's sarcoma it is not possible to separate the influence of chemotherapy (vincristine, actinomycin D, cyclophosphamide, and doxorubicin with irradiation) from irradiation alone as these treatments relate to local control. In the prechemotherapy era it was not uncommon to achieve local control in 65% to 75% of the patients with doses of 4500 to 6000 rad, but only 10% to 15% of the patients were cured. For those patients who presented with metastases or developed metastases, cure was rarely reported. When irradiation was combined with effective drug therapy, local control increased from 80% to 95% (Johnson and Pomeroy; Chabora and associates). When doses of 6000 rad were combined with multiagent chemotherapy, severe local tissue damage was noted (Tefft and associates). Perez and associates reported the results of treatment of 187 patients entered in the Intergroup Ewing's Study. Twenty-two of twenty-five local failures occurred in the first 24 months. Local control was achieved in 87% of patients with doses of 4000 to 6000 rad. For twenty-one patients given at least 6000 rad and nine patients given lower doses with regimens that included doxorubicin, there were no local recurrences. One third of the entire group of patients developed distant metastases. In an analysis of dose response the preliminary review of this study concluded that the final reduced volume should be given at least 5500 rad in conjunction with the appropriate adjuvant drug regimen.

These preliminary results of a large clinical trial clearly indicate an improvement in median survival, disease-free survival, and local control attributable to a combined modality approach. Routine use of computed tomography for periodic definition of tumor volume, particularly at the time of considering boost doses, should be encouraged. This is especially true for the primaries in the pelvis. In those patients who develop metastases, good palliation invariably follows properly planned irradiation.

Malignant lymphoma

Malignant lymphoma of bone arises from the lymphoid cells normally present in the marrow. The malignant cell is identical to its nodal counterpart and exhibits a similar radiosensitivity. The lesion originating in bone, however, has distinctive characteristics that justify its consideration separately from both Ewing's tumor of bone and generalized malignant lymphoma involving bone secondarily. Patients with the latter are generally older and usually die within 1 year of bone involvement. In contrast, malignant lymphoma of bone does not necessarily involve lymph nodes, appears at an average of 34 years of age (Francis and associates), and carries a relatively good prognosis. Pain is a constant first symptom and is frequently a chief complaint. It may be severe but is usually described as a moderate or mild ache.

The radiographic findings may be suggestive of the diagnosis but are never diagnostic. Both medullary and cortical bone destruction are invariably present. The location of destruction within the bone is of no help. Periosteum may be elevated and perforated, with extensive infiltration of adjacent soft tissues. Lymph node metastases are not infrequent. McCormack and associates reported regional node metastases in six of their thirty-two patients. If untreated, the tumor is moderately aggressive locally and kills with generalized metastases.

TECHNIQUE. Malignant lymphoma of bone exhibits the same relative radiosensitivity as malignant lymphoma of nodal origin. After irradiation, it regresses rapidly and is controlled with moderate doses. Because of this local radiocurability, radiotherapy can offer the same local control rate as radical surgery; yet the involved extremity or bone segment can be preserved. For this reason radiotherapy is the treatment of choice. A lymphangiogram is indicated as a part of the pretreatment evaluation in most patients. The node areas should be irradiated with generous margins if adenopathy is present.

The techniques of irradiation are identical to those discussed for Ewing's tumor. Since extension in the medullary cavity cannot be accurately determined from the films, and since periosseous soft tissues are frequently infiltrated beyond the limits of palpable disease, large volumes must be routinely irradiated just as for Ewing's tumor. Computed tomography is useful in defining the extension from primary bone sites. The entire length of an involved long bone should be irradiated. Doses of 4000 to 5000 rad in 4 to 5 weeks are considered optimum for local control.

PROGNOSIS AND RESULTS. These lesions are seen to respond well both on physical examination and radiographically. Within 1 month bone repair may be evident, and it is usually obvious by 3 months. The cortical bone is slowly replaced. Eventually the density of the cortex may be greater than that of previously uninvolved bone (Fig. 21-11). In contrast to the prognosis in patients with generalized malignant lymphoma with secondary bone involvement, patients with primary malignant lymphoma of bone have a relatively good prognosis. Complete cure of more than 50% of patients and local control in a greater number are expected from irradiation alone.

In those patients not cured, significant palliation is given. With doses mentioned previously to the volumes suggested, local recurrence will be uncommon and patients may live comfortably and usefully many years before they die from dissemination. Once widespread, chemotherapy should be tried, but its role is otherwise poorly defined.

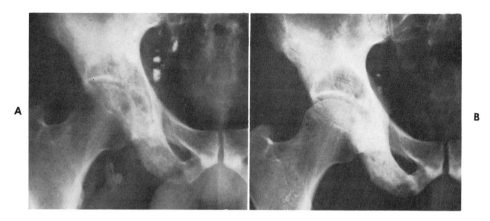

Fig. 21-11. Reticulum cell sarcoma of the ischium in 29-year-old man. **A,** Film made after bone biopsy and lymphangiogram. Dose of 4000 rad (^{60}Co) in 5 weeks was given to the hemipelvis. **B,** Film made 22 months after completion of therapy. Note increased density of ischium and incomplete repair at biopsy site. (Courtesy Dr. L. Topouzian.)

Multiple myeloma

The many interesting and controversial features of multiple myeloma have provoked a voluminous literature on the various aspects of this disease. The malignant plasma cell of multiple myeloma is thought to arise from the primitive reticulum cells of the marrow and rarely from extramedullary reticulum cells. In the former, the marrow invariably shows extensive destruction. Later the cortex may likewise be absorbed. These destructive changes account for the major initial symptoms. Pain, most often in the ribs or low back, weakness, weight loss, anemia, and thrombocytopenia are commonly present. Pathologic fractures occur in about 50% of the patients. Extraosseous spread may produce a variety of findings secondary to pressure from a tumor mass or destruction or infiltration by plasma cells. Lesions of almost every abdominal and thoracic organ have been reported. Similarly, neurologic signs and symptoms are common from infiltrative lesions or pressure from masses or fractures. Lichtenstein states that the only difference between the large and small cell tumors is one of maturity of the cell of origin.

The radiographic changes in multiple myeloma are not diagnostic. The commonly described discrete osteolytic defects may be found in patients with other diseases (hyperthyroidism, certain primary bone tumors, and carcinoma metastatic from the breast or thyroid). Occasionally in multiple myeloma, an osseous defect will be produced that has the soap-bubble appearance of a giant cell tumor of bone. The severe diffuse marrow destruction so characteristic of this disease may be reflected as nothing more than an osteoporosis.

An ideal treatment for multiple myeloma would selectively destroy the malignant plasma cells. The large number of therapeutic agents that have been used with this aim is a measure of the limited effectiveness of existing methods. Except for experimental procedures, the treatment is now centered around the use of local palliative irradiation, whereas the drugs melphalan (Alkeran) and cyclophosphamide are the systemic agents of choice. Recent interest has focused on combination chemotherapy.

General supportive measures are extremely important in the care of these patients. This includes relief of pain with analgesics, ambulation, and blood replacement. Nursing care associated with their multiple fractures is also essential. There is an occasional patient with this disease who is asymptomatic. It is questionable whether available techniques contribute to increased longevity. Therefore the question of whether an asymptomatic patient should be treated cannot be answered.

TECHNIQUE. The myeloma cells exhibit radiosensitivity similar to that of the lymphocytes in histiocytic lymphoma of bone. The usual diffuse involvement of bone marrow in multiple myeloma, coupled with this radiosensitivity, forbids cure by irradiation. Attempts at total body irradiation with internal emitters have not proved beneficial. The higher doses permitted with local irradiation frequently provide definite benefit. However, the optimum dose-time levels for local irradiation of multiple myeloma are not well established. We believe a tissue dose of 2000 rad in 2 to 3 weeks is a minimum. Doses of this level are simple to give. A generous margin around the zone of suspected involvement should be included in the field. In selected patients with limited areas of involvement, a more aggressive approach and doses approaching 4000 rad may be justified. This is especially true as the median survival improves with combination chemotherapy.

Demineralization of vertebral bodies is invariable in multiple myeloma. As a consequence, vertebral collapse with all of its sequelae is not infrequent. Such fractures occurred in 48% of ninety-seven patients. If cord compression occurs, either with or without fracture, early surgical decompression followed by appropriate immobilization and irradiation may be of great value.

PROGNOSIS AND RESULTS. Although an occasional long-term survival will be encountered, the majority of patients with multiple myeloma will die within 4 years of the time the diagnosis is made. In a large series of patients receiving an alkylating agent with prednisone, the median survival ranged from 12 and 23 months, and in the group who responded to this combination therapy, the median survival ranged between 32 and 36 months (Alexanian and associates, 1972). In an update of the SWOG trials the addition of vincristine to an alkylating agent prednisone combination has brought the median survival up to 34 months for all patients receiving treatment (Alexanian and associates, 1977). In view of the response of selected patients with advanced disease and bone pain to high increment hemibody radiotherapy, a consideration of some form of external beam total body irradiation as an adjuvant in early disease may be justified in a clinical trial. Either local or hemibody irradiation usually results in excellent pain relief. Unfortunately, in the final stages of disease the anemia and widespread painful areas preclude successful palliation by any form of treatment other than narcotic analgesics.

The pain relief provided by local irradiation may be incomplete or of short duration. However, some degree of relief is the rule, and striking relief of pain with recalcification, union of a fracture, or alleviation of pressure symptoms is not infrequent.

Solitary plasma cell tumors of bone

Myeloma confined to a single bone is unusual. Most of the patients with what initially appears to be a solitary myeloma will eventually develop other lesions and will die with typical multiple myeloma. For this reason Carson and associates have applied the term *apparent solitary plasma cell tumor* to these lesions. Some of the patients show no new foci for 6 to 9 years, and a small number may never develop additional lesions. For this reason we believe one should routinely attempt eradication of the apparent solitary myeloma. Surgical excision has been advocated for the accessible lesions. Since the lesions are radiosensitive and locally radiocurable, the problem is not unlike that presented in Ewing's tumor of bone. Doses of 3500 to 4000 rad to the lesion in 4 weeks are required. These lesions are not common, and it is impossible to be more specific regarding either treatment or prognosis.

Extramedullary plasma cell tumors

Extramedullary plasma cell tumors are a heterogeneous group of lesions, some of which appear to be the first manifestations of multiple myeloma, whereas others behave like benign tumors. It is not easy to separate the two by conventional microscopy. If only one type of light immunoglobulin chains, such as kappa or lambda, is formed by the tumor cells, their monoclonal (and presumably neoplastic) origin can be assumed. This can be tested simply and reliably with immunofluorescence or immunoperoxidase techniques even from formalin-fixed paraffin-embedded material. In Hellwig's extensive review, sixty-five of 128 lesions originated in the upper air passages, forty-seven in the conjunctiva, four in lymph nodes, and thirteen in other organs. Of the sixty-five in the upper air passages, thirty-five were apparently localized and thirty were locally invasive. However, two patients reported by Howarth had definite bone destruction yet showed good response to irradiation. Similarly, three of Carson and associates' patients show that despite bone destruction, these tumors can be locally controlled with irradiation. We believe that these tumors of the upper air passages should be irradiated with the aim of controlling the local disease. Doses recommended are similar to those described for the apparent solitary plasma cell tumor. Plasma cell lesions of the conjunctiva appear to be entirely different in their behavior. They are benign lesions, and simple excision will suffice.

Histiocytosis X (eosinophilic granuloma, Hand-Schüller-Christian disease, and Letterer-Siwe disease)

Eosinophilic granuloma, Hand-Schüller-Christian disease, and Letterer-Siwe disease represent, in the order listed, progressively greater degrees of bone and visceral destruction. This is not meant to imply that there is transition from one disease to another. On the contrary, there is good evidence that eosinophilic granuloma rarely if ever is transformed into either of the other diseases. The etiology of the diseases is unknown, but in many respects the areas appear to have an inflammatory origin. Well-differentiated histiocytes and eosinophils are common to each type, and microscopically one cannot usually distinguish one disease from the other two.

Clinically, eosinophilic granuloma is usually a single lesion, but there may be multiple areas of involvement. About a third to a fourth of the patients will have multiple lesions. The skull is the most frequent site of involvement, but the ribs, femur, vertebrae, pelvis, mandible, and humerus may also be involved.

The lesions of eosinophilic granuloma have been controlled by irradiation or surgery, and in a few instances spontaneous regression has occurred. However, we believe that, with few exceptions, the treatment of choice is irradiation. About 1000 rad in 1 week is usually sufficient. With this low dose, the technique of irradiation is simple. Complete restitution of bone will be seen on follow-up radiographs after such a dose.

Hand-Schüller-Christian disease is known for the triad of exophthalmos, diabetes insipidus, and osteolytic defects in the skull. The triad is not always present, and other parts of the skeleton are usually also involved. It is treated with the same doses as recommended for eosinophilic granuloma. Unfortunately, diabetes insipidus does not respond to hypothalamic irradiation.

Letterer-Siwe disease is frequently fatal. Irradiation should be directed to the symptom-producing lesions initially. The most one can expect is temporary regression. Survival is related to age at onset. In Lucaya's series only 23% of neonates survived, whereas of those between 2 and 36 months of age 66% survived, and beyond 36 months all children survived.

RADIOTHERAPY FOR ANEURYSMAL BONE CYST

Aneurysmal bone cyst, a benign lesion of bone, has distinct radiologic and pathologic features. There is typically an extraosseous soft tissue extension outlined by a thin rim of new bone. The mass usually contains irregular trabeculations. Pathologically, cavernous spaces without an endothelial lining are the dominant feature. Giant cells are present in the solid portions of the lesion (Dahlin, 1967). The same confusion that makes evaluation of the management of giant cell tumors difficult applies to aneurysmal bone cysts.

Curettement or local resection are not uniformly successful. Nobler and associates reviewed the results of treatment of thirty-three patients with aneurysmal bone cyst. There was recurrence in eight of twenty-six cases selected for surgery and in only one of six cases selected for irradiation. Additionally, five surgical failures were controlled by irradiation. There was no instance of sarcomatous degeneration.

Such results justify irradiation of surgically inaccessible lesions and further suggest that irradiation may be the treatment of choice in all cases. A minimum tumor dose of 2500 rad is recommended.

REFERENCES

Alexanian, R., Bonnet, J., Gehan, E., Haut, A., Hewlett, J., Lane, M., Monto, R., and Wilson, H.: Combination chemotherapy for multiple myeloma, Cancer **30:**382-389, 1972.

Alexanian, R., Salmon, S., Bonnet, J., Gehan, E., Haut, A., and Weick, J.: Combination therapy for multiple myeloma, Cancer **40:**2765-2771, 1977.

Aspin, N., and Johns, H. E.: The absorbed dose in cylindrical cavities within irradiated bone, Br. J. Radiol. **36:**350-362, 1963.

Baclesse, F.: Quelques remarques sur les tumeurs à myéloplaxes et leur traitement radiothérapique considéré à longue échéance, J. Radiol. Electrol. **26:**41-46, 1944-1945.

Baker, S. L.: Metastatic tumours of bone, J. Fac. Radiologists **1:**245-256, 1950.

Barnhard, H. J., and Geyer, R. W.: Effects of x-radiation on growing bone, Radiology **78:**207-214, 1962.

Barr, J. S., Lingley, J. R., and Gall, E. A.: The effect of roentgen irradiation on epiphyseal growth, Am. J. Roentgenol. **49:**104-115, 1943.

Baserga, R., Lisco, H., and Cater, B.: The delayed effects of external gamma irradiation on the bones of rats, Am. J. Pathol. **39:**455-472, 1961.

Beck, J. C., Wara, W. M., Boyill, E. G., Jr., and Phillips, T. L.: The role of radiation therapy in the treatment of osteosarcoma, Radiology **120:**163-165, 1976.

Berman, H. L.: The treatment of benign giant-cell tumors of the vertebre by irradiation, Radiology **83:**202-207, 1964.

Bonarigo, B. C., and Rubin, P.: Nonunion of pathologic fracture after radiation therapy, Radiology **88:**889-898, 1967.

Bonfiglio, M.: The pathology of fracture of the femoral neck following irradiation, Am. J. Roentgenol. **70:**449-459, 1953.

Bradshaw, J. D.: The value of x-ray therapy in the management of osteoclastoma, Clin. Radiol. **15:**70-74, 1964.

Buschke, F., and Cantril, S. T.: Roentgentherapy of benign giant cell tumor of bone, Cancer **2:**293-315, 1949.

Caceres, E., and Zaharia, M.: Massive preoperative radiation therapy in the treatment of osteogenic sarcoma, Cancer **30:**634-638, 1972.

Cade, S.: Giant cell tumour of bone, J. Bone Joint Surg. **31-B:**158-160, 1949.

Cahan, W. G., Woodward, H. G., Higinbotham, N. L., Stewart, F. W., and Coley, B. L.: Sarcoma arising in irradiated bone, Cancer **1:**3-29, 1948.

Carson, C. P., Ackerman, L. V., and Maltby, J. D.: Plasma cell myeloma, Am. J. Clin. Pathol. **25:**849-888, 1955.

Chabora, B. M., Rosen, G., Cham, W., D'Angio, G. J., and Tefft, M.: Radiotherapy in Ewing's sarcoma, Radiology **120:**667-671, 1976.

Cohen, D. M., Dahlin, D. C., and MacCarty, C. S.: Vertebral giant-cell tumor and variants, Cancer **17:**461-472, 1964.

Cohen, L.: Dose, time and volume parameters in irradiation therapy of Kaposi's sarcoma, Br. J. Radiol. **35:**485-488, 1962.

Compere, E. L.: Diagnosis and treatment of giant cell tumors of bone, J. Bone Joint Surg. **35-A:**822-830, 1953.

Cruz, M., Coley, B. L., and Stewart, F. W.: Post-radiation bone sarcoma, Cancer **10:**72-88, 1957.

Dahl, B.: La théorie de l'ostéoclasie et le comportement des ostéoclastes vis à vis du bleu trypan et vis à vis de l'irradiation aux rayons X, Acta Pathol. Microbiol. Scand., suppl. 26, pp. 234-239, 1936.

Dahlin, D. C.: Bone tumors, ed. 2, Springfield, Ill., 1967, Charles C Thomas, Publisher.

del Regato, J. A., and Spjut, H. J.: Ackerman and del Regato's cancer: diagnosis, treatment, and prognosis, ed. 5, St. Louis, 1977, The C. V. Mosby Co.

del Regato, J. A.: Malignant tumors of bone. In del Regato, J. A., and Spjut, H. J.: Ackerman and del Regato's cancer: diagnosis, treatment, and prognosis, ed. 5, St. Louis, 1977, The C. V. Mosby Co.

Ellis, F.: Treatment of osteoclastoma by irradiation, J. Bone Joint Surg. **31-B:**268-280, 1949.

Evans, H. L., Ayala, A. G., and Romsdahl, M. M.: Prognostic factors in chondrosarcoma of bone, Cancer **40:**181-831, 1977.

Francis, K. C., Higinbotham, N. L., and Coley, B. L.: Primary reticulum cell sarcoma of bone, Surg. Gynecol. Obstet. **99:**142-146, 1954.

Francis, K. C., Phillips, R., Nickson, J. J., Woodward, H. Q., Higinbotham, N. L., and Coley, B. L.: Massive preoperative irradiation in the treatment of osteogenic sarcoma in children, Am. J. Roentgenol. **72:**813-818, 1954.

Freeman, A. I., Sachatello, C., Gaeta, J., Shah, N. K., Wang, J. J., and Sinks, L. F.: An analysis of Ewing's tumor in children at Roswell Park Memorial Institute, Cancer **29:**1563-1569, 1972.

Hatcher, C. H.: The development of sarcoma in bone subjected to roentgen or radium irradiation, J. Bone Joint Surg. **27:**179-195, 1945.

Hayashi, S., and Suit, H. D.: Effect of fractionation

of radiation dose on callus formation at site of fracture, Radiology **101**:181-186, 1971.

Heller, M.: Bone. In Bloom, W., editor: Histopathology of irradiation, New York, 1948, McGraw-Hill Book Co.

Hellwig, C. A.: Extramedullary plasma cell tumors observed in various locations, Arch. Pathol. **36**: 95-111, 1943.

Hinkel, C. L.: The effect of roentgen ray upon the growing long bones of albino rats, Am. J. Roentgenol. **47**:439-457, 1942.

Hinkel, C. L.: The effect of roentgen rays upon the growing long bones of albino rats, Am. J. Roentgenol. **49**:321-348, 1943.

Hustu, H. O., Pinkel, D., and Pratt, C.: Treatment of clinically localized Ewing's sarcoma with radiotherapy and combination chemotherapy, Cancer **30**:1522-1527, 1972.

Jenkin, R. D. T., Rider, W. D., and Sonley, M. J.: Ewing's sarcoma: a trial of adjuvant total-body irradiation, Am. J. Roentgenol. **96**:151-155, 1970.

Jenkin, R. D. T., Allt, W. E. C., and Fitzpatrick, P. J.: Osteosarcoma: an assessment of management with particular reference to primary irradiation and selective delayed amputation, Cancer **30**:393-400, 1972.

Johnson, E. W., and Dahlin, D. C.: Treatment of giant-cell tumor of bone, J. Bone Joint Surg. **41-A**:895-904, 1959.

Johnson, R. E., and Pomeroy, T. C.: Evaluation of therapeutic results in Ewing's sarcoma, Am. J. Roentgenol. **123**:583-587, 1975.

Kember, N. F.: Cell survival and radiation damage in growth cartilage, Br. J. Radiol. **40**:496-505, 1967.

Kolar, J., Vraber, R., and Chyba, J.: Arthropathies after irradiation, J. Bone Joint Surg. **49A**:1157-1166, 1967.

Koletsky, S., Bonte, F. J., and Friedell, H. L.: Production of malignant tumors in rats with radioactive phosphorus, Cancer Res. **10**:129-138, 1950.

Kriss, J. P., Bierman, H. R., Thomas, S. F., and Newell, R. R.: Treatment of multiple myeloma with radioactive iodine and radioactive iodinated serum albumin, Radiology **65**:241-248, 1955.

Lacassagne, A., and Vinzent, R.: Sarcomes provoqué chez des lapins par l'irradiation d'abcès a Streptobacillus caviae, Compt. Rend. Soc. Biol. **100**:249-251, 1929.

Lacassagne, A., and Gricouroff, G.: Action des radiations sur les tissues, Paris, 1941, Masson et Cie.

Lee, E. S., and Mackenzie, D. H.: Osteosarcoma:

a study of the value of preoperative megavoltage radiotherapy, Br. J. Surg. **51**:252-274, 1964.

Lichtenstein, L.: Bone tumors, ed. 5, St. Louis, 1977, The C. V. Mosby Co.

Longheed, M. N., and Brown, B. S. J.: Comparison of effect of cobalt-60 and 250 kv. radiation on the bones of the rat, Radiology **78**:278-280, 1962.

Looney, W. B., Hasterlik, R. J., Brues, A. M., and Skirmont, E.: A clinical investigation of the chronic effects of radium salts administered therapeutically (1915-1931), Am. J. Roentgenol. **73**:1006-1037, 1955.

Looney, W. B., and Colodzin, M.: Late follow-up studies after internal deposition of radioactive materials, J.A.M.A. **160**:1-3, 1956.

Lovisatti, N.: Il comportamento del callo di frattura nelle ossa irradiate, Radiol. Med. **18**:1-8, 1931.

Lucaya, J.: Histiocytosis X, Am. J. Dis. Child. **121**: 289-295, 1971.

Lynch, A. C., Sullivan, R., and Dahlin, D. C.: Pathologic fractures of femur treated at Mayo Clinic (1950-1959), Arch. Surg. **90**:127-132, 1965.

Martland, H. S.: The occurrence of malignancy in radioactive persons, Am. J. Cancer **15**:2435-2516, 1931.

McCormack, L. J., Ivins, J. C., and Dahlin, D. C.: Primary reticulum cell sarcoma of bone, Cancer **5**:1182-1192, 1952.

McGavran, M. H., and Spady, H.: Eosinophilic granuloma of bone, J. Bone Joint Surg. **42-A**: 979-992, 1960.

Meredith, W. J.: Some aspects of supervoltage radiation therapy, Am. J. Roentgenol. **79**:57-63, 1958.

Meyerding, H. W.: Benign and malignant giant cell tumors of bone; diagnosis and results of treatment, J.A.M.A. **117**:1849-1855, 1941.

Murphy, W. T., and Berens, D. L.: Late sequelae following cancerocidal irradiation in children: a report of three cases, Radiology **58**:35-42, 1952.

Neuhauser, E. B., Wittenborg, M. H., Berman, C. Z., and Cohen, J.: Irradiation effects of roentgen therapy on the growing spine, Radiology **59**: 637-650, 1952.

Nobler, M. P., Higinbotham, N. L., and Phillips, R. F.: The cure of aneurysmal bone cyst, Radiology **90**:1185-1192, 1968.

Parker, F., and Jackson, H.: Primary reticulum cell carcinoma of bone, Surg. Gynecol. Obstet. **68**: 45-53, 1939.

Perez, C. A., Razek, A. A., Tefft, M., Newbit, M., Omer Burgert, E., Jr., Kissane, J., Vietti, T., and Gehan, E. A.: Analysis of local tumor control in Ewing's sarcoma, Cancer **40**:2864-2873, 1977.

Phillips, T. L., and Sheline, G. E.: Bone sarcomas

following radiation therapy, Radiology **81**:992-996, 1963.

Pifer, J. W., Hempelman, L. H., Dodge, H. J., and Hodges, F. J. II.: Neoplasms in the Ann Arbor series of thymus irradiated children: a second survey, Am. J. Roentgenol. **103**:13-18, 1968.

Pratt, C., Shanks, E., Hustu, O., Rivera, G., Smith, J., and Mahesh Kuman, A. P.: Adjuvant multiple drug chemotherapy for osteosarcoma of the extremity, Cancer **39**:51-57, 1977. ·

Regaud, C.: Sur la sensibilite du tissu osseux normal vis-a-vis de rayons X et gamma et sur le mecanisme de l'osteoradionecrose, C. R. Soc. Biol. **87**:629-632, 1922.

Regen, E. M., and Wilkins, W. E.: The influence of roentgen irradiation on the rate of healing of fractures and the phosphatase activity of the callus of adult bone, J. Bone Joint Surg. **18**:69-79, 1936.

Reinhard, E. H., Moore, C. V., Bierbaum, D. S., and Moore, S.: Radioactive phosphorus as a therapeutic agent, J. Lab. Clin. Med. **31**:107-218, 1946.

Richards, W. G., Coleman, F. C., and Irving, N. W.: Giant cell tumor of bone involving the fifth lumbar vertebra, J.A.M.A. **163**:731-733, 1957.

Roberts, J. E.: Dosage in clinical practice. In Carling, E. R., Windeyer, B. W., and Smithers, D. W., editors: Practice in radiotherapy, London, 1955, Butterworth & Co., Ltd.

Rosen, G., Murphy, M. L., Huvos, A. G., Gutierrez, M., and Marcove, R. C.: Chemotherapy, en bloc resection, and prosthetic bone replacement in the treatment of osteogenic sarcoma, Cancer **37**:1-11, 1976.

Rosenthal, L., and Marvin, J. F.: The effect of roentgen-ray quality on bone growth and cortical bone damage, Am. J. Roentgenol. **77**:893-898, 1957.

Royster, R. L., King, E. R., Ebersole, J., DeGiorgi, L. S., and Levitt, S. H.: High dose, preoperative supervoltage irradiation for osteogenic sarcoma, Am. J. Roentgenol. **114**:536-543, 1972.

Rubin, P., Andrews, J. R., Swarm, R., and Gump, H.: Radiation induced dysplasia of bone, Am. J. Roentgenol. **82**:206-216, 1959.

Saenger, E. L., Silverman, F. N., Sterling, T. D., and Turner, M. E.: Neoplasia following therapeutic irradiation for benign conditions in childhood, Radiology **74**:889-904, 1960.

Sagerman, R. H., Cassady, J. R., Tretter, P., and Ellsworth, R.: Radiation induced neoplasia following external beam therapy for children with retinoblastoma, Am. J. Roentgenol. **105**:529-535, 1969.

Schajowicz, F., Ackerman, L. V., and Sissons, H. A.: Histological typing of bone tumors. International histological classification of tumors, No. 6, Geneva, 1972, World Health Organization.

Shanks, W.: The treatment of bone sarcoma, J. Bone Joint Surg. **35-B**:3-5, 1953.

Sissons, H. A.: Experimental study of local irradiation on bone growth. In Mitchell, J. S., Holmes, B. E., and Smith, C. L., editors: Progress in radiobiology, Edinburgh, 1956, Oliver & Boyd.

Spiers, F. W.: Effective atomic number and energy absorption in tissues, Br. J. Radiol. **19**:52-63, 1946.

Spiers, F. W.: Symposium: Radiotherapeutic physics; dosage in irradiated soft tissue and bone, Br. J. Radiol. **24**:365-370, 1951.

Splittler, A. W., Batch, J. W., and Rutledge, B. A.: Whole body irradiation on the healing of fresh fractures, Arch. Surg. **68**:93-104, 1954.

Stampfli, W. P., and Kerr, H. D.: Fractures of the femoral neck following pelvic irradiation, Am. J. Roentgenol. **57**:71-83, 1947.

Stephenson, W. H., and Cohen, B.: Post-irradiation fractures of the neck of the femur, J. Bone Joint Surg. **38-B**:830-845, 1956.

Stewart, J. W., and Dische, S.: Effect of radiotherapy on bone marrow in ankylosing spondylitis, Lancet **2**:1063-1069, 1956.

Tefft, M., Lattin, P. B., Jereb, B., Chamb, W., Ghavimi, F., Rosen, G., Exelby, P., Marcove, R., Murphy, M. L., and D'Angio, G. J.: Treatment of rhabdomyosarcoma and Ewing's sarcoma of childhood: acute and late effects on normal tissue following combination therapy with emphasis on the role of irradiation combined with chemotherapy, Cancer **37**:1201-1213, 1976.

Tudway, R. C.: Radiotherapy for osteogenic sarcoma, J. Bone Joint Surg. **43-B**:61-67, 1961.

Walter, J.: Giant-cell lesions of bone: osteoclastoma and giant-cell tumour variants, Clin. Radiol. **11**:114-124, 1960.

Whitehouse, W. M., and Lampe, I.: Osseous damage in irradiation of renal tumors in infancy and childhood, Am. J. Roentgenol. **70**:721-729, 1953.

Williams, R. R., Dahlin, D. C., and Ghormley, R. K.: Giant cell tumor of bone, Cancer **7**:764-773, 1954.

Wilson, C. W.: The effects of x-rays on the uptake of phosphorus[32] by the knee joint and tibia of six-weeks-old mice: relation of depression of uptake to x-ray dose, Br. J. Radiol. **29**:571-574, 1956.

Windeyer, B. W., and Woodyatt, P. B.: Osteoclastoma, J. Bone Joint Surg. **31-B**:252-267, 1949.

Woodward, H. Q.: Some effects of roentgen rays on mouse bone, Radiat. Res. **1**:567, 1954.

Woodward, H. Q., and Coley, B. L.: The correlation of tissue dose and clinical response in irradiation of bone tumors and of normal bone, Am. J. Roentgenol. **57**:464-471, 1947.

Woodward, H. Q., and Spiers, F. W.: The effects of x-rays of different qualities on the alkaline phosphatase of living mouse bone, Br. J. Radiol. **26**:38-46, 1953.

22

The brain, spinal cord, and pituitary gland

RESPONSE OF THE NORMAL NERVOUS SYSTEM TO IRRADIATION

The adult central nervous system is relatively radioresistant. In 1945 Peirce and associates stated "There is no clinical evidence so far to cause us to hesitate to increase the tumor dose where possible to 10,000 or 15,000 R. The limitation will be that of the scalp and possibly the vascular structure of the skull."* Their factors of treatment were 200 kv, an hvl of 2 mm Cu, a target-skin distance of 50 cm, and 100 to 150 R per day per field. Since 1945, evidence has accumulated to indicate that the normal adult brain, brain stem, and spinal cord can be damaged in a significant proportion of patients by considerably lower doses, but nerve tissue must still be classed as relatively radioresistant. As is true of many other relatively radioresistant tissues, the damage to nerve tissue may be slow in making its appearance, and once damage has occurred the patient recovers slowly and incompletely. At present we can recognize three phases in the radiation response of the central nervous system— an acute phase of meningoencephalitis, a period of apparent normalcy, and a period of late nerve cell damage and vascular change.

ACUTE CHANGES. The first phase is obvious shortly after large doses to the brain. Edema of all intracranial structures develops, and cerebrospinal fluid pressure increases. The severity of these changes is proportional to the dose. With single doses of 6000 R delivered to the monkey's whole brain (250 kvp; hvl, 1.4 mm Cu; TSD, 35 cm), the immediate response is so severe that death usually follows within 55 hours (Ross and associates). Edema of the meninges and brain and an increase in the production of cerebrospinal fluid occur. A pressure cone at the foramen magnum has been found frequently after such doses and probably is a major factor in causing early death. Preceding death, there is progressive inactivity of the animal with shivering, poor coordination, loss of pupillary light reflex, both tonic and clonic seizures, blindness, ataxia, paraplegia, and partial facial paralysis (Ross and associates). Rectal temperature decreases until death. Electroencephalographic abnormali-

---

*From Peirce, C. B., Cone, W. V., Elvidge, A. E., and Tye, J. G.: Radiology **45:**247-252, 1945.

ties consist of intermittent spiking and seizure patterns, together with slowing of activity and augmented amplitude. It is a surprising fact that transient electroencephalograph changes are produced by doses as low as 1 R whole head irradiation (Sams and associates). Such changes appear within seconds of the exposure, and their magnitude and duration are dependent on the dose. Such spiking usually begins in the cortex and ultimately involves all levels of the brain.

Some of the physiologic changes leading up to death after high doses have been studied by Clemente and Holst. The normal blood-brain barrier is selectively impermeable to certain substances. Trypan blue is such a substance. Subsequent to its intravenous injection it can normally be found in all tissues except the central nervous system. After doses of radiations mentioned previously, the barrier is selectively damaged so that trypan blue permeates into the hypothalamus and medulla. Clemente and Holst regard this as a vascular injury in which the sequence of events is edema caused by a protein-free transudate, perivascular leukocytic infiltration, and finally penetration of protein-bound vital dyes into the brain stem. Needless to say, death follows. However, despite a single dose of 10,000 R, Nair and Roth were unable to demonstrate an increased blood-brain barrier permeability to ^{131}I-labeled serum albumin, but there was an increased permeability to ^{35}S-labeled sodium sulfate. They found permeability changes to be subtle in nature and to vary from one region of the brain to another, as just indicated. Bering and associates have tabulated the reported effects of a variety of acute experiments, and their review should be consulted for more details on this phase of radiation response.

Early microscopic studies reveal neuron destruction to be rather diffuse but maximal in the brain stem and least in the cerebral cortex and cerebellum (Clemente and Holst). Astrocytic destruction seems sharply localized to areas of trypan blue permeation. Myelin of the central nervous tissues appears particularly sensitive to radiation damage, and changes in its optical activity can be measured after doses of therapeutic levels (Reynolds). Progressive demyelinization may require a year to reach its maximum. Axon degeneration follows myelin degeneration or neuron death.

Studies made of the behavior of animals after whole brain irradiation reveal that relatively small doses (200 R) can produce detectable changes (Zeleny). These changes in behavior are predominantly inhibiting processes. In contrast to these studies of whole brain irradiation, there have been numerous studies of high-dose localized irradiation (Bering and associates). It is obvious that irradiation of a critical area might have lethal effects, whereas a high dose to a larger but less critical volume might produce surprisingly little effect. Such areas are the same for irradiation as for other destructive agents and need not be discussed here.

The importance of each of these changes in brain tissues remains unknown, but it seems probable that during the early acute phase of radiation response to high doses, blood vessels, nerve cells, and glial cells are injured directly. In addition, the vascular changes so clearly demonstrated by the studies with trypan blue likely contribute to the further cell degeneration. Doses of 600 to 3000 rad directed to the spinal cord enhance both monosynaptic and polysynaptic reflex activity (Sato and Austin). This is associated with changes in membrane permeability and possibly with an increase in the amplitude of the intracellular spike response. This increase in activity of the spinal reflex system is manifested by spinal cord convulsions in rats given various doses of total body irradiation. The degree of response is dose-dependent and is greater in young animals (Vernadakis and associates).

Behavioral studies in rodents have proved that relatively low doses of radiations given at relatively low dose rates do produce immediate behavioral changes. Radiations apparently stimulate the autonomic nervous system either directly or indirectly to produce avoidance responses (Arbit).

Redmond and associates recorded the cerebrospinal fluid pressure in healthy dogs for 14 days after whole brain irradiation. Midbrain single doses of 1000, 2000, or 4000 R were administered. There was no significant elevation of cerebrospinal fluid pressure at any of the dose levels tried. Hakansson was able to measure the ventricular pressure of three patients with brain tumors before, during, and after irradiation. Fields were not larger than 10×10 cm, and exposure doses were 200 to 400 R. No significant pressure elevation occurred, but his patients exhibited symptoms classically attributed to acute radiation effects. It appears that symptoms occur as a direct consequence of irradiation of the brain and are not secondary to elevated cerebrospinal fluid pressure at the dose levels mentioned before. Regardless of the effect, the clinically immediate danger of high daily doses of radiations in the therapy of brain tumors justifies our practice of fractionation. With the usual daily therapeutic doses, these acute effects are well tolerated by the patient.

Some children who are treated for central nervous system prophylaxis following induction of remission from acute leukemia (brain dose of 1800 to 2400 rad with intrathecal methotrexate) will develop a transient encephalopathy shortly after completion of irradiation. The clinical picture is characterized by lethargy and somnolence. There are no other specific neurologic findings, and the cerebrospinal fluid is normal. This entity is distinct from the more severe neurologic complications of intrathecal methotrexate. In children observed for more than 5 years there has been no return of this clinical picture or any change from a normal neurologic status. It should be noted, however, that in approximately one third of all children given cranial prophylaxis there may be late changes seen on CT brain scans consisting mainly of ventricular dilatations (Peylan-Ramu and associates). Whether irradiation alone in these doses will produce either encephalopathy or late mild hydrocephalus is not clearly known.

CHRONIC CHANGES. With single doses of 1500 to 2000 rad (factors as mentioned before) to the monkey's whole brain, some of the animals will live beyond the previously described acute phase. A 6- to 24-month latent period of relative normalcy precedes the delayed sclerotic and necrotic changes. During the period of apparent normalcy there are nevertheless functional and behavioral changes, as have been described. The higher the dose, the younger the patient, and the larger the volume, the shorter will be the period of apparent normalcy. Large ports and high doses in patients lead to steady deterioration in mental status (Bailey and associates). There is no question but that vascular occlusions are caused by such radiations. However, Bailey has concluded that infarctions account for only a relatively small part of the total radiation injury; Arnold and associates describe this late necrosis after high doses as being "strikingly selective for white matter." It occurs predominantly in the path of the beam, begins as a demyelinization, and progresses to a necrosis of all the constituents of white matter (Arnold and associates). The cortex is least affected. The Betz cells are particularly resistant. The brain stem is again the most susceptible portion of the brain. Usually, vascular occlusion and subendothelial fibrous connective tissue proliferation of small and medium vessels are seen in the areas of necrosis. As just stated, coexistence of vascular changes and necrosis does not justify the assumption that a cause-and-effect relationship exists between them. In fact, necrosis has been described in the absence of these vascular changes (Wachowski and Chenault; Arnold and associates).

The neurologic signs and symptoms will naturally depend on which areas of the brain are involved in these changes, the dose, and the interval between irradiation and examination. When excessive doses are delivered through relatively large ports, the asymptomatic period is followed by progressive "general paresis," leading to death (Wachowski and Chenault). Rottenberg and associates reviewed six patients who developed cerebral necrosis following irradiation of extracranial neoplasms. A latent period of 4 to 31 months preceded the development of signs and symptoms of a mass lesion within the contiguously irradiated brain. Two of their six patients were successfully treated by craniotomy and resection of the necrotic mass. Since cerebral necrosis is usually fatal and pathologic examination is necessary for diagnosis, craniotomy with resection should be considered for such patients. Both systemically administered methotrexate and vincristine as well as intrathecal methotrexate may reduce the tolerance of brain tissue to irradiation.

The more common requirement in radiotherapy is the irradiation of a portion of the brain or spinal cord. Just as in neurosurgery injury of certain areas is compatible with a useful life, so in radiotherapy the magnitude of the dose must be tailored to the limitations imposed by the area involved by cancer. High doses can be given to the frontal lobes, certain portions of the temporal lobes, and even to the occipital portions of the cerebral hemispheres. On the other hand, similar high doses delivered to the motor areas, brain stem, and spinal cord may produce severely disabling or lethal changes. The brain stem with its vital centers and greater sensitivity may limit the dose delivered to centrally located lesions demanding irradiation of this area. Boden (1948, 1950) has clearly described the clinical consequences of brain stem and spinal cord irradiation (Fig. 22-1). He also defined the tolerance of the brain stem and spinal cord from a review of his own material. At the same time he cited published evidence that the tolerance of the brain is probably similar (Table 22-1). This is in contrast to the findings in laboratory animals described previously. With small fields of 10 × 7 cm or less, tissue doses up to 4300 rad in 17 days or their biologic equivalent seem to be tolerated by the cord, brain stem, and brain with little

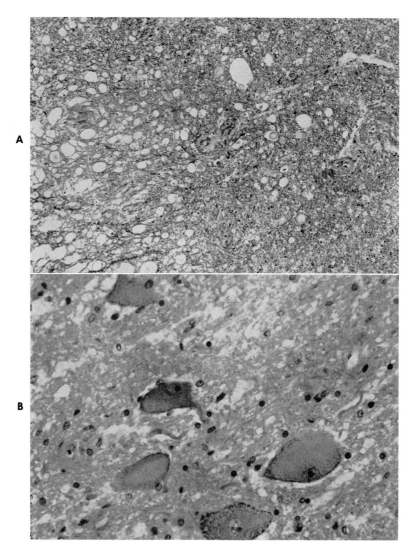

Fig. 22-1. Radiation damage of spinal cord after administration of calculated minimum of 4900 rad in 17 days. **A** shows myelomalacia of a nonspecific type. **B,** High-power enlargement showing signs of nonspecific injuries of neurons. Surrounding tissues as described for **A.**

or no danger of significant clinical change. Dynes and Smedal independently found a similar tolerance of the thoracic region of the spinal cord. With large fields of 20 × 10 cm, tissue doses up to 3200 rad in 17 days or their biologic equivalent seem to be safe. When doses higher than these are used, there will be a definite risk of late radiation encephalitis or myelitis. Of forty-one patients given doses of about 4300 rad or higher in 17 days with small fields, eleven (25%) developed clinical signs and symptoms of central nervous system damage (Boden, 1950). The damage was usually fatal. The clinical findings in seven patients with brain stem damage were also reported. The damage appears 1 to 20 months after irradiation. The irradiated zone

Table 22-1. Patients developing postirradiation changes in the central nervous system; dosage in terms of roentgens in 17 days overall time*

Author	Case	Tumor dose R/days	Equivalent dose/17 days	Site irradiated
Small fields				
Wachowski and Chenault	5	8693/58	6600	Cerebrum
Wachowski and Chenault	2	8910/84	6200	Cerebrum
Wachowski and Chenault	3	8809/87	6050	Cerebrum
Boden	2.1	6050/17	6050	Brain stem
Boden	2.3	5860/17	5860	Brain stem
Stevenson and Eckhardt		6000-8000/75	4300-5710	Cord
Boden	2.2	5860/17	5680	Brain stem
Boden	2.6	5550/17	5550	Brain stem
Boden	2.4	5450/17	5450	Brain stem
Wachowski and Chenault	6	6150/32	5350	Cerebrum
Boden	1.2	2224/single	5230	Cord
Boden	1.3	5200/17	5200	Cord
Wachowski and Chenault	1	7758/105	5150	Cerebrum
Boden	2.7	4900/17	4900	Brain stem
Wachowski and Chenault	4	6403/58	4850	Cerebrum
Boden	1.1	2000/single	4700	Cord
Pennybacker and Russell		1885/single	4470	Cerebrum
Boden	2.5	4500/19	4400	Brain stem (medium fields)
Boden	2.8	4900/32	4250	Cord (vascular accident)
Large fields				
Scholz and Hsu		4320/3	6450	Cerebrum
Greenfield	1	6320/43	5140	Cord, 1000 kv
Smithers and associates		5800/39	4830	Cord
Boden	1.6	4320/17	4320	Cord
Boden	1.4	3936/17	3936	Cord
Boden	1.5	4210/38	3500	Cord
Boden	2.9	3500/17	3500	Cord
Greenfield	2	4750/89	3290	Cord, 1000 kv ⎰ lessened bone
Greenfield	3	4450/83	3150	Cord, 1000 kv ⎱ absorption

*Modified from Boden, G.: J. Fac. Radiologists **2**:79-94, 1950.
4500 R in 17 days to a *small field* has been selected as the maximum tolerated dose to the brain stem and the cord; 3500 R in 17 days to a *large field* has been selected as the maximum tolerated dose to the brain stem and cord.

accounts for the neurologic abnormalities. At the time of the late reaction, spinal fluid is not under pressure, but the protein may be slightly elevated. Death usually follows.

RADIATION INJURY OF THE SPINAL CORD. Lesions of the spinal cord may have a shorter latent period than those of the brain stem. It is now fairly well established that there are two distinct types of radiation injury to the spinal cord. The first is an early transient myelopathy characterized by paresthesia, and the second is the late irreversible injury terminating in paresis or paralysis.

Early transient myelopathy. The subjective complaint of electric shock radiating down the back and over the extremities after neck flexion is the only clinical feature of transient radiation-induced myelopathy. This phenomenon is referred to as "Lhermitte's sign of electrical paresthesia." It occurs 2 to 4 months after irradiation of the cervical cord and persists for several months. The appearance of this sign is easily overlooked by the physician, and consequently its true incidence is unknown. Fletcher and Million reported four instances of radiation myelitis in 112 patients treated for cancer of the nasopharynx. It is interesting that three of the four had a fatal outcome and in only one case was the process self-limited. Jones reported seven cases of transient myelitis seen during a 5-year period in which there were no cases of progressive radiation myelopathy. He emphasizes the difficulty of determining the incidence of transient myelitis, but it is likely to be a more frequent complication than the permanent type. Jones has reviewed the pathogenesis and neuroanatomic basis for transient radiation myelopathy. He postulates that irradiation inhibits myelin production by the oligodendroglia. The latent period reflects the lack of a direct effect on preformed myelin, the symptomatic period reflects relative demyelinization, and clinical recovery is associated with increased myelin synthesis. Although clinical verification is lacking, there is experimental evidence to support the concept that radiations suppress myelin synthesis (Innes and Carsten; Schjeide and associates).

Late irreversible injury. Lhermitte's sign may be the first indication of the onset of a permanent dysfunction, but irreversible changes are preceded by a longer latent period than the transient response. There is no recovery; signs and symptoms increase in severity and finally simulate partial or complete cord transection. Dynes and Smedal reported an average latent period of 23 months. The findings may resemble those of a Brown-Séquard syndrome. Early, Romberg's sign may be positive along with a loss of vibration sense. Radiographs are normal, spinal fluid pressure is normal, no obstruction in the canal can be demonstrated, the fluid protein is normal, and no unusual cells are seen in the fluid. Death results from ascending urinary tract infection or from pneumonia (Boden).

It is worth noting that, with the exception of children with medulloblastomas, all the patients with radiation-induced brain stem and spinal cord damage were treated for cancer outside of the central nervous system. In almost every case the damage could have been avoided if the tolerance of the central nervous system had been appreciated and the technique had been modified to shield the spinal cord after a dose of 5000 rad in 5½ weeks. The greatest danger arises from poorly directed converging beams or thoughtlessly administered, poorly fractionated high doses through a single posterior port. With fractionation of 7 to 8 weeks or more, doses of 6000 rad are usually well tolerated (Vaeth). Data collected by Phillips and Buschke indicate that 5000 rad in 5 weeks to 6000 rad in 7 weeks are tolerated by the thoracic spinal cord (Table 22-2). Abbatucci and associates discovered twelve patients with cervical myelopathy out of 1715 treated for head and neck cancers. They concluded that doses to the cervical cord of under 5500 rad (27 fractions, 37 days) carried no risk of damage but that spinal cord injury was almost inevitable with doses greater than

Table 22-2. Collected data relating NSD and thoracic spinal cord myelitis*

NSD range	Patients with myelitis
Less than 1000	0/8
1000-1250	0/6
1250-1500	2/12
1500-1750	8/19
1750-2000	2/4

*Modified from Phillips, T. L., and Buschke, F.: Am. J. Roentgenol. **105**:659-664, 1969.

7000 rad (35 fractions, 49 days). In almost every recorded instance of spinal cord myelopathy, unconventional fractionation schemes have been employed. Wollin and Kagan have shown that the size of the daily dose and overall treatment time are important factors in the development of radiation myelitis. Their work lends support to the recommendation for daily doses less than 200 rad when the spinal cord is included in the treatment volume.

PERIPHERAL NERVES. Peripheral nerves withstand high doses of radiations (Gerstner and associates; Bachofer and associates). Whether they be in the cervical region, chest, or pelvis, treatment is never limited because of the tolerance of peripheral nerves. The only exception may be seen in damage to pelvic nerves after [198]Au injections for cancer of the cervix. Griffith and Pendergrass demonstrated similar radioresistance in the sympathetic nerves. High doses of radiations can produce extensive fibrotic changes in the connective tissue surrounding peripheral nerves. With time these tissues may contract, and nerve paralysis will result from the constricting pressure. This has been reported most often in the brachial plexus after irradiation for carcinoma of the breast (Mumenthaler).

THE DEVELOPING NERVOUS SYSTEM. In contrast to the moderately high doses tolerated by the adult nervous system, early during the period of organogenesis the brain and spinal cord are the most sensitive tissues in the embryo (Russell). Doses delivered during some diagnostic procedures are probably sufficiently high to produce significant changes during this period. Neuroblasts continue their migration later in the fetus. These cells are highly sensitive, so behavioral changes can result from low doses. Rugh and Wohlfromm have shown that the lowest $LD_{50/30}$ values for irradiated mouse embryos occur during the period of most active differentiation of the nervous system, and most neonatal deaths are associated with marked abnormalities of the brain.

GUIDE FOR TOLERANCE OF THE BRAIN IN IRRADIATING BRAIN TUMORS. We have tried to organize a scale of radiation tolerance based on the combination of the apparent radiosensitivity of the area in question and the relative functional importance of the area. Mendelsohn has severely, but justly, criticized the clinical data available on which we set normal tissue tolerance limits for the central nervous system. Admittedly we have much to learn about each of these factors, and many brain tumors will involve tissues in several areas. Nevertheless, we have found such a scale useful in directing our thinking. We prefer to avoid fractionation schemes that exceed the equivalent of 900 rad per week given in 5 fractions.

1. Vital areas in the brain stem are moderately radiosensitive. Radiation-induced damage results in either severe disability or death. Therefore, regardless of the aim of therapy, the upper limit of dose for this area is set at 5400 rad in 6 weeks.

2. Other selected areas are of major functional importance but are not essential for life. We place the motor cortex in this category. Radiosensitivity of this area seems to be significantly less than that of the brain stem. The dose limit when cure seems possible has been set at 6000 rad in 7 weeks.

3. Finally, certain areas are of apparently less functional importance. We place the frontal and occipital portions of the cerebrum in this category. High doses can be given to these areas with acceptable sequelae. The dose limit is therefore set at 6000 to 7000 rad in 7 to 8 weeks.

MALIGNANT TUMORS OF THE BRAIN AND SPINAL CORD

As discussed previously, none of the mature elements of the normal central nervous system is particularly radiosensitive. Few of the tumors arising in these tissues are sufficiently radiosensitive to be curable. However, unless a brain tumor happens to be limited to one of the polar regions of the brain, its complete surgical removal is rarely accomplished. Radiotherapy is usually advocated because the neurosurgeon knows complete excision is impossible. Yet, with few exceptions, irradiation is no more successful than surgery.

Kernohan and Sayre's histogenic classification is simple and rational (Table 22-3). From a prognostic viewpoint it helps in separating the slow and rapidly growing tumors. The gliomas are divided into four groups—astrocytomas, ependymomas, oligodendrogliomas, and medulloblastomas. The astrocytomas and the ependymomas are subdivided into four grades each of increasing mitotic activity and with progressively poorer prognosis. The gliomas are thought to arise through malignant transformation of the adult glial tissues. Not infrequently in a given tumor there is evidence of differentiation toward more than one type of glial cell. In the well-differentiated gliomas one can recognize the cell of origin, but in the less differentiated gliomas the cell of origin may not be identifiable and may have a variety of forms, hence the term *glioblastoma multiforme.*

In general, Grade 1 gliomas have sharply defined margins, enlarge slowly, and after incomplete excision may not show evidence of recurrence for 2 to 4 years. Indeed cystic cerebellar astrocytomas may be amenable to complete surgical excision. In contrast, glioblastoma multiforme may have indefinite margins, may infiltrate widely and early, and usually kills the patient within a year.

Aside from these histologic differences, it is well to remember that the prognosis is also dependent on the site of the lesion. Lesions of identical or similar cell types exhibit different growth characteristics in various sites. Gliomas of the optic nerve, basal ganglia, and cerebral hemisphere carry different prognoses.

Except to say that most of the gliomas respond poorly to irradiation, it is extremely difficult to evaluate their radiosensitivity. Improvement resulting from decompression or the administration of steroids may occur during the period of irradiation and may mask the response to irradiation. It is indeed likely that a dose of radiation sufficient to eradicate all malignant cells in an astrocytoma would be associated with a proportion of brain necrosis. Thus the benefits of irradiation must be judged by comparing survival of patients with malignant astrocytomas treated by surgery alone to the survival of those treated by surgery with irradiation.

Table 22-3. Histogenic classification of gliomas*

Differentiated types	Undifferentiated types and common classical names†	Highly anaplastic types
Grade 1 astrocytoma	Grades 2 and 3 (astroblastoma and spongioblastoma unipolare)	
Grade 1 ependymoma	Grades 2 and 3 (ependymoblastoma, neuroepithelioma, and medulloepithelioma)	Grades 3 and 4 glioblastoma multiforme Medulloblastoma
Oligodendroglioma	Oligodendroblastoma	

*Modified from Kernohan, J. W., and Sayre, G. P.: Tumors of the central nervous system, Armed Forces Institute of Pathology, Section X, Fascicles 35 and 37, Washington, D.C., 1952.
Mixed lesions containing various proportions of all cell types also occur. These, too, may be differentiated or undifferentiated.
†For extensive lists of synonyms, see Kernohan and Sayre.

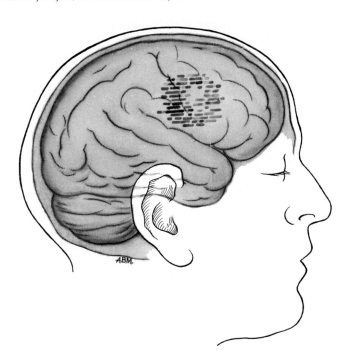

Fig. 22-2. Surface anatomy of brain shown in relation to external landmarks. Abnormal findings of a brain scan are schematically superimposed for comparison.

Not the least problem in irradiating brain tumors has been the difficulty of defining the limits of the lesion. Until brain scans became available, it was necessary to proceed with the limited information provided by neurologic angiographic, and neurosurgical exploration. Rarely was the radiation oncologist provided with all dimensions and the precise location of the cancer. With isotope and computed tomography (CT) brain scans, we can define location, size, and shape of the cancer in a high proportion of cases (Fig. 22-2). We believe beams can be tailored to the dimensions of the cancer. A randomized study reported by Ramsey and Brand verifies this belief and substantiates the rationale of treating limited volumes in patients with positive brain scans. They found that a higher dose delivered to smaller volumes resulted in a longer survival than a lesser dose in those patients who received whole brain irradiation. Caldwell and Aristizabal, on the other hand, found no such correlation between survival and total dose using a variety of fractionation schemes. With the availability of CT brain scans there is now perhaps even less reason to consider whole brain irradiation for primary tumors except in those instances when irradiation of the entire cerebral spinal fluid axis is planned as in the case of medulloblastoma or when seeding from other cell types is expected.

Astrocytomas

The astrocytomas, including glioblastomas multiforme, compose about two thirds of all malignant brain tumors. Astrocytomas may be either solid or cystic and usually present rather well-defined borders. Within this group there are several variants. The two major groups are those composed of fibrillary astrocytes with fine short thick processes and those composed of cytoplasmic astrocytes with rather short thick processes. Neither of these cell types in any of its arrangements is particularly radiosensitive. Grades 1 and 2 astrocytomas carry a relatively good prognosis and have not been routinely referred for postoperative irradiation even when known residual tumor is present. We believe that the greatest benefit of irradiation can be demonstrated in these low-grade tumors. Sheline has shown a significant improvement in survival attributable to postoperative irradiation following incomplete resection of Grades 1 and 2 astrocytomas (Table 22-4). Most of the irradiated patients were given doses between 5000 and 5500 rad. Of those patients with Grade 1 tumors, 25% survived 5 years without irradiation and 58% with irradiation. Of those patients

Table 22-4. Survival of patients after incomplete resection of Grades I and II astrocytomas*

Procedure	Number of patients	Survival (%)		
		5 years	10 years	20 years
Surgery alone	37	19	11	0
Surgery and irradiation	71	46	35	23

*Modified from Sheline, G. E.: Cancer **39**:873-871, 1977.

with Grade 2 lesions, there were no survivors treated by surgery alone when excision was incomplete and a 25% survival in the group given postoperative irradiation at the doses mentioned.

Glioblastoma multiforme

The term glioblastoma multiforme includes all Grades 3 and 4 malignant astrocytomas and, as a group, these are the most treacherous of all brain tumors. They may occur at any age and in almost any location, although they are most commonly found in the frontal, parietal, and temporal lobes during middle age. The interval from the onset of symptoms to diagnosis is usually brief. They usually kill within a matter of months. Taveras and associates directed a study specifically toward answering the question of the value of postoperative irradiation for these tumors. Of their entire group of 425 patients, only seven lived 5 years or longer. However, irradiation increased the ratio of survival in all categories. Similar results have been reported by Ley and associates, by Roth and Elvidge, and from our own institution by Jelsma and Bucy.

Andersen reported the results of a randomized clinical trial of postoperative irradiation for glioblastoma multiforme. The trial included 108 patients, and half were assigned to receive 4500 rad following surgical decompression and partial resection. At the end of 1 year none of the patients treated with surgery only had survived; however, 19% of those who received postoperative irradiation survived.

Trials of high LET irradiation have been undertaken at the several neutron therapy facilities in the United States. The rationale for such efforts is obvious; however, it would appear that brain tolerance once again remains the dose-limiting factor in efforts to destroy glioblastoma multiforme. The use of metronidazole as a radiosensitizer has been reported by Urtasun and associates. In their small group of patients treated by irradiation with metronidazole there appears to be a significant increase in median survival. An expanded trial with this approach is underway.

The use of nitrosourea compounds as an adjunct to radiation treatment of glioblastoma multiforme has not been as impressive. Solero and associates summarized several clinical trials of the nitrosourea compounds and also reported their own experience in a trial of BCNU and CCNU used with 5000 rad delivered to the whole brain postoperatively. Median survivals were 10.5 months with irradiation alone, 12 months with irradiation with BCNU, and 16 months with irradiation with CCNU. Certainly the 5000 rad dose of irradiation is less than that commonly employed when irradiation alone is used postoperatively.

Location of the lesion within the brain is important in determining prognosis. Those patients with frontal lobe tumors have a better survival than those with tumors of the parietal lobe when extensive resection, corticosteroids, and postoperative irradiation are employed.

TECHNIQUE. Brain scans (either CT or radionuclide) permit good localization of the anatomic extent of the tumor. The tendency of these tumors to invade the corpus callosum and the opposite hemisphere has led to a need for homogeneous irradiation of at least the demonstrable tumor volume and often the whole brain. In most instances opposing lateral ports readily encompass this volume. Russell and Rubenstein estimate the frequency of multifocal glioblastoma multiforme to be at least 6%. We do not believe, however, that this frequency alone justifies whole brain irradiation in all cases. A tissue dose of 5400 to 7000 rad in 6 to 8 weeks for small volumes and more commonly 6000 rad for larger volumes is probably the upper limit, but we are guided by the content of the volume, as discussed previously. The RTOG malignant glioma studies have all employed whole brain irradiation for the first 5000 or 6000 rad followed by a reduced volume boosting dose where permissible.

Ependymomas

Ependymomas, like astrocytomas, are graded from 1 to 4 according to their pleomorphism. A variety of histologic types is recognized, but no prognostic significance is attached to them. These tumors arise from the ventricular lining and the cells lining the central canal of the spinal cord. However, by the time the diagnosis is made, infiltration of brain substance usually masks the site of origin. For this reason, on gross examination they may be difficult to differentiate from astrocytomas. Seeding of the subarachnoid space is known to occur (Fig. 22-3), but there is no agreement in the literature as to either the frequency of this phenomenon or its significance. In reviewing the findings in seventy patients, Kricheff and associates reported only one instance of clinically evident seeding of the spinal cord. Phillips and associates reported only two instances of clinically evident seeding from their group of forty-two patients. Formerly we concluded that seeding was infrequent and

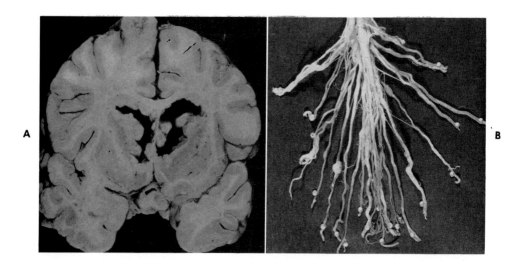

Fig. 22-3. A, Postmortem specimen demonstrating multiple nodules of ependymoma lining lateral ventricles. **B,** Postmortem specimen illustrating seeding of ependymoma to cauda equina. Such seeding was demonstrated in nine of fourteen cases reported by Sagerman et al. (From Sagerman, R. H., et al.: Radiology **84:**401-408, 1965.)

did not irradiate the entire cerebrospinal axis. However, two consecutive cases showed seeding. This prompted us to reevaluate the need for irradiation of the entire cerebrospinal axis in all cases. Such an approach was taken with the realization that the number of patients available was too small to evaluate the validity of this approach. Recently Salazar and associates reviewed the outcome of twenty-eight patients with primary intracranial ependymomas and nineteen with spinal cord primaries. They concluded that the primary tumor site should receive a dose of 5000 rad. They restrict cerebral spinal axis irradiation to those cases with high-grade tumors. For those patients with low-grade ependymomas arising in the infratentorial space we would include the cervical spinal area in the primary volume of irradiation. Ependymomas may present as a primary intraspinal lesion. In the review of seventy-four histologically verified ependymomas reported by Barone and Elvidge, twenty-seven had an intraspinal origin. Ependymomas arising in the spinal cord tend to be of low grade and have a better long-term prognosis than those arising within the brain. Of their forty-seven patients with intracranial ependymomas, there was no instance of subarachnoid seeding. We employ the technique and dose recommendations used in the treatment of medulloblastoma (p. 602).

PROGNOSIS AND RESULTS. Phillips and associates reported an overall 5-year survival of 40% (fourteen of thirty-five patients). If those who died in the immediate postoperative period are excluded, the 5-year survival was 56%. Of the ten patients who received low-dose irradiation (less than 3300 rad) or no postoperative irradiation, only one survived 5 years. If vigorous postoperative irradiation was administered (greater than 4300 rad), four of five patients with supratentorial tumors and nine of ten patients with infratentorial tumors survived 5 years (87% overall 5-year survival in this group of fifteen patients). Salazar and associates noted a similar experience with the survival of only one of ten patients treated with less than 4500 rad, whereas ten of the eighteen patients with doses of above 4500 rad survived. We believe that the primary tumor site should be given a dose of 5400 rad in 6 weeks, and in those instances in which seeding is likely, 3000 to 3500 rad should be delivered to the spinal cord to the level of S_2. This dose dependence supports the view that ependymoma is radiocurable. Bouchard and Pierce reported a 58% 5-year survival for those who survived surgery and received postoperative irradiation.

OLIGODENDROGLIOMAS

Oligodendrogliomas are infrequent. The differentiated types are usually slow-growing and, after incomplete surgical excision, may take years to kill. The few published reports suggest that they are moderately radiosensitive types, although these reports deal with small numbers of patients collected over a period of years and with changing techniques. Sheline and associates (1964) reported the results of treatment of thirty-two patients with oligodendroglioma, twenty-six of whom survived the immediate postoperative period. Only four of thirteen patients (31%) treated by surgery alone survived 5 years, whereas eleven of thirteen (85%) who received postoperative irradiation survived 5 years, and six of eleven patients survived 10 years.

Shenkin reported the results of treatment of fifteen patients with verified oligoden-drogliomas. All but four had recurrence, and one of the four died 5 months after surgery. Eight of the eleven who had recurrence were irradiated with remission of symptoms lasting from 8 to 54 months. He recommends delay of irradiation until there is clear evidence of recurrence. In his four cases not receiving postoperative irradiation, recurrence was evident in 13 to 40 months, and in each case a remission was obtained after irradiation. Although delayed treatment may be a reasonable alternative to the hazards of high-dose irradiation in children, we recommend immediate curative radiotherapy when there is a likelihood that tumor was left behind. Maximum tolerated doses are used as outlined previously.

Gliomas of optic nerve, hypothalamus, pons, and brain stem

Tumors of the optic nerve, hypothalamus, pons, and brain stem present a widely variable pattern of behavior. This has led to great uncertainty as to the method of management of these tumors. The term glioma is used as a morphologic description, since the true histologic nature of the tumor cannot be known until after the decision to proceed with surgical excision or, ultimately, at the time of postmortem examination. Biopsy or excision at the time of craniotomy may be deemed impossible or, in the case of those tumors of the optic nerve, unacceptable in view of the anticipated surgical sequelae. The radiation oncologist must then make his recommendations without a histologic diagnosis. This problem is most apparent in the management of gliomas of the optic nerve and chiasm. Such lesions diagnosed in childhood are frequently associated with multiple neurofibromatosis. Surgical therapy demands a major loss of vision. Irradiation of the same tumor must be undertaken with no real assurance that the course of the disease will be modified or that long-term survival can be attributed to the treatment given. Hoyt and Baghdassarian reviewed the long-term behavior in thirty-six *children* with optic glioma. They concluded that optic glioma of childhood is nonmalignant and self-limited and that the visual impairment present does not necessarily progress. There is little meaningful evidence in the literature to support routine irradiation of the true optic glioma in children.

In our own experience there is little if any evidence to support irradiation of gliomas that involve only the optic nerve or chiasm in children. The results of treatment are indistinguishable from the results of observation only. If, however, there is hydrocephalus or evidence of extension of the chiasmatic glioma into the diencephalon posteriorly, then irradiation is recommended. Doses of 5400 rad in 6 weeks are recommended to the defined tumor volume. Progressive optic gliomas in adults do require irradiation.

Unfortunately, "gliomas" of the pons and brain stem do not have such a favorable natural history as do those of the optic nerves. Tumors in this region may present with cranial nerve signs, ataxia, or cortical spinal tract involvement with or without the presence of increased intracranial pressure. These lesions may extend to involve the cerebral peduncles. Although rarely biopsied, they are for the most part malignant astrocytomas. Attempts to control these lesions by irradiation justify serious consideration. Urtasun found an almost uniformly good response in patients with pontine glioma who were given doses of 3000 to 4500 rad in a period of 4 to 5 weeks. Two of his twelve patients remained free of disease for 5 years. Sheline and associates (1965) reported initial improvement after irradiation in fifteen of twenty-one patients with unbiopsied tumors of the pons, medulla, or brain stem. Five patients are living over 5 years. Similar results have been reported by others (Liebner and associates; Lassman and Arjona). Panitch and Berg reviewed forty cases of brain stem tumors; twenty-eight patients were given doses of 3500 to 5000 rad in 4 to 8 weeks. The average survival was 47 months for the irradiated patients, versus 15 months for the untreated patients. A more interesting observation was that of the twenty-one of twenty-eight patients irradiated who showed improvement, the average survival was 61 months, whereas in those who showed no response to therapy, the average survival was less than 6 months. Greenberger and associates have shown the difference in survival following irradiation between tumors arising in the thalamus and midbrain versus those that arise in the brain stem (57% vs 38%).

SUMMARY. We do not recommend irradiation of children with uncomplicated optic nerve gliomas, although in those cases with extension beyond the optic radiations a more aggressive tumor may be anticipated and irradiation given with the hope of growth restraint. In tumors of the brain stem and pons, large parallel opposing portals are used to encompass the known limits of the tumor and extended anteriorly and superiorly to the limits of the cerebral peduncles and posteriorly and inferiorly to include the upper three cervical segments. A dose of 5400 rad in 6 weeks is delivered to this large volume at the rate of 900 rad per week. The treatment aims may be modified if a precise histologic diagnosis is available.

Medulloblastomas

Medulloblastomas are highly malignant tumors, usually arising from the vermis of the cerebellum or laterally in the cerebellar hemispheres. Growth of the tumor usually invades and compresses the fourth ventricle, resulting in an obstructive hydrocephalus. The tumor readily gains access to the cerebrospinal fluid, and metastasis by this route is extremely common (Fig. 22-4). Occasionally this seeding may give rise to the first sign of disease, but more often the presenting picture is one of a posterior fossa space-occupying lesion. Spread beyond the cranial spinal axis has been attributed to surgical intervention or shunting procedures employed to relieve the hydrocephalus, or both. Although medulloblastoma occurs in both children and adults, it is most frequently seen in childhood.

The management of medulloblastomas is based on the fact that surgery is notoriously unsuccessful in the removal of these lesions and on the fact that they are radiosensitive. After craniotomy for biopsy and decompression, irradiation is indicated.

TECHNIQUE. Regardless of the apparent extent of the tumor, the entire brain and the contents of the spinal subarachnoid space should be irradiated as soon after surgery as is practical. Care should be taken to include the base of the brain and to protect the eyes. In the treatment of the cord, the second sacral segment is taken as the inferior boundary. Although the beam width need rarely exceed 4 to 5 cm in the

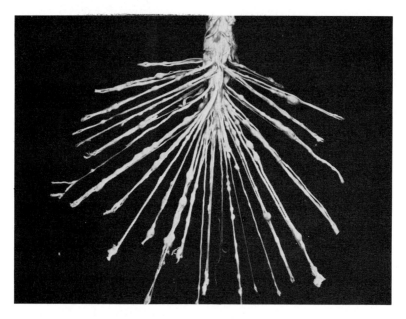

Fig. 22-4. Metastases to spinal cord and nerves by way of the spinal fluid of a cerebellar medulloblastoma. Such "seeding" demands routine irradiation of spinal column in these patients. (From Kernohan, J. W.: Bull. Los Angeles Neurol. Soc. **8:**1-10, 1943.)

thoracic and upper lumbar region, we have found it necessary to employ a field 5 to 7 cm wide at the level of the cauda equina (Fig. 22-5).

We have preferred to treat the spinal subarachnoid space from the inferior sacral border up to the level of the lateral brain port with a single posterior portal. The entire brain is treated by means of opposed lateral portals with the inferior margin of one portal at C_3 and the inferior margin of the other portal at C_7. On alternate treatment days the upper margin of the spine port abuts the lower margin of the lateral brain port, that is, either C_3 or C_7. This technique provides uniform dose distribution in the region of the cervical junctions (Fig. 22-5). A similar technique has been described by Van Dyk and associates. Hemopoietic depression is monitored by white blood cell counts. It is rarely necessary to interrupt treatment because of hemopoietic depression when total weekly doses of 750 to 900 rad are employed. We have favored postoperative myelograms in all patients with medulloblastoma. If spinal masses are seen on the myelogram, an additional dose can be delivered to those sites. We have found this technique useful for other situations that require craniospinal irradiation.

The dose to the primary tumor and known areas of seeding may be taken to 5400 rad with the fractionation scheme previously described. The dose to the spinal cord should be 3000 to 3500 rad in 4 to 4½ weeks unless there is evidence of seeding as shown on a myelogram, in which case the dose to that volume would be taken to 5400 rad. The dose to the spinal cord has frequently been less with no measurable

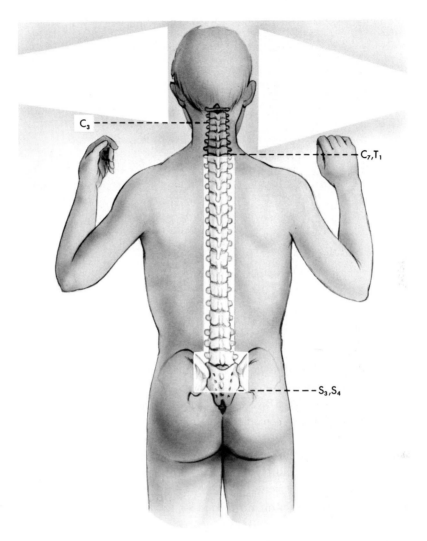

Fig. 22-5. Ports used for cranial spinal irradiation. Upper margin of spinal port abuts inferior margin of appropriate lateral port, that is, either C_3 or C_7.

decrease in survival. Lampe and MacIntyre used a lower total dose in a shorter treatment time but revised their technique to a more highly fractionated program in an attempt to reduce the incidence of sequelae (Smith and associates). With doses of 3000 to 3500 rad to the vertebral bodies, growth impairment must be anticipated. Growth restraint of other organs anterior to the spine (aorta, heart, gonads, thyroid, larynx, etc.), should be considered when photon beams are used (Chapter 24). With recommended doses to the brain in treatment of medulloblastoma, there are undoubtedly effects on the growing bones of the skull. This is especially true in the bones of the base of the skull, which are preformed in cartilage, but to our knowledge there are no reports of disturbance in skull growth. This may in part be due to the

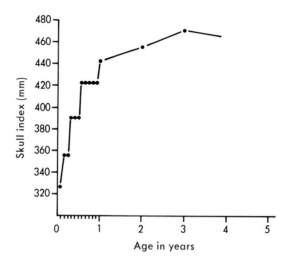

Fig. 22-6. Growth of skull is calculated by sum of greatest length, height, and width in millimeters obtained from series of 262 children as correlated with age. During the first year of life there is a rapid growth in skull size, which plateaus at about the age of 2. There is a slow rate of growth after this age until adulthood. (Modified from Austin, J. H. M., and Gooding, C. A.: Radiology **99:**641-646, 1971.)

rapid growth of the skull in the first year or two of life and the few cases available for evaluation in this age group (Fig. 22-6).

PROGNOSIS AND RESULTS. Several factors seem to be related to prognosis. Patients who present or develop spinal subarachnoid metastases are not frequently cured. Chatty and Earle reported a longer survival in patients over 15 years of age compared to those 15 and under and further noted that the primary location of the lesion influenced survival. Those patients with a tumor in the cerebellar hemisphere survived longer than those with midline lesions. Unfortunately, none of these factors can be of assistance in determining the need for irradiation. The median age for the cured patients in Smith's series was 8 years, compared with 5 years for his entire series. Of seven patients treated by Paterson, five lived 5 years or longer. In a more recent group, eleven of seventeen were alive and free of disease after 3 years. Smith and associates treated a total of thirty-eight patients, eleven of whom were living at 5 years. Five of the eleven were without serious sequelae. Eight of these thirty-eight patients were treated with a more highly fractionated technique. Five of these eight were living at 5 years. Two of the five were without serious sequelae. Tice has reported similar survival rates (six of twenty patients living at 5 years without high-dose sequelae), and Bloom and associates reported a 32% 5-year survival rate in sixty-eight unselected cases. A 5-year survival rate of 25% to 40% can be expected with medulloblastoma. We are beginning to see reports of survivals greater than 60% of patients treated more than 5 years ago with techniques described here. Cumberlin and associates have reported the experience of the University of California at San Francisco and have noted that since adoption of current cranial spinal techniques employing doses of at least 5000 rad to the posterior fossa, survival at 5 years has improved significantly (six of seven patients versus only two of twelve patients with lesser doses). One factor that appears to influence reported survival data is the difficulty of certain distinctions between true medulloblastomas and cerebellar sarcomas and, on rare occasions, intracranial neuroblastomas (Russell and Rubenstein). Bouchard has demonstrated the superior prognosis and enhanced radiosensitivity of the sarcomas. He reported a 26% 5-year survival for medulloblastoma and a 58% 5-year survival for cerebellar sarcoma.

Recent trials with adjuvant vincristine and cyclophosphamide have not shown significant improvement in survival compared to irradiation alone. The possible contribution of radiosensitizers for this tumor remains to be evaluated.

The frequency with which this treatment produces gonadal sterilization in the female is not known. Scattered radiations to male or female gonads probably produce significant genetic changes, but the seriousness of this is also unknown. At present we must accept it as a risk of curative attempts.

Carcinoma metastatic to the brain

Between 5% and 10% of all cancers will at some stage in their course metastasize to the central nervous system. The incidence varies according to tumor type and location of the primary lesion. No sites or types are exempted. Bronchogenic carcinoma is the most common offender and accounts for nearly a third of all brain metastases (Chao and associates). Carcinoma of the breast is the second most common offender. Cancers of the gastrointestinal tract, kidney, nasopharynx, and sinuses compose most of the remainder.

The signs and symptoms of metastasic brain lesions are not significantly different from those of primary brain lesions. When symptoms and brain scans permit accurate localization of the metastases, when the cell type is such that response to irradiation is likely, and when life expectancy is otherwise of the order of 2 months or more, we recommend palliative irradiation. We recommend whole brain irradiation in selected patients with metastatic carcinomas that cannot be localized and in leukemias, rare lymphomas, and metastases from seminomas or tumors of similar radiosensitivity (Chapter 20). The majority of cases have multiple metastatic deposits, and whole brain irradiation is necessary. Minimum doses of 3000 to 4000 rad in 3 to 4 weeks have generally been recommended. Experience has led us to favor 3000 rad to the whole brain in 10 fractions over 12 elapsed days for metastases from most lung cancers. In the case of isolated metastases to the brain from cancers of the breast we consider doses of 5000 rad reasonable for long-term palliation. We have seen no serious sequelae with 300 rad to the whole brain on the first day of treatment, even in patients who have not had craniotomy or similar decompression.

Results from such palliative irradiation will, of course, depend on the selection of patients treated. Chao and associates reported that 63% of their patients received symptomatic relief. At times relief is unpredictable and may be striking, with disappearance or decrease of headaches, vomiting, visual abnormalities, paralysis, convulsions, and, in fact, any of the signs and symptoms associated with an expanding intracranial lesion. Localization of the area of involvement with brain scans permits us to tailor our technique more specifically to the volume of involvement and makes this type of treatment more useful, with minimal sequelae. Many of these patients live for months, and a few live for years. As a result of irradiation they may be continent and will be able to care for themselves, and some will return to their former occupation. All too often the patient with brain metastases is in a preterminal condition, and brain irradiation is not effective in altering the patient's condition.

Carcinoma metastatic to the spine

As is the case in brain metastases, bronchogenic carcinoma frequently spreads to the spinal cord. Cancer of the breast and the other lesions mentioned are also seen frequently as extradural metastases. The earliest signs and symptoms must be detected and prompt treatment instituted if recovery from neurologic deficits is to be successful. Posttreatment recovery is directly related to the degree of involvement. Bansal and associates reported 78% recovery with moderate paresis and 23% recovery with marked paresis. They recommend immediate decompressive laminectomy and postoperative irradiation. Khan and associates reported worthwhile results in 40% of eighty-two patients treated with radiations alone. Doses of 1500 to 2500 rad in 10 to 20 days were used in their successful cases. Neither reported a poor prognosis in patients with sphincter loss.

We recommend a vertebral dose of 2500 to 4000 rad in usual daily fractions in those patients selected for treatment. Decompressive laminectomy is usually reserved for those patients who show rapid deterioration, and it is always followed by irradiation. Millburn and associates reported the successful treatment of a cord lesion with a single dose of 1000 rad. In theory such a rapid technique has some advantages as well as disadvantages when compared to conventional fractionation, and it deserves a clinical trial especially for the near terminal patient.

RESPONSE OF THE NORMAL PITUITARY GLAND TO IRRADIATION

The pituitary gland is composed of nerve and glandular tissues. The anterior part arises from an evagination of the primitive buccal cavity. The radiosensitivity of the anterior portion does not simulate that of the oral cavity, however. The posterior part arises from tissues from the region of the third ventricle. Most of the studies on the effects of radiations on the pituitary gland refer to damage of the anterior portion.

The normal adult pituitary gland is relatively radioresistant. Tissue doses of 3000 to 5000 rad in 3 to 5 weeks produce no significant signs of hypopituitarism in man. Early attempts with x rays to decrease function of the normal adult pituitary gland were thought to have failed, even with doses as high as 10,000 rad (Kelly and associates). Damage to neighboring nerves and the base of the brain prevented attempts to carry the dose still higher. High well-localized doses have been given by placing radioactive sources in the sella turcica and by using carefully collimated and precisely directed beams of deuterons or protons (Tobias and associates; McCombs). These studies have greatly clarified the effects of radiations on the pituitary gland. They may be summarized as follows:

1. All cell types in the normal pituitary gland appear to be equally affected by a given dose of radiations.
2. The pituitary gland of a young animal is more radiosensitive than that of an adult; that is, after pituitary irradiation in young animals, the pituitary gland, testis, adrenal gland, prostate, thyroid, and seminal vesicles fail to reach their anticipated weights with doses that produce almost no changes in the adult pituitary gland (Tobias and associates). Diabetes insipidus has not been reported as occurring in these animals.
3. Single doses of 30,000 rep (deuterons) to the adult rat's pituitary gland produce immediate changes indistinguishable from those of complete surgical hypophysectomy. Smaller doses produce less severe changes both in the pituitary gland and its target organs. Changes that do occur with these decreased doses are delayed in making their appearance (Tobias and associates). These findings have been confirmed in man (McCombs).
4. There is no evidence that the pituitary gland can recover from any of the radiation-induced changes.
5. There are now several reports in the literature documenting hormone deficiencies in patients irradiated for primary brain tumors or cancers of the nasopharynx (Fuks and associates; Richards and associates; Samaan and associates; de Schryver and associates; Wara and associates). In all instances the areas of the pituitary gland and hypothalamus received doses that equaled or exceeded those normally recommended for pituitary adenomas. The most common picture was that of growth hormone deficiency with arrest of growth, although in some patients gonadotropin, ACTH, and TSH levels were reduced. We have now seen two children treated for medulloblastoma in whom growth was arrested and growth hormone levels were markedly reduced. One logically would wish to avoid pituitary irradiation in the young, particularly with doses greater than 3500 rad; however, the requirements of treating sarcomas in the nasopharynx or middle ear or irradiation of that region for primary brain tumors usually make this an unrealistic aim of treatment. It is thus imperative that in children at risk for developing pituitary deficiencies after some latent period this risk be recognized and disturbances detected early so that replacement therapy can be instituted in the survivors. Similar though less frequent changes will develop in adults.

Almost every disease even remotely associated with pituitary function has at some time or another been treated by pituitary irradiation. Sterility, hypertension, diabetes insipidus, poorly controlled diabetes mellitus, thyroid and thymic disorders, and dysmenorrhea have been treated with various doses of radiations to the pituitary gland. The fact that clinical improvement sometimes followed this treatment may be explained with the current availability of pituitary hormone assays. For instance galactorrhea and/or amenorrhea with resultant sterility may be related to the secretion of prolactin by microadenomas that could have responded to the doses of radiation employed. It is in fact the very existence of such endocrine assays that has led to the recognition of microadenomas in the pituitary gland. Although the functional classification of pituitary adenomas based on endocrinologic evaluation is valuable both in consideration and evaluation of results, we have elected to continue the use of the traditional description of pituitary adenomas for the purpose of discussion.

TUMORS OF THE PITUITARY GLAND
Pituitary adenomas

Pituitary adenomas comprise about 10% of all intracranial neoplasms. They produce symptoms both by pressure on neighboring structures and by either increasing or decreasing pituitary hormonal secretions. Although pituitary adenomas are ordinarily classified according to the cells responsible for the dominant clinical features, a significant proportion of these tumors present a mixture of cell types. This has become increasingly clear as the means for identifying increases or decreases in pituitary function have become more available.

CHROMOPHOBE ADENOMAS. About 80% of all pituitary tumors are classified as chromophobe adenomas. They affect sexes equally, are most frequent at 30 to 50 years of age, and usually produce sellar enlargement. However, the size of the sella is not a reliable guide to the size of the tumor. Extrasellar extension into the hypothalamus or posterior fossa may not be diagnosed on the routine skull films. Angiograms, ventriculograms, and CT scans are especially helpful. Hormonal deficiencies usually do not occur until about three fourths of the gland is destroyed. The more common and disturbing symptoms are visual deficits from pressure on the optic chiasma or tracts, headaches, and pressure on the floor of the third ventricle and on the hypothalamus. The role of radiotherapy in the management of chromophobe adenoma is to shrink the tumor mass and relieve the pressure. The optimum technique and results have been analyzed by Chang and Pool and are summarized in Table 22-5. These results have been substantiated by Pistenma and associates.

We do not believe that surgery and irradiation should be considered competitive in the treatment of chromophobe adenomas. It is impossible to accurately compare these two modalities with any recent series. The worst lesions are invariably treated by combining the advantages of both modalities.

ACROMEGALY (EOSINOPHILIC ADENOMA). Acromegaly is a consequence of a long-standing hypersecretion of pituitary growth hormone. The secretion rarely returns to normal without treatment. The myth that such hyperfunction "burns itself out" has been disproved. Even if the gross clinical features seem to be static, the growth hormone level remains elevated without effective treatment. A wide spectrum of serious metabolic and endocrine defects combine to shorten life. The decrease in longevity is most often a consequence of cardiovascular changes, including hypertension.

Along with treating the patient's endocrinopathies, it is essential to decrease the growth hormone level by destroying the adenoma. Many destructive agents have

Table 22-5. Results of irradiation of chromophobe adenoma*

Author	Treatment	Percentage with improved vision	Period of observation
Horrax	Irradiation alone		
	4000 R/3.5 weeks	88 (58 of 66)	1-6 years
	Postoperative irradiation		
	4000 R/3.5 weeks	72 (18 of 25)	5 years
Correa and Lampe	Irradiation alone		
	2-2500 R/2.5-3.5 weeks	44 (12 of 27)	
	3-3500 R/3-4 weeks	60 (20 of 33)	
	4000 R/4-4.5 weeks	79 (23 of 29)	1-5 years
	Postoperative irradiation		
	2-3000 R/3-3.5 weeks	53 (8 of 15)	
	4000 R/4-4.5 weeks	76 (13 of 18)	
Emmanuel	Irradiation alone		
	4000 R/4 weeks	75 (12 of 16)	4 years
	Postoperative irradiation		
	4000 R/4 weeks	92 (38 of 41)	
Bouchard	Irradiation alone		
	4-4500 R/5-6 weeks	71 (20 of 28)	
	Postoperative irradiation		
	4-4500 R/5-6 weeks	82 (25 of 28)	5-20 years
Chang and Pool	Irradiation alone		
	3-3900 R/4 weeks	75 (30 of 40)	1-13 years
	4-5000 R/5 weeks	90 (38 of 42)	1-12 years
	Cases selected for irradiation alone†		
	2-2900 R/3 weeks	43 (3 of 7)	
	3-3900 R/4 weeks	56 (34 of 61)	1-13 years
	4-5000 R/5 weeks	78 (40 of 51)	1-12 years
	Postoperative irradiation		
	3-5000 R/3-5 weeks	88 (37 of 42)	1-13 years

*Modified from Chang, C. H., and Pool, J. L.: Radiology **89:**1005-1016, 1967.
These selected results demonstrate the improvement attributable to currently recommended doses.
†This category includes all patients initially selected for irradiation. Seventy-seven of the 216 patients available for follow-up were radiation failures subsequently treated by surgery.

been tried, including surgery, cryosurgery, implantation of radioactive sources, and heavy particle and x-irradiation. None of the currently available methods of treatment is both uniformly successful and without risk. If more than slight visual loss or progressive visual loss is present, prompt hypophysectomy is indicated. Otherwise, the only acceptable criterion for improvement is a decrease in the serum growth hormone. The aim should be to restore the level to as near normal as possible. No clinical improvement can be expected unless the level falls below 50 millimicrograms per milliliter. The growth hormone may not reach its lowest level for 3 or 4 years, so a long follow-up is necessary. Roth and associates reported that 4000 to 5000 rad in 3 to 4 weeks reduced plasma growth hormone in nineteen of twenty acromegalic patients. In 4 years the mean decrease in hormone level was 76% (60% to 89%). Similar results have been obtained by Lawrence and associates. Whether other currently available modalities are equal or superior in terms of risks and effectiveness is uncertain. The hazards of nerve damage after using the Bragg peak of the proton beam were emphasized by Dawson and Dingman. In our opinion, external megavoltage radiation therapy continues to be a superior method for decreasing growth hormone in the acromegalic patient.

CUSHING'S DISEASE. Primary pituitary tumors associated with Cushing's syndrome are infrequent and respond moderately to radiotherapy (Levitt and associates; Orth and Liddle; Aristizabal and associates). Patients with these tumors must be distinguished from those with Cushing's syndrome from other causes. Once the pituitary tumor is known to be the cause of Cushing's syndrome, we have accepted the recommendations of Aristizabal and associates and proceeded with pituitary irradiation. Doses of 4500 to 5000 rad in 4 to 5 weeks cured 25% of the patients and produced partial benefit in another 25%. Those not improved by radiotherapy are considered for surgery.

TECHNIQUE FOR IRRADIATING PITUITARY ADENOMAS. The external landmarks of the sella turcica and any extrasellar extension are easily defined from films taken in the treatment position. Except for extensive lesions, 5 × 5 cm ports are adequate. For chromophobe adenoma a tissue dose of 4500 to 5000 rad in 4 to 5 weeks is safe and in most instances adequate. Parallel opposing lateral ports coupled with a single anterior port are satisfactory. Hemorrhage is a frequently mentioned risk of irradiation, but it is also known to occur spontaneously. Just how much this complication may be increased by irradiation is unknown. In the report of Chang and Pool, three of 226 patients initially selected for irradiation were proved at surgery to have intracapsular hemorrhage. Sudden changes in vision demand immediate consideration of operative intervention. A three- or four-port technique or a rotational technique assist in reducing the dose to normal structures.

MICROADENOMAS OF THE PITUITARY GLAND. Now that functional disorders of the pituitary gland are being recognized and classed by their hormonal production, and now that transsphenoidal hypophysectomy is detecting microadenomas of the pituitary gland, the precise role of postoperative irradiation in these instances awaits clarification. At the present time we would prefer to follow patients who have had successful surgical procedures and to irradiate only those with persistent functional abnormalities or persistent elevation of the abnormal hormones. There is no evidence to suggest that lower doses than those recommended by Chang and Pool would be appropriate for treating microadenomas.

Craniopharyngiomas

Craniopharyngiomas arise from evagination of the embryonic gut. Histologically, these benign tumors may vary in appearance from cysts lined with a squamous epithelium to solid tumors resembling adamantinoma. The tumor usually appears before the age of 20 years and expands slowly, producing symptoms due to the pressure on neighboring structures. Surgical excision is usually incomplete because of these associated structures. Postoperative irradiation is frequently tried. Craniopharyngiomas are not particularly radiosensitive lesions. As doses to these lesions have increased, so have cure rates increased. Kramer and associates recommend biopsy and cyst aspiration followed by irradiation with doses of 5500 rad in 5 weeks for children and 7000 rad in 7 weeks for adults. In their first series all six children have survived from 13 to 15 years, whereas three of four adults have died at 2, 10, and 14 years after treatment. In their recent series of sixteen patients, eleven have survived from 6 months to 8 years. With this control rate, we follow their recommended doses. Careful definition of volume and rotational techniques are necessary to avoid persistence or necrosis or both with the doses recommended.

CHORDOMAS

Chordomas arise from notochordal remnants. These rare tumors occur intracranially in about half of reported instances. Other sites are in the cervical, lumbar, and dorsal spine, as well as in the sacrococcygeal region, the latter being the most frequent extracranial site. In the case of lesions arising in the sacrococcygeal region, complete surgical excision has been attempted. Local recurrence after surgery is common. Since more than subtotal removal of intracranial chordoma is highly unlikely, postoperative irradiation has been tried, with some encouraging results. Kamrin and associates reviewed this subject and recommended biopsy and decompression as necessary, followed by vigorous irradiation. Doses that approach the tolerance of the volume irradiated are recommended. Despite the absence of significant survival data, Higinbotham and associates concluded that irradiation offers an improved quality of survival.

NEUROBLASTOMAS

Neuroblastomas usually arise from the adrenal medulla, or similar tissue along the aorta, or in the posterior portion of the mediastinum. The tumors are composed of malignant neurons, which in tissue culture can be shown to possess neurites. They appear almost exclusively in children, are rapidly growing, and metastasize early. They are radiosensitive. Occasionally, there have been reports of lesions that have changed spontaneously from neuroblastoma to benign ganglioneuroma (Kissane and Ackerman). Some tumors will show areas of well-differentiated ganglioneuroma and these so-called "ganglioneuroblastomas" have a better prognosis. Children's Cancer Study Group A has proposed this staging system for neuroblastoma:

Stage I	Tumor confined to the organ or structure of origin
Stage II	Tumors extending in continuity beyond the organ or structure of origin but not crossing the midline; regional lymph nodes on the homolateral side may be involved
Stage III	Tumors extending in continuity beyond the midline; regional lymph nodes may be involved bilaterally
Stage IV	Remote disease involving skeleton, organs, soft tissues, distant lymph node groups, etc.
Stage IV-S	Patients who would otherwise be Stage I or II, but who have remote disease confined only to one or more of the following sites: liver, skin, or bone marrow (without radiographic evidence of bone metastases on complete skeleton survey)

Table 22-6. Two-year survival data for neuroblastoma*

Stage I	4 of 5 (80%)
Stage II	9 of 15 (60%)
Stage III	1 of 8 (13%)
Stage IV	4 of 56 (7%)
Stage IV-S	12 of 16 (75%)
ALL STAGES	30 of 100 (30%)

*Modified from Evans, A. E., D'Angio, G. J., and Randolph, J.: Cancer **27**:374-378, 1971.

Evans and associates demonstrated the influence of age at diagnosis on survival. Eighteen of twenty-two (82%) children less than 1 year of age survived, whereas only six of fifty-nine (10%) over 2 years of age survived. Even the presence of bone marrow or liver involvement in infancy does not significantly worsen prognosis.

TECHNIQUE. Optimum doses for neuroblastoma are rather indefinite. We believe that if there are no signs of distant metastases, even a large primary lesion should be treated to a tissue dose of 2000 to 3000 rad with appropriate fractionations. Ports should be generous. If the disease has metastasized widely, hemibody techniques should be considered.

PROGNOSIS AND RESULTS. Much of the data that supported a curative role for radiation therapy in the treatment of neuroblastoma was based on results in treating Stages I and II tumors and in many instances Stage IV-S (five of twenty-seven patients with liver metastases reported by Priebe and Clatworthy). It is now clear that most of these patients have a good survival that cannot be attributed to irradiation. Similarly in that group of patients there is no evidence that chemotherapy contributes to the favorable prognosis. The greatest contribution to the control of disease would be in Stage III patients with gross residual. Although we now realize that many of these patients have microscopic dissemination at time of diagnosis, there should be a group whose disease is truly localized and their survival might be attributed to irradiation. Approximately 30% of Stage III patients will be cured by combinations of local irradiation and multiagent chemotherapy. This figure has not changed in a meaningful sense over the past three decades. When metastasis does occur it is usually to lymph nodes and bones. There is no question of the palliative value of irradiation in patients with disseminated neuroblastoma, but unlike Wilm's tumor this disease has not yielded to aggressive multiple modal therapy. The commonly employed chemotherapeutic agents include cyclophosphamide, vincristine, and DTIC. Representative survival data are shown in Table 22-6. Perhaps because of improved staging procedures there is a shift of survival between Stage II and III patients with a slight improvement in both categories but no dramatic changes otherwise.

REFERENCES

Abbatucci, J. S., Delozier, T., Quint, R., Roussel, A., and Brune, D.: Radiation myelopathy of the cervical spinal cord: time, dose and volume factors, Int. J. Radiat. Oncol. Biol. Phys. 4:239-248, 1978.

Adler, H., and Kaplan, G.: Improvement of osseous changes in the sella turcica following irradiation for a pituitary tumor, Radiology 66:856-858, 1956.

Anderson, A. P.: Postoperative irradiation of glioblastomas, Acta Radiol. 17:475-484, 1978.

Arbit, J.: The autonomic nervous system and avoidance conditioning to ionizing radiation. In Haley, T. J., and Snider, R. S., editors: Response of the nervous system to ionizing radiation, Boston, 1964, Little, Brown & Co.

Aristizabal, S., Caldwell, W. L., Avila, J., and Mayer, E. G.: Relationship of time-dose factors to tumor control and complications in the treatment of Cushing's disease by irradiation, Int. J. Radiat. Oncol. Biol. Phys. 2:47-54, 1977.

Arnold, A., Bailey, P., Harvey, R. A., Haas, L. L., and Laughlin, J. S.: Changes in the central nervous system following irradiation with 23 Mev x-rays from the betatron, Radiology 62:37-47, 1954.

Austin, J. H. M., and Gooding, C. A.: Roentgenographic measurement of skull size in children, Radiology 99:641-646, 1971.

Bachofer, C. S., Gautereaux, M. E., and Kaack, S. M.: Relative sensitivity of isolated nerves to Co^{60} gamma rays. In Haley, T. J., and Snider, R. S., editors: Response of the nervous system to ionizing radiation, Boston, 1964, Little, Brown & Co.

Bailey, O. T., Woodward, J. S., and Putnam, T. J.: Tissue reactions of the human frontal white matter to gamma radiation. In Haley, T. J., and Snider, R. S., editors: Response of the nervous system to ionizing radiation, Boston, 1964, Little, Brown & Co.

Bailey, P.: Intracranial tumors, Springfield, Ill., 1948, Charles C Thomas, Publisher.

Bansal, S., Brady, L. W., Olsen, A., Faust, D. S., Osterholm, J., and Kazem, I.: The treatment of metastatic spinal cord tumors, J.A.M.A. 202:686-688, 1967.

Barone, B. M., and Elvidge, A. R.: Ependymomas: a clinical survey, J. Neurosurg. 33:428-438, 1970.

Bering, E. A., Bailey, O. T., Fowler, F. D., Dillard, P. H., and Ingraham, F. D.: The effect of gamma radiation on the central nervous system.

II. The effect of localized irradiation from tantalum 182 implants, Am. J. Roentgenol. 74:686-701, 1955.

Bloom, H. J. G., Wallace, E. N. K., and Henk, J. M.: The treatment and prognosis of medulloblastoma in children, Am. J. Roentgenol. 105:43-62, 1969.

Boden, G.: Radiation myelitis of the cervical spinal cord, Br. J. Radiol. 21:464-469, 1948.

Boden, G.: Radiation myelitis of the brain stem, J. Fac. Radiologists 2:79-94, 1950.

Bouchard, J., and Pierce, C. B.: Radiation therapy in the management of neoplasms of the central nervous system, with a special note in regard to children: twenty years experience, 1939-1958, Am. J. Roentgenol. 84:610-628, 1960.

Bouchard, J.: Radiation therapy of tumors and diseases of the nervous system, Philadelphia, 1966, Lea & Febiger.

Caldwell, W. L., and Aristizabal, S. A.: Treatment of glioblastoma multiforme—a review, presented at the 58th Scientific Assembly, Radiological Society of North America, Chicago, 1972.

Chang, C. H., and Pool, J. L.: The radiotherapy of pituitary chromophobe adenomas: an evaluation of indication, technique, and result, Radiology 89:1005-1016, 1967.

Chao, J. H., Phillips, R., and Nickson, J. J.: Roentgen-ray therapy of cerebral metastases, Cancer 7:682-689, 1954.

Chatty, E. M., and Earle, K. M.: Medulloblastoma: a report of 201 cases with emphasis on the relationship of histologic variants to survival, Cancer 28:977-983, 1971.

Clemente, C. D., and Holst, E. A.: Pathological changes in neurons, neuroglia and blood brain barrier induced by x-irradiation of heads of monkeys, Arch. Neurol. Psychiatr. 71:66-79, 1954.

Correa, J. N., and Lampe, I.: The radiation treatment of pituitary adenomas, J. Neurosurg. 19:626-631, 1962.

Cumberlin, R. L., Luk, K. H., Wara, W. M., Sheline, G. E., and Wilson, C. B.: Medulloblastoma treatment, results, and effect on normal tissue, Cancer 43:1014-1020, 1979.

Dawson, D. M., and Dingman, J. F.: Hazards of proton-beam pituitary irradiation, N. Engl. J. Med. 282:1434, 1970.

deSchryver, A., Ljunggren, J. G., and Baryd, I.: Pituitary function in long-term survival after radiation therapy of nasopharyngeal tumors, Acta Radiol. (Ther.) 12:497-508, 1973.

Dohan, F. C., Raventos, A., Boucot, N., and Rose,

E.: Roentgen therapy in Cushing's syndrome without adenocortical tumor, J. Clin. Endocrinol. **17**:8-32, 1957.

Dyke, C. G., and Davidoff, L. M.: Roentgen treatment of diseases of the nervous system, Philadelphia, 1942, Lea & Febiger.

Dynes, J. B., and Smedal, M. I.: Radiation myelitis, Am. J. Roentgenol. **83**:78-87, 1960.

Edmonds, M. W., Simpson, W. J., and Meakin, J. W.: External irradiation of the hypophysis for Cushing's disease, Can. Med. Assoc. J. **107**:860-862, 1972.

Emmanuel, I. G.: Symposium on pituitary tumors. 3. Historical aspects of radiotherapy, present treatment technique and results. Clin. Radiol. **17**:154-160, 1966.

Evans, A. E., D'Angio, G. J., and Randolph, J.: A proposed staging for children with neuroblastoma, Cancer **27**:374-378, 1971.

Fletcher, G. H., and Million, R. R.: Malignant tumors of the nasopharynx, Am. J. Roentgenol. **93**:44-55, 1965.

Fuks, Z., Glatstein, E., Marsa, G. W., Bagshaw, M. A., and Kaplan, H. S.: Long-term effects of external radiation on the pituitary and thyroid glands, Cancer **37**:1152-1161, 1976.

Gerstner, H. B., Orth, J. S., Richey, E. O.: Effect of high intensity x-radiation on velocity of nerve conduction, Am. J. Physiol. **180**:232-236, 1955.

Gerstner, H. B., Pickering, J. E., and Dugi, A. J.: Sequelae after application of high intensity x-radiation to the head of rabbits, Radiat. Res. **2**:219-226, 1955.

Greenberger, J. S., Cassady, J. R., and Levene, M. B.: Radiation therapy of thalamic, midbrain and brain stem gliomas, Radiology **122**:463-468, 1977.

Greenfield, M. M., and Stark, F. M.: Postirradiation neuropathy, Am. J. Roentgenol. **60**:617-622, 1948.

Griffith, J. G., and Pendergrass, E. P.: A study of the effect of irradiation upon the lumbar sympathetic ganglia in rats, Radiology **23**:463-465, 1934.

Hakansson, C. H.: Effect of irradiation of brain tumors on ventricular fluid pressure, Acta Radiol. (Ther.) **6**:22-32, 1967.

Haley, T. J., and Snider, R. S., editors: Response of the nervous system to ionizing radiation, Boston, 1964, Little, Brown & Co.

Hamwi, G. J., Skillman, T. G., and Tufts, K. C.: Acromegaly, Am. J. Med. **29**:690-699, 1960.

Hayes, T. P., Davis, R. A., and Raventos, A.: The treatment of pituitary chromophobe adenomas, Radiology **98**:149-153, 1971.

Higinbotham, N. L., Phillips, R. F., Farr, H. W.,

and Hustu, H. O.: Chordoma: thirty-five year study at Memorial Hospital, Cancer **20**:1841-1850, 1967.

Horrax, G., Smedal, M. I., Trump, J. G., Granke, R. C., and Wright, K. A.: Present day treatment of pituitary adenomas: surgery versus x-ray therapy, N. Engl. J. Med. **252**:524-526, 1955.

Horrax, G.: Treatment of pituitary adenomas: surgery versus radiation, Arch. Neurol. Psychiatr. **79**:1-6, 1958.

Hoyt, W. F., and Baghdassarian, S. A.: Optic glioma of childhood, Br. J. Ophthalmol. **53**:793-798, 1969.

Innes, J. R. M., and Carsten, A.: A demyelinating or malacic myelopathy and myodegeneration—delayed effects of localized x-irradiation in experimental rats and monkeys. In Haley, T. J., and Snider, R. S., editors: Response of the nervous system to ionizing radiation, Boston, 1964, Little, Brown & Co.

Jelsma, R., and Bucy, P. C.: Glioblastoma multiforme: its treatment and some factors affecting survival, Arch. Neurol. **20**:161-171, 1969.

Jones, A.: Transient radiation myelopathy (with reference to Lhermitte's sign of electrical paraesthesia), Br. J. Radiol. **37**:727-744, 1964.

Kamrin, R. P., Potanos, J. N., and Pool, L.: An evaluation of the diagnosis and treatment of chordoma, J. Neurol. Neurosurg. Psychiatry **27**:157-165, 1964.

Kelly, K. H., Felsted, E. T., Brown, R. F., Ortega, P., Bierman, H. R., Low-Beer, B. V. A., and Shimken, M. G.: Irradiation of the normal human hypophysis in malignancy: report of three cases receiving 8,100-10,000 R tissue dose to the pituitary, J. Natl. Cancer Inst. **11**:967-983, 1951.

Kernohan, J. W., and Sayre, G. P.: Tumors of the central nervous system, Armed Forces Institute of Pathology, Section X, Fascicles 35 and 37, Washington, D.C., 1952.

Khan, F. R., Glicksman, A. S., Chu, F. C. H., and Nickson, J. J.: Treatment by radiotherapy of spinal cord compression due to extradural metastasis, Radiology **89**:495-500, 1967.

Kissane, J. M., and Ackerman, L. V.: Maturation of tumors of the sympathetic nervous system, J. Fac. Radiologists **7**:109-114, 1955.

Kleinberg, D. L., Noel, G. L., and Frantz, A. G.: Galactorrhea: a study of 235 cases, including 48 with pituitary tumors, N. Engl. J. Med. **296**:589-600, 1977.

Kramer, S., Southard, M., and Mansfield, C. M.: Radiotherapy in the management of craniopharyngiomas, Am. J. Roentgenol. **103**:44-52, 1968.

Kricheff, I. I., Becker, M., Schneck, S. A., and

Taveras, J. M.: Intracranial ependymomas, Am. J. Roentgenol. **91**:167-175, 1964.

Lampe, I., and MacIntyre, R. S.: Experiences in the radiation therapy of medulloblastoma of the cerebellum, Am. J. Roentgenol. **71**:659-668, 1954.

Lassman, L. P., and Arjona, V. E.: Pontine gliomas of childhood, Lancet **1**:913-915, 1967.

Lawrence, A. M., Pinsky, S. M., and Goldfine, I. D.: Conventional radiation therapy in acromegaly, Arch. Intern. Med. **128**:369-377, 1971.

Lawrence, J. H., and Tobias, C. A.: Heavy particles in medicine, progress in atomic medicine, New York, 1965, Grune & Stratton, Inc.

Levitt, S. H., Prather, C. A., and Bogardus, C. R.: Radiation therapy for primary pituitary tumors associated with Cushing's syndrome, Clin. Radiol. **21**:47-51, 1970.

Ley, A., Ley, A., Jr., Guitart, J. M., and Oliveras, C.: Surgical management of intracranial gliomas, J. Neurosurg. **19**:365-374, 1962.

Liebner, E. J., Pretto, J. I., Hochhauser, M., and Kassaraba, W.: Tumors of the posterior fossa in childhood and adolescence, Radiology **82**:193-201, 1964.

McCombs, R. K.: Proton irradiation of the pituitary and its metabolic effect, Radiology **68**:797-811, 1957.

Millburn, L., Hibbs, G. G., and Hendrickson, F. R.: Treatment of spinal cord compression from metastatic carcinoma, Cancer **21**:447-452, 1968.

Moore, D. H., and Mendelsohn, M. L.: Optimal treatment levels in cancer therapy, Cancer **30**:97-106, 1972.

Mumenthaler, M.: Brachial plexus, paralysis following irradiation: report of eight personal observations, Schweiz. Med. Wochenschr. **94**:1069-1075, 1964.

Nair, V., and Roth, L. J.: A pharmacological assessment of the changes in the central nervous system following x-irradiation. In Haley, T. J., and Snyder, R. S., editors: Response of the nervous system to ionizing radiation, Boston, 1964, Little, Brown & Co.

Orth, D. N., and Liddle, G. W.: Result of treatment in 108 patients with Cushing's syndrome, N. Engl. J. Med. **285**:243-285, 1971.

Panitch, H. S., and Berg, B. O.: Brain stem tumors of childhood and adolescence, Am. J. Dis. Child **119**:465-471, 1970.

Paterson, E., and Farr, R. F.: Cerebellar medulloblastoma: treatment by irradiation of the whole central nervous system, Acta Radiol. **39**:323-336, 1953.

Paterson, R., Tod, M., and Russell, M.: The results of radium and x-ray therapy in malignant disease, Edinburgh, 1950, E. & S. Livingstone, Ltd.

Peirce, C. B., Cone, W. V., Elvidge, A. E., and Tye, J. G.: Roentgen therapy of primary neoplasms of the brain and brain stem, Radiology **45**:247-252, 1945.

Pendergrass, E. P., Hodes, P. J., and Groff, R. A.: Intracranial complications following irradiation for carcinoma of the scalp, Am. J. Roentgenol. **43**:214-225, 1940.

Pennybacker, J., and Russell, D. S.: Necrosis of brain due to radiation therapy; clinical and pathological observations, J. Neurol. Neurosurg. Psychiatry **11**:183-198, 1948.

Peylan-Ramu, N., Poplack, D. G., Pizzo, P. A., Adornato, B. T., and Di Chiro, G.: Abnormal CT scans of the brain in asymptomatic children with acute lymphocytic leukemia after prophylactic treatment of the central nervous system with radiation and intrathecal chemotherapy, N. Engl. J. Med. **298**:815-818, 1978.

Phillips, T. L., Sheline, G. E., and Boldrey, E.: Therapeutic considerations in tumor affecting the central nervous system: ependymomas, Radiology **83**:98-105, 1964.

Phillips, T. L., and Buschke, F.: Radiation tolerance of the thoracic spinal cord, Am. J. Roentgenol. **105**:659-664, 1969.

Pistenma, D. A., Goffinet, D. R., Bagshaw, M. A., Hanbery, J. W., and Eltringham, J. R.: Treatment of chromophobe adenomas with megavoltage irradiation, Cancer **35**:1574-1582, 1975.

Priebe, C. J., and Clatworthy, H. W.: Neuroblastoma: evaluation of the treatment of 90 children, Arch. Surg. **95**:538-545, 1967.

Ramsey, R. G., and Brand, W. N.: Radiotherapy of glioblastoma multiforme, J. Neurosurg. **39**:197-202, 1973.

Redmond, D. E., Rinderknecht, R. H., and Hudgins, P. T.: The effect of total-brain irradiation on cerebrospinal fluid pressure, Radiology **89**:727-732, 1967.

Reynolds, L.: Newer investigations of radiation effects and their clinical applications, Am. J. Roentgenol. **55**:135-152, 1946.

Richards, G. E., Wara, W. M., Grumbach, M. M., Kaplan, S. L., Sheline, G. E., and Conte, F. A.: Delayed onset of hypopituitarism: sequelae of therapeutic irradiation of central nervous system, eye, and middle ear tumors, J. Pediatr. **89**:553-559, 1976.

Richmond, J. J.: Radiotherapy of intracranial tumours in children, J. Fac. Radiologists **4**:180-189, 1953.

Ross, J. A. T., Leavitt, S. R., Holst, E. A., and

Clemente, C. D.: Neurological and electroencephalographic effects of x-irradiation on the head of monkeys, Arch. Neurol. Psychiatr. **71:** 238-249, 1954.

Roth, J. G., and Elvidge, R.: Glioblastoma multiforme: a clinical survey, J. Neurosurg. **17:**736-750, 1960.

Roth, J., Gorden, P., and Brace, K.: Efficacy of conventional pituitary irradiation in acromegaly, N. Engl. J. Med. **282:**1385-1391, 1970.

Rottenberg, D. A., Chernik, N. L., Deck, M. D. F., Ellis, F., and Posner, J. B.: Cerebral necrosis following radiotherapy of extracranial neoplasms, Ann. Neurol. **1:**339-357, 1977.

Rugh, R., and Wohlfromm, M.: Prenatal x-irradiation and postnatal mortality, Radiat. Res. **26:**493-506, 1965.

Russell, D. S., and Rubenstein, J. L.: Pathology of tumors of the nervous system, London, 1963, Edward Arnold Ltd.

Russell, L. B.: The effects of radiation on mammalian prenatal development. In Hollaender, A., editor: Radiation biology, New York, 1954, McGraw-Hill Book Co.

Sagerman, R. H., Bagshaw, M. A., and Hanberg, J.: Considerations in the treatment of ependymoma, Radiology **84:**401-408, 1965.

Salazar, O. M., Rubin, P., Bassano, D., and Marcial, V. A.: Improved survival of patients with intracranial ependymomas by irradiation: dose selection and field extension, Cancer **35:**1563-1573, 1975.

Samaan, N. A., Bakdash, M. M., Cadero, J. B.: Hypopituitarism after external irradiation; evidence for both hypothalamic and pituitary origin, Ann. Intern. Med. **83:**771-777, 1975.

Sams, C. F., Aird, R. B., Adams, G. D., and Ellman, G. L.: Electrophysiological changes of the central nervous system to response to low-level radiation. In Haley, T. J., and Snider, R. S., editors: Response of the nervous system to ionizing radiations, Boston, 1964, Little, Brown & Co.

Sato, M., and Austin, G.: Acute radiation effects on mammalian synaptic activities. In Haley, T. J., and Snider, R. S., editors: Response of the nervous system to ionizing radiation, Boston, 1964, Little, Brown & Co.

Schjeide, O. A., Yamazaki, J., Haack, K., Ciminelli, E., and Clemente, C. D.: Biochemical and morphological aspects of radiation inhibition of myelin formation, Acta Radiol. **5:**185-203, 1966.

Scholz, W., and Hsu, Y. K.: Late damage from roentgen irradiation of the human brain, Arch. Neurol. Psychiatr. **40:**928-936, 1938.

Sheline, G. E., Goldberg, M. B., and Feldman, R.: Pituitary irradiation for acromegaly, Radiology **76:**70-75, 1961.

Sheline, G. E., Boldrey, E., Karlsberg, P., and Phillips, T. L.: Therapeutic considerations in tumors affecting the central nervous system: oligodendrogliomas, Radiology **82:**84-89, 1964.

Sheline, G. E., Phillips, T. L., and Boldrey, E.: The therapy of unbiopsied brain tumors, Am. J. Roentgenol. **93:**664-670, 1965.

Sheline, G. E.: Radiation therapy of brain tumors, Cancer **39:**873-881, 1977.

Shenkin, H. A.: The effect of roentgen-ray therapy on oligodendrogliomas of the brain, J. Neurosurg. **22:**57-59, 1965.

Smith, D. E.: Central nervous system. In Ackerman, L. V.: Surgical pathology, ed. 4, St. Louis, 1968, The C. V. Mosby Co.

Smith, R. A., Lampe, I., and Kahn, E.: Prognosis of medulloblastoma in children, J. Neurosurg. **18:**91-97, 1961.

Smithers, D. W., Clarkson, J. R., and Strong, J. A.: Roentgen treatment of cancer of the esophagus, Am. J. Roentgenol. **49:**606-634, 1943.

Solero, C. L., Monfardini, S., Brambilla, C., Vaghi, A., Valagussa, P., Morello, G., and Bonadonna, G.: Controlled study with BCNU vs. CCNU as adjuvant chemotherapy following surgery plus radiotherapy for glioblastoma multiforme, Cancer Clin. Trials **2:**43-48, 1979.

Stevenson, L. D., and Eckhardt, R. E.: Myelomalacia of cervical portion of the spinal cord, probably result of roentgen therapy, Arch. Pathol. **39:**109-112, 1945.

Taveras, J. M., Thompson, H. G., and Pool, J. L.: Should we treat glioblastoma multiforme? Am. J. Roentgenol. **87:**473-479, 1962.

Tice, G. M.: Treatment and prognosis of medulloblastoma, J.A.M.A. **182:**629-631, 1962.

Tobias, C. A., Van Dyke, D. C., Simpson, M. E., Anger, H. O., Huff, R. L., and Koneff, A. A.: Irradiation of the pituitary of the rat with high energy deuterons, Am. J. Roentgenol. **72:**1-21, 1954.

Urtasun, R. C.: ^{60}Co radiation treatment of pontine gliomas, Radiology **104:**385-387, 1972.

Urtasun, R. C., Band, P. R., Chapman, J. D., and Feldstein, M. L.: Radiation plus metronidazole for glioblastoma, N. Engl. J. Med. **296:**757, 1977.

Vaeth, J.: Radiation-induced myelitis. In Buschke, F.: Progress in radiation therapy, vol. 3, New York, 1965, Grune & Stratton, Inc.

Van Dyk, J., Jenkin, R. D. T., Leung, P. M. K., and Cunningham, J. R.: Medulloblastoma: treatment technique and radiation dosimetry, J. Radiat. Oncol. Biol. Phys. **2:**993-1005, 1977.

Vernadakis, A., Geel, S., and Timiras, P. S.: Effects of whole-body x-radiation on spinal cord convulsions in rats. In Haley, T. J., and Snider, R. S., editors: Response of the nervous system to ionizing radiation, Boston, 1964, Little, Brown & Co.

Wachowski, T. J., and Chenault, H.: Degenerative effects of large doses of roentgen rays on the human brain, Radiology 45:227-246, 1945.

Wara, W. M., Richards, G. E., Grumbach, M. M., Kaplan, S., Sheline, G. E., and Conte, F. A.: Hypopituitarism after irradiation in children, Int. J. Radiat. Oncol. Biol. Phys. 2:549-552, 1977.

Wollen, M., and Kagen, A. R.: Modification of biological dose to normal tissue by daily fractionation, Acta Radiol. 15:481-492, 1976.

Zeleny, V.: The influence of local x-ray irradiation on functional processes in the central nervous system. In Mitchell, J. S., Holmes, B. E., and Smith, C. L., editors: Progress in radiobiology, Edinburgh, 1956, Oliver & Boyd, Ltd.

23

Radiotherapy of selected soft tissue tumors

A large number of tumors fall in the category of tumors of the soft tissues. Stout's classification (1953) includes about forty benign types and over twenty malignant varieties. Pack and Ariel (1958) include an even greater number of tumor types. We presently use a slightly modified version of the World Health Organization classification of soft tissue tumors.* Radiotherapy has undoubtedly been tried on most of these growths, but only a few will be discussed. Many types, because of their poor radiosensitivity, are not radiotherapy problems. Some have been discussed in Chapter 20. Others have been discussed in the various sections dealing with the organs with which the tumors are most frequently associated.

BENIGN DISEASES OF SOFT TISSUES
Wound healing; keloids and keloid formation

There is ample evidence in the older literature suggesting that irradiation promotes wound healing of certain infected wounds. However, there is no clear-cut evidence that the healing of a clean surgical wound is accelerated by irradiation. In fact, all evidence suggests that irradiation decreases the rate of healing in ordinary surgical incisions. Lawrence and associates and Nickson and associates reviewed this subject and reported their findings in rats. Tensile strength across an abdominal incision was used as an index of wound healing. Both single and fractionated doses of radiations carried to near epidermicidal levels decrease the rate of subsequent wound healing. This is noticeable even when the irradiation is performed 12 weeks prior to surgery (Fig. 23-1). It can be seen from Fig. 23-1 that the ultimate tensile strengths of the incisions in control and experimental animals are the same. Similar slow healing of intestinal anastomosis is produced by preoperative irradiation of abdominal cancers (Crowley and associates). Such interference with the wound healing should not be a cause for extensive delays of necessary surgery. When tension is likely to be put on such a wound, sutures should be left in longer and greater care

---

*W.H.O. International Reference Center for Histologic Diagnosis of Soft Tissue Tumors (Franz Enzinger, editor), Armed Forces Institute of Pathology.

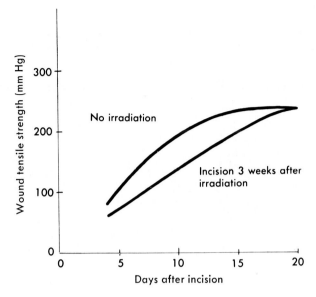

Fig. 23-1. Effects of preoperative irradiation on wound healing in rats (500 R air every 2 days for four treatments starting 3 weeks before incision; 100 kv; hvl, 1.8 mm Al). (Modified from Nickson, J. J., et al.: Surgery **34:**859-862, 1953.)

should be taken in initiating physical activity. The complications of combined irradiation and surgery are discussed on p. 48.

When irradiation follows surgery by 8 to 10 days, no significant abnormality in tensile strength can develop. There is, however, a striking suppression of scar formation (Fig. 23-2). This is the rationale for the use of irradiation as a keloid-preventing measure.

In contrast to the rather minor effect of recent irradiation on wound healing, a year or more after cancerocidal doses tissue vitality may be severely impaired. A surgical wound may then be extremely slow in healing, or the trauma of making an incision may initiate necrosis. This complication was discussed in Chapters 1 and 2. Obviously, deep tissues are also damaged.

A keloid is a hyperplastic scar in which there is an overproduction of hyaline collagenous tissue. The epithelium covering a keloid is thin and atrophic, tolerates trauma poorly, and, if broken, heals slowly. Except for this thin epithelium, a keloid 1 year or older is not particularly radiosensitive. In fact, if through necessity an old keloid is included in a treatment field during the irradiation of a deep-seated tumor, the thin epithelium will be the first to desquamate and the last to heal. Its poor tolerance may be a factor in determining ports and skin doses. Under these circumstances the fibrous tissue of the keloid will show little or no change. In contrast, irradiation will produce varying degrees of regression in a newly formed pink keloid. The regression will usually be incomplete.

The fibroblasts in a fresh wound of an individual who forms keloids are highly

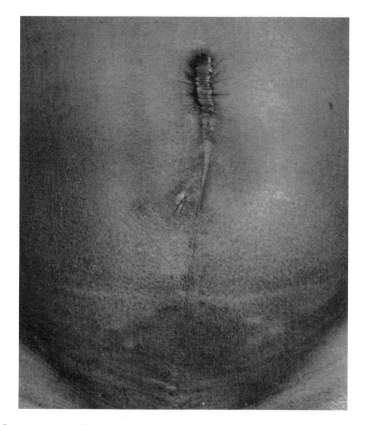

Fig. 23-2. Demonstration of the effectiveness of irradiation in suppressing keloid formation. On laparotomy the patient proved to have an inoperable carcinoma of the endometrium. During subsequent lower abdominal irradiation only half of the recent incision was included in the field. Large keloid formed in upper unirradiated portion. No keloid formed in irradiated lower portion. Skin dose was 2400 rad in 5 weeks (much higher than is actually necessary for keloid prevention). (W. U. neg. 53-1993.)

radiosensitive (Fig. 23-2). Doses of 1000 rad in 1 to 5 days suppress the abnormal proliferation of these fibroblasts. Because already-developed keloids respond so poorly to irradiation, our treatment usually consists of excision followed within 3 days by the first of a series of three or four daily x-ray treatments of 300 to 400 rad (surface) each. This dose is probably near the upper limit of the required level. Noticeable permanent skin changes should be avoided. Since we are directing our treatment to the dermis as well as to the skin, radiations produced at 100 kv with 2 mm Al filters are desirable. Care should be taken to include the suture holes.

The risk of subsequent skin cancer must be realized, and for this reason, we would avoid treating children or young adults except in unusual circumstances.

Hemangiomas

Hemangiomas appear in several forms. Capillary (strawberry nevus) and cavernous hemangiomas are the only types considered for irradiation. They are usually

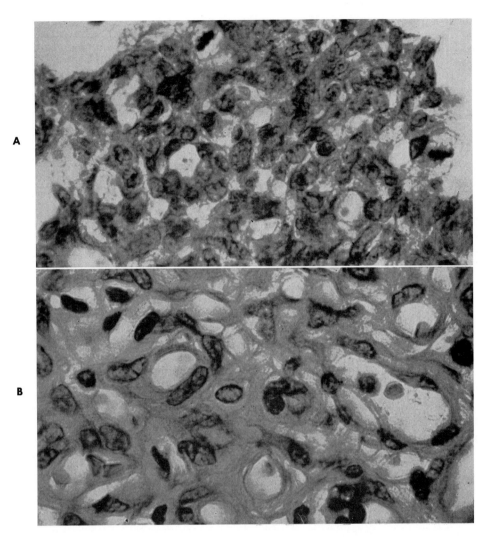

Fig. 23-3. A, Photomicrograph of highly cellular capillary hemangioma in infant 1 month old. Note mitotic figures and solid masses of cells. (magnification ×480) **B,** Photomicrograph of capillary hemangioma in infant 1 year old. Note vascular channels, decreased cellularity, and increased connective tissue. (magnification ×480.) (From Ackerman, L. V., and Rosai, J.: Surgical pathology, ed. 5, St. Louis, 1974, The C. V. Mosby Co.)

present at or soon after birth and may occasionally grow over a period of several weeks. They are characteristically bright red and slightly raised. Exertion may make them swell and become redder. Capillary hemangiomas are highly cellular with many mitotic figures. A large proportion of these lesions will lose their cellular character spontaneously and progressively become fibrotic (Fig. 23-3). Through this process over 90% will regress, and most will disappear entirely over a period of 2 to 3 years. When routine irradiation, dry ice, steroids, or escharotics are used, this spontaneous regression can easily be misinterpreted as a favorable response. The important and still unanswered question is: Just how effective are these techniques in producing regression in lesions not destined to regress spontaneously? Until the answer to this question is known, treatment, if any, must be administered in such a fashion that it produces no permanently noticeable sequelae. Damage to the skin, gonads, bone, eyes, and breasts (Fig. 11-1) must be considered during the treatment of capillary or cavernous hemangiomas.

If all capillary and cavernous hemangiomas are observed, there will be a few that fail to regress spontaneously. It soon becomes obvious that these few lesions also respond poorly to irradiation. The argument against this wait-and-see policy is that with observation the number of relatively resistant lesions increases. Existing studies do not enable us to evaluate these aspects of hemangiomas.

TECHNIQUE. We have preferred to observe most capillary and cavernous hemangiomas. There are no serious objections to using irradiation in critical sites (that is, lesions of the airway or gastrointestinal tract) if it is carried out with the precautions and knowledge presented previously. A dose of 250 to 300 rad (treatment factors depending on site) may be given to the lesion when first seen. This can be repeated in 4 to 6 weeks if there has been no regression. Although still further irradiation is frequently recommended, we believe that radiation-induced regression will be produced in few, if any, additional lesions. The risk of damage to normal structures in children with hemangiomas increases rapidly with higher doses. Many cavernous hemangiomas have lymphangiomatous elements. They usually respond to the same therapy as the hemangiomas.

In rare instances thrombocytopenia is seen in association with cavernous hemangiomas. Although the exact mechanism of this form of thrombocytopenia is not clear, we have observed rapid recovery of the platelet count in an infant after resection of a cavernous hemangioma of the right lobe of the liver. Duncan and Halman suggest that irradiation of the hemangioma may be effective in correcting the thrombocytopenia.

Other types of hemangiomas of the skin, subcutaneous tissues, bone, and almost every organ of the body require much greater doses of radiations. Except for symptom-producing lesions of vertebral bodies or other surgically inaccessible sites, they are usually better treated by other methods.

MALIGNANT TUMORS OF SOFT TISSUE

Although there is uniform agreement that only an occasional malignant tumor of soft tissue is radiocurable, there is general agreement that significant radiation-induced growth restraint can frequently be achieved. Doses sufficient to produce growth restraint of these tumors are rather high, and at times results are poor. Nevertheless, until we have a means of separating the responsive sarcomas from the poorly responsive sarcomas, these rather high doses must be delivered in all situations justifying attempted growth restraint or even cure. del Regato has reviewed the justification for treating these tumors and emphasized the occasional and sometimes unexpected favorable response.

With regrowth of sarcomas, whether or not the tissues have been irradiated, some of the most massive tissue necroses encountered in medicine occur. If high doses of radiations have been given and there is regrowth of tumor, radiotherapy may be suggested as the cause of such massive necrosis. The possibility that this situation may occur should be realized before irradiation is given and must be accepted as a part of the course of the incurable cancer patient.

Rhabdomyosarcoma

Rhabdomyosarcoma is recognized in several histologic forms—pleomorphic, alveolar, and embryonal—as well as the morphologic variant of embryonal rhabdomyosarcoma, botryoid (Horn and Enterline). These uncommon tumors are predominantly seen in children, although they can occur at any age. In children the embryonal type is most common about the head and neck, and the botryoid variant is most often found in the urogenital tract. Pleomorphic rhabdomyosarcoma is said to predominate in the adult. It is now a very rare neoplasm, since it appears evident that most cases of pleomorphic rhabdomyosarcoma in the past would now be reclassified as malignant fibrous histiocytoma. Three fourths of head and neck lesions occur in children 12 years of age or younger (Dito and Batsakis). Sutow and associates reviewed the cases of seventy-eight children with rhabdomyosarcoma, fifty-four of whom had localized disease at the time of diagnosis. The median time between diagnosis and local recurrence or metastasis for those children with localized disease was 9.5 months. Of this group, 28% remained free of disease at 5 years, whereas none of the twenty-four children with locally advanced or metastatic disease at diagnosis survived more than 30 months. Excluding sarcoma botryoides of the vagina, the site of origin with the best prognosis was in the orbital tumor—42% survived 5 years. The poorest survival was in the group of patients with primaries in other sites of the head and neck—14% survived 5 years. There were no survivors in the group with alveolar rhabdomyosarcoma. Jones and associates reviewed sixty-two cases of orbital rhabdomyosarcoma seen over a long period at the Institute of Ophthalmology of the Presbyterian Hospital and Columbia University College of Physicians. The average age in this group was 8 years with a range of 3.5 months to 41 years. Exophthalmos was always the first sign of disease. Approximately two thirds of the cases were embryonal types, and more than half of these patients survived after a variety of treatment modalities. In a series of eighty-eight patients with head and neck lesions reported by Masson and Soule, thirty-three had metastases to regional lymph nodes. The preliminary report of the Rhabdomyosarcoma Study reviewing 308 eligible patients indicates that, except for primary sites in the extremities or genitourinary tract, lymph node metastases are not common in rhabdomyosarcoma. Hematogenous spread to lung, bone, and other organs is a common feature of either the natural or the treated course of the disease. Liebner reported his experience with eighteen consecutive children with rhabdomyosarcoma of the head and neck treated to cure. All were treated in combination with actinomycin D, but only four recent cases received combination therapy with maintenance therapy. Local control was achieved in 89% with a 5-year survival of 67%. Unfortunately, tumors at other sites usually require irradiation of large volumes.

Edland has attempted to define optimum time-dose relationships for embryonal rhabdomyosarcomas. In twenty patients local control by irradiation was obtained in eleven sites (six primary and five metastatic) with doses greater than 5000 rad in 5 weeks. The likelihood of control was greatest with a dose of 6000 rad in 6 weeks. These doses are not well tolerated by large volumes, but generally they can be given in cases of head and neck primaries with acceptable risks. Similar evidence of local radiocurability was presented by Cassady and associates in a review of orbital rhabdomyosarcomas. Nine of ten patients who were given doses of about 5000 rad in 5 weeks had no evidence of local recurrence during a minimal observation period of 15 months. Liebner found control most frequent with doses of 1600 to 1750 rets when given with actinomycin D.

Despite the possibility of local tumor control by irradiation, a long survival, free of disease, is rare except for orbital lesions. In the absence of a specific cure, permanent control of the primary site and symptomatic metastases by irradiation with the doses mentioned should provide significant palliation.

As noted before, failure is most frequently the result of distant metastases. With the recognition that certain drug combinations can produce complete response in metastatic disease, a clinical trial of adjuvant therapies was organized in the form of the Intergroup Rhabdomyosarcoma Study. Although this trial is ongoing, a preliminary report has been issued. Since the size of tumor and complexities of treatment vary so much from site to site in the body, a single staging system has been difficult to employ. The Intergroup Rhabdomyosarcoma Study has adopted a clinical grouping classification that essentially relates to the bulk of the tumor and presence or absence of metastases at the time treatment is to be defined.

Clinical grouping of rhabdomyosarcoma employed by The Intergroup Rhabdomyosarcoma Study

Group I   Localized disease, completely resected (regional nodes not involved); confined to muscle or organ of origin and with contiguous involvement-infiltration outside the muscle organ of origin, as through fascial planes (includes both gross inspection and microscopic confirmation of complete resection)

Group II   Includes—

1. Grossly resected tumor with microscopic residual disease (in which the surgeon believes that he has removed all the tumor, but the pathologist finds tumor at the margin of resection); there should be no evidence of gross residual tumor or any clinical or microscopic evidence of regional node involvement
2. Regional* disease, completely resected (all tumor completely resected with no microscopic residual)
3. Regional disease with involved nodes, grossly resected, but with evidence of microscopic residual

Group III   Those with incomplete resection or biopsy with gross residual disease

Group IV   Patients with metastatic disease present at onset (lung, liver, bones, bone marrow, brain, and distant muscle and nodes)

---

*Regional nodes involved and/or extension of tumor into adjacent organ.

This clinical grouping is clearly influenced by the site of the primary lesions, that is, most extremity lesions might be in Group I or II, whereas most head and neck lesions would be in Group III. The preliminary report suggests that both local control and median survival are being improved by combined modality therapy. The report by Jereb with a smaller number of children supports the conclusion of a prolonged disease-free survival in children receiving irradiation and multidrug therapy.

Fibrosarcoma

Fibrosarcoma is a tumor made up of fibroblasts, variable collagen production, and a characteristic herringbone pattern of growth. Of the malignant soft tissue tumors this is the one most amenable to histologic grading. Grade I tumors grow slowly, recur, and metastasize late (Broders and associates). The more undifferentiated tumors grow more rapidly, recur more frequently, and metastasize sooner. Most fibrosarcomas do not fall into this category. Lymph node metastases are infrequent. Pulmonary metastases will develop in about 20% of all patients. The incidence of postoperative local recurrence is high: 56% of the operable cases in Pack and Ariel's series (1952) and 42.3% and 75.6%, respectively, for differentiated and undifferentiated lesions in Stout's series (1953).

Fibrosarcomas are not generally regarded as being sufficiently radiosensitive to be radiocurable. Surgery is the treatment of choice, and it must be radical if local recurrences are to be avoided.

Doses of 4000 to 4500 rad in 4 weeks will frequently produce regression, but with these doses regrowth invariably occurs. For any operable lesion, surgery is the unquestioned treatment of choice. The high incidence of local recurrence has prompted attempts to follow the operative procedure with irradiation. To our knowledge there is no evidence that routine postoperative irradiation has increased the survival rate. If persistence is known to be present or suspected, vigorous irradiation with doses of 5000 to 6000 rad in 6 weeks or longer should be given. Few cures have been obtained by irradiation alone. Perry and Chu found there was no fibrosarcoma that failed to regress if the tissue dose was at least 3400 rad in 23 days. The regression lasted from 2 to 8 months. Windeyer and associates treated twenty-two patients with a curative intent (6000 to 8500 rad in 5 to 9 weeks) and obtained complete tumor regression in fourteen. There was local recurrence in six of the fourteen. Of thirty-four patients observed for more than 5 years after irradiation, seventeen survived without evidence of tumor. This result is comparable to that obtained by surgery; however, longer observation is necessary for this type of sarcoma, for many patients will live over 5 years with their disease. For those patients with inoperable tumors or those who categorically refuse surgery, an aggressive approach with irradiation may result in long-term control for some.

Synovial sarcoma

Despite its name, synovial sarcoma rarely arises directly from synovial membrane but develops commonly near joints. Less common sites of occurrence are the abdominal wall and pharynx. A biphasic pattern of growth with glandular and spindle components are characteristic of this tumor. Tumors made up predominantly of spindle cells may be difficult to distinguish from fibrosarcoma.

These tumors may appear encapsulated but do not invade locally. They may be either cystic or solid. Synovial sarcomas usually metastasize hematogenously. Sixty-five percent of Pack and Ariel's patients (1950) developed pulmonary metastases, and 19% developed regional lymph node metastases. In patients with these sarcomas, just as in those with fibrosarcomas, postoperative local recurrences are frequent. Ariel and Pack have emphasized that with conservative surgery, 70% of the lesions will recur locally, although with more radical therapy they reported six of twenty-five patients living and well after 5 years. Haagensen and Stout also emphasize this strong tendency to recur locally and to metastasize and the resulting poor prognosis. Of forty-two patients reported earlier by Pack and Ariel (1950), eight were asymptomatic at least 5 years; two of these eight were definitely cured by irradiation, and two others had irradiation after what was thought to have been inadequate surgery. Their doses were apparently low by most modern standards. Berman has made a plea for routine local excision followed by postoperative irradiation with tumor doses of 4500 rad in 4 to 5 weeks. He also argues for irradiation of the regional lymph nodes even when they are not involved clinically. In view of the relatively radioresistant nature of synovial sarcoma, we do not believe the radical approach of Ariel and Pack should be abandoned for the local excision plus irradiation of Berman. When radiotherapy is to be administered with a curative aim, doses higher than those recommended by Berman should be given. Just what can be accomplished with modern vigorous irradiation alone is unknown, but we do not hesitate to recommend tissue doses of 5500 to 6500 rad in 6 weeks or more for those patients with known inoperable persistent disease. Suit and associates reported minimal 2-year disease-free survival in ten of fifteen patients treated by simple excision and radiation with doses ranging from 6300 to 7000 rad.

Liposarcomas

As the name implies, liposarcomas appear to be composed of embryonal fat cells. The tumor may originate in any site but most frequently appears in the retroperitoneal, popliteal, and gluteal regions. It infiltrates neighboring structures. These lesions may rarely arise from lipomas and may have multicentric foci of origin. However, it is always a problem clinically to decide whether a second area of involvement is a new primary lesion or a metastasis. Some liposarcomas closely resemble lipomas and have very little potential for metastasis. On the other hand, the round cell liposarcoma, a very cellular tumor made up of small, round lipoblasts, is characterized by frequent hematogenous spread.

Myxoid liposarcoma, the most common member of the group, is a richly vascularized oligocellular tumor with abundant mucoid matrix. It is characterized by a tendency to recur locally but rarely metastasizes. Intermediate forms may be found. Pleomorphic liposarcoma carries a high incidence of recurrence and metastases as does round cell liposarcoma. It may be difficult to distinguish from malignant fibrous histiocytoma.

In a review of 103 liposarcomas from the retroperitoneum and lower extremities, Enzinger and Winslow (1962) noted an 85% and 77% 5-year survival for well-differentiated and myxoid liposarcomas respectively; by contrast, the 5-year survival for round cell liposarcoma was only 18% and that for pleomorphic liposarcoma was 21%.

Thus grading of liposarcoma by a combination of cell type and pattern of growth is not only feasible but mandatory. A simple unqualified diagnosis of liposarcoma is unacceptable.

Surgical removal is the treatment of choice in patients with operable liposarcomas. However, local recurrence is common in all but those patients in whom amputation is required.

Liposarcomas present a wide variation in radiosensitivity. Some of the tumors we have irradiated have regressed rapidly and become impalpable with less than 1000 rad, but we have seen other tumors that have shown little change after 3000 rad in 3 weeks. Perry and Chu reported that all patients getting at least 2900 rad to the tumor (fractionation not given) showed shrinkage of the tumor. Beneficial effects lasted for an average of 10.7 months, with myxoliposarcoma showing a more frequent favorable response than other types. Friedman and Egan gave doses up to 9000 rad in 50 days to liposarcomas, with control in some. However, the high incidence of sequelae associated with these dose levels makes us favor radical surgery from the start if it is practical. As Friedman and Egan have pointed out, additional information is necessary before we can establish optimum dose-time levels for liposarcoma. Pack and Ariel (1950) employed preoperative irradiation at one time (dose and factors not given). They reported that 60% of the patients showed regression and 15% showed complete clinical regression of the tumor. There are a few patients cured with radiotherapy alone and a much larger number cured by a combination of surgery with wide-field postoperative irradiation.

Most liposarcomas arise in deep-seated muscle planes adjacent to or infiltrating neurovascular bundles, and many present in the retroperitoneal space, making total excision difficult. When tumor is left behind under these conditions, recurrence is certain.

In view of the previously mentioned response and the tendency for liposarcomas to recur, we advocate wide-field postoperative irradiation where excision has been performed. We do not advocate irradiation of a stump when amputation is required. Doses should be the maximum tolerated by the tumor volume. This is 5500 to 6500 rad or more in 5 to 6 weeks to the popliteal areas and rarely this much to the retroperitoneal tissues. The contribution of postoperative irradiation to the cure rate also remains to be defined.

Kaposi's sarcoma

Kaposi's sarcoma usually arises in the skin, but it has been reported as arising in almost all tissues. The cutaneous lesions are usually bluish red, enlarge slowly, and

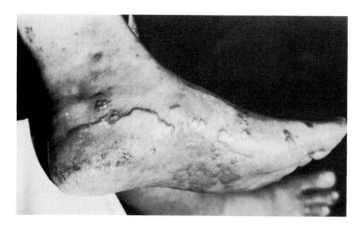

Fig. 23-4. Kaposi's sarcoma involving left foot. Satellite nodules can be seen on ankle.

coalesce with other skin lesions (Fig. 23-4). The areas may ulcerate and become infected and bleed. Death usually follows involvement of many organs and is usually ascribed to the debilitating effects of the previously mentioned complications. Most patients will live with their disease for many months, and some will live 5 to 10 years.

The nodules are radiosensitive. Cohen performed a time-dose analysis on sixty-five lesions. He concluded that an adequate dose consisted of 1000 rad single dose or 2500 rad in 4 weeks for an entire extremity. He pointed out that higher doses for an entire extremity are associated with frequent (25%) ischemic gangrene. Superficial radiations are adequate for skin nodules, whereas ^{60}Co or megavoltage beams can be used for more deeply situated lesions. The conduct of therapy is tailored to the extent of the disease. As the disease progresses, the depression of hemopoietic tissues will generally demand cessation of irradiation. It should be recognized, however, that with the doses just suggested, Cohen and associates achieved local control with no subsequent regional or distant extension in 35% of their patients. Holecek and Harwood recently reported an experience with single doses of 800 rad to large fields, and in one instance the large field included hemibody irradiation. They observed complete disappearance of disease in ten of twelve patients treated with this technique. Duration of response varied from 1 to 10 years. Such an approach indeed seems appropriate in view of the multicentricity of lesions in typical patients with Kaposi's sarcoma. (For other aspects of this interesting disease see Cook and Keen; Cook; and Ackerman [1962].)

Other soft tissue sarcomas

Malignant fibrous histiocytoma, malignant hemangiopericytoma, and alveolar soft part sarcomas are but several of the uncommon types of soft tissue sarcomas that from time to time confront the radiation oncologist. In a group of thirty-three patients with malignant fibrous histiocytoma reviewed by Soule and Enriquez, ten patients died of metastases and three died as a result of recurrent or inoperable retroperitoneal tumors. Five-year survival was 65% for the whole group. Suit and associates using combined surgery and radiotherapy had ten of eighteen patients surviving disease-free for greater than 24 months. In a review by McMaster and associates, twenty-five of thirty-two malignant hemangiopericytomas metastasized, and only one of their patients available for 5-year analyses survived free of disease. Even in those lesions with borderline malignancy the incidence of metastases was 37%, and local recurrence after limited excision was high. Certainly in these two highly malignant types of sarcomas current results with surgical excision and even attempts at postoperative irradiation produce few cures. At the present time we would advocate vigorous attempts by surgery and irradiation to achieve local control along with the principles of adjuvant chemotherapy which were discussed in current considerations of treatment of rhabdomyosarcoma.

Alveolar soft part sarcoma, although more indolent in nature than malignant hemangiopericytoma, has a great predilection toward distant metastases and local recurrence. The principle of surgical excision followed by irradiation if surgery is not complete should be employed.

REFERENCES

Ackerman, L. V., and Wheeler, P.: Liposarcoma, South. Med. J. **35**:156-160, 1942.

Ackerman, L. V.: Symposium on Kaposi's sarcoma. Concluding remarks, Acta Unio Internat. Contra Cancrum **18**:510-511, 1962.

Ariel, I. M., and Pack, G. T.: Synovial sarcoma, N. Engl. J. Med. **268**:1272-1275, 1963.

Berman, H. L.: The role of radiation therapy in the management of synovial sarcoma, Radiology **81**:997-1002, 1963.

Cassady, J. R., Sagerman, R. H., Tretter, P., and Ellsworth, R. M.: Radiation therapy for rhabdomyosarcoma, Radiology **91**:116-120, 1968.

Cohen, L.: Dose, time and volume parameters in irradiation therapy of Kaposi's sarcoma, Br. J. Radiol. **35**:485-488, 1962.

Cohen, L., Palmer, P. E. S., and Nickson, J. J.: Treatment of Kaposi's sarcoma by radiation, Acta Unio Internat. Contra Cancrum **18**:502-508, 1962.

Cook, J.: The treatment of Kaposi's sarcoma with nitrogen mustard, Acta Unio Internat. Contra Cancrum **18**:494-501, 1962.

Cook, J., and Keen, P.: Surgery in the treatment of Kaposi's sarcoma, Acta Unio Internat. Contra Cancrum **18**:492-493, 1962.

Crowley, L. G., Christopher, J. A., Nelsen, T., and Bagshaw, M.: Effect of radiation on canine intestinal anastomoses, Arch. Surg. **97**:423-428, 1968.

del Regato, J. A.: Radiotherapy of soft-tissue sarcomas, J.A.M.A. **185**:216-218, 1963.

Dito, W. R., and Batsakis, J. G.: Rhabdomyosarcoma of the head and neck, Arch. Surg. **84**:582-588, 1962.

Duncan, W., and Halman, K. E.: Giant hemangioma with thrombocytopenia, Clin. Radiol. **15**:224-231, 1964.

Edland, R. W.: Embryonal rhabdomyosarcoma, Am. J. Roentgenol. **93**:671-685, 1965.

Enzinger, F. M., and Winslow, D. J.: Liposarcoma; a study of 103 cases, Virchows Arch. (Pathol. Anat.) **335**:367-388, 1962.

Feder, B. H., Shramek, J. H., and Ikeda, T. S.: Large-field radiotherapy in lethal midline granuloma, Radiology **81**:293-299, 1963.

Friedman, M., and Egan, J. W.: Irradiation of liposarcoma, Acta Radiol. **54**:225-238, 1960.

Haagensen, C. D., and Stout, A. P.: Synovial sarcoma, Ann. Surg. **120**:826-842, 1944.

Holecek, M. J., and Harwood, A. R.: Radiotherapy of Kaposi's sarcoma, Cancer **41**:1733-1738, 1978.

Horn, R. C., Jr., and Enterline, H. T.: Rhabdomyosarcoma: a clinicopathological study and classification of 39 cases, Cancer **11**:181-199, 1958.

Jereb, B., Cham, W., Lattin, P., Exelby, P., Ghavimi, F., D'Angio, G. J., and Tefft, M.: Local control of embryonal rhabdomyosarcoma in children by radiation therapy when combined with concomitant chemotherapy, Int. J. Radiat. Oncol. Biol. Phys. **1**:217-225, 1976.

Jones, I. S., Reese, A. B., and Kraut, J.: Orbital

rhabdomyosarcoma: an analysis of 62 cases, Am. J. Ophthalmol. **61**:721-736, 1966.

Laborde, S.: Le traitement des angiomes chez les enfants, Paris, 1956, Masson et Cie.

Lawrence, W., Jr., Nickson, J. J., and Warshaw, L. M.: Roentgen rays and wound healing, Surgery **33**:376-384, 1953.

Lieberman, P. H., Foote, F. W., Stewart, F. W., and Berg, J. W.: Alveolar soft-part sarcoma, J.A.M.A. **198**:1047-1051, 1966.

Liebner, E. J.: Embryonal rhabdomyosarcoma of head and neck in children, Cancer **37**:2777-2786, 1976.

Lister, W. A.: The natural history of strawberry nevi, Lancet **1**:1429-1434, 1938.

Masson, J. K., and Soule, E. H.: Embryonal rhabdomyosarcoma of the head and neck, Am. J. Surg. **110**:585-591, 1965.

Maurer, H. M., Moon, T., Donaldson, M., Fernandez, C., Gehan, E. A., Hammond, D., Hays, D. M., Lawrence, W., Jr., Newton, W., Ragab, A., Raney, B., Soule, E. H., Sutow, W. W., and Tefft, M.: The Intergroup Rhabdomyosarcoma Study—a preliminary report, Cancer **40**:2015-2026, 1977.

McMaster, M. J., Soule, E. H., and Ivinns, J. C.: Hemangiopericytoma, Cancer **36**:2232-2244, 1975.

Merrill, M. D.: Roentgen therapy in Wegener's granulomatosis, Am. J. Roentgenol. **85**:96-98, 1961.

Nickson, J. J., Lawrence, W., Jr., Rachwalsky, I., and Tyree, E.: Roentgen rays and wound healing; fractionated irradiation; experimental study, Surgery **34**:859-862, 1953.

Pack, G. T., and Ariel, I. M.: Synovial sarcoma (malignant synovioma); report of 60 cases, Surgery **28**:1047-1084, 1950.

Pack, G. T., and Ariel, I. M.: Fibrosarcoma of soft tissue, Surgery **31**:443-478, 1952.

Pack, G. T., and Pierson, J. C.: Liposarcoma; a study of 105 cases, Surgery **36**:687-712, 1954.

Pack, G. T., and Ariel, I. M.: Tumors of the soft tissues, New York, 1958, Harper & Row, Publishers.

Perry, H., and Chu, F. C.: Radiation therapy in the palliative management of soft tissue sarcomas, Cancer **15**:179-183, 1962.

Smith, L. H., and Vickery, A. L.: Rapidly progressive uremia in patients with pneumonia, sinitis, otitis, and arthritis, N. Engl. J. Med. **269**:206-215, 1963.

Soule, E. H., and Enriquez, P.: A typical fibrous histiocytoma, malignant fibrous histiocytoma, malignant histiocytoma, and epitheloid sarcoma—a comparative study of 65 tumors, Cancer **30**:128-143, 1972.

Stout, A. P.: Liposarcoma, the malignant tumor of lipoblasts, Ann. Surg. **119**:86-107, 1944.

Stout, A. P.: Tumors of the soft tissues. Armed Forces Institute of Pathology, Section XI, Fascicle 5, Washington, D.C., 1953.

Suit, H. D., Russell, W. O., and Martin, R. G.: Sarcoma of soft tissue: clinical and histopathologic parameters and response to treatment, Cancer **35**:1478-1483, 1975.

Sutow, W. W., Sullivan, M. P., Ried, H. I., Taylor, H. G., and Griffith, K. M.: Prognosis in childhood rhabdomyosarcoma, Cancer **25**:1384-1390, 1970.

Wigley, J. E., Ress, D. L., and Symmers, W. S.: Kaposi's idiopathic haemorrhagic sarcoma, Proc. R. Soc. Med. **48**:449-450, 1955.

Wildermuth, O.: Lethal midline granuloma, Radiology **78**:269-271, 1962.

Windeyer, B., Dische, S., and Mansfield, C. M.: The place of radiotherapy in the management of fibrosarcoma of the soft tissues, Clin. Radiol. **17**:32-40, 1966.

24

Childhood cancers

The primary intent of radiation therapy is the destruction of a cancer with the preservation of tissues in the irradiated volume. In the treatment of childhood cancers, this intent is rarely met without compromise. In an attempt to deliver a dose sufficient to destroy a cancer, tissue growth or organ function may be arrested or impaired (Fig. 24-1). On the other hand, the delivery of a dose that will not interfere with growth or function may be totally inadequate to destroy the cancer selected for irradiation. The degree of impairment of growth is, of course, a function of the anticipated total growth (Fig. 24-2). This amplification phenomenon would be best illustrated in the eventual growth of an infant with medulloblastoma treated with a curative dose of radiations compared to an adolescent successfully treated with the same dose. This problem is most obvious and has been generally appreciated in its effect on arrest of bone growth that is preformed in cartilage, but as is pointed out in each chapter of this book, all organs and their supporting tissues suffer some degree of dose-dependent growth restraint. Our knowledge of the sequelae of irradiation of childhood cancers is based to a large extent on those tissues for which we have adequate information regarding the effects of treatment. In some instances, ignorance of the effects on other tissues may lead to more serious sequelae than those we anticipated. A perfect example of this situation is the treatment of the orbit (for retinoblastoma or orbital sarcomas) in which the significance of postirradiation cataract may diminish in comparison to irreparable corneal opacification from epithelial damage or as a sequelae of failure to provide a "dry eye" with proper lubrication. Examples of such failure to anticipate sequelae of childhood irradiation are common and ongoing (see Fig. 13-7).

Techniques and fractionation appropriate for adult or postadolescent patients cannot be transferred indiscriminately to children unless the effects of radiations on children are fully appreciated and the sequelae judged absolutely necessary when weighed against alternative lifesaving procedures. Despite these problems, radiation therapy plays a major part in the management of childhood cancer.

Although cancer is the second leading cause of death in children, its absolute incidence permits few radiation oncologists to see a significant number of childhood cancers in any year. The sites and relative frequency of childhood cancers seen at Children's Memorial Hospital, Chicago, during a 20-year period are shown in Table

631

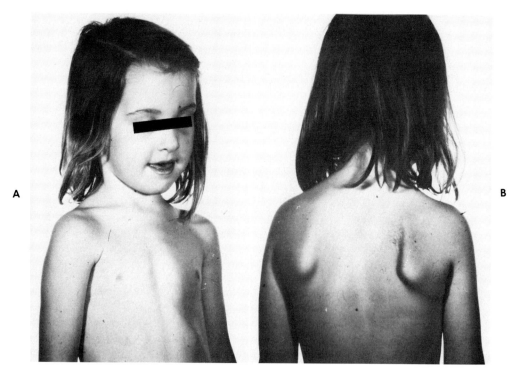

Fig. 24-1. A 4½-year-old girl, 33 months after irradiation of an upper thoracic neuroblastoma with anterior and posterior opposed ports, orthovoltage. Note atrophy of right pectoralis major muscle, **A,** and similar changes of the trapezius, rhomboid, and infraspinatous muscles, **B.**

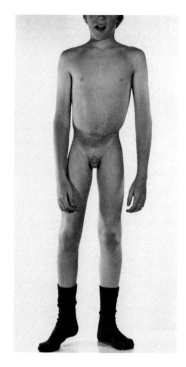

Fig. 24-2. An 11-year-old boy given approximately 2000 rad to midpelvis at age 1 month, using anterior and posterior opposed orthovoltage beams. Treatment was given after complete resection of a sacrococcygeal neuroblastoma.

Table 24-1. Tumor registry, solid tumors 1951-1970, Children's
Memorial Hospital, Chicago

Type	Number		Percent	
Brain		164		21.1
Sympathetic nervous system		117		15.1
Kidney		117		15.1
Wilms'	114		14.7	
Others	3		0.4	
Lymphoma		96		12.4
Lymphosarcoma	61		7.9	
Hodgkin's disease	26		3.4	
Reticulum cell sarcoma	7		0.9	
Unclassified lymphoma	2		0.2	
Connective and other soft tissue tumors		71		5.3
Bone		33		4.2
Histiocytosis—group		26		3.4
Eye		18		2.3
Thyroid		16		2.1
Sacral coccygeal teratoma		16		2.1
Peritoneum and retroperitoneal tissue		14		1.8
Liver and intrahepatic ducts		13		1.7
Pituitary and craniopharyngeal duct		12		1.5
Spinal cord		11		1.4
Ovary, fallopian tube, broad ligament		11		1.4
Respiratory system		9		1.2
Cranial nerves (optic tract glioma)		9		1.2
Testis		9		1.2
Ill-defined sites		8		1.0
Pelvis, pelvic viscera, rectovaginal septum	7		0.9	
Abdomen	1		0.1	
Bladder		7		0.9
Pineal		6		0.8
Meninges		5		0.6
Cerebral	3		0.4	
Spinal	2		0.2	
Buccal cavity and pharynx		4		0.5
Melanoma		2		0.2
Malignant neoplasm of skin		2		0.2
Suprarenal		2		0.2
Stomach		1		0.1
Unspecified female genital organs		1		0.1
TOTAL		800		

24-1. During this 20-year period, 306 cases of leukemia were registered, and of those, 271 were seen in the period between 1961 and 1970. Currently 40 new cases of acute leukemia are seen there each year.

It can be seen that even in institutions with large numbers of children with cancer there are certain uncommon types and, all too often, no collective experience has been published to provide guidelines in either the selection of the modality or expectations of a given modality of treatment.

Table 24-2. Doses recommended for the National Wilms' Tumor Study showing the relationship to the age of the child

Age	Total tumor dose
Birth to 18 months	1800-2400 rad
19 to 30 months	2400-3000 rad
31 to 40 months	3000-3500 rad
41 months or older	3500-4000 rad

As in the case of adults, children come in a variety of ages and sizes and with various degrees of comprehension and communication skills. Beyond this, the similarity disappears and the special responsibility of treating children cannot be taken lightly. Some childhood cancers, such as retinoblastoma, are unique to the young age group. Others, including Wilms' tumor and neuroblastoma, are rarely seen beyond adolescence. Still others, such as Hodgkin's disease, may be commonly shared by children and adults, and finally others common in the adult population, including adenocarcinoma of the breast and multiple myeloma, are rarely seen in childhood. Malignant brain tumors, perhaps because of the earlier morphologic maturation of the brain, share some features with the adult forms, but this in no way implies that the treatment of childhood brain tumors can simply be undertaken without regard for the sequelae of radiations on the child as a whole.

The critical treatment factors in the irradiation of childhood cancers are total dose and fractionation. It is accepted practice in the treatment of Wilms' tumor to adjust the total dose given prophylactically to the tumor bed according to the age of the child. Table 24-2 shows the dose recommendations of the National Wilms' Tumor Study. The implication is that in the younger children treated with curative attempts, fewer sequelae are acceptable than in the older children treated with the same intent. Or, expressed another way, the younger the child, the greater the damage of a given dose. To our knowledge there are no reports of a threshold dose for failure of local control in the present combined management of Wilms' tumor over the range of dose shown in Table 24-2. On the contrary, even large multiple pulmonary metastases can be eradicated with doses of 1200 to 1400 rad combined with the same dose of actinomycin D employed in prophylactic treatment of the primary tumor. It is apparent that the doses selected express the radiation tolerance of the volume treated (both lungs or upper abdomen) and are not a reflection of altered radiosensitivity dependent on the location of the tumor mass in different sites or organs. This point is amplified in a personal letter from Dr. J. del Regato to one of us (W. T. M.).

All that we know about dosage in radiotherapy of malignant tumors is that, all other conditions remaining the same, the higher the dose the greater the chance of success. We have also empirically established that some tumors, like lymphosarcomas, Hodgkin's disease, neuroblastomas, etc. may require a relatively lesser amount to be completely destroyed, but this amount is never reduced by half and this view is only an impression, not verified by a controlled experiment.

I agree that it is not proper to expect the same tumor in small children can be cured by a

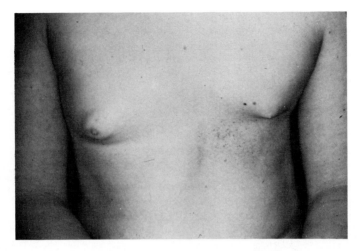

Fig. 24-3. An 18-year-old girl treated for massive Ewing's tumor arising from symphysis pubis at age 11 and a solitary pulmonary metastasis to left lower lobe at age 12. Excess gonadotropic hormone was demonstrated at age 13, and she was given estrogen to stimulate breast maturation. There is no palpable breast tissue beneath irradiated left areola. Note hypoplasia of left nipple and areola. Dose to left breast was 3300 rad in 18 days. Compare to Fig. 11-1.

smaller dose. What is obvious, however, is that the risks to be taken in the irradiation of growing children are greater and that consequently the maximum dose referred above can be reduced accordingly. Under normal circumstances this could imply that there would be a lesser chance of cure. The fact is, however, that in most instances we over dose because we can afford it.

A factor involved in all of this, which is seldom spoken about these days when we appear mesmerized by *dose,* is the first that in the treatment of malignant tumors in children an advantage is to be gained by fractionating the treatment over a longer period than used in an adult. There is a lot to be said in the avoidance of injury which results from fractionation and in the tumors found in children large or even moderate doses are not necessarily the basis of success.*

Other tumors in children do not give us the same opportunity to reduce dose according to age (Fig. 24-3). Such is the case with embryonal rhabdomyosarcomas of the orbit, which fortunately is rarely seen in infancy, and with Ewing's tumor. In these instances we are able to take advantage of greater fractionation. Similarly, the treatment of Hodgkin's disease in children provides ample opportunity to maximize the benefits of fractionation. In the case of medulloblastoma, after earlier trials of high-dose, short-course irradiation, current techniques employ high-dose, long fractionation schemes (Chapter 19).

In general, orthovoltage beams have no place in the treatment of childhood cancers. The skin- and bone-sparing properties of megavoltage beams make them preferable, yet we have no assurance that the higher dose in depth in techniques

*From del Regato, J. A.: Personal communication, 1971.

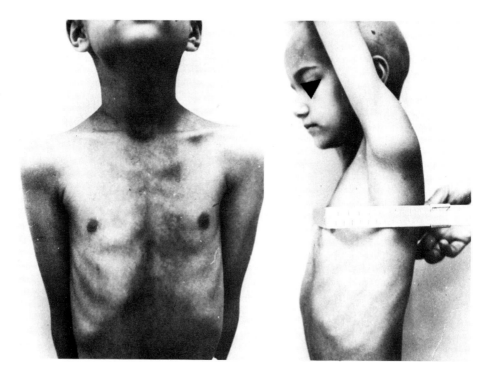

Fig. 24-4. Exit skin changes in a 9-year-old girl given cranial spinal irradiation for a medulloblastoma with a 4 mev photon beam (see Fig. 22-5 for description of technique). Significant doses are delivered to structures anterior to spinal cord.

that employ single field arrangements will produce fewer sequelae to normal tissues deep to the volume of interest. This is of special interest in the current techniques of craniospinal irradiation for leukemia or medulloblastoma (Fig. 24-4). With extended-field techniques employed in treatment of leukemia, lymphomas, and certain primary tumors of the central nervous system, the difference in active bone marrow distribution between children and adults must be appreciated (Chapter 20). The frequent combination of irradiation and chemotherapy in which both modalities may depress the bone marrow makes careful monitoring of the combined effects necessary. A close collaboration between the radiation oncologist and chemotherapist is essential in every instance.

Farber has described the traditional course of "sequential" therapy wherein a child with cancer was passed from surgeon to radiotherapist to chemotherapist, and in this sequence a fatal outcome was almost inevitable. More often than not, such a tradition persists in the management of adult cancers, but fortunately a combined approach is now common in the management of childhood cancer. Thus, when a preoperative diagnosis is established in the child, consultation between radiation and medical oncologists is readily available to the surgeon. This approach has reached its zenith in the care of the child with Wilms' tumor and should serve as a model for treatment planning. Farber has demonstrated an almost threefold increase in survival of children with Wilms' tumor whose entire treatment was given in an institution with adequate experience in treating childhood cancers. Although the processes of referral may explain some failures, the lack of experience in treating childhood cancers remains the most likely cause of failure.

The more common cancers in childhood as well as the reported effects of ionizing radiations on selected normal tissues are to be found in other parts of this book as well as the rationale, technique, and results of irradiation. This chapter is intended to provoke the radiation oncologist who would undertake the treatment of childhood cancers to review his own experience, treatment plans, and approach to the problem.

REFERENCE

Farber, S.: Solid tumors of children: historical background and perspectives in the total care of childhood cancer. In Oncology 1970, Proceedings of the Tenth International Cancer Congress, Chicago, 1971, Year Book Medical Publishers, Inc.

Index

639